MEDICINE FOR
EXAMINATIONS

Commissioning Editor: Laurence Hunter
Project Development Manager: Helen Leng
Project Manager: Nancy Arnott
Designer: Erik Bigland

MEDICINE FOR
EXAMINATIONS

R.J. Epstein MD PhD
Deputy Director, National Cancer Centre
Singapore

FOURTH EDITION

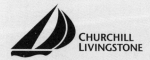
CHURCHILL
LIVINGSTONE

EDINBURGH LONDON NEW YORK OXFORD PHILADELPHIA ST LOUIS SYDNEY TORONTO 2003

CHURCHILL LIVINGSTONE
An imprint of Elsevier Science Limited

First edition 1985
Second edition 1990
Third edition 1996
Fourth edition 2003

ISBN 0443070474

British Library Cataloguing in Publication Data
A catalogue record for this book is available from the British
Library

Library of Congress Cataloging in Publication Data
A catalog record for this book is available from the Library of
Congress

Note
Medical knowledge is constantly changing. Standard safety
precautions must be followed, but as new research and
clinical experience broaden our knowledge, changes in
treatment and drug therapy may become necessary or
appropriate. Readers are advised to check the most current
product information provided by the manufacturer of each
drug to be administered to verify the recommended dose, the
method and duration of administration, and contraindications.
It is the responsibility of the practitioner, relying on
experience and knowledge of the patient, to determine
dosages and the best treatment for each individual patient.
Neither the Publisher nor the author assumes any liability for
any injury and/or damage to persons or property arising from
this publication.

 ELSEVIER SCIENCE your source for books,
journals and multimedia
in the health sciences

www.elsevierhealth.com

The
publisher's
policy is to use
paper manufactured
from sustainable forests

Printed in China

CONTENTS

The format of this new edition of MFE has changed substantially. Four new chapters have been created to reflect the growing importance of *HIV-related Disease*; *Sexual and Reproductive Medicine*; *Palliative Care, Rehabilitation and Gerontology*; and *Statistics, Evidence-based Medicine, and Clinical Trials*. In addition, the beginning of each chapter now includes separate sections on *Emergencies* and *Common or Classic Cases*. The range of new information is immense, and I will not attempt to summarize it.

All efforts have been made to check the accuracy of drug dosages and other therapeutic recommendations in this book. Some of the drugs mentioned in the text are not available world-wide but are cited as examples of use only. It is recommended, therefore, that physicians consult other sources prior to prescribing any course of therapy mentioned in the book.

Any errors or oversimplifications in the text are my own responsibility. I will be grateful to any reader who takes the trouble to feed back (whether positively or negatively) about the book (MFE.feedback@elsevier.com); this applies equally to general impressions and to specific queries and comments.

Singapore 2003

R.J.E.

ACKNOWLEDGEMENTS

Many of the improvements to this fourth edition of *Medicine for Examinations* have been contributed by readers and colleagues (please keep those comments coming!). I would like particularly to thank Bhupinder Mann, Sandeep Rajan, Philip Eng, Ian Turner and Mark Thomas for their thoughtful suggestions; Laurence Hunter, Sian Jarman, Helen Leng and Isobel Black for their outstanding editorial and production support; and to Anne, Julia, Catherine, Helen and Alec for their constant forgiveness.

CHAPTER 1

Cancer

Physical examination protocol 1.1   You are asked to examine a patient who has recently presented with metastatic disease of unknown primary etiology

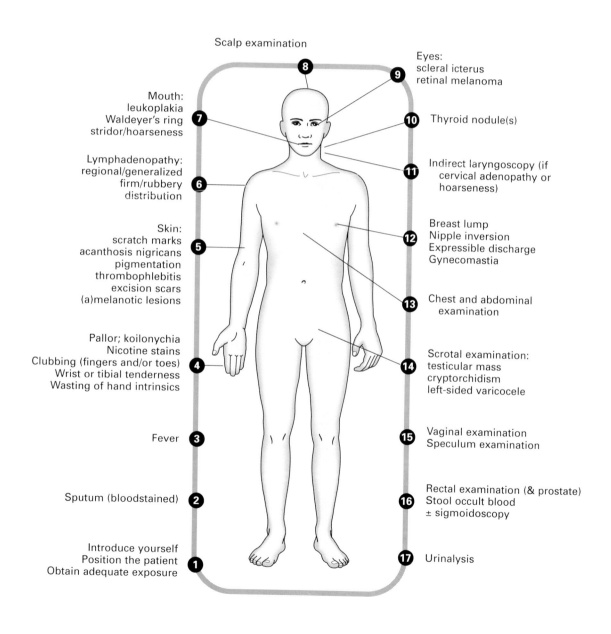

Scalp examination

Eyes:
scleral icterus
retinal melanoma

Mouth:
leukoplakia
Waldeyer's ring
stridor/hoarseness

Thyroid nodule(s)

Indirect laryngoscopy (if
cervical adenopathy or
hoarseness)

Lymphadenopathy:
regional/generalized
firm/rubbery
distribution

Skin:
scratch marks
acanthosis nigricans
pigmentation
thrombophlebitis
excision scars
(a)melanotic lesions

Breast lump
Nipple inversion
Expressible discharge
Gynecomastia

Chest and abdominal
examination

Pallor; koilonychia
Nicotine stains
Clubbing (fingers and/or toes)
Wrist or tibial tenderness
Wasting of hand intrinsics

Scrotal examination:
testicular mass
cryptorchidism
left-sided varicocele

Fever

Vaginal examination
Speculum examination

Sputum (bloodstained)

Rectal examination (& prostate)
Stool occult blood
± sigmoidoscopy

Introduce yourself
Position the patient
Obtain adequate exposure

Urinalysis

Diagnostic pathway 1.1   This patient has ascites. What is the most likely cause?

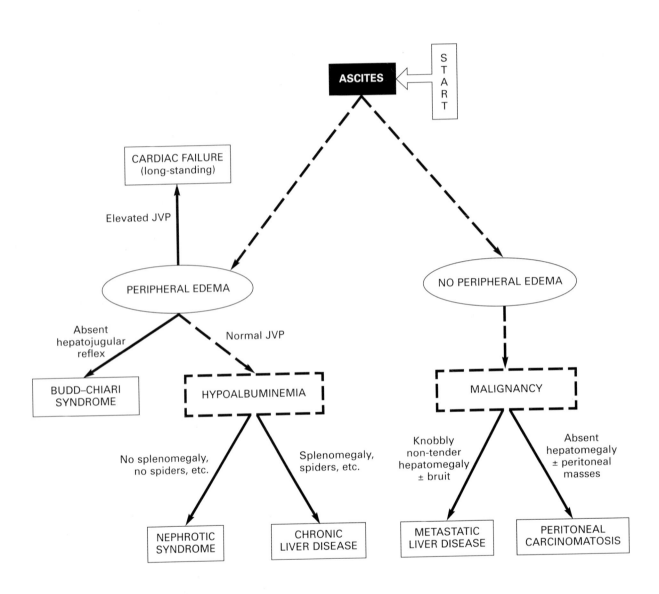

COMMON AND CLASSIC CANCER PROBLEMS

Common cancer problems in clinical practice
1 Refractory pleural effusion or ascites
2 Thromboembolic disease
3 Progressive bony metastases with fracture and/or cord compression

Classic cancer problems in medical exams
1 Obstructive jaundice
2 Superior vena caval obstruction
3 Meningeal carcinomatosis

CANCER EMERGENCIES

See also: Febrile neutropenia, disseminated intravascular coagulation (p. 139)

Spinal cord compression: presentation and action
1 Patients may be known to have extensive bone metastases; previous courses of radiotherapeutic 'patch-welding' are common
2 Onset of paraparesis or urinary symptoms is usually preceded by pain. Increasing pain should raise suspicion of impending cord compression
3 Confirm the diagnosis with MRI scanning *before* the weekend. If compressive lesions at multiple levels are demonstrated, surgery is usually not appropriate
4 Commonest primary tumors are breast (25%), lung (15%), prostate (10%) and myeloma (10%). Rarely, TB can also present in this way
5 Refer for immediate surgical decompression if
 — Paraplegia or incontinence has not supervened, *and*
 — Prognosis following surgery is reasonable*, *and*
 — The primary pathology is unknown, *or*
 — Tumor is probably radioresistant (e.g. melanoma), *or*
 — The tumor has progressed following or during irradiation
6 Refer for immediate radiotherapy if
 — The tumor is at least moderately radiosensitive, *and*
 — Corticosteroids have already been commenced, *and*
 — Neither surgery nor chemotherapy is indicated
7 Refer for initial cytotoxic therapy‡ (rarely) if
 — The tumor is likely to be highly chemosensitive, *and*
 — The neurologic deficit is neither serious nor fulminant, *or*
 — Both surgery and radiotherapy are contraindicated
8 Corticosteroids should be commenced immediately in any suspected case of cord compression, and be discontinued only after investigations have excluded the diagnosis

* i.e. disease is not (say) both extensive and heavily pretreated with chemotherapy and radiotherapy

‡ Note that it is often difficult to administer effective tumorilytic doses of cytotoxic therapy if patients with widespread bony metastases have had previous courses of radiotherapy to the spine; in such cases, myelosuppression is often dose limiting

Approach to the patient with hypercalcemia
1 The mainstay of management is IV saline, approximately 1 L every 3–4 h*. Furosemide (frusemide) promotes calcium excretion, and may be added if concerns over cardiac or renal compromise
2 Adjunctive measures include
 — Cessation of iatrogenic precipitants, e.g. tamoxifen (p. 19), vitamins A or D
 — Mobilization if feasible, ensuring adequate analgesia and fracture prevention
3 Specific hypocalcemic drugs
 — Bisphosphonates (osteoclast inhibitors)
  • Pamidronate infusion (acute, or regular monthly)‡
  • Oral clodronate (maintenance daily)
 — Calcitonin
4 Treat the underlying malignancy
5 Evaluate prospects for survival *before* embarking upon definitive intervention; terminal hypercalcemia may not require treatment

* Patients with symptomatic hypercalcemia usually have a fluid deficit of 3–6 L
‡ May also be infused every 3–4 weeks for treatment of metastatic bone pain and/or prevention of pathologic fractures

Approach to the patient with superior vena caval obstruction
1 Confirm the diagnosis with CXR or CT showing mediastinal widening
2 If the primary histological diagnosis is not known, this should be sought by either bronchoscopic biopsy (if lung primary suspected) or mediastinoscopy; careful evaluation for peripheral adenopathy may spare invasive diagnostic procedure
3 Note that a small proportion (5%) of cases arise due to benign lesions (e.g. retrosternal goiter, aortic aneurysm)
4 Obstruction due to SCLC or lymphoma may be best treated with systemic chemotherapy in the first instance
5 Although often described as an emergency, most SVC obstructions present subacutely and can be managed non-urgently. Steroids can be administered prior to irradiation
6 Intravenous lines used for cytotoxic therapy should not be sited in the arms

Approach to the patient with cytotoxic drug extravasation
1 Stop the infusion and aspirate residual unabsorbed drug from the extravasated region
2 Apply local cooling or warming packs
 Cooling: anthracyclines, paclitaxel, nitrogen mustard
 Warming: vinca alkaloids, etoposide

3 Antidotes

— vincas, etoposide, paclitaxel:	hyaluronidase 150 U/mL, infiltrated subcutaneously
— cisplatin, nitrogen mustard:	sodium thiosulfate 4% (inject before removing needle)
— doxorubicin, mitomycin:	dimethyl sulfoxide (DMSO) 50% solution topically

CLINICAL ASSESSMENT OF THE CANCER PATIENT

ASSESSMENT OF THE SYMPTOMATIC PATIENT

The palpable lump: how to describe it
1 **S**: **s**ite, **s**ize, **s**hape
2 **F**: **f**irmness, **f**luctuation, **f**ixation
3 **T**: **t**exture, **t**emperature, **t**enderness

Triple assessment of the symptomatic breast*
1 Physical examination, esp.
   — Clinical lump assessement (as above)
   — Skin or nipple involvement
   — Regional adenopathy
2 Mammogram
   — Two views: mediolateral + craniocaudal
   — Compression views of any abnormality
   — Ultrasound of palpable (mammo-negative) or suspected cystic lesions
3 Tissue diagnosis
   — Fine-needle aspiration cytology‡
   — Trucut percutaneous biopsy
   — Excision biopsy

* NB: Mammography in the evaluation of symptomatic breast disease (lumps) is purely adjunctive, i.e. a negative examination is *unhelpful* and provides *no* reassurance (15–20% of palpable carcinomas are mammogram-negative)
‡ Complicated by false-negatives; in general, a negative aspirate may need to be followed by a biopsy

Initial approach to the patient with colorectal symptoms*
1 Patients presenting with colorectal symptoms other than rectal bleeding
   — Digital rectal examination (DRE) followed by sigmoidoscopy
2 Patients presenting de novo with rectal bleeding
   — DRE followed by colonoscopy (± proctoscopy)

* Due to its high false-negative rate, fecal occult blood testing (p. 402) is an *inappropriate* test for patients with colorectal symptoms

DIFFERENTIAL DIAGNOSES IN THE CANCER PATIENT

Differential diagnosis of fever in the cancer patient
1 Infective
   — Septicemia, esp. if neutropenic*: absolute neutrophil count (ANC) < 0.5 × 10^9/L
   — Intermittent bacteremias (e.g. from central line)

   — Localized infections, e.g. pneumonia (incl. aspiration), abscess, cellulitis, UTI
   — Viremia, esp. CMV following marrow transplant
   — HIV complication in AIDS-associated neoplasms
2 Intrinsic‡
   — Lymphoma
   — Retroperitoneal tumors (e.g. renal cell carcinoma)
   — Metastatic liver disease
3 Iatrogenic
   — Drug-induced (e.g. gemcitabine, taxanes, interferon, ATRA¶, antibody therapies)
   — Transfusion-associated

* Usually due to endogenous GI tract flora, although most often culture-negative
‡ i.e. disease manifestation; a diagnosis of exclusion
¶ All-*trans*-retinoic acid, used in acute promyelocytic leukemia (p. 148)

Differential diagnosis of confusion in the cancer patient
1 Metabolic
   — Hypercalcemia
     • With bone metastases (e.g. Ca breast, myeloma)
     • PTHrP-mediated (squamous cell cancers)
   — Hyponatremia (e.g. SIADH in small-cell lung cancer)
   — Hypoglycemia (e.g. insulinoma, hepatoma, renal cell carcinoma)
   — Hypopituitarism/-adrenalism (e.g. post-cranial irradiation, sellar tumor)
   — Hyperviscosity (e.g. in macroglobulinemia)
   — Renal failure (e.g. cervix cancer) or liver failure (multiple liver metastases)
2 Hypoxic, esp.
   — Pulmonary emboli
   — Progressive lymphangitic carcinomatosis
3 Septic, esp.
   — Pneumonia
   — Meningitis (e.g. cryptococcal)
   — Progressive multifocal leucoencephalopathy (p. 167)
4 Tumor-related
   — Paraneoplastic dementia (diagnosis of exclusion)
   — Limbic encephalitis (short-term memory loss, mood change)
   — Cerebral metastases, esp. with edema or obstructive hydrocephalus
5 Iatrogenic
   — Opiates (common)
   — Steroids (common)
   — Ifosfamide, procarbazine

Differential diagnosis of vomiting in the cancer patient
1 Gastrointestinal obstruction
   — Peritoneal carcinomatosis (e.g. Ca ovary/colon, lobular Ca breast)
   — Primary gastrointestinal tumors (e.g. linitis plastica)
2 Raised intracranial pressure due to intracranial metastases
   — Cerebral edema (responds to steroids)
   — Ventricular obstruction (responds to shunting)

3 Metabolic
  — Hypercalcemia
  — Uremia due to obstructive uropathy
  — Adrenal insufficiency
4 Iatrogenic
  — Chemotherapy (incl. anticipatory)
  — Opiates

Differential diagnosis of alopecia in the cancer patient
1 Total alopecia
  — Whole-brain cranial irradiation
  — Drugs, esp. anthracyclines, taxanes, alkylators
2 Asymmetric alopecia
  — Post-craniotomy (for brain tumor)

PRESENTATIONS OF LUNG TUMORS

Symptoms and signs of lung tumors
1 Local endobronchial symptoms
  — Chronic cough
  — Fever due to post-obstructive pneumonia
  — Hemoptysis
  — Stridor
2 Local extrabronchial obstructive presentations
  — Superior vena caval obstruction (esp. SCC, small-cell)
  — Chylous pleural effusion (rare*)
3 Syndromes due to nerve palsies
  — Hoarseness (recurrent laryngeal nerve compression, esp. left-sided primaries)
  — Hemidiaphragmatic paralysis (phrenic nerve palsy)
  — Horner's syndrome (see below)
4 Metastatic presentations
  — Serosal spread: pleural effusion, pericardial tamponade
  — Other: jaundice, convulsions, weight loss
5 Paraneoplastic syndromes (see below)

* May in theory still be associated with curable disease, unlike most malignant pleural effusions

Classic presentations of lung tumor subtypes
1 Non-small-cell lung cancer ($\rightarrow$ 80%: SCC, adenoCa, large-cell)
  — Hypertrophic pulmonary osteoarthropathy (HPO), clubbing
  — Non-metastatic hypercalcemia (esp. SCC) due to PTHrP
2 Small-cell lung cancer ($\rightarrow$ 20%; SCLC)
  — Metastases at presentation
  — Leucoerythroblastic anemia
  — Cerebral metastases, meningeal carcinomatosis
  — SIADH* (due to 1° tumor or intracranial spread)
  — Ectopic ACTH syndrome (hypokalemia, weakness, pigmentation, weight loss)
  — Eaton–Lambert (myasthenic) syndrome
  — Extensive mediastinal involvement‡
  — SVC obstruction
  — Rapid but transient response to chemotherapy
3 Bronchioloalveolar cell carcinoma
  — Copious clear sputum (may affect non-smokers)
  — Respiratory insufficiency ± pulmonary infiltrate

4 Bronchial adenoma (usually a carcinoid tumor; p. 7)
  — Hemoptysis with normal CXR (tumor usually central)
  — Recurrent chest infections (e.g. abscess, pneumonia)¶
  — Incidental CXR finding in a non-smoker
  — Brisk hemorrhage if biopsied (highly vascular)

* DDx = Syndrome of increased atrial natriuretic peptide (ANP)
‡ DDx = Lymphoma, germ-cell tumor
¶ Due to bronchial obstruction

Predominant localization of lung tumor subtypes
1 Central
  — Small-cell lung cancer
  — Squamous cell carcinoma
  — Bronchial adenoma
2 Peripheral
  — Adenocarcinoma*
  — Large cell carcinoma

* Metastasis from other primary site may require exclusion if no luminal lesion visualized at bronchoscopy

Superior sulcus (Pancoast) syndrome
1 Components
  — Superior sulcus tumor, and
  — Upper extremity pain, and
  — Neurologic deficit
2 Cause(s)
  — Superior pulmonary sulcus/thoracic inlet tumors (usually at least T_3 stage)
  — > 90% due to non-small-cell lung cancer; complicates < 5% lung cancers
3 Upper extremity pain
  — Shoulder or axillary pain due to invasion of pleura, vertebrae, ribs
  — C_8/T_{1-2} radicular pain (may mimic ulnar nerve distribution) due to invasion of lower trunks of brachial plexus
4 Neurologic deficit:
  — Horner's syndrome (ipsilateral ptosis, miosis, anhidrosis) caused by invasion of inferior cervical (stellate) ganglion or paravertebral sympathetic chain
  — C_8/T_{1-2} sensory loss (esp. medial forearm) and/or interossei wasting
5 Associated clinical signs worsening the prognosis
  — Supraclavicular or axillary adenopathy
  — Hoarseness, hemidiaphragmatic elevation (see above)
6 CXR
  — Early-stage tumors may not be detected (CT or MRI may be needed)
  — Erosion of first and second ribs may be seen
  — May reveal cervical rib, TB (i.e. pain, neuro deficit not always due to cancer)

PRESENTATIONS OF GASTROINTESTINAL TUMORS

Classical presentations of colorectal cancer
1 Distal (left-sided) colon tumors
  — Changed bowel habit
  — Rectal bleeding

2　Transverse colon tumors
  — Obstruction
  — Perforation
3　Proximal (right) colon tumors
  — Iron-deficiency anemia
  — Hereditary non-polyposis colorectal cancer
    (p. 22)
4　Other (rare) presentations
  — *Strep. bovis* endocarditis or bacteremia
  — *Clostridium septicum* myonecrosis

Clinical presentations of pancreatic cancer

1　'Head' tumors
  — Common
    • Progressive jaundice
    • Back pain (due to invasion of celiac plexus)
  — Classical
    • Palpable nontender gallbladder (Courvoisier's
      sign)
2　'Tail' tumors
  — Common
    • Weight loss
    • Diabetes mellitus
  — Classical
    • Endogenous depression (*angor animi*)
    • Migratory thrombophlebitis (Trousseau's
      syndrome)

Clinical presentations of gastric cancer

1　Common
  — Weight loss
  — Epigastric discomfort
2　Classical
  — Troisier's sign (enlargement of Virchow's node)
  — Sister Mary Joseph nodule (umbilical mass)
  — Blumer's (prerectal) shelf on digital
    examination
  — Krukenberg tumors (ovarian metastases) at
    laparotomy
  — Acanthosis nigricans (symmetric pigmented
    warty skin lesions → axillae, pubis, neck,
    umbilicus)

Clinical presentations of primary liver tumors

1　Hepatoma
  — Common
    • Onset of ascites in a previously stable
      cirrhotic
    • Unexplained weight loss in an alcoholic
    • Tender hepar with bruit (DD_x: alcoholic
      hepatitis)
  — Uncommon
    • Polycythemia
    • Dysproteinemia
    • Porphyria
  — Investigations
    • HBsAg, HCV serology
    • AFP (elevated in 75%)
    • Lipiodol CT
2　Hepatic adenoma (→ young women)
  — Intraperitoneal rupture in a woman taking oral
    contraceptives for > 5 years
3　Hepatoblastoma (→ infants only)
  — Clubbing; precocious puberty

PRESENTATIONS OF GYNECOLOGIC AND GENITOURINARY TUMORS

Symptoms and signs of choriocarcinoma

1　Hyperemesis gravidarum
2　Hemorrhagic metastases → hemoptysis, stroke
3　Painful gynecomastia (in males)
4　Rare: mild hyperthyroidism (HCG shares TSH β-
  subunit)
5　Metastatic presentation usual (cf. seminoma)

Symptoms and signs of cervical carcinoma

1　Majority detected by Pap smear of *asymptomatic*
  patients
2　Presentations of advanced disease:
  — Vaginal discharge or bleeding
  — Fistulas (e.g. rectovaginal → pneumaturia)*
  — Pelvic pain (advanced disease)
  — Obstructive uropathy (frequently terminal)

* Often iatrogenic, e.g. post-radiotherapy

Symptoms and signs of ovarian tumors

1　Adenocarcinoma*
  — Abdominal fullness due to ascites
  — Bowel obstruction due to peritoneal
    carcinomatosis
2　Stromal tumors (rare)

— Fibroma, thecoma	→	Meigs' syndrome
— *Struma ovarii*	→	thyrotoxicosis
— Granulosa cell tumor	→	vaginal bleeding
— Sertoli–Leydig tumor‡	→	virilization

* Early disease? *no* symptoms
‡ Formerly termed arrhenoblastoma

Symptoms and signs of renal cell carcinoma

1　Common
  — Incidental finding on CT scan
  — Hematuria
  — Weight loss
  — Flank pain
  — Flank mass
  — Anemia
2　Uncommon
  — Polycythemia (5%)
  — Fever; thromboembolism
  — Left-sided varicocele presenting in adult male
  — Hypercalcemia (may be non-metastatic)
  — Non-metastatic liver dysfunction (Stauffer's
    syndrome)

HEAD AND NECK TUMORS

The solitary thyroid nodule: factors favoring malignancy

1　Positive family history of medullary thyroid cancer
2　Past history of low-dose neck irradiation, esp. in
  childhood
3　Clinical features: hard nodule, lymphadenopathy
4　Elevated serum thyroglobulin (papillary/follicular
  cancer); elevated serum calcitonin (medullary
  carcinoma)

5 Cold nodule on scintigraphy; solid lesion on ultrasound
6 Expression of the variant hyaluronate receptor (CD44) isoform CD44v6, together with the β-galactosil-binding protein galectin-3

Symptoms and signs of head and neck cancers
1 Non-healing mouth ulcer
2 Neck lump
3 Rhinorrhea, nasal stuffiness
4 Odynophagia
5 Hoarse voice
6 Cranial nerve (e.g. bulbar) palsy

NEUROENDOCRINE TUMORS

Multiple endocrine neoplasia (MEN): the clinical spectrum
1 Multiple endocrine neoplasia type I (MEN1)
— **P**arathyroid adenoma/hyperplasia (in 90%)
— **P**ituitary adenoma (60%)
— **P**ancreatic and/or duodenal/gastric neuroendocrine tumors, e.g.
• insulinomas (rarely metastasize; treat by enucleation)
• gastrinomas (often metastasize; rarely cured)
• carcinoids (thymic, usually invasive; gastric, usually not)
• glucagonomas, VIPomas, lipomas, thymomas, PPomas, somatostatinomas
2 Multiple endocrine neoplasia type IIa (MEN2A)
— Pheochromocytoma*
— Medullary carcinoma of the thyroid
— Parathyroid hyperplasia (in 50%; generally subclinical)
— Gliomas, meningiomas
3 Multiple endocrine neoplasia type IIb (MEN2B): similar to IIa, but
— Hyperparathyroidism rare
— Marfanoid habitus
— Mucosal neuromas (protruding lips, gut gangliomas)

NB: MEN1 adenomas may often be managed medically, whereas MEN2 adenomas are best removed by surgery
* Also seen in von Hippel–Lindau syndrome

Medullary thyroid carcinoma (MTC): features
1 75% are sporadic (no family history of MEN2)
2 *Familial* MTC may be either
— Isolated familial MTC (least aggressive type)
— MTC with type IIa MEN
• Pheochromocytoma, parathyroid adenoma
— MTC with type IIb MEN (rarest and most aggressive)
• 'Mucosal neuroma' syndrome (± pheo-, etc.)
3 Familial transmission is autosomal dominant:
— 90% get MTC by age 60
— 50% develop hyperparathyroidism
4 Clinical presentation*
— Lumps in neck
— Watery diarrhea (due to high calcitonin levels)
— Flushing (less marked than in carcinoid syndrome)

5 Screen family members of index cases using
— DNA analysis *if* a germline mutation affecting the *Ret* gene is confirmed
6 Biochemical screening tests (pentagastrin-stimulated calcitonin, *or* calcium- or alcohol-stimulated calcitonin) now *only* indicated *if*
— Familial MTC and no *Ret* mutation detectable, *or*
— Annual surveillance of *Ret*-positive MEN/MTC family member who refuses prophylactic thyroidectomy
7 Prognosis: in general, worse than other differentiated thyroid cancer (e.g. papillary)
— Calcitonin < 1000 pg/mL: 95% cure
— Calcitonin > 10 000 pg/mL: 5% cure

* Calcium remains *normal* despite gross elevation of calcitonin

Carcinoid syndrome: features
1 Primary tumors arise most often in the GI tract (esp. ileum, appendix, stomach, rectum) or bronchi
2 Humoral symptoms (carcinoid syndrome) usually imply metastatic disease, esp. liver
3 Symptoms are most often due to serotonin (5HT), but may also be due to neuropeptide K, neurokinin A, substance P, ACTH, somatostatin, dopamine, gastrin, or histamine*
4 Symptoms include
— flushing (in 90%, esp. in foregut tumors)
— diarrhea (in 70%; secretory)
— abdominal pain (in 40%; due to obstruction, hepatomegaly or gut ischemia)
— facial telangiectasia (in 25%)
— wheezing (in 15%)
— symptoms of valvular lesions‡ (right-sided in 20%, left-sided in 5%)
— pellagra (in 5%)
5 Elevated 24-h urinary level of the serotonin metabolite 5-hydroxyindoleacetic acid (5-HIAA) is almost 100% specific for the diagnosis, esp. for midgut primary tumors. Another useful serum marker is chromogranin A (esp. for hindgut and foregut tumors), which is also elevated in other neuroendocrine tumors including pheochromocytoma and neuroblastoma
6 Extent of disease may be scintigraphically imaged using either ^{123}I-MIBG or ^{111}In-labelled octreotide
7 Octreotide improves flushing and diarrhea
8 *Therapeutic* administration of ^{131}I-MIBG, ^{111}In-octreotide or ^{90}Y-octreotide may cause tumor shrinkage
9 Surgical metastasectomy or liver transplantation may be considered in selected patients

* But note that rectal carcinoids usually secrete glucagon
‡ The anorectic drugs fenfluramine and dexfenfluramine interfere with normal serotonin metabolism and cause identical heart valve lesions

PATTERNS OF NEUROLOGIC DEFICIT IN CANCER

Common presentations of intracranial neoplasms
1 Headaches
— Morning esp.; ± diplopia, projectile vomiting

— May be associated with visual blurring, papilledema, diplopia

2 Convulsions
— May be focal or associated with residual deficit (hemiparesis, aphasia)

3 Cranial nerve deficit
— May be mixed or false-localizing
— May include homonymous/bitemporal hemianopia, CN VI (abducens) palsy, Parinaud's syndrome

4 Personality change
— Including amnesia, dementia

Clinical features of meningeal carcinomatosis

1 Commonest causes
— Small-cell lung cancer
— Breast cancer
— Melanoma

2 Presentation
— Cranial nerve deficits
— Disseminated or mixed deficits (e.g. upper and lower motor neuron lesions)
— Bizarre sensory disturbances (e.g. jaw numbness)

3 Diagnosis
— CSF cytology (positive for malignant cells*)
— ↑ CSF protein ± ↓ CSF glucose
— MRI may confirm nodules within spinal canal or meninges

4 Approach to management
— Intrathecal chemotherapy (usually methotrexate)
— Irradiation of affected neuraxis segment
— Systemic chemotherapy (may penetrate meningeal deposits)

* NB: CSF examination may need to be repeated several times for diagnosis

Cerebrovascular manifestations of malignant disease

1 Intracranial hemorrhage
— Leukemia (e.g. DIC in acute promyelocytic leukemia)
— Bleeding metastases (melanoma, choriocarcinoma)

2 TIAs/cerebral infarction
— Leukemia (DIC, or leukostasis: WCC > 100 000)
— Waldenström's macroglobulinemia (hyperviscosity)
— Non-bacterial endocarditis

3 Sagittal sinus thrombosis
— DIC (e.g. in Ca breast/prostate, APL)

Clinical features of myasthenic (Eaton–Lambert) syndrome

1 Commonest cause
— Small-cell lung cancer
— IgG autoantibodies to presynaptic P/Q type voltage-gated calcium channels

2 Symptoms
— Weakness; myalgias, paresthesiae
— Impotence; dry mouth

3 Signs
— Minimal wasting; hyporeflexia
— Ocular/bulbar sparing

4 Diagnosis
— Negative edrophonium (Tensilon) test
— Post-tetanic facilitation on EMG

5 Treatment
— Ablation of underlying malignancy
— Corticosteroids, plasmapheresis
— Diaminopyridine, guanidine HCl*

6 Prognosis
— Better than non-myasthenic SCLC patients
— Autoantibodies may slow tumor growth by blocking calcium influx

* Both enhance acetylcholine release at neuromuscular junction

Back pain: features suggesting malignant etiology*

1 Past history of cancer
2 Insidious onset, progressive course, worse at night
3 Thoracic or upper lumbar nerve root distribution
4 Disseminated sites of vertebral tenderness
5 Signs of multiple and/or bilateral nerve root lesions
6 Coexisting upper motor neuron signs
7 Sphincter dysfunction, perianal anesthesia, leg weakness

* NB: Back pain due to spinal cord compression of malignant origin is a medical emergency which may require rapid treatment to prevent permanent neurologic sequelae (p. 3)

INVESTIGATING MALIGNANT DISEASE

TUMOR MARKERS

Diagnostic significance of tumor markers*

1 AFP
— Non-seminomatous germ-cell tumors (80%)
• i.e. Teratocarcinomas and embryonal cell carcinomas
• Very high AFP levels correlate with poor prognosis (pp. 19–20)
— Hepatoma (75% have levels > 500 ng/mL)
• Minor elevations (high CEA:AFP ratio) occur in liver metastases
• In *high-risk* populations (e.g. HBV+ Chinese), minor elevations (> 100 ng/mL) indicate a 30–40% risk of hepatoma within 5 years
• Mild elevations also seen in hepatitis and cirrhosis

2 βHCG
— Choriocarcinoma (100%)
— Non-seminomatous germ-cell tumors (50%)
— Seminoma (10% only; elevation is typically mild)

3 CEA
— Levels above 10 ng/mL are fairly specific for cancer, esp. colorectal cancer, but also gastric, pancreatic, hepatobiliary, breast, ovarian and lung cancer
— Often within normal limits in early-stage cancers; hence, useless for screening. High levels generally indicate metastatic disease, esp. in liver; measurement is therefore justified as part of preoperative colorectal cancer staging

— Smaller rises (5-10 ng/mL) occur in smokers, inflammatory bowel disease, liver and lung disease

4 Prostate-specific antigen (PSA)
   — Elevated in 95% primary prostate cancers
   — Levels reflect degree of extraprostatic extension
   — Elevation in asymptomatic patients may indicate need for transrectal ultrasound and/or needle biopsy

5 Alkaline phosphatase
   — Elevations may signify metastasis to bone or liver; in bone disease the enzyme is heat-labile ('bone burns') and there is no elevation of GGT
   — Bone-derived enzyme is marker of osteoblastic activity; correlates with ^{99m}Tc bone scan
   — Placental isoenzyme (PLAP) is elevated in 50% of seminomas and dysgerminomas, and is a sensitive marker for (rare) extragonadal germ-cell tumors

6 Calcitonin
   — Medullary carcinoma of the thyroid
   — Invaluable in screening, diagnosis *and* follow-up‡

7 Thyroglobulin
   — Papillary/follicular thyroid cancer
   — Useful in follow-up

8 Paraprotein
   — B-cell neoplasm, esp. myeloma
   — Useful in diagnosis *and* follow-up
   β2-Microglobulin
   — Myeloma (in follow-up)

9 ESR
   — Hodgkin's, myeloma
   — Useful in follow-up (and as a clue to myeloma diagnosis)

10 Urinary 5-HIAA
   — Carcinoid syndrome
   — Useful in diagnosis *and* follow-up

11 Urinary/plasma catecholamines¶
   — Pheochromocytoma
   — Useful in diagnosis and screening, less so in follow-up

12 Ca 125
   — Ovarian cancer (esp. non-mucinous; cf. inhibin)
   — Positive in 80% cases; predicts recurrence in 75%
   — Not specific for ovarian Ca; can indicate serosal spread of other Ca

13 Ca 15-3
   — Breast cancer
   — Elevated in 75% metastatic cases (cf. CEA ~ 60%)

14 Ca 19-9
   — Rises in response to cholestasis
   — Elevations in the apparent absence of cholestasis suggest Ca pancreas (also biliary system, stomach, colon)
   — > 10 000 U/mL indicates distant metastases; > 1000 U/mL indicates lymph node spread; < 100 U/mL favors possibility of curative pancreatic cancer resection

15 Inhibin
   — Ovarian tumors, esp.
     • Granulosa-cell tumors (also have ↑ plasma estradiol)
     • Mucinous ovarian adenocarcinomas

* Note that only AFP, β-HCG and PSA are therapeutically useful (and hence routinely indicated) in the work-up of unknown primary malignancies (see below)
‡ But has become less useful since the advent of *Ret* gene mutation scanning (p. 23)
¶ Incl. plasma normetanephrine and metanephrine, and urinary vanillylmandelic acid (VMA)

Clinical utility of CEA
1 Immunohistochemical CEA detection
   — Diagnostic distinction of undifferentiated carcinoma (if +) from poorly differentiated lymphoma, germ-cell tumor or amelanotic melanoma (−)
2 Serum CEA measurement
   — Monitoring efficacy of therapy
   — Following up post-surgical colorectal patients: rising CEA levels may indicate resectable disease recurrence (e.g. a solitary liver metastasis)

Prognostic vs predictive factors
1 Prognostic factors
   — Used to estimate the *natural history* of the disease as defined by likely overall survival, relapse-free survival, pattern of metastasis, severity of clinical deficits, etc.; e.g.
     • morphologic tumor differentiation is prognostic in breast cancer
     • young age predicts for aggressive locoregional recurrence in breast cancer
2 Predictive factors
   — Used to predict the *therapeutic response* of the disease to given interventions, e.g.
     • estrogen receptor (ER) predicts for breast cancer response to tamoxifen
     • young age predicts for adjuvant benefit of cytotoxic therapy in breast cancer

CANCERS OF UNKNOWN PRIMARY

Metastases from unknown primary: investigative rationâle
1 Diagnosis of treatable disease, esp.
   — Hormone-responsive disease
   — Chemosensitive disease
2 Prevention of complications related to occult primary (e.g. bowel obstruction)
3 Avoidance of iatrogenic morbidity in resistant disease
4 Prognostic clarification

Prognosis of unknown primary cancers
1 More favorable factors
   — Female
   — Performance status 0–1
   — Presents with lymphadenopathy alone
   — Histology: SCC or poorly differentiated
2 Less favorable factors
   — Male
   — Performance status ≥ 2
   — Presents with ≥ 2 sites of disease, esp. liver, lung, bone
   — Histology: adenocarcinoma

Unknown primary diagnoses requiring active exclusion
1 Chemocurable or chemosensitive tumors, esp.
   — Non-Hodgkin's lymphoma
   — Germ-cell tumors
   — Neuroendocrine tumors (incl. SCLC)
   — Ovarian cancer
2 Hormone-sensitive tumors
   — Breast cancer
   — Prostate cancer
   — Endometrial cancer
   — Thyroid cancer

Post-biopsy evaluation of metastatic disease from unknown primary
1 Well-differentiated adenocarcinoma*
   — Hormone receptor (ER/PR) immunocytochemistry in females
   — Bilateral mammography (irrespective of ER/PR)
   — Plasma PSA in males
2 Well-differentiated squamous cell carcinoma
   — Inspection of cervix, anus, genitals, mouth, vocal cords, scalp and skin
   — CXR (± CT, barium swallow)
3 Carcinoma in cervical nodes
   — CXR; sputum cytology (most reliable in SCLC)
   — Thyroid scan + needle biopsy
   — ENT exam: indirect laryngoscopy ± examination under anesthesia (EUA) with blind biopsies from nasopharynx, base of tongue
4 Retroperitoneal/mediastinal mass, or multiple pulmonary metastases, in a young male
   — AFP, β-HCG, PLAP (plasma *and* immunohistochemistry)
   — ± Testicular ultrasound
   — Blood film, differential, marrow (exclude lymphoma, T-cell leukemia)
   — Tumor cytogenetic analysis for isochromosome 12p
5 Anaplastic tumor
   — Plasma AFP and β-HCG
   — Plasma CEA
   — Exclude undifferentiated lymphoma (monoclonal light chains and other lymphoid lineage markers, e.g. leukocyte common antigen, LCA)
   — Exclude undifferentiated melanoma (S-100, melanin, tyrosinase)
   — Exclude sarcoma (vimentin)

* Consider endoscopy if GI primary suspected *and* management affected

PATHOLOGIC EVALUATION

Histopathologic characterization of tumor tissue
1 Light microscopy
   — Signet ring cells (favor gastric primary)
   — Melanin (melanoma)
   — Mucin
     • Common in gut/lung/breast/endometrial cancer
     • Less common in ovarian cancer
     • Rare in renal cell or thyroid cancer
   — Psammoma bodies
     • Ovarian cancer (mucin +)
     • Thyroid cancer (mucin –)
2 Immunoperoxidase
   — AFP, β-HCG, ± PLAP (p. 9)
   — PSA
   — CEA, cytokeratin, EMA (carcinomas)
   — Leukocyte common antigen (lymphomas)
   — Neuron-specific enolase (neuroblastoma, SCLC)
   — Thyroglobulin (follicular thyroid carcinoma)
   — Calcitonin (medullary thyroid carcinoma)
   — S-100, vimentin, tyrosinase (melanoma)
   — Vimentin (sarcomas)
   — Desmin, muscle-specific actin (rhabdomyosarcoma)
   — Factor VIII antigen (angiosarcoma)
3 Surface immunoglobulin
   — Anti-light chain monoclonal antibodies
   — Phenotypic T-cell markers (e.g. CD4)
4 Hormone receptor immunocytochemistry (Ca breast)
5 Electron microscopy
   — Distinguishes
     • Adenocarcinoma and mesothelioma
     • Spindle-cell tumors (sarcomas, melanoma, SCC)
     • Small round-cell tumors (see below)
   — May identify
     • Amelanotic melanoma (melanosomes)
     • Carcinoids (neurosecretory granules)
     • Undifferentiated lymphomas, histiocytosis X

Differential diagnosis of small round-cell tumors
'LEMON':
1 **L**ymphoma
2 **E**wing's tumor; rhabdomyosarcoma
3 **M**edulloblastoma
4 **O**at-cell (small-cell) carcinoma
5 **N**euroblastoma, primitive neuroectodermal tumor (PNET)

STAGING OF SOLID TUMORS

Staging of testicular germ-cell tumors
1 Stage I   — Involvement limited to testis
2 Stage II — Abdominal nodal involvement
3 Stage III — Mediastinal involvement, *and/or*
             — Supraclavicular node involvement, *and/or*
             — Lung parenchyma involvement
4 Stage IV — Extranodal, extrapulmonary disease

Adverse prognostic features in testicular germ-cell tumors
1 Bulky disease
   — Infradiaphragmatic tumor mass > 10 cm diameter
   — Supradiaphragmatic tumor mass > 5 cm diameter
2 Extragonadal primary tumor, esp. 1° mediastinal disease
3 AFP > 10 000 ng/mL; β-HCG > 50 000 mIU/mL

4 Non-pulmonary visceral spread (esp. to liver, bone, CNS), *or*
   Pulmonary metastases: > 20 tumors, or > 3 cm diameter
5 Unfavorable histology (e.g. pure choriocarcinoma)

Histologic subtypes of testicular tumors
1 Seminoma (dysgerminoma)   — 40%
2 Non-seminomatous germ-cell tumors
     Mixed embryonal/teratoma   — 40%
     Pure embryonal carcinoma   — 12%
     Pure teratoma   — 7%
     Pure choriocarcinoma   — 1%

Staging of colorectal carcinoma
1 Duke's A
   — Confined to (sub)mucosa
   — > 90% 5-year survival
   — No proven survival benefit with adjuvant chemotherapy
2 Duke's B
   — Spread through muscularis layer
   — 70–85% 5-year survival
   — Probable survival benefit with adjuvant chemotherapy
3 Duke's C
   — Involvement of local nodes
   — 30–60% 5-year survival
   — Definite survival benefit with adjuvant chemotherapy
4 Duke's D
   — Distant metastases
   — < 5% 5-year survival
   — No survival benefit with adjuvant chemotherapy

Staging of cervical cancer
1 FIGO stage 0— Carcinoma in situ
2 FIGO stage 1— Confined to cervix
3 FIGO stage 2— Extends to upper vagina or parametrium
4 FIGO stage 3— Extends to lower vagina/pelvic sidewall
5 FIGO stage 4— Extends beyond true pelvis

Staging of small-cell lung cancer
1 Limited disease
   — Confined to hemithorax
   — Includes ipsilateral supraclavicular nodes
   — Can be encompassed within a single radiotherapy port
2 Extensive disease
   — Spread beyond hemithorax
   — Includes ipsilateral pleural effusion
   — Cannot be encompassed within a single radiotherapy port

BREAST CANCER EVALUATION AND STAGING

TNM staging*: breast cancer as an example
1 **T** = tumor
   — T1: tumor < 2 cm diameter
   — T2: tumor 2 cm diameter
   — T3: tumor fixed to pectoralis muscle/fascia‡
   — T4: tumor involving chest wall or skin; includes
      • Peau d'orange
      • Dermal lymphatic invasion ('inflammatory' Ca)
2 **N** = nodes
   — N0 = impalpable nodes (± negative histology)
   — N1 = mobile axillary adenopathy (positive histology)
   — N2 = matted/fixed axillary nodes
   — N3 = supraclavicular or internal mammary adenopathy
3 **M** = metastases
   — M0 = no evidence of metastases
   — M1 = distant metastases

* Note that many important variables relevant to choice of therapy (e.g. hormone receptor status) are *not* included in this classification system
‡ But note that T3 is not always stage III

Clinical approach to mammographic findings
1 Minimally suspicious abnormality in an asymptomatic (screened) patient with negative findings on physical examination
   — Repeat the mammogram in 6 months
2 Architectural distortion, mass or microcalcifications of uncertain significance
   — Needle (wire) localization under X-ray followed by excision biopsy
3 Suspicious (linear or branching) microcalcifications, or clinically occult mass lesion
   — Stereotactic breast biopsy (may use Mammotome™)
4 Clinical mass associated with a normal mammogram
   — Biopsy (fine needle aspirate, core or excision)

Axillary nodal staging of primary breast cancer
1 Although axillary staging is an informative *prognostic* measure, node-negative patients still have a 20–30% risk of dying from breast cancer (depending upon other variables such as tumor size). The prognostic accuracy of axillary staging is less in medial quadrant tumors (which tend to metastasize to internal mammary or supraclavicular nodes). Nodal status is not highly *predictive* (p. 9) since node-negative patients derive almost as much benefit from adjuvant treatment as do node-positive patients
2 Patients with 1–3 nodes involved have a slightly worse outlook than node-negative patients, whereas those with 4–9 nodes do worse again
3 Patients with 10 or more involved nodes are likely to die from breast cancer despite standard adjuvant treatments. Whether such patients benefit from such treatments in terms of disease-free or overall survival remains uncertain
4 Although the risk of axillary recurrence is lessened by routine dissection of the axilla, such recurrences may be amenable to salvage surgery; the net benefit of prophylactic dissection in terms of local control is therefore small. Nodes do not limit metastatic spread
5 Dye can be injected into the breast to identify the first lymph node draining the breast lymphatics.

Selective resection of this *sentinel node* permits reliable characterization of nodal metastatic status, obviating the need for further node dissection in negative patients

6 Morbidity from axillary dissection is significant; the commonest residua are pain and limitation of shoulder movement

7 Nodal surgery is not indicated in pure carcinoma in situ

8 Combination of dissection and axillary radiotherapy is contraindicated due to the high incidence of lymphedema

MANAGING MALIGNANT DISEASE

(See also Chapter 11, Palliative care)

MANAGEMENT OF PREMALIGNANT CONDITIONS

Premalignant conditions susceptible to cancer chemoprevention

1 Oral cancer
   — Treat leukoplakia patients with 13-*cis*-retinoic acid
2 Breast cancer
   — Treat high-risk patients with tamoxifen or raloxifene
3 Colorectal cancer
   — Treat high-risk individuals with COX2 inhibitors and/or folic acid or calcium supplements

Potential indications for surgery in premalignant conditions

1 Orchiopexy in children with testicular maldescent
   Orchidectomy in adolescents or adults with cryptorchidism
   Bilateral orchidectomy in testicular feminization
2 Oophorectomy in Turner's syndrome (incl. mosaics)
3 Colectomy in familial polyposis or in long-standing ulcerative colitis with severe dysplasia
4 Prophylactic mastectomy in high-risk *BRCA1/2* carriers (controversial)
5 Thyroidectomy for MEN2 family carriers (i.e. *Ret* mutation-positive) in childhood

TREATMENT STRATEGIES

Extent of disease: influence on treatment

1 Local treatments
   — Surgery
   — Radiotherapy
2 Systemic treatments
   — Cytotoxic chemotherapy
   — Biotherapy (e.g. hormone therapy, bisphosphonates, antibodies, cytokines)

Therapeutic approaches in oncology

1 Neoadjuvant
   — Initial (upfront, presurgical) systemic therapy of locally advanced disease aimed at downstaging, thus expediting local R_x
2 Adjuvant
   — Prophylactic (e.g. post-surgical) treatment of presumed micrometastases
3 Radical
   — Maximal local treatment, usually with curative intent
4 Palliative (Ch. 11)
   — Specific antitumor treatment administered without anticipated survival prolongation, but with hope of improved quality of life
5 Symptomatic (Ch. 11)
   — Non-specific measures only; no anticancer efficacy

Malignancies curable with chemotherapy

1 70–95% cure rate
   — Testicular teratoma or seminoma
   — Choriocarcinoma (in women)
   — Hodgkin's disease
   — Wilms' tumor
2 40–60% cure rate
   — Acute lymphoblastic leukemia (in childhood)
   — Burkitt's lymphoma (endemic variety)
   — Non-Hodgkin's lymphoma (diffuse large-cell)
3 20–30% cure rate
   — Acute lymphoblastic leukemia (in adults)
   — Acute myeloblastic leukemia

Advanced malignancies highly responsive to palliative chemotherapy

1 Lymphomas, chronic leukemias, myeloma
2 Breast cancer
3 Ovarian cancer
4 Lung cancer, esp. small-cell
5 Colorectal cancer
6 Head and neck cancer, esp. nasopharyngeal

Malignancies in which adjuvant chemotherapy improves survival

1 Breast cancer
2 Colorectal cancer (Dukes stage C, or B2)
3 Wilms' tumor, osteogenic sarcoma, embryonal rhabdomyosarcoma

Malignancies curable with radiotherapy

1 Seminoma
2 Hodgkin's disease stages IA and IIA (unless bulky)
3 Early-stage head/neck tumors (incl. laryngeal or lingual SCC)
4 Early-stage carcinoma of the cervix or bladder
5 Non-melanomatous skin cancer (if surgery contraindicated)

Malignancies treated with chemoradiation*

1 Squamous cell carcinoma of the cervix
2 Squamous cell carcinoma of the vulva
3 Squamous cell carcinoma of the anus
4 Squamous cell carcinoma of the head and neck (incl. laryngeal or lingual SCC)

5 Squamous cell carcinoma of the lung‡

* i.e. Concomitant chemotherapy and radiotherapy
‡ Actually, any non-small-cell lung cancer!

Malignancies responsive to hormonal manipulation
1 Breast cancer (p. 19)
2 Prostate cancer (p. 20)
3 Endometrial cancer (progestogens)
4 Papillary/follicular thyroid cancer ($T_4 \rightarrow$ TSH suppression)

Malignancies that may undergo spontaneous regression
1 Neuroblastoma (esp. stage IV S)
2 Kaposi's sarcoma (endemic variety)
3 Renal cell carcinoma (*rarely*, metastases may regress after removing primary)
4 Melanoma

Malignancies generally resistant to treatment
1 Gastrointestinal adenocarcinomas, esp. pancreas
2 Renal cell carcinoma
3 Melanoma
4 Mesothelioma
5 Hepatoma

Prognosis of treated malignancies*
1 Breast cancer
  Bladder cancer } 60% 5-year survival
  SCC cervix
2 Colorectal cancer }
  Prostate cancer } 40% 5-year survival
3 Ovarian cancer } 30% 5-year survival
4 Pancreatic cancer
  Gastric cancer
  Esophageal cancer } 5% 5-year survival
  Lung cancer

* For all stages of disease and all causes of death

MECHANISMS OF CYTOTOXIC ACTIVITY AND RESISTANCE

Classification of common chemotherapeutic agents
1 Alkylators (i.e. add methyl groups to DNA)
  — Cyclophosphamide, ifosfamide
  — Nitrogen mustard (mechlorethamine), melphalan (phenylalanine mustard), busulfan
  — Platinum derivatives (carboplatin, cisplatin)
2 Intercalators (i.e. crosslink DNA strands)
  — Anthracyclines (daunorubicin, doxorubicin, epirubicin)
  — Anthraquinones (mitoxantrone)
3 Nitrosoureas (alkylate and crosslink DNA)
  — BCNU, CCNU, streptozotocin
4 Spindle toxins (poison the microtubular contractile system)
  — Vinca alkaloids: vinorelbine, vincristine, vinblastine
  — Yew bark derivatives: paclitaxel (Taxol™), docetaxel

5 Topoisomerase inhibitors (inhibit DNA-untangling enzymes)
  — Topoisomerase I inhibitors (e.g. irinotecan, topotecan)
  — Topoisomerase II inhibitors: podophyllotoxin derivatives (e.g. etoposide)
6 Antimetabolites (spuriously incorporated into replicating DNA)
  — Purine analogs
    • Azathioprine, 6MP, 6TG
  — Enzyme inhibitors and chain terminators
    • Methotrexate ($\rightarrow$ dihydrofolate reductase)
    • Hydroxyurea, fludarabine ($\rightarrow$ ribonucleotide reductase, DNA polymerase)
    • 5-FU, capecitabine, ralitrexed ($\rightarrow$ thymidylate synthetase)
    • Gemcitabine* ($\rightarrow$ cytidine synthetase)
    • Deoxycoformycin ($\rightarrow$ cytosine deaminase)
7 Antitumor antibiotics (variable mechanisms of action)
  — Bleomycin, mitomycin C, dactinomycin
8 Protein synthesis inhibitors (block translation)
  — L-asparaginase

* A cytosine arabinoside analog

Mechanisms of tumor resistance to cytotoxic drugs
1 General
  — Tumor heterogeneity: genetic instability of primary tumor $\rightarrow$ clonal loss of sensitive tumor cells leading to dominant outgrowth of drug-resistant clones
  — Small growth fraction: many tumors replicate no faster than normal tissues, and thus have ample time to repair chemotherapy-induced DNA damage
2 Specific
  — Increased drug efflux (amplification of multidrug transporter genes)
  — Enhanced lesion repair (e.g. induction of DNA alkyltransferase activity)
  — Gene amplification (e.g. of the *DHFR* gene during methotrexate therapy)

THERAPEUTIC USE OF CYTOTOXIC DRUGS

Points to discuss with patients prior to commencing treatment
1 Prognosis with and without treatment
2 Probability of therapeutic benefit (cure, complete or partial remission, disease-free interval, symptoms)
3 Risks of infertility/teratogenicity/premature menopause; availability of sperm banking
4 Likely severity of alopecia; availability of wig-making
5 Likely severity and duration of nausea; prophylactic drugs
6 Need for allopurinol (in hematologic malignancies)
7 Requirement for regular blood tests
8 Urgent significance of fever or bruising/bleeding
9 Rationâle of clinical trials and informed consent
10 Long-term risk of second malignancy, esp. in good-prognosis disease treated with alkylating agents ± radiotherapy

Clinical assessment of the patient commencing treatment
1 Assessment and documentation of disease extent
   — Measurement (and/or photography) of visible lesions
   — Radiographic corroboration
   — Measurement of tumor markers
   — Invasive staging *if* stage-specific therapy exists
2 Assessment of vital organ function
   — Left ventricular function (pre-doxorubicin)
   — Renal function, e.g. creatinine clearance (pre-platinum)
3 Assessment of immune status (in leukemia, transplantation)
   — CXR
   — Viral (CMV, HSV, hepatitis B) and toxoplasma serology
4 Assessment of venous access
   — Consideration of an implantable infusion port/catheter
5 Assessment of psychological adjustment to disease, and to disease- and treatment-related disability

Chemotherapeutic agents often used for solid tumors
1 Germ-cell tumors
   — Bleomycin, etoposide, cisplatin (BEP): first-line
   — Vinblastine, ifosfamide, cisplatin (VIP): salvage/pretransplant
2 Small-cell lung cancer
   — Topoisomerase inhibitors (etoposide > topotecan), cisplatin
   — Doxorubicin, cyclophosphamide, vincristine
   Non-small-cell lung cancer
   — Paclitaxel, carboplatin
   — Gemcitabine, vinorelbine
3 Breast cancer
   — Doxorubicin *or* epirubicin (± cyclophosphamide and/or 5-FU)
   — Docetaxel *or* paclitaxel
   — Vinorelbine, gemcitabine, capecitabine
   — Cyclophosphamide, methotrexate, 5-FU (CMF)
4 Ovarian cancer
   — Cisplatin *or* carboplatin (see below)
   — Paclitaxel
   — Chlorambucil *or* cyclophosphamide
   — Topotecan (in platinum-resistant disease)
5 Choriocarcinoma
   — Methotrexate, dactinomycin
6 Osteosarcoma
   — Methotrexate, doxorubicin, cisplatin
7 Colorectal cancer
   — 5-FU + calcium folinate
   — Irinotecan, oxaliplatin
8 Adrenocortical carcinoma
   — Mitotane (*o,p*-DDD)
9 Langerhans cell histiocytosis ('histiocytosis X')
   — Etoposide

Cytotoxic drugs often administered orally
1 Capecitabine
2 Cyclophosphamide, chlorambucil, busulfan
3 Etoposide
4 Corticosteroids

Hair-sparing cytotoxic drugs
1 Gemcitabine
2 Capecitabine
3 Vinorelbine
4 Platinum derivatives

Relatively non-myelosuppressive cytotoxics
1 Cisplatin (cf. carboplatin)
2 Bleomycin
3 Vincristine (cf. vinblastine, vinorelbine)
4 Methotrexate *with* folinate rescue
5 L-Asparaginase

Cisplatin or carboplatin?
1 Testicular germ-cell tumors
   Head and neck cancers, bladder cancer
   — Cisplatin (more effective)
2 Ovarian cancer
   — Carboplatin (more convenient)
3 Poor bone marrow reserve, esp. leukocytes
   — Cisplatin
4 Pre-existing renal failure, heart failure or hearing impairment
   — Carboplatin
5 Lung cancer
   — No difference in efficacy

Drug therapies that tend to be expensive
1 Any newly licensed anticancer agent (e.g. imatinib)
2 Recombinant products (e.g. growth factors)
3 Humanized monoclonal antibodies (e.g. rituximab, trastuzumab)
4 Chronic oral drugs (e.g. hormone antagonists, bisphosphonates)
5 New adjunctive drugs for symptom control (e.g. antiemetics)

MORBIDITY OF CYTOTOXIC THERAPY

Common problems limiting use of cytotoxic therapy
1 Myelosuppression
   — Alkylators, anthracyclines, nitrosoureas
   — Vinblastine, vinorelbine
   — Ara-C
2 Nausea
   — Cisplatin
   — Anthracyclines, alkylating agents
   Diarrhea
   — Irinotecan
   Typhilitis (neutropenic necrotizing enterocolitis)
   — Docetaxel (and other myelosuppressives)
3 Total alopecia
   — Anthracyclines, taxanes
   — Etoposide, ara-C, cyclophosphamide (IV)
4 Mucositis, stomatitis
   — Irinotecan
   — 5-FU, methotrexate, bleomycin
   — Anthracyclines
5 Pulmonary fibrosis
   — Bleomycin, busulfan (dose-related)
   — Methotrexate, cyclophosphamide (idiosyncratic)

6 Radiation recall reactions
  — Anthracyclines, dactinomycin
  — Methotrexate, bleomycin, 5-FU
7 Myalgias
  — Taxanes, esp. paclitaxel
8 Infusional vessel toxicity
  — Anthracyclines (extravasation necrosis)
  — Vincas, esp. vinorelbine (phlebitis)
9 Neurotoxicity
  — Vincas, taxanes, cisplatin
10 Cardiotoxicity
  — Trastuzumab (Herceptin)
  — Anthracyclines* (cardiac failure or arrhythmias)
  — Taxanes; cyclophosphamide (myopericarditis)
  — 5-FU (coronary spasm or arrhythmias)

* Usually at cumulative doses > 240 mg/m²; risk may be reduced using the EDTA-like iron chelator dexrazoxane

Skin reactions following chemotherapy
1 Hand–foot syndrome (palmar–plantar desquamation)
  — Capecitabine (+ other thymidylate synthetase inhibitors)
2 Photosensitivity
  — Bleomycin, procarbazine, vinblastine
3 Pigmentation
  — Busulfan, doxorubicin
4 Nail changes
  — Docetaxel

Chemotherapy of the jaundiced patient
1 Drugs that *may* be administered at near-full dose
  — Gemcitabine (caution if significant transaminitis)
  — Ifosfamide (with MESNA and hydration)
  — Nitrogen mustard
2 Drugs that should be avoided or heavily dose-reduced
  — Anthracyclines
  — Cyclophosphamide
  — Taxanes
  — Vincas

Relative contraindications to anthracycline therapy*
1 Left ventricular dysfunction (ejection fraction < 50%) or arrhythmia
2 Concomitant administration of trastuzumab (Herceptin, anti-*Erb*B2)
3 Other cardiac risk factor(s), esp. if also combined with history of mediastinal or left chest irradiation, and/or with concomitant use of cyclophosphamide or taxane
4 Deep jaundice or severe transaminitis (> 4 times upper limit of normal)
5 Frail and/or elderly patient
6 Morbid fear of hair loss

* Cumulative doses (esp. above 240 mg/m²) are associated with cardiotoxicity

Drug interactions with cytotoxic therapy
1 Azathioprine, oral 6-MP
  — 4-fold potentiation by allopurinol (inhibits drug catabolism by xanthine oxidase)
2 Methotrexate
  — Potentiated by aspirin, NSAIDs (see below)
3 Procarbazine
  — Hypertension on tyramine ingestion (MAO inhibitor)
4 Cyclophosphamide
  — Activated in liver (hence, potentiated) by enzyme inducers (e.g. barbiturates)

Methotrexate toxicity: precipitants, potentiation and prevention
1 Precipitants (drugs competing for renal tubular secretion)
  — Aspirin: displaces drug from plasma protein binding
  — Probenecid, phenylbutazone, trimethoprim
2 Potentiation
  — Concurrent radiotherapy
  — Third-space sequestration in effusions or ascites
3 Prevention (esp. in high-dose regimens)
  — Forced diuresis (intravenous prehydration)
  — Urinary alkalinization
  — Oral folinic acid (calcium folinate) rescue*

* Note that whereas folinic acid *rescues* methotrexate toxicity on normal cells, its combination with thymidylate synthesis inhibitors such as 5-FU serves to *enhance* tumor cell killing

Which antiemetic for the vomiting patient?
1 Chemoreceptor trigger zone-induced emesis (e.g. due to chemotherapy)
  — Acute (< 3 days) nausea: 5-HT₃ receptor blockers (ondansetron, granisetron)
  — Prolonged (> 3 days) nausea: metoclopramide, domperidone, haloperidol
2 Raised intracranial pressure, cranial irradiation, distension of liver capsule, ureters, etc.
  — Dexamethasone + cyclizine infusion
3 Intestinal obstruction*
  — Octreotide
  — Metoclopramide

* e.g. associated with opioid use

SECOND PRIMARY NEOPLASMS

Neoplastic disorders often complicated by second malignancy
1 Hodgkin's disease, non-Hodgkin's lymphoma
2 Multiple myeloma (melphalan)
3 Polycythemia vera (chlorambucil, ³²P)

Cytotoxic agents predisposing to second malignancies
1 Alkylating agents (e.g. chlorambucil, melphalan)
  — Associated with 5q- and 7q- deletions
2 Etoposide (VP-16)
  — Causes 11q23 and 21q22 translocations
3 Mitoxantrone; other intercalators
4 Nitrosoureas; procarbazine
5 Platinum drugs
6 Azathioprine*

* Azathioprine is partly converted to thioguanine which is in turn methylated; the mutagenic alkylguanine lesions which result may lead to *post-transplant* malignancies

Cytotoxic-induced malignancies
1 Acute non-lymphocytic leukemia*
   — esp. Myelomonocytic
2 Non-Hodgkin's lymphoma
   — Post-transplant/-Hodgkin's
3 SCC (skin, cervix)
   — Post-transplant
4 TCC (bladder)
   — Post-cyclophosphamide
5 Miscellaneous adenocarcinomas and soft-tissue
   sarcomas
   — Colon, lung, bone, thyroid

* Up to 5% incidence within 10 years, esp. if also treated with
radiotherapy. Myelodysplastic syndrome (MDS; p. 160) is a
common antecedent

Radiation-induced malignancies
1 Thyroid tumors
   — After low-dose external radiation (e.g. skin
     irradiation for acne)
   — *Not* seen after ¹³¹I therapy
2 Myeloma, non-lymphocytic leukemias
   — AML (7q-)
   — CML (*not* CLL)
3 Breast cancer
   — e.g. following radiotherapy for Hodgkin's
     disease
4 Lung cancer, esp. SCLC
   — e.g. in Hiroshima survivors
5 Osteo-/soft tissue sarcoma
   — e.g. chest wall sarcomas after breast cancer
     irradiation
6 Skin tumors
   — e.g. after scalp irradiation for ringworm
7 CNS tumors (meningiomas, other neural tumors)
   — After low-dose (1–2 Gy) scalp irradiation for
     tinea capitis

Hormone-induced neoplasms
1 Hepatocellular carcinoma	— Androgenic anabolic steroids
2 Hepatic adenoma	— Combined oral contraceptive
3 Endometrial carcinoma	— Exogenous estrogens; tamoxifen
4 Breast cancer Prostate cancer	— Endogenous estrogens, HRT — Endogenous androgens
5 Clear-cell vaginal carcinoma	— Maternal diethylstilbestrol

THROMBOTIC DISORDERS IN CANCER

Predispositions to thromboembolism in cancer patients
1 Prior surgery
2 Immobilization
3 Metastatic disease
4 Intravenous chemotherapy
5 Hormone therapy

Risk factors for upper limb thrombosis* in cancer patients
1 Axillary or mediastinal tumor masses

2 Central venous line in situ
3 Intravenous chemotherapy (including adjuvant)

* Including arterial thrombosis

PRINCIPLES OF RADIATION THERAPY

Modes of radiotherapy administration
1 External beam
   — Superficial (25–150 kV)
     • Limited penetration
     • Used for skin cancers (BCC, SCC)
   — Orthovoltage (250–350 kV)
     • Moderate penetration
     • Used to palliate painful bone metastases
     • Skin toxicity may be a problem
   — Megavoltage (> 1 MV; usually 4–10 MV)
     • Produced by cobalt machines or linear
       accelerators
     • Excellent penetration ('skin-sparing'
       radiation)
2 Brachytherapy (interstitial)
   — Unsealed sources
     • ³²P (polycythemia vera)
     • ¹³¹I (Graves' disease, differentiated thyroid
       cancer)
     • ¹³⁷Cs (cesium: Ca cervix)
   — Sealed sources
     • ¹⁹²Ir (iridium: e.g. head and neck tumors)

Determinants of radiation-induced toxicity
1 Volume irradiated
2 Tissue/organ irradiated
3 Fraction size (i.e. dose per treatment session)
4 Total dose

Normal tissue tolerance: radiation dose thresholds*
1 Brain
   — 40 Gy
2 Heart, small intestine
   — 30 Gy
3 Liver, lung, kidney
   — 20 Gy
4 Whole body
   — 3–5 Gy

* = the 5% injury risk for an 'average' treatment volume and
fractionation

Common problems following therapeutic irradiation*
1 Acute local toxicity
   — Skin erythema, desquamation, photosensitivity
   — Hair loss (usually transient)
   — Mucositis: xerostomia, esophagitis, cystitis
2 Acute systemic toxicity (radiation sickness)
   — Fatigue and malaise
   — Nausea, anorexia
3 Late toxicity caused by endarteritis obliterans, e.g.
   — Radiation nephritis
   — Radiation pneumonitis
   — Radiation myelopathy (cord ischemia)
   — ↓ Hemopoietic reserve (compromising
     chemotherapy)

4 Following mantle irradiation (Hodgkin's)
   — Hypothyroidism (30% within 20 years)
   — Graves' disease, thyroiditis, carcinoma
5 Following cranial irradiation
   — Intellectual deterioration, somnolence (esp. children)
   — Hypopituitarism due to hypothalamic damage
     • Low GH, high prolactin, low FSH/LH
     • Low free T_4 without $\uparrow$ TSH
6 Mutagenicity
   — Leukemia, (esp.) after megavoltage therapy or ^{32}P
   — CNS tumors after neuraxis irradiation for ALL

* NB. *Late* toxicity (e.g. stricture, second malignancy) is a major concern in *radical* treatment, but less so (or not at all) in *palliative* treatment

Problems following abdominal or pelvic irradiation
1 Nausea, esp. following abdominal irradiation (e.g. for ovarian cancer, seminoma, lymphoma)
   — Management: antiemetics (p. 15)
2 Diarrhea, esp. following radical pelvic irradiation (for gynecological or genitourinary malignancies)
   — Management: loperamide, codeine, low-residue diet
3 Tenesmus, rectal bleeding (radiation proctitis)
   — Management: prednisolone suppositories
4 Urinary frequency/dysuria
   — Management: exclude infection; anticholinergics; alkalinizers; cystoscopy
5 Vaginal discharge ± cervicitis
   — Management: exclude *Candida, Trichomonas* spp.
   Vaginal adhesions or stenosis
   — Management: treat with dilators
6 Nephrotoxicity (dose-related)
   — Management: prevent by shielding

MANAGEMENT OF LUNG CANCER

Contraindications to thoracotomy for lung cancer*
1 Evidence of local extrapulmonary invasion‡
   — Hoarseness, bovine cough (laryngeal nerve palsy) *or* phrenic nerve palsy)
   — Superior vena caval obstruction; dysphagia
   — Horner's (± Pancoast's) syndrome
   — Pleural effusion (unless chylous)
2 Evidence of mediastinal involvement¶
   — Carinal widening on chest X-ray
   — Positive mediastinoscopy
3 Evidence of distant spread§
   — Positive liver/bone/brain scan/marrow/CSF
4 Inability to tolerate surgery
   — Age: > 65 (for pneumonectomy), > 70 (for lobectomy)
   — FEV_I < 1.5 L (pneumonectomy) or < 1.0 L (lobectomy)
   — P_aCO_2 > 45 mmHg *unless* due to distal collapse
   — Pulmonary hypertension ± cor pulmonale
   — Anesthetic risk factors (e.g. ischemic heart disease)
   — Technical problems: tumor < 2 cm from carina on bronchoscopy

* Only 10% of patients are found suitable for surgery on initial assessment, and of these only a minority prove resectable; *paraneoplastic syndromes* (p. 5) per se are *not* contraindications
‡ Best evaluated by CT
¶ If no clinical or CT evidence of advanced disease, preoperative mediastinoscopy is indicated
§ Small cell histology on biopsy or sputum cytology is usually predictive of distant spread

Favorable prognostic features in non-small-cell lung cancer
1 Age < 60 with normal lung function
2 No weight loss
3 Right-sided tumor with no demonstrable spread
4 Well-differentiated histology
5 Removable by single lobectomy

Adverse prognostic features in small-cell lung cancer
1 Weight loss
2 Extensive disease (p. 11), esp. CNS/liver/marrow spread
3 Failure to achieve complete remission with chemotherapy

Therapeutic modalities in small-cell lung cancer
1 Combination chemotherapy: curative intent in patients with limited-stage disease (p. 11), palliative if adverse prognosis
2 Prophylactic cranial irradiation for patients achieving complete remission following cytotoxic treatment
3 Mediastinal irradiation for all patients with limited disease, usually starting after one cycle of chemotherapy. Patients achieving complete remission of bulky mediastinal disease may also benefit from mediastinal irradiation

Therapeutic modalities in non-small-cell lung cancer
1 Stage II or IIIA disease: mediastinoscopy negative, or positive only for microscopic involvement of mediastinal lymph nodes
   — Induction chemoradiotherapy followed by surgery
2 Stage IIIB disease: macroscopic (N2) mediastinoscopic disease or CT-staged N3 or T4 disease
   — Concurrent chemoradiotherapy ± surgery
3 Advanced disease: distant metastases; vertebral lysis, venous obstruction, subclavian arterial involvement, widespread nodal disease or extensive nerve root destruction; or significant cardiopulmonary disease
   — Radiotherapy for local symptomatic palliation
   — Palliative chemotherapy for progressive multifocal disease

MANAGEMENT OF BREAST CANCER

Precursor lesions in breast cancer: in situ carcinoma
1 Ductal carcinoma in situ (DCIS; intraductal carcinoma)
   — Different histologic subtypes (e.g. comedo-DCIS) and grades

— Gives rise to invasive cancer (infiltrating ductal carcinoma) in 30%
— Often associated with suspicious mammographic microcalcifications (p. 11)
— Microcalcifications may be needle-localized under X-ray, then excised
— Prognosis for recurrence varies directly with the excision margin
— Extensive intraductal carcinoma (EIC) may necessitate mastectomy
— Both radiotherapy and tamoxifen reduce the risk of post-operative local recurrence of DCIS

2 Lobular carcinoma in situ (LCIS)
— Not precancerous per se; rather, a marker of increased cancer risk in *both* breasts
— Incidence of subsequent invasive cancer ~ 1%/year
— Subsequent tumors may be ductal in origin (i.e. *not* usually lobular carcinomas)
— Subsequent tumors may *not* arise from LCIS region
— Manage with close clinical and mammographic follow-up

Prognostic considerations in breast cancer

1 Relapse may occur several decades after diagnosis
2 The post-surgical risk of relapse and *relapse-free survival* is best predicted by the number of axillary node metastases (and, to a lesser extent, by tumor size)
3 The *post-relapse survival* (i.e. length of survival after disease recurrence) is best predicted by the clinical response to hormonal manipulation. The average post-relapse survival is currently 18 months
4 Relapses within 12 months of completing primary treatment generally indicate a poor outlook (exception: relapse within the breast or axillary nodes may still be curable)

Variables influencing choice of local treatment

1 Prerequisites for omitting post-lumpectomy irradiation*
— Axillary lymph node negativity, *and*
— Absence of lymphatic or vascular invasion (LVI), *and*
— Clear (> 2 mm) resection margins‡, *and*
— Small tumor (e.g. < 1 cm, detected by mammography)
2 Indications for mastectomy
— Diffuse multifocal carcinoma *or* extensive intraductal carcinoma (EIC)
— Unacceptable cosmetic result from breast conservation¶
— Contraindication to radiotherapy (e.g. pregnancy)
— Patient preference

* In general, post-lumpectomy radiotherapy reduces the overall risk of local recurrence from 25% to 5%. Hence, almost all lumpectomy patients currently get radiotherapy.
‡ Re-excision (± radiotherapy) is also an option if technically feasible
¶ i.e. relatively large tumor; better cosmesis (if desired) achieved with immediate reconstruction

Breast cancer in pregnancy: management considerations

1 No role is proven for abortion in modifying the natural history of the disease
2 Surgery appears to be tolerated by mother and fetus at any stage of pregnancy
3 Chemotherapy is contraindicated in the first trimester and best postponed if possible until after delivery. Few teratogenic effects are well documented, however
4 Ionizing radiation should be avoided throughout pregnancy
5 Subsequent pregnancies are not contraindicated, but mothers should realize that their life expectancy remains reduced

LOCAL TREATMENT OF BREAST CANCER

Management of locally recurrent breast cancer

1 Intramammary (post-lumpectomy) recurrence
— Mastectomy
2 Chest wall recurrence* (e.g. post-mastectomy)
— Palliative systemic therapy
3 Nodal recurrence
— Isolated axillary relapse
  • Dissection and/or irradiation
— Supraclavicular/internal mammary nodes
  • Palliative systemic therapy and/or radiotherapy

* Same prognostic significance as distant metastases

Indications for post-mastectomy irradiation

1 T_3 or T_4 stage primary tumor
2 Mastectomy specimen reveals involved (or ≤ 1 mm) margins
3 Heavy axillary nodal involvement (≥ 4 nodes positive)

Post-mastectomy reconstructive surgery for primary breast cancer

1 Varieties
— Silicone implant
— Latissimus dorsi flap
— TRAM (trans-rectus abdominus muscle) flap
2 May be carried out either at the time of mastectomy, or subsequently
3 Relatively contraindicated for bad prognosis (e.g. heavily node-positive) disease

SYSTEMIC TREATMENT OF BREAST CANCER

Choice of adjuvant systemic therapy in breast cancer

1 Premenopausal*
— Adjuvant cytotoxic therapy, *and*
— Adjuvant oral hormonal therapy (if ER+) *or*
— Ovarian ablation (if ER+ *and* chemotherapy is declined)
2 Post-menopausal
— Adjuvant oral hormonal therapy if ER+
— Consider cytotoxic chemotherapy if ER−

* In practice, includes patients menstruating normally *or* plasma FSH < 20 *or* age < 60 years

Indications for chemotherapy (> hormones) in breast cancer

1 Inflammatory* primary carcinoma
2 Aggressive relapse (e.g. metastatic liver disease or lymphangitic pulmonary spread)
3 Any ER-negative metastatic disease
4 Any metastatic disease with no response to an adequate (6-week) trial of hormonal therapy

* Clinical T_4 presentation defined histopathologically by dermal lymphatic involvement

Predictors of drug sensitivity in breast cancer

1 ER/PR-positive, *Erb*B2-negative
   — Likely sensitive to hormone therapy (e.g. tamoxifen)
2 ER/PR-negative, *Erb*B2-positive
   — More likely sensitive to anthracycline-based chemotherapy regimens

HORMONAL TREATMENT OF BREAST CANCER

Estrogen receptor (ER) status and hormone responsiveness

1 About 50% of primary breast tumors are ER+
2 About 50% of ER+ tumors respond to hormonal treatment*
3 About 50% of ER+ tumors have progesterone receptors (PR)
4 About 50% more responses are seen in tumors which are both ER+ and PR+ (i.e. 75% will respond)
5 About 50% of tumors responding to tamoxifen will respond to a second-line hormonal manipulation on relapse

* cf. < 5% for ER– tumors

Factors favoring response to hormonal manipulation

1 ER(PR)+
2 High ER absolute level (e.g. > 100 fmol/mg protein) or cellularity (e.g. > 90%)
3 Response to previous hormonal manipulation
4 Long relapse-free interval following resection of primary
5 Metastatic disease confined to bone/soft tissue/pleura/lymph nodes
6 Post-menopausal status; increasing age

Varieties of hormonal manipulation in breast cancer

1 All patients
   — Tamoxifen (an antiestrogen or SERM, selective estrogen receptor modifier)
2 Premenopausal patients
   — LHRH analogs (medical oophorectomy)
   — Oophorectomy (by laparoscopy or radiotherapy)
3 Post-menopausal patients
   — Aromatase inhibitors (block aromatization of androstenedione to estrone in fat), e.g. anastrozole, letrozole
4 Progestogens (medroxyprogesterone, megestrol acetate)
   — Bind progesterone receptors (many side-effects, esp. weight gain)
5 Androgens, estrogens (rarely used now)

Clinical features of flare reactions to hormonal interventions

1 Most commonly seen now with tamoxifen (the commonest hormonal intervention) but formerly reported most often after androgens or estrogens; affects about 1% of patients
2 Usually presents 3 days to 3 weeks after initiating treatment; typically occurs in setting of widespread bone metastases
3 Manifests with
   — Subacute worsening of bone pain (may be severe)
   — Hypercalcemia
4 Alkaline phosphatase may rise and bone scan worsen; this reflects osteoblast activation rather than disease progression
5 Treatment consists of analgesia; reversing hypercalcemia; and continuing hormonal medication where possible. Initiation of chemotherapy may be indicated
6 Flare occurrence predicts *neither* failure *nor* efficacy of treatment

MANAGEMENT OF TESTICULAR GERM-CELL NEOPLASMS

Surgical considerations in testis tumors

1 Orchidectomy of *any* undiagnosed testicular mass should be undertaken via a transinguinal (not scrotal) approach; this reduces tumor spread to inguinal nodes
2 Tumor markers (AFP, β-HCG) should be sent prior to surgery for *any* undiagnosed testicular mass
3 Retrograde ejaculation and sterility may complicate para-aortic lymphadenectomy for suspected stage II disease, esp. if *bilateral* lymphadenectomy is performed
4 Surgical debulking of residual (post-chemotherapy) tumor is recommended in non-seminomatous germ-cell tumors (NSGCT): one-third will yield residual carcinoma, one-third will yield differentiated teratoma and one-third will yield fibrosis
5 Resection of pulmonary metastases may be of value in selected patients

Diagnostic considerations in testis tumors

1 Computed tomographic (CT) scanning of abdomen and chest is the staging procedure of choice; > 50% of NSGCT patients have metastases at presentation (cf. seminoma)
2 Residual abdominal lymph node enlargement on CT scanning following chemotherapy may signify benign differentiated teratoma rather than tumor persistence. If tumor markers have returned to normal, surgical exploration is indicated to exclude residual disease

3 Persistent elevation of markers (even in the absence of radiographic disease recurrence) is an indication for recommencement of radical cytotoxic therapy

4 The plasma half-life of AFP is 5 days while that of β-HCG is 30 h; the *rate of decline* of these markers can therefore be used to *predict* the success or otherwise of therapy administered with curative intent. If β-HCG level on day 22 is > 0.5% pretreatment, response will be incomplete

5 Elevated serum AFP excludes a diagnosis of pure seminoma. However, 5–10% of seminomas have elevated β-HCG (i.e. indicating choriocarcinomatous elements)

Therapeutic considerations in testis tumors

1 Tumor markers should be assayed after any therapeutic intervention (if elevated pretreatment) to assess response and need for further treatment

2 Sperm banking should be offered prior to initiation of cytotoxic therapy, although patients may already be too azoospermic for preservation of fertility

3 There is an increased incidence of neoplasia in the remaining testicle; clinical/ultrasound monitoring may be of value

4 Radiotherapy may be curative in stage I (para-aortic field) and II (dog-leg field) seminomas. Stage I disease is usually managed with surveillance, i.e. no chemo until and unless relapse (in 15%)

5 Platinum-based chemotherapy (cisplatin) is the most effective modality in teratoma (> stage I) and in seminoma (> bulky stage II); combination bleomycin, etoposide and cisplatin (BEP) is standard for both histologies. Surveillance (no chemo) in stage I and II NSGCT is associated with 15% and 50% relapse rate respectively.

6 Cure rates are > 90% for seminomas (all stages) and > 85% for NSGCT (all stages)

MANAGEMENT OF PROSTATE CANCER

Prostatic carcinoma: available endocrine therapies

1 Testicular (LH-dependent) androgen ablation
— Long-acting LHRH analogs, incl.
• Buserelin, goserelin, leuprorelin
• Induce continuous LH release leading to LH receptor downregulation, with suppression of testosterone secretion after 3–4 weeks
— Not thrombogenic (no ↓ AT-III; cf. estrogens) but may cause disease flare (p. 19)

2 Antiandrogens
— Non-steroidal antiandrogens
• Flutamide, nilutamide, bicalutamide
→ Block androgen receptors (AR), thus preventing LHRH-induced flare if used beforehand
→ Hence, block peripheral effects of adrenal (LH-independent) androgens
→ Compensatory ↑ plasma LH/testosterone
— Progestational antiandrogens
• Cyproterone acetate: LH-reducing (progestational) *and* AR-blocking

(antiandrogen) effects; hence, opposes both testicular and adrenal androgens

3 Complete androgen blockade
— Due to combined LHRH agonist + pure antiandrogen
— Testicular and adrenal androgens effectively blocked

4 Estrogens
— Diethylstilbestrol (DES)
• Acts by inhibiting LHRH secretion
• Plasma testosterone declines to castrate levels
• Cardiovascular and sexual side-effects limit popularity

5 Bilateral orchidectomy
— Efficacy and cost-effectiveness remain unsurpassed
• Popularity limited by psychological factors

Efficacy of first-line endocrine treatment for prostate cancer

1 Benefits
— Pain relief (in 75%)
— Lower incidence of ureteric obstruction
— Fewer neurologic complications

2 Limitations
— No significant survival prolongation (30–36 months)

THYROID CANCER TREATMENT

Management of papillary/follicular thyroid carcinoma

1 Subtotal thyroidectomy (if tumor < 1 cm diam.; else total)

2 Radioiodine (30 mCi ^{131}I) ablation of remnant (therapeutic scan) if high risk of relapse
— Incomplete excision *or* demonstrable metastases
— Large primary tumor mass *or* extension beyond capsule
— Aggressive histology: poorly differentiated follicular; diffuse sclerosing papillary, tall-cell or columnar cell; Hurthle cell
— Elevated plasma thyroglobulin levels > 3 months post-operatively or during T_4 suppressive therapy

3 Long-term TSH suppression using thyroxine (~200 μg/day)

4 Monitoring of disease
— Serum thyroglobulin (> 2 μg/L suggests recurrence)
— Whole-body iodine uptake scanning (= diagnostic scan); requires either T_4 withdrawal or administration of recombinant TSH to stimulate iodine uptake

Management of medullary carcinoma of the thyroid

1 Total thyroidectomy (i.e. as for anaplastic carcinoma)

2 Exclusion of pheochromocytoma, parathyroid tumor (p. 7)

3 Family screening: screen for *Ret* gene mutations

4 Octreotide

MANAGEMENT OF GYNECOLOGIC AND GENITOURINARY TUMORS

Indications for hysterectomy
1 Persistent cervical dysplasia in a patient older than 40 who has undergone previous cone biopsy or excision with positive resection margins
2 Biopsy-proven leiomyomata (fibroids) contributing to a uterine size greater than 14 weeks' gestation in a premenopausal patient older than 40 with persistent bleeding or pain despite optimal hormonal treatment
3 Undiagnosed uterine bleeding in a symptomatically anemic patient younger than 40 who has received a biopsy and optimal hormonal treatment

Management of ovarian cancer
1 Staging
 — CT
 — Ca-125
 — Surgery
2 Systemic cytotoxic therapy
 — Surgical resection
 — Adjuvant chemotherapy: carboplatin + paclitaxel

Management of bladder carcinoma
1 Superficial tumors
 — Cystoscopic fulguration, transurethral resection
 — Intravesical agents (prophylactic or therapeutic)
  • BCG ($\rightarrow$ antitumor T-cell response)
  • Mitomycin C, doxorubicin
2 Invasive tumors
 — Radical cystectomy (ileal bladder) ± adjuvant cisplatin
 — Partial cystectomy + radical irradiation
3 Extensive disease
 — Palliative irradiation (i.e. for symptoms)
 — Cytotoxic therapy (e.g. MVAC)

Management of metastatic renal cell carcinoma
1	Surgery	Isolated secondaries can be resected if technically possible
2	Adjuvant therapy	Oral thalidomide (unproven benefit)
3	Palliative therapy	Interferon-α and/or interleukin-2 (20% response) Gemcitabine, vinorelbine, 5-FU (15% response)
4	Investigational	Non-myeloablative marrow transplantation (NBMT) Dendritic cell therapy

MANAGEMENT OF METASTATIC CANCER

Approach to the patient with a malignant pleural effusion
1 Confirm the diagnosis by pleurocentesis and cytology. If not symptomatic, consider systemic management alone
2 If symptomatic, consider admission for pleurodesis (e.g. using talc or bleomycin) at first presentation. If pleurodesis is attempted after repeated failures of aspiration attempts to remove all the fluid, loculation will usually prevent success
3 Refractory or loculated effusions may be best managed with an indwelling soft catheter (Cope loop)

Approach to treating the jaundiced patient
1 Use ultrasound/CT to determine whether the jaundice reflects extrahepatic obstruction
2 If so, attempt stent passage via ERCP. If ERCP not possible, consider percutaneous transhepatic cholangiography (PCTHC) and extracorporeal biliary drainage
3 If jaundice relieved, commence optimal anticancer treatment. If jaundice not relieved, use cytotoxic drugs not metabolized by the liver (p. 15)

Approach to the patient with a single brain metastasis
1 Assess the maximum life expectancy suggested by the extent of extracranial disease
2 If this maximum life expectancy is 1 year or greater, consider radiosurgery, gamma-knife ablation or surgical removal of the metastasis in preference to palliative whole-brain irradiation

Approach to the colorectal cancer patient with a single liver metastasis
1 Determine the extent of surgery required for removal of the metastasis
2 If suitably confined (e.g. to adjacent segments of one lobe), remove the metastasis
3 Value of intra-arterial chemotherapy for unresectable colonic metastases is not proven
4 Value of post-surgical 'adjuvant' chemotherapy is not (yet) proven

Management of progressive bony metastases
1 Bilateral cortical erosion on X-ray of long bone (esp. femur)
 — Pin prophylactically
 — Irradiate following surgical fixation
2 Bone pain without gross cortical erosion
 — Systemic treatment, esp. if hormone-responsive disease
 — Palliative irradiation
3 Intractable pain in resistant, terminal disease
 — Strontium, other osteotropic radioisotopes
 — Hemibody irradiation
 — Regular morphine (p. 288)

UNDERSTANDING MALIGNANT DISEASE

INHERITED CANCER SUSCEPTIBILITY SYNDROMES

Familial syndromes of intestinal polyps due to *APC* mutations
1 Familial adenomatous polyposis (FAP)
 — Colorectal carcinomas (+ gastric, duodenal)
2 Gardner's syndrome
 — Small and large intestinal Ca, mesodermal tumors (e.g. jaw fibromas)

3 Turcot's syndrome
— Colonic adenomatosis and brain tumors

Non-APC familial syndromes of intestinal polyps
1 Hereditary non-polyposis colorectal cancer (HNPCC)
— Colorectal carcinomas esp. right-sided, flat (fewer polyps than FAP)
— Endometrial, gastric, urinary tract cancers
— Due to mutations of mismatch repair (*MLH1* in 70%) genes
2 Peutz–Jeghers syndrome
— Small intestinal hamartomatous polyps
— Perioral and finger pigmentation
— Due to mutations of the *LKB1* gene
3 Juvenile polyposis
— Colonic adenomatous polyps
— Due to mutations of the *SMAD4* or PTEN genes

Familial syndromes predisposing to multiple malignancies
1 Familial breast cancer (autosomal dominant inheritance pattern)
— *BRCA1* mutations
  • Premenopausal breast cancer, esp. bilateral
  • Ovarian cancer (50% lifelong risk; accounts for 5% of all cases)
  • Due to mutations of *BRCA1* on chromosome 17q
— *BRCA2* mutations
  • Early breast cancer, including male
  • Ovarian cancer (20% lifelong risk)
  • Prostate cancer
  • Due to mutations of *BRCA2* on chromosome 13q
2 Li-Fraumeni syndrome
— Soft tissue sarcoma, melanoma, glioma
— Leukemias
— Breast cancer
— Adrenocortical cancer
— Gastrointestinal and lung cancer
  • Due to mutations of the *p53* (or *Chk2*) gene on chromosome 17p
3 Gorlin's (basal cell nevus) syndrome
— Multiple BCCs, medulloblastoma, intestinal polyps
  • Due to mutations of the *Patched* gene on chromosome 9q
4 Familial melanoma syndrome
— Melanoma (incl. retinal melanoma), pancreatic cancer, breast cancer
  • Due to mutations of *CDKN2A* (p16^{INK4}) on 9p, or rarely *CDK4* (12q)
5 Von Hippel–Lindau syndrome
— Retinal and cerebellar hemangioblastomas; pheochromocytomas and islet cell tumors; and renal cell carcinomas
  • Due to mutations of the *VHL* gene on chromosome 3p
6 Von Recklinghausen's disease (neurofibromatosis)
— Neurofibromas, meningiomas, acoustic neuromas, neurosarcomas
  • Due to mutations of the GAP-like *NF1* gene, or else the *NF2* gene
7 Familial retinoblastoma
— Bilateral retinoblastoma (in early life)
— Osteosarcoma (in survivors)
  • Due to mutations of the retinoblastoma susceptibility (*Rb*) gene on 13q
8 Cowden's syndrome
— Glioma, follicular thyroid cancer, breast and prostate cancer, head and neck cancer
  • Due to mutations affecting the lipid phosphatase PTEN

Premalignant syndromes of chromosomal instability
·1 Xeroderma pigmentosum
— Ultraviolet light sensitivity
— Prone to skin SCCs
— Due to mutations of nucleotide excision repair (*NER*) genes
— Other *NER*-defective syndromes include Cockayne's and trichothiodystrophy
2 Ataxia telangiectasia
— X-radiation sensitivity
— Prone to leukemias and lymphomas esp.
— Due to mutations of the *ATM* gene (a nuclear protein kinase that modifies *p53*)
3 Fanconi's anemia
— DNA crosslinking drug sensitivity
— Prone to leukemias
4 Bloom's syndrome
— Oncogenic virus sensitivity
— Prone to leukemias

ONCOGENES AND TUMOR SUPPRESSORS

Cytogenetic aspects of tumor evolution
1 Hereditary retinoblastoma/osteosarcoma
— 13q deletion leading to loss of *Rb* gene heterozygosity
2 Wilms' tumor
— 11p deletion
— Associated with aniridia/hemihypertrophy (WAGR syndrome) due to adjacent gene deletions
3 Lymphoma
— Burkitt's lymphoma
  • 8:14 translocation affecting *Myc*
— Low-grade non-Hodgkin's lymphoma
  • t(14:18) *Bcl2* translocation in > 80%
— Other
  • t(11:14), (3:14), (2:5)
4 Chronic myeloid leukemia
— 9:22 translocation affecting *Abl*
5 Small-cell lung cancer
— 3p14–23 deletion* (> 90%)
6 Germ-cell tumors
— Isochromosome 12p in > 80%
7 Sarcomas
— Ewing's tumor
  • t(11q;22q) in 90% cases
— Synovial sarcoma‡
  • t(X:18)(p11:q11)
— Alveolar rhabdomyosarcoma
  • t(2:13)
— Liposarcoma
  • t(12:16)

* Also seen in almost 100% bronchial carcinoids
‡ Patients with fusions of *SYT* (chromosome 18) to the *SSX2* gene (on chromosome Xp11) have less metastasis and survive significantly longer than those with fusions of *SYT* to *SSX1*.

Critical oncogenes in cancer development

1 Cellular oncogenes (proto-oncogenes) are normal regulatory genes, some of which are homologous to retroviral oncogenes. Constitutively activating mutations may confer cell-transforming properties on such genes (i.e. they become dominant oncogenes)
2 Putative mechanisms of oncogene action include
   — Cellular immortalization (e.g. *Myc*)
   — Transformation of immortalized cells (e.g. *Ras, Src*)
   — Growth factor agonism, (e.g. *Sis* (PDGF-B))
   — Growth factor receptor signalling (e.g. EGFR, *Erb*B2)
3 Disease associations of oncogene activation include
   — *Abl* gene activation in chronic myeloid leukemia*
   — *Sis* overexpression in myelofibrosis
   — N-*Myc* amplification in neuroblastoma, retinoblastoma
   — L-*Myc* amplification in small-cell lung cancer
   — *Erb*B2 amplification in breast/ovarian cancer
   — EGFR amplification in squamous cell cancers, gliomas
   — Cdk4 amplification/activation in melanoma, sarcomas
   — *Ret* activation in papillary or medullary thyroid cancer

* The *Abl* tyrosine kinase is inhibited by the drug imatinib, a kinase inhibitor, with therapeutic benefit

Tumor suppressor genes (recessive oncogenes) in cancer development

1 Most common cancers arise via the accumulation of common genetic mistakes. These mistakes affect critical growth-control genes which are generically termed *tumor suppressor genes* (TSGs)
2 The retention of a single TSG allele may suffice to prevent neoplastic transformation. *Loss of heterozygosity* (LOH) for a particular TSG allele within a tumor, however, implicates that gene as a likely contributor to the malignant phenotype
3 Tumor suppressor gene mutations may underlie many tumors, e.g.
   — Retinoblastoma, osteosarcomas (*Rb*)
   — Li–Fraumeni syndrome (*p53*)
   — Familial breast/ovarian cancer (*BRCA1, BRCA2*)
   — Neurofibromatosis (*NF1, NF2*)
   — Wilms' tumor (*WT1*)
   — Lobular breast cancer, diffuse gastric cancer (E-cadherin)
   — Colorectal and gastric cancers (TGF-βII receptor)

Genetic changes in colorectal cancer evolution

1 Hereditary genetic defects
   — Familial adenomatous polyposis (FAP)
      • *APC* (adenomatous polyposis coli) mutations
   — Hereditary non-polyposis colorectal cancer (HNPCC)
      • DNA mismatch repair genes (e.g. *hMLH1, hMSH2*)
2 Defects seen in hyperplastic epithelium
   — DNA hypomethylation (leads to tumor suppressor gene inactivation)
3 Defects seen in adenomas and/or carcinomas
   — K-*Ras* mutation
   — *SMAD4* deletion or TGF-βII receptor mutation
   — *p53* mutations

Genetic changes in thyroid cancer evolution

1 Medullary carcinoma of the thyroid with MEN2A
   — Chromosome 10 mutations affecting the extracellular domain of the *Ret* receptor tyrosine kinase*, leading to constitutive (ligand-independent) activation
2 Medullary carcinoma of the thyroid with MEN2B
   — Mutations affecting the intracellular (catalytic) domain of *Ret*, leading to tyrosine phosphorylation of abnormal substrates
3 Papillary thyroid cancer (PTC)
   — Chromosome 10 translocations resulting in formation of Ret fusion proteins with a variety of other genes (e.g. H4), leading to several constitutive Ret/PTC products
4 Follicular thyroid cancer (FTC)
   — *Ras* (and other) gene mutations

* cf. parathyroid adenomas in MEN1: due to *Menin* gene mutations on chromosome 11q13

Genetic changes in neuroblastoma evolution

1 Favorable (chemosensitive) disease
   — High TrkA (nerve growth factor receptor) expression
   — Absent N-*Myc* gene amplification
   — Triploid karyotype
2 Unfavorable (chemoresistant) disease*
   — Low TrkA expression
   — N-*Myc* amplification (> 3 gene copies)
   — Pseudodiploid karyotype

* Often present with hepatomegaly prior to age 4 weeks

REVIEWING THE LITERATURE: CANCER

1.1   Prostate Cancer Trialists' Collaborative Group (2000) Maximum androgen blockade in advanced prostate cancer. Lancet 355: 1491–1498

      Meta-analysis of 27 randomized studies showing that addition of an antiandrogen (e.g. flutamide) to androgen-suppressive therapy (e.g. LHRH agonists) improves survival by 2–3% plus or minus 5%.

1.2   Hartmann LC et al (1997) G-CSF in severe chemotherapy-induced afebrile neutropenia. N Engl J Med 336: 1776–1780

      Routine administration of G-CSF to afebrile patients with severe neutropenia did reduce the duration of neutropenia, but did not affect the number of days in hospital, use of antibiotics, or proportion of culture-positive infections.

1.3 Fuchs CS et al (1999) Dietary fiber and the risk of colorectal cancer and adenoma in women. N Engl J Med 340: 169–176

Schatzkin A et al (2000) Lack of effect of a low-fat, high-fiber diet on the recurrence of colorectal adenomas. N Engl J Med 342: 1149–1155

Sinha R et al (1999) Well-done, grilled red meat increases the risk of colorectal adenomas. Cancer Res 59: 4320–4324

The role of dietary composition in influencing the risk of colorectal neoplasia is accepted, but the preventative efficacy of (attempts at) dietary modification in midlife remains controversial.

1.4 Sorensen HT et al (1998) The risk of a diagnosis of cancer after primary deep venous thrombosis or pulmonary embolism. N Engl J Med 338: 1169–1173

This review of over 25 000 cases of DVT or pulmonary embolism documented a 30% increased risk of cancer relative to national incidence rates. Pancreatic cancer, ovarian cancer, hepatoma and glioma were most strongly associated. Of those patients identified to have cancer within 12 months follow-up of thromboembolism, 40% were already incurable due to metastases. The authors conclude that routine aggressive investigation of DVT/PE patients for occult malignancy is not worthwhile.

1.5 Soutter WP et al (1997) Invasive cervical cancer after conservative therapy for cervical intraepithelial neoplasia (CIN). Lancet 349: 978–980

Although outpatient treatment of CIN reduced invasive cancer risk by 95%, the absolute risk of the latter remained 5–fold elevated to the general population, indicating the need for careful long-term follow-up.

1.6 Quasar Collaborative Group (2000) Comparison of fluorouracil with additional levamisole, higher-dose folinic acid, or both, as adjuvant chemotherapy for colorectal cancer: a randomised trial. Lancet 355: 1588–1596

Neither levamisole nor higher-dose folinic acid made any difference to survival in this landmark study of 5000 patients. Anybody out there like to admit they were wrong?

1.7 Pieterman RM et al (2000) Preoperative staging of non-small-cell-lung cancer with positron-emission tomography. N Engl J Med 343: 254–261

More accurate staging of local and distant metastatic disease was possible due to PET. This improves the 'stage-specific survival' of patients evaluated in this way compared to routine (less sensitive) staging.

1.8 Elsaleh H et al (2000) Association of tumour site and sex with survival benefit from adjuvant chemotherapy in colorectal cancer. Lancet 355: 1745–1750

Survival benefits of adjuvant chemotherapy were strongly skewed towards patients with right-sided tumors and/or those with microsatellite instability (MSI), with the latter two variables tending to vary together as in full-blown HNPCC (p. 22). This trend may reflect the fact that MSI-positive tumors are less likely to harbor *p53* mutations.

1.9 Slamon DJ et al (2001) Use of chemotherapy plus a monoclonal antibody against HER2 for metastatic breast cancer that overexpresses HER2. N Engl J Med 344: 783–792

In metastatic patients already receiving conventional chemotherapy, the addition of this targeted antibody improved response rates and durations, but at the cost of appreciable cardiotoxicity.

1.10 Druker BJ et al (2001) Activity of a specific inhibitor of the Bcr-Abl tyrosine kinase in the blast crisis of chronic myeloid leukemia and acute lymphoblastic leukemia with the Philadelphia chromosome. N Engl J Med 344: 1038–1042

van Oosterom AT et al (2001) Safety and efficacy of imatinib (STI571) in metastatic gastrointestinal stromal tumours: a phase I study. Lancet 358: 1421–1423

Two studies showing the remarkable effectiveness and tolerability of the Abl (Kit, PDGF receptor) tyrosine kinase inhibitor, imatinib.

1.11 Henderson MA et al (2001) Parathyroid hormone-related protein production by breast cancers, improved survival, and reduced bone metastases. J Natl Cancer Inst 93: 234–237

Study of 367 breast cancer patients, in whom 72% exhibited immunohistochemically detectable PTHrP (which was also associated with estrogen receptor expression). These latter patients had only half the risk of death from breast cancer, compared with PTHrP-negative patients.

CHAPTER 2

Cardiology

Physical examination protocol 2.1   You are asked to examine the patient's cardiovascular system

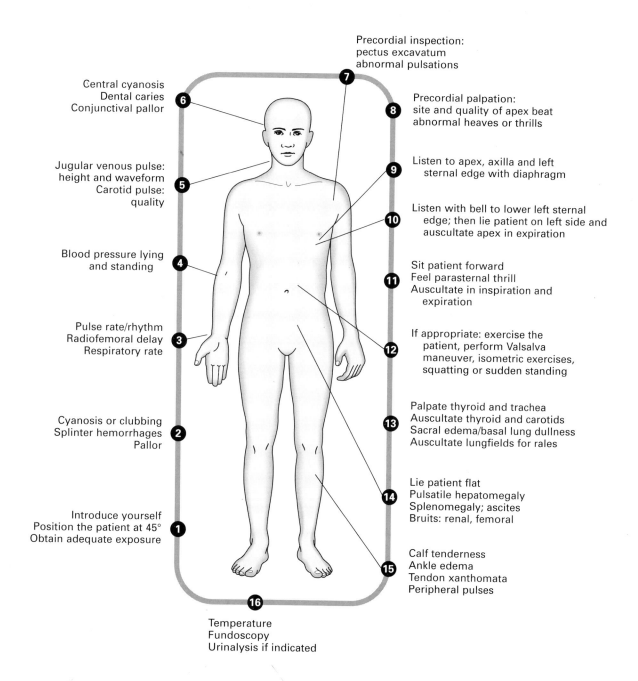

Precordial inspection:
pectus excavatum
abnormal pulsations

Central cyanosis
Dental caries
Conjunctival pallor

Precordial palpation:
site and quality of apex beat
abnormal heaves or thrills

Jugular venous pulse:
height and waveform
Carotid pulse:
quality

Listen to apex, axilla and left
sternal edge with diaphragm

Listen with bell to lower left sternal
edge; then lie patient on left side and
auscultate apex in expiration

Blood pressure lying
and standing

Sit patient forward
Feel parasternal thrill
Auscultate in inspiration and
expiration

Pulse rate/rhythm
Radiofemoral delay
Respiratory rate

If appropriate: exercise the
patient, perform Valsalva
maneuver, isometric exercises,
squatting or sudden standing

Palpate thyroid and trachea
Auscultate thyroid and carotids
Sacral edema/basal lung dullness
Auscultate lungfields for rales

Cyanosis or clubbing
Splinter hemorrhages
Pallor

Lie patient flat
Pulsatile hepatomegaly
Splenomegaly; ascites
Bruits: renal, femoral

Introduce yourself
Position the patient at 45°
Obtain adequate exposure

Calf tenderness
Ankle edema
Tendon xanthomata
Peripheral pulses

Temperature
Fundoscopy
Urinalysis if indicated

Physical examination protocol 2.2   You are asked to examine a patient with refractory hypertension

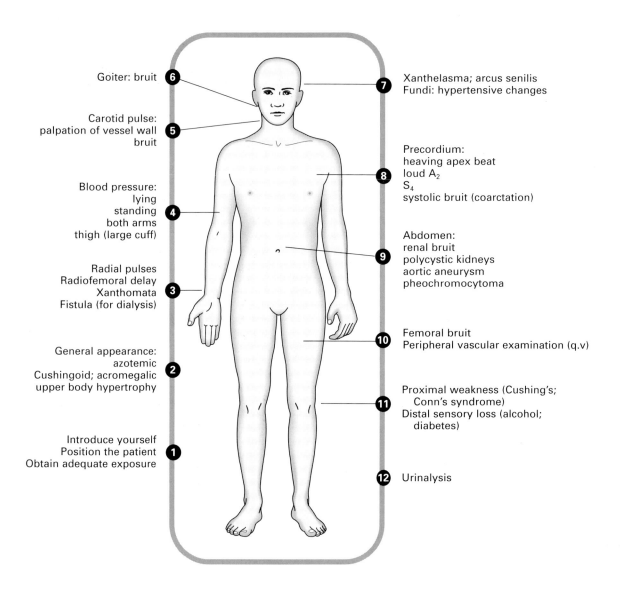

Goiter: bruit **6**

Carotid pulse:
palpation of vessel wall
bruit **5**

Blood pressure:
lying
standing
both arms
thigh (large cuff) **4**

Radial pulses
Radiofemoral delay
Xanthomata
Fistula (for dialysis) **3**

General appearance:
azotemic
Cushingoid; acromegalic
upper body hypertrophy **2**

Introduce yourself
Position the patient
Obtain adequate exposure **1**

7 Xanthelasma; arcus senilis
Fundi: hypertensive changes

8 Precordium:
heaving apex beat
loud A_2
S_4
systolic bruit (coarctation)

9 Abdomen:
renal bruit
polycystic kidneys
aortic aneurysm
pheochromocytoma

10 Femoral bruit
Peripheral vascular examination (q.v)

11 Proximal weakness (Cushing's;
Conn's syndrome)
Distal sensory loss (alcohol;
diabetes)

12 Urinalysis

Physical examination protocol 2.3 You are told that the patient is known to have aortic incompetence, and are asked to examine him from that point of view

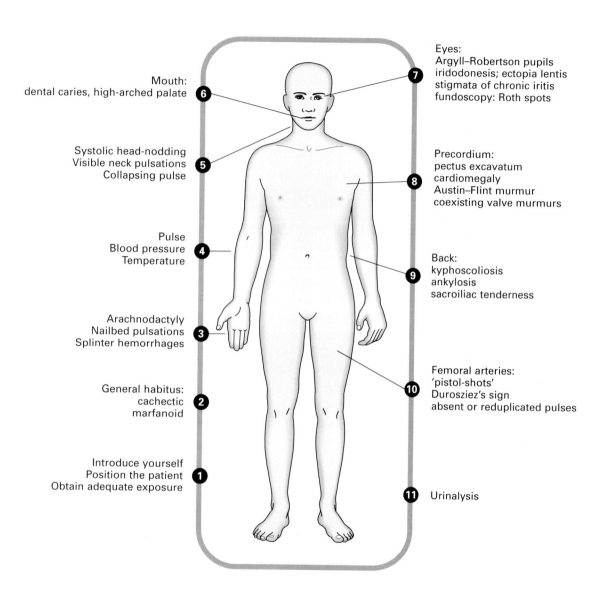

Mouth:
dental caries, high-arched palate **6**

7 Eyes:
Argyll–Robertson pupils
iridodonesis; ectopia lentis
stigmata of chronic iritis
fundoscopy: Roth spots

Systolic head-nodding
Visible neck pulsations
Collapsing pulse **5**

8 Precordium:
pectus excavatum
cardiomegaly
Austin–Flint murmur
coexisting valve murmurs

Pulse
Blood pressure
Temperature **4**

9 Back:
kyphoscoliosis
ankylosis
sacroiliac tenderness

Arachnodactyly
Nailbed pulsations
Splinter hemorrhages **3**

General habitus:
cachectic
marfanoid **2**

10 Femoral arteries:
'pistol-shots'
Durosziez's sign
absent or reduplicated pulses

Introduce yourself
Position the patient
Obtain adequate exposure **1**

11 Urinalysis

Physical examination protocol 2.4 You are asked to examine the patient looking specifically for signs of bacterial endocarditis

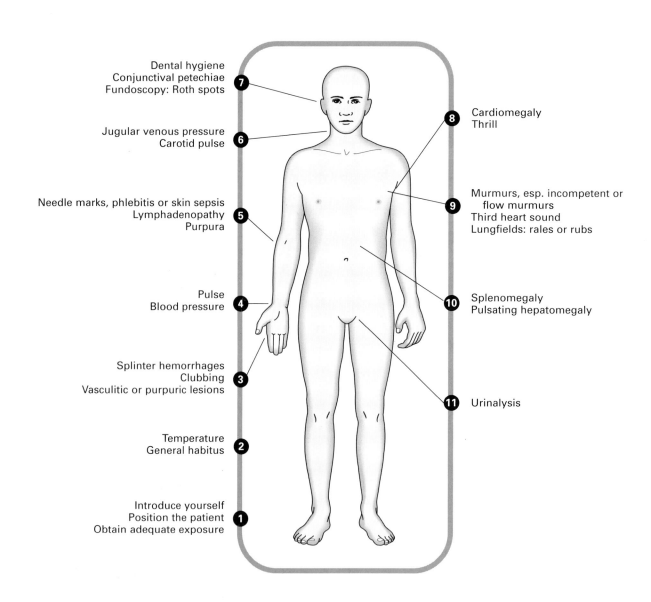

Dental hygiene
Conjunctival petechiae
Fundoscopy: Roth spots — **7**

8 — Cardiomegaly
Thrill

Jugular venous pressure
Carotid pulse — **6**

Needle marks, phlebitis or skin sepsis
Lymphadenopathy
Purpura — **5**

9 — Murmurs, esp. incompetent or
flow murmurs
Third heart sound
Lungfields: rales or rubs

Pulse
Blood pressure — **4**

10 — Splenomegaly
Pulsating hepatomegaly

Splinter hemorrhages
Clubbing
Vasculitic or purpuric lesions — **3**

11 — Urinalysis

Temperature
General habitus — **2**

Introduce yourself
Position the patient
Obtain adequate exposure — **1**

Physical examination protocol 2.5   You are asked to examine the patient's peripheral vascular system

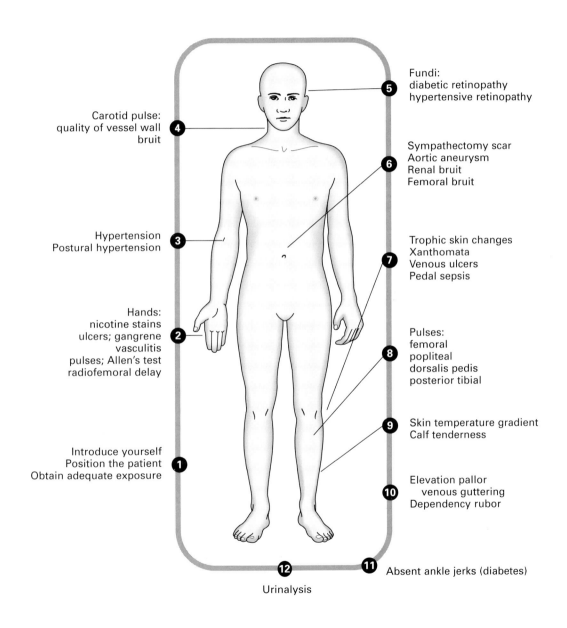

Carotid pulse:
quality of vessel wall
bruit — **4**

Fundi:
5 diabetic retinopathy
hypertensive retinopathy

Sympathectomy scar
6 Aortic aneurysm
Renal bruit
Femoral bruit

Hypertension
Postural hypertension — **3**

Trophic skin changes
7 Xanthomata
Venous ulcers
Pedal sepsis

Hands:
nicotine stains
ulcers; gangrene
vasculitis
pulses; Allen's test
radiofemoral delay — **2**

Pulses:
8 femoral
popliteal
dorsalis pedis
posterior tibial

Skin temperature gradient
9 Calf tenderness

Introduce yourself
Position the patient
Obtain adequate exposure — **1**

Elevation pallor
10 venous guttering
Dependency rubor

12   **11** Absent ankle jerks (diabetes)

Urinalysis

Diagnostic pathway 2.1   This patient has a fundoscopic abnormality. How would you characterize this?

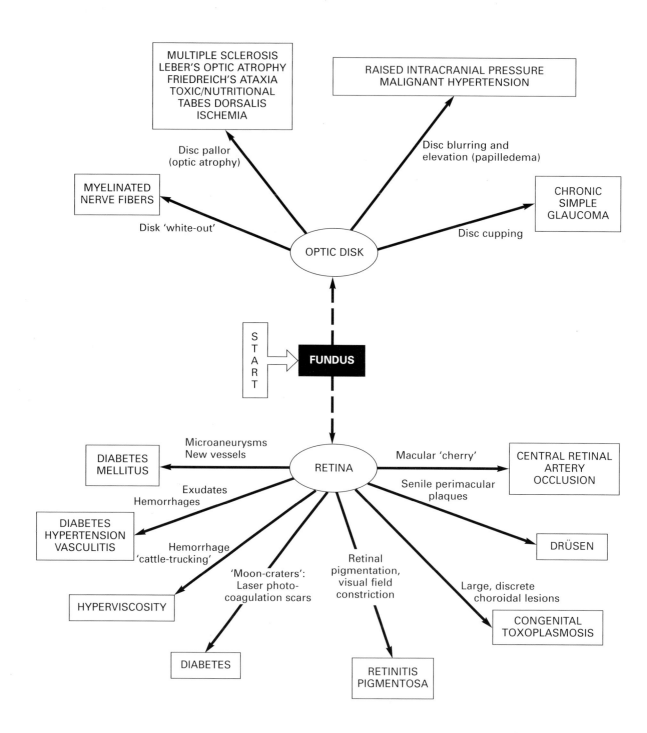

MULTIPLE SCLEROSIS
LEBER'S OPTIC ATROPHY
FRIEDREICH'S ATAXIA
TOXIC/NUTRITIONAL
TABES DORSALIS
ISCHEMIA

RAISED INTRACRANIAL PRESSURE
MALIGNANT HYPERTENSION

Disc pallor
(optic atrophy)

Disc blurring and
elevation (papilledema)

MYELINATED
NERVE FIBERS

CHRONIC
SIMPLE
GLAUCOMA

Disk 'white-out'

Disc cupping

OPTIC DISK

START

FUNDUS

Microaneurysms
New vessels

Macular 'cherry'

DIABETES
MELLITUS

RETINA

CENTRAL RETINAL
ARTERY
OCCLUSION

Exudates
Hemorrhages

Senile perimacular
plaques

DIABETES
HYPERTENSION
VASCULITIS

Hemorrhage
'cattle-trucking'

DRÜSEN

HYPERVISCOSITY

'Moon-craters':
Laser photo-
coagulation scars

Retinal
pigmentation,
visual field
constriction

Large, discrete
choroidal lesions

CONGENITAL
TOXOPLASMOSIS

DIABETES

RETINITIS
PIGMENTOSA

COMMON AND CLASSIC CARDIOVASCULAR PROBLEMS

Common cardiac problems in clinical practice
1 Hypertension
2 Angina
3 Exertional dyspnea

Classic cardiac problems in clinical exams
1 Mitral and/or aortic valve disease
2 Cardiac failure/cardiomyopathy
3 Atrial fibrillation

CARDIAC EMERGENCIES

Differential diagnosis of acute life-threatening dyspnea
1 Pulmonary embolism
2 Acute myocardial infarction (and/or failure, rupture)
3 Cardiac tachyarrhythmia
4 Asthma and/or anaphylaxis
5 Pneumonia
6 Pericardial tamponade
7 Massive gastrointestinal hemorrhage

Possible indications for transferring an inpatient to the coronary care unit
1 Cardiac arrest *or* ventricular tachyarrhythmia
2 Acute myocardial infarction
3 Cardiogenic shock (systolic BP < 90 mmHg)* *or* cardiac tamponade
4 Pulse rate < 40/min *or* > 140/min

* 80% in-hospital mortality; cf. myocardial infarction without heart failure, 6% in-hospital mortality

Possible indications for transferring an inpatient to the intensive care unit*
1 Respiratory arrest *or* threatened airway (esp. if absent gag reflex)
2 Oxyhemoglobin saturation < 90% on 50% oxygen via mask
3 Respiratory rate < 8/min (respiratory acidosis) *or* > 40/min
4 Loss of consciousness *or* status epilepticus

* Other factors to consider include age, prognosis, bed status, etc.

CLINICAL ASSESSMENT OF THE CARDIAC PATIENT

THE CARDIOVASCULAR HISTORY

Assessment of cardiorespiratory capacity
1 NYHA I — Dyspneic only on severe exertion
2 NYHA II — Dyspneic walking up hills or stairs
3 NYHA III — Dyspneic walking on a level surface
4 NYHA IV — Dyspneic at rest

Assessment of angina severity
1 Grade I — Angina on strenuous/prolonged exertion
2 Grade II — Angina on climbing two flights of stairs
3 Grade III — Angina walking one block on the level
4 Grade IV — Angina at rest

Pain: how to describe it
1 When?
   — First onset?
   — Duration of individual episodes?
   — Periodicity?
2 Where?
   — Site of origin?
   — Radiation?
   — Effect of different postures?
3 How?
   — Severity?
   — Nature?
   — Exacerbating and relieving factors?

Characteristics of atypical angina
1 Not substernal in location
2 Not heavy, dull or tight in quality
3 Not induced, worsened or otherwise related to exertion or emotion
4 Not relieved by nitrates

THE PULSE

Describing pulse character
1 Volume
   — Low/full
   — Alternans
   — Paradoxical (reduces on inspiration)
2 Upstroke
   — Normal
   — Slow/brisk

Clinical varieties of pulse character
1 Paradoxical
   — Tamponade/constrictive pericarditis
   — Severe asthma
   Alternans
   — Severe left ventricular failure
2 Collapsing
   — Aortic incompetence
   — Patent ductus arteriosus ('big' pulse)
   Jerky
   — Hypertrophic cardiomyopathy (HOCM)
3 Plateau
   — Aortic valvular stenosis (diagnostic)
4 Bisferiens
   — Mixed aortic valve disease

Differential diagnosis of unequal radial pulses
1 Atheroma
2 Proximal coarctation
3 Cervical rib
4 Takayasu's arteritis
5 Dissecting aneurysm

The irregularly irregular pulse: differential diagnosis
1 Atrial fibrillation
2 Sinus arrhythmia
3 Multiple atrial or ventricular premature beats
4 Atrial tachycardia or atrial flutter with varying block

Clinical signs of atrial fibrillation
1 Irregularly irregular pulse in time and amplitude
2 Absent 'a' waves in jugular venous pulse
3 Variation in intensity of first heart sound
4 Signs of mitral valve disease, cardiomyopathy, thyrotoxicosis

Analysing the jugular venous pulse (JVP)
1 Raised or not?
  — Measure height above sternal angle
2 If raised, is it fixed?
  — Stand the patient up
    • Fixed: SVC obstruction
  — Elicit hepatojugular reflux
    • Absent: IVC obstruction, Budd–Chiari
3 Is the 'a' or 'v' wave dominant?
  — Palpate contralateral carotid artery

Interpreting elevated 'a' and 'v' waves in the JVP
1 Normal
  — 'a' wave: (right) atrial systole
  — 'v' wave: venous filling
2 Abnormal 'a' wave
  — Absent: atrial fibrillation
  — Giant*: tricuspid/pulmonary stenosis
  — Solitary: complete heart block
3 Cannon waves (= large 'a' waves)
  — Atrial contraction against closed tricuspid valve
    • Regular: nodal rhythm
    • Irregular: complete heart block, ectopics
4 Systolic (ventricular) waves‡
  — Tricuspid incompetence

* Associated with right atrial S_4.
‡ *Not* 'v' waves; indicate 'ventricularization' of right atrium, and associated with pulsatile liver

Subclinical abnormalities of the JVP 'x' and 'y' descents
1 Definitions
  — 'x' descent: systolic collapse (atrial relaxation)
  — 'y' descent: diastolic collapse (tricuspid opening)
2 Rapid 'y' descent
  — Tricuspid incompetence, constrictive pericarditis
3 Slow/absent 'y' descent
  — Tricuspid stenosis, cardiac tamponade
4 Rapid 'x' descent
  — Constrictive pericarditis, cardiac tamponade

THE PRECORDIUM

Cardiac significance of a left thoracotomy scar*
1 Mitral valvotomy
2 Repair of aortic coarctation or PDA
3 Pneumonectomy, splenectomy or gastrectomy

* cf. sternotomy scar

Reasons for failure to palpate the apex beat
1 Emphysema, obesity
2 Poor technique
3 Pericardial disease
  — Effusion, constriction
4 Dextrocardia
  — Any cause, incl. right pneumonectomy

Palpable heart sounds
1 Palpable S_1
  — 'Tapping' apex beat (mitral stenosis)
2 Palpable S_4
  — 'Double' apex beat (HOCM/severe aortic stenosis)
  — Left ventricular aneurysm
3 Palpable P_2
  — Pulmonary hypertension

Quality of the apex beat*
1 Heaving (sustained): LV pressure load
  — Aortic stenosis, long-standing hypertension
2 Hyperdynamic, displaced: LV volume load
  — Mitral/aortic incompetence, patent ductus arteriosus
3 Dyskinetic
  — Left ventricular aneurysm
4 Displaced to right
  — Dextrocardia, right pneumonectomy
5 Impalpable (see above)

* NB: As with real estate, *location* of apex is more important than quality

THE HEART SOUNDS

Conditions causing a soft first heart sound
1 Large pericardial effusion
2 Severe mitral regurgitation
3 Mitral stenosis with rigid valve
4 Cardiomyopathy, left ventricular failure
5 First-degree heart block (intensity varies)

Conditions causing a loud first heart sound
1 Mitral stenosis with mobile valve
2 Sinus tachycardia (e.g. thyrotoxicosis)
3 Short P-R interval
  — Wolff–Parkinson–White syndrome
  — Lown–Ganong–Levine syndrome

Splitting of the second heart sound
1 Physiological
  — Single S_2 in expiration
  — A_2 pre-P_2 appears on inspiration
2 Split, widens on inspiration
  — RBBB
3 Split, paradoxical
  — i.e. P_2 pre-A_2; widens on expiration
  — LBBB
4 Widely split, fixed
  — ASD
5 Narrow split with loud P_2 ($\gg A_2$)
  — Pulmonary hypertension
6 Wide split with soft P_2
  — Pulmonary stenosis

7 Loud A_2
   — Systemic hypertension
8 Single S_2 (inaudible A_2)
   — Calcific aortic stenosis
  Single S_2 (inaudible P_2)
   — Obesity, emphysema

Differential diagnosis of the fixed split second heart sound

1 Atrial septal defect (ASD)
   — Secundum (60%) or primum (30%)
2 Partial anomalous pulmonary venous drainage
   — Associated with ASD (10%)
3 Misdiagnosis
   — Opening snap (mitral stenosis) simulating P_2
   — Midsystolic click (mitral valve prolapse) simulating A_2

Characterization of third heart sounds

1 Genuine S_3
   — Low-pitched, localized
   — Best heard with bell at apex, patient on left side
2 Other 'third sounds'
   • Opening snap in mitral stenosis
   • Fixed split second sound in atrial septal defect
   • Mitral valve prolapse: systolic click simulating S_2
   — High-pitched sounds heard all over precordium

MURMURS OF THE HEART

Features of an 'innocent' murmur

1 **S**ystolic ejection murmur
2 **S**hort (duration < 50% systole)
3 **S**oft, low-pitched and well-transmitted
4 **S**upine position best for auscultation
5 **S**ingle S_2 during expiration while standing
6 **S**atisfactory (normal) ECG and CXR

Characteristics of a venous hum*

1 Low-pitched sound best heard when sitting up
2 More common on right side, esp. in subclavian region
3 Increases during inspiration (often continuous)
4 Louder in diastole
5 Maximal with head turned away; abolished by finger pressure over internal jugular vein

* Usually in children

Differential diagnosis of continuous murmurs

1 Patent ductus arteriosus ('machinery' murmur)
2 Pulmonary flow murmur, cervical venous hum
  AV fistula; ruptured sinus of Valsalva aneurysm
  'Mammary soufflé' (pregnancy)
3 Pseudocontinuous murmur (mixed aortic valve disease)

Causes of a late systolic murmur

1 Mitral (or tricuspid) valve prolapse
2 'Secondary' (ischemic) mitral prolapse
   — Papillary muscle dysfunction
   — Ruptured mitral chorda tendineae
3 Hypertrophic cardiomyopathy

Systolic sounds associated with myocardial infarction

1 Papillary muscle dysfunction or partial rupture (common)
   — Apical pansystolic murmur, no thrill; clinically stable
  Ruptured chorda tendineae (uncommon, serious)
   — Loud apical murmur (mitral regurgitation) + thrill
  Complete papillary muscle rupture (uncommon, often fatal)
   — Loud apical murmur, prominent thrill; usually fatal
2 Ruptured interventricular septum (common, often operable)
   — Loud medial murmur (VSD), thrill+++
3 Functional mitral incompetence due to cardiac dilatation
4 Pulmonary systolic murmur*
5 Pericardial rub
   — Transmural infarction
   — Dressler's syndrome
6 Aortic incompetence
   — Secondary to aortic dissection, esp. after inferior infarct

* Think of pulmonary embolism

Dire prognosticators in valvular heart disease

1 Syncope, angina: aortic stenosis
2 Pulmonary edema: aortic stenosis/regurgitation, mitral stenosis
3 Aortic dissection: aortic regurgitation
4 Refractory heart failure: mitral regurgitation
5 Acute deterioration: all

MITRAL STENOSIS (MS)

Signs of valve mobility in mitral stenosis

1 Loud S_1
2 Opening snap*

* If S_2–OS gap easily audible, stenosis *not* severe; see below

Radiographic features of mitral stenosis

1 PA film
   — Straight (or convex) left heart border*
   — Double shadow of left atrium behind right atrium
   — Splaying of subcarinal angle greater than 90°
   — Dilated upper lobe veins
   — Prominent pulmonary conus
   — Pulmonary hemosiderosis
2 Lateral
   — Left atrial/right ventricular enlargement
   — Valvular calcification‡
   — McCallum's patch (left atrial calcification)
   — Esophageal indentation on barium swallow

* *Unless* auricle removed at valvotomy
‡ Calcification of the mitral annulus is associated with 2-fold stroke risk

M-mode echocardiography* in mitral stenosis

1 Thickened leaflets; calcification
2 Left atrial enlargement

3 Loss of 'A' point, if in atrial fibrillation
4 Excursion of anterior leaflet less than 20 mm
5 Anterior position of posterior leaflet throughout diastole
   — Most *specific* sign
6 Reduced EF slope
   — Semi-quantitative for *severity*

* M-mode little used now in most centers

Indicators of severity in mitral stenosis
1 Symptoms
2 Signs
   — Length of diastolic murmur
   — Proximity of opening snap to S_2
   — Signs of pulmonary hypertension/congestion
   — Functional pulmonary incompetence (Graham Steell murmur) or tricuspid incompetence
3 CXR
   — Left atrial/right ventricular enlargement
   — Pulmonary hypertension and congestion
4 ECG
   — Atrial enlargement
   — Right ventricular strain pattern
5 Echo
   — M-mode: flattening of EF slope
   — Severity best quantitated by Doppler or 2-D echo
6 Catheter
   — Mitral valve gradient
   — Elevated right heart pressures
   — Decreased cardiac output during exercise

Severity of mitral stenosis assessed by 2-D echocardiography
1 Cross-sectional valve area > 2.5 cm^2
   — Asymptomatic
2 Cross-sectional valve area 1.5–2.5 cm^2
   — Symptoms on exercise only (mild)
3 Cross-sectional valve area 0.5–1.5 cm^2
   — Symptoms at rest (think of valvuloplasty)
4 Cross-sectional valve area < 0.5 cm^2
   — Severe stenosis (think of valve replacement)

Contraindications to valvotomy/valvuloplasty
1 Lack of symptoms
2 Significant mitral incompetence
3 Low chance of success*
   — Rigid valve
   — Heavily calcified leaflets (on echo, fluoroscopy)
4 Suspicion of left atrial thrombus

* esp. with balloon valvuloplasty

Indications for surgery in mitral stenosis
1 Progressive symptomatic deterioration due to pulmonary congestion in the absence of identifiable reversible factors
2 Recurrent embolic episodes

Mitral stenotic diastolic murmur: differential diagnosis
1 Flow murmur due to volume overload (like Austin Flint)
   — Severe mitral regurgitation
   — VSD, PDA
   — Renal failure with fluid overload (functional AR)

2 Austin Flint murmur
   — Non-stenotic mitral flow murmur
   — Due to severe aortic incompetence
3 Graham Steell murmur
   — Pulmonary incompetent murmur ($\uparrow$ on inspiration)
   — Due to severe MS causing pulmonary hypertension
4 Carey-Coombs murmur
   — Non-stenotic mitral flow murmur
   — Occurs in rheumatic valvulitis
5 Tricuspid flow murmur with secundum ASD
6 Left atrial myxoma

Signs favouring an Austin Flint murmur
1 Cardiomegaly* (apex *not* tapping)
2 Soft S_1
3 No opening snap ($\pm S_3$)
4 ECG → left ventricular dominance
5 Echo → flutter on anterior mitral valve leaflet, posterior diastolic motion of posterior valve leaflet

* NB: Right ventricular dilatation (e.g. due to MS) can also cause apical displacement; may be tricky to distinguish clinically

MITRAL REGURGITATION (MR)

Signs of dominant MR in mixed mitral valve disease
1 Soft S_1
2 Left ventricular enlargement with thrusting apex
3 ECG → left ventricular hypertrophy + left axis deviation

Clinical assessment of severity in mitral regurgitation*
1 Degree of left ventricular enlargement
2 Mid-diastolic flow murmur
3 Thrill; murmur intensity; loud P_2; basal creps

* NB: Presence of S_3 does *not* correlate well with MR severity

Causes of mitral regurgitation
1 Rheumatic
2 Infective endocarditis
3 Mitral valve prolapse and/or Marfan's syndrome
4 Functional (left ventricular dilatation)
5 Ischemic
   — Papillary muscle dysfunction
   — Ruptured chorda tendineae
6 Rheumatoid arthritis, ankylosing spondylitis
7 Associations
   — 1° ASD
   — Hypertrophic cardiomyopathy
8 Congenital

Signs favoring acute rather than chronic mitral regurgitation
1 Acute onset of symptoms
2 Loud, short bruit (esp. in young male) radiating well to base
3 Other signs
   — Sinus tachycardia
   — Large 'a' wave
   — Minimally displaced apex beat

— Right ventricular heave with apical systolic thrill
— Normal intensity S_1; S_4; loud P_2

LEFT ATRIAL MYXOMA

Diagnostic clues to left atrial myxoma
1 Symptoms
   — Constitutional symptoms (esp. in females; occasionally familial)
   — Sudden onset; episodic
   — Postural
2 Signs
   — Pansystolic murmur; may be postural
   — Mid-diastolic murmur
   — Loud or soft S_1; ± 'tumor plop'
   — Sinus rhythm
3 Investigations
   — Normal CXR
   — Left atrial mass on 2-D echocardiogram*
   — Positive embolus histology

* But note that 15% of cardiac myxomas arise from the *right* atrium

Echocardiographic differential diagnosis of left atrial myxoma
1 Left atrial thrombus
2 Large mitral valve vegetation (e.g. staphylococcal, fungal)
3 Ruptured chorda tendineae
4 Thick or redundant valve leaflets (e.g. in SLE)
5 Cyst (hydatid or pericardial)
6 Other tumor (e.g. sarcoma, lymphoma, teratoma, lipoma)

MITRAL VALVE PROLAPSE (MVP)

Clinical associations of mitral valve prolapse
1 Marfan's syndrome; Ehlers–Danlos syndrome
2 Ostium secundum atrial septal defect
3 Wolff–Parkinson–White syndrome ± SLE

Maneuvers intensifying the murmur
1 Sudden standing
2 Valsalva (phases 2 and 3)

Maneuvers intensifying the click
1 Squatting
2 Isometric handgrip

Significance and timing of the midsystolic click
1 Caused by sudden tension on the chorda tendineae on stretching of the billowing valve
2 Sound occurs after beginning of carotid upstroke

ECG associations of mitral valve prolapse
1 Non-specific ST–T wave changes, esp. in inferior leads
2 Frequent atrial or ventricular ectopic beats
3 Prolonged $Q-T_c$; episodic ventricular tachycardia
4 Wolff–Parkinson–White syndrome (type A)

5 False-positive stress test*

* More likely *only* because this is a low-risk group

Approach to management of mitral valve prolapse
1 Incidental finding, asymptomatic patient
   — Reassure, follow up
2 Atypical (non-anginal) chest pain *or* Exertional chest pain and/or dyspnea
   — Stress test
3 'Funny turns', ECG ST–T wave changes, prolonged $Q-T_c$
   — Holter monitor
4 Significant degree of associated mitral regurgitation
   — Antibiotic prophylaxis

AORTIC REGURGITATION (AR)

Eponymous signs associated with aortic regurgitation
1 Quincke's
   — Capillary pulsation visible on nail compression
2 Corrigan's (pulse)
   — Collapsing pulse
3 Corrigan's (sign)
   — Visible carotid systolic pulsation
4 DeMusset's
   — Systolic head nodding
5 Austin Flint (murmur)
   — Functional mitral diastolic flow murmur
6 Durosziez's
   — To-and-fro bruit audible on lightly compressing femoral arteries with diaphragm
7 Traube's
   — Systolic 'pistol-shots' heard over femoral arteries
8 Marfan's (syndrome), Argyll Robertson (pupils)
   — Etiologic associations

Clinical indicators of severity in chronic aortic regurgitation
1 Presence of symptoms
2 Pulse character, pulse pressure
   Absolute value of diastolic blood pressure
3 Degree of cardiomegaly
4 S_3; Austin Flint murmur; length of diastolic murmur

Indicators of severity in acute aortic regurgitation*
1 Symptoms and signs of pulmonary venous congestion
2 Secondary mitral valve dysfunction
   — Soft S_1
   — Austin Flint murmur; premature closure of mitral valve on echo

* e.g. due to infective endocarditis, ruptured chorda
NB: Pulse pressure may *not* be wide despite severe (acute) aortic regurgitation

Indications for valve replacement in aortic regurgitation
1 Symptoms
2 Declining exercise tolerance on stress testing
   Fall in ejection fraction on exercise gated blood pool scan

3 Increasing heart size on CXR
4 Development of left ventricular strain pattern on ECG
5 Echocardiogram showing left ventricular end-diastolic diameter greater than 7 cm

Causes of aortic incompetence
1 Valvulitis
— Rheumatic
2 Infective endocarditis
— Rheumatoid arthritis
3 Aortitis
— Syphilis
— Ankylosing spondylitis
4 Annuloaortic ectasia
— Marfan's syndrome
— Atheroma
5 Hypertension
6 Bicuspid aortic valve
7 Aortic dissection; trauma
8 Fluid overload in renal failure

Predictors of heart failure following aortic valve surgery
1 Symptoms preoperatively
2 Echo
— Fractional shortening less than 25%
— Left ventricular end-systolic diameter > 55 mm
3 Gated blood pool scan
— Left ventricular dysfunction
— Fall in ejection fraction on exercise

AORTIC STENOSIS (AS)

Indicators of severity in aortic stenosis
1 Symptoms (see below)
2 Pulse character (slowly rising, 'plateau')*
Pulse pressure (narrow)
3 Signs of left ventricular failure, including S_3
4 Thrill
5 S_2: soft, single, or paradoxically split
Presence of S_4; long, late-peaking murmur
6 Cardiac catheter
— Systolic transvalvular gradient > 50 mmHg
(in presence of normal left ventricular function‡)

* NB: Systolic hypertension does *not* exclude severe stenosis. Pulse pressure width is unreliable in elderly patients, while murmurs may become inaudible in patients with cardiac failure. Accurate assessment may thus be *impossible* without catheterization.
‡ The transvalvular gradient may decline in left ventricular dysfunction

Prognosis: symptom-related actuarial outcome of aortic stenosis
1 Exertional angina
— Death within 3 years (if untreated)
2 Effort syncope
— Death within 2 years
3 Exertional dyspnea
— Death within 1 year
4 Overt cardiac failure
— Death within 6 months

Indications for surgery in aortic stenosis prior to symptoms
1 Severe valvular calcification, *and*
2 Rapid increase in aortic jet velocity

Signs of dominant aortic stenosis in mixed aortic valve disease
1 Minimal cardiomegaly
2 Anacrotic pulse and narrow pulse pressure
3 S_4; no S_3

Causes and differential diagnosis of aortic stenosis
1 Valvular
— Rheumatic
— Calcific (degenerative)
— Congenital bicuspid valve
— Congenital aortic stenosis (with ejection click)
2 Subvalvar
— Hypertrophic cardiomyopathy
— Congenital subaortic membranous stenosis
3 Supravalvar
— Congenital aortic coarctation
— Congenital supravalvar aortic stenosis with or without elfin facies and hypercalcemia

NB: Aortic stenotic murmurs may be simulated by pulmonary outflow bruits, esp. pulmonary stenosis

TRICUSPID VALVE DISEASE

Diagnostic clues to tricuspid stenosis*
1 History
— Unexplained spontaneous symptomatic improvement in patient with known mitral stenosis
2 Examination
— Giant 'a' waves but no parasternal heave or loud P_2
— Diastolic murmur increases on inspiration
— Hepatomegaly with presystolic pulsation
3 Investigations
— Clear CXR despite marked venous engorgement
— Isolated right atrial enlargement on CXR and ECG
4 Definitive diagnosis
— Echocardiography (makes the above redundant)

* Rare as hen's teeth, but anyhow ...

Tricuspid incompetence: distinction from mitral incompetence
1 Murmur increases on inspiration
2 Murmur does not radiate well to axilla
3 Systolic waves and steep 'y' descents in jugular venous pulse
4 Pulsatile liver
5 Right (not left) ventricular enlargement *if* isolated lesion
6 Etiological stigmata
— Cyanosis and fixed split S_2: Ebstein's anomaly
— Nodular hepar, telangiectasia: carcinoid syndrome
— Needle marks: intravenous drug abuse

NB: Tricuspid valve lesions most commonly occur *with* other valvular lesions

INVESTIGATING CARDIOVASCULAR DISEASE

CHEST X-RAYS

Differential diagnosis of pulmonary plethora
1 Atrial septal defect
2 Ventricular septal defect
3 Patent ductus arteriosus (i.e. any left-to-right shunt)

Differential diagnosis of pulmonary oligemia
1 Pulmonic valvular stenosis
2 Pulmonary atresia
3 Primary pulmonary hypertension (peripheral oligemia)
4 Massive pulmonary embolism
5 Any right-to-left shunt
   — Fallot's tetralogy, transposition
   — Eisenmenger syndrome

Differential diagnosis of enlarged cardiac silhouette
1 Cardiomyopathy
2 Multiple valvular defects
3 Ischemic heart disease with aneurysm
4 Complex congenital heart disease with RV enlargement
5 Pericardial effusion

The 'normal' chest X-ray: checklist
1 Patient's name; film date; correct siding
2 Adequate inspiration; optimal exposure; clavicles centered
3 Transradiancy of both lungfields (?mastectomy, Swyer-James)
4 *Actively* look for
   — Retrocardiac mass
   — Valvular calcification
   — Rib resection/notching/erosions/fractures
   — Small pneumothorax, effusion
   — Gastric air bubble on right (*situs inversus*)
   — Nipple shadow (absent on lateral)
5 Assess bones
   — Osteoporosis (outer two-thirds of clavicle)
   — Lytic lesions (e.g. myeloma, breast cancer)

Indications for additional X-ray views
1 Lateral
   — Request routinely
2 Decubitus
   — To confirm whether 'effusion' layers out (i.e. to exclude pleural thickening or loculation)
3 Expiratory
   — To confirm or exclude pneumothorax
4 Erect
   — To look for gas under diaphragm (suspected perforation of abdominal hollow viscus)
5 Apical lordotic
   — Suspected TB

ECHOCARDIOGRAPHY

Echocardiographic features of left ventricular dysfunction
1 Left ventricular enlargement; wall thickness
2 Reduced fractional shortening
3 Paradoxical septal motion
4 'B' notch; reduced EF slope
5 Premature aortic valve closure or reduced valve opening

Differential diagnosis of paradoxical septal motion
1 Congestive cardiomyopathy
2 Ischemic heart disease, esp. septal infarction
3 Right ventricular volume overload (e.g. ASD)
4 Conduction disturbance
   — LBBB
   — WPW
   — Right ventricular pacing
5 Post-CABG

Asymmetric septal hypertrophy: differential diagnosis
1 Hypertrophic cardiomyopathy (incl. asymptomatic relatives*)
2 Infarction of left ventricular free wall
3 Rarely: LVH due to hypertension or valvular aortic stenosis‡

* i.e. these people have HOCM even if they don't think so
‡ i.e. probably HOCM in fact

Potential indications for transesophageal echocardiography
1 Diagnosis of thoracic aortic dissection
   — Investigation of choice (result in 15 min)
2 Suspected left atrial thrombus or cardiogenic embolism
   — Commonest indication
3 Assessment of vegetations or abscesses in endocarditis
4 Evaluation of prosthetic valve dysfunction (esp. mitral) or mitral valvuloplasty
5 Intraoperative assessment of LV function
6 Technically suboptimal transthoracic echocardiogram

Transthoracic better than transesophageal echocardiography?
1 Mitral or aortic stenosis
2 Mitral valve prolapse
3 Left ventricular thrombus

Valve surgery indicated by echo alone: prerequisites
1 Young patient (< 30 years)
2 Single valve involvement (esp. mitral)
3 Consistent clinical picture
4 Technically unequivocal echocardiogram

NUCLEAR CARDIOLOGY

Clinical utility of 'hot-spot' (^{99m}Tc pyrophosphate) scanning*

1 Suspected infarct with negative enzymes (e.g. late presentation)
2 Suspected infarct with equivocal enzymes (e.g. post-surgery, intramuscular injection)
3 Suspected infarct with non-diagnostic ECG
   — Previous infarction
   — Pacemaker in situ
   — LBBB, WPW
4 Suspected right ventricular (or true posterior) infarct

* NB: Acute utility is limited, since may take 48 h to become positive

Indications for 'cold-spot' myocardial perfusion scanning*

1 Preangiographic evaluation of 'intermediate' chest pain
   — Non-diagnostic stress ECG
   — Male with atypical chest pain and positive stress ECG
   — Female with chest pains and positive stress ECG
2 Post-angiography
   — To ascertain exact site of ischemia in patient with multivessel disease, some of which are ungraftable
   — To assess functional significance of stenoses seen at angiography and adequacy of collateral circulation
   — To assess the viability of myocardium apparently jeopardized by stenosis at angiography
3 Angioplasty patients
   — To assess site of ischemia pre-PTCA
   — To check for development of restenosis post-PTCA
4 Post-bypass assessment of chest pain
   — Graft occlusion vs post-(peri)cardiotomy syndrome
   — Graft occlusion vs chest wall pain
   — Graft occlusion vs ungrafted stenosis
5 Stress (exercise or adenosine) testing in asymptomatic patients, incl. post-bypass patients
   — Presence or absence of reversible perfusion defect predicts further infarct or early mortality
6 Prior to thrombolytic therapy
   — To assess extent of jeopardized myocardium
   — ^{99m}Tc has superseded thallium in this context

* Usually uses thallium (^{201}Tl), but sometimes other tracers; scan becomes positive (i.e. revealing cold spot) within 4 h of infarct, unlike 'hotspot'

Value of gated cardiac blood pool scanning

1 Assessment of left ventricular function prior to
   — Valve replacement
   — CABG
   — Heart transplant
2 Distinguishing global cardiomyopathy from segmental ventricular dysfunction*

* Rarely indicated; cardiomyopathy may also be segmental

CARDIAC CATHETERIZATION

Rationâle in valvular heart disease

1 To define the nature and severity of the suspected lesion
2 To detect coexisting valvular lesions
3 To assess left ventricular function
4 To determine the state of the coronary arteries
5 To assess pulmonary vascular resistance and/or pulmonary capillary wedge pressure

Other indications for cardiac catheterization

1 Detection and quantification of shunts
2 Electrophysiologic studies
3 Endomyocardial biopsy*
   — Cardiomyopathy/myocarditis
   — Intracardiac tumor
   — Post-transplant

* Precise role remains to be clarified

Indications for coronary angiography

1 Typical angina refractory to medical therapy
2 Typical angina and/or myocardial infarction in a patient younger than 40 years
3 Angina following myocardial infarction
4 Strongly positive exercise test
5 Atypical chest pain
   — In a male with a positive stress test
   — In a female with a positive exercise thallium scan

Morbidity of cardiac catheterization

1 Brachial or femoral arterial occlusion
2 Coronary dissection; aortic dissection; tamponade
3 Left ventricular perforation
4 Cerebral embolism
5 Complete heart block, esp. if pre-existing RBBB
6 Ventricular dysrhythmias*
7 Hypotension, pulmonary edema*
8 Death, esp. if left main disease (mortality 2/1000)

* Frequency reduced if low-osmolality contrast agents used (expensive)

EXERCISE STRESS (ECG) TESTING

Indications for exercise testing

1 Diagnosis of ischemic heart disease where the diagnosis cannot be made on clinical grounds (e.g. atypical pain)
2 Investigation of suspected exercise-induced arrhythmias
3 Objective evaluation of symptoms (and/or degree of incapacity) in patients with known coronary artery disease
4 Assessment of patients following myocardial infarction
   — Submaximal (symptom-limited) test prior to discharge
   — Maximal test 6 weeks later (prior to return to work)
5 Assessment of 'at-risk' individuals prior to exercise program

Exclusion criteria for exercise testing
1 Recent prolonged ischemic chest pain
2 Known severe left main coronary artery disease
3 Severe hypertension, cardiac failure or aortic stenosis
4 Debility
5 Relative
  — Recurrent ventricular tachyarrhythmias
  — LBBB
  — WPW; LV strain pattern on resting ECG
  — Digoxin R_x in previous week ($\rightarrow$ false-positive)

Indicators of test positivity
1 Development of angina (esp. within first 3 min)
2 Inability to achieve workload > 5 Mets*, or to continue exercise > 6 min
3 2 mm downward-sloping ST segment depression
  — Onset at heart rate < 120/min, *or* within first 3 min; *or*
  — Post-test duration > 6 min; *or*
  — Seen in multiple leads
4 Failure of blood pressure to rise (remains < 130 mmHg) despite increasing workload and pulse rate
5 Failure of heart rate to exceed 120/min (off β-blockers), or < 85% of age-predicted rate
6 Delayed decrease in heart rate during first minute post-exercise

* A Met is a (metabolic) unit of work (O_2 utilization @ 3.5 mL/kg/min)

Indicators for aborting test
1 Dizziness, leg pains, severe dyspnea and/or angina
2 Fall in systolic blood pressure of more than 10 mmHg
3 Sustained ventricular tachyarrhythmias

Associations of false-positive tests
1 Low-risk patient populations, e.g.
  — Female (general)
  — Mitral valve prolapse
2 Conditions which cause ischemia without vascular disease
  — Anemia
  — Post-prandial
  — Valve stenosis, hypertension
  — Myxedema
3 Conditions causing ECG changes (see also Exclusions above)
  — Hypokalemia
  — Hyperventilation
  — Cardiomyopathy
  — Recent digoxin R_x (cf. β-blockers: false-negative)

ELECTROCARDIOGRAPHY (ECG)

Common cardiac rhythm anomalies in athletes
1 Sinus arrhythmia
2 Sinus bradycardia
3 First-degree heart block
4 Wenckebach phenomenon
5 Junctional rhythm

ECG effects of carotid sinus massage (CSM)
1 Left CSM $\rightarrow$ atrioventricular (AV) node
  Right CSM $\rightarrow$ sinoatrial (SA) node
2 Sinus tachycardia
  — Transient slowing
3 Paroxysmal junctional (AV nodal re-entry) tachycardia
  — Termination (sinus rhythm)
4 Atrial tachycardia/flutter/fibrillation
  — Slowing (AV block), may be abrupt
5 Wenckebach phenomenon
  — Slowing (AV nodal block) *if* intra-His block
6 Tachycardia-dependent bundle branch block
  — Disappearance of block
7 Bradycardia-dependent bundle branch block
  — Appearance of block
8 Demand pacemaker
  — Reinitiation of pacemaker rhythm
9 Ventricular tachycardia
  — No effect (*rarely* reverts)
10 WPW
  — Increased delta wave on ECG
  — Termination of tachycardia *or* no effect

Causes of a low-voltage ECG
1 Pulmonary emphysema
2 Cardiomyopathy ± ischemia, amyloid
3 Myxedema
4 Pericardial effusion ($\rightarrow$ electrical alternans)
5 Incorrect calibration

Voltage criteria for left ventricular hypertrophy
1 None is absolute
2 $S(V_1) + R(V_6) > 35$ mm
3 Any R > 25 mm; any R + any S > 45 mm
4 R(lead 1) > 20 mm
  R(aVl) > 13 mm if cardiac axis normal
  R(aVl) > 16 mm if there is left axis deviation

Diagnostic criteria for right ventricular hypertrophy
1 Dominant R wave in V_1; $R(V_1)$ amplitude > 7 mm
2 Diagnosis supported by T-wave inversion in V_{1-4} ('strain')
3 Exclusion of other causes of tall $R(V_1)$
  — RBBB
  — WPW type A
  — Dextrocardia
  — Posterior infarction
  — Hypertrophic cardiomyopathy

Left anterior hemiblock: diagnosis and significance
1 Left axis deviation without other cause (LBBB, LVH)
2 Small 'q' in lead I, small 'r' in III
3 May mask inferior infarct

Left posterior hemiblock: diagnosis and significance
1 Axis to the right of +100° without other cause
2 Small 'r' in I, small 'q' in III
3 May mask anterior infarct

Complete heart block: important causes
1 Lenègre's disease: sclerodegeneration of conduction system

2 Lev's disease: fibrocalcareous encroachment onto the conduction system; often associated with calcific aortic stenosis and preceded by first-degree heart block
3 Ischemic heart disease; inferior infarct
4 Digoxin toxicity, esp. when associated with ischemia
5 Congenital (proximal block, narrow QRS)
6 Surgical (e.g. AVR or for congenital heart disease)

Criteria for pathological Q wave in standard lead III
1 Duration of Q greater than 0.04 sec
2 Presence of Q (aVf) > 0.02 sec in duration
3 Presence of Q in lead II
4 Q(III) > 2.5 mm amplitude*

* Unless R(III) > 5 mm and P(III) upright; does *not* disappear on inspiration

Pathological Q waves*
1 Transmural myocardial injury (indeterminate age)
   — Myocardial infarction
   — Myocarditis
   — Cardiac contusion
2 Cardiomyopathy
   — HOCM
   — Myocarditis
3 WPW
4 Recording artefact
   — Dextrocardia
   — Reversed limb leads
   — High lead placement

* Differential diagnosis = deep (not pathological) 'Q' waves

Causes of an elevated ST segment
1 Ischemia
   — Acute myocardial infarction
   — Coronary spasm (may be microvascular)
2 Pericarditis
3 Ventricular aneurysm
4 Early repolarization (normal variant, e.g. in vagotonic individual)

Non-specific ST–T wave changes: some causes
1 Ischemic heart disease
2 Post-tachycardia
3 Hyperventilation; anxiety
4 Postprandial; cold drinks
5 Mitral valve prolapse
6 Subarachnoid hemorrhage*
7 Smoking
8 Pheochromocytoma
9 Digoxin therapy and/or hypokalemia

* Causes deep 'T' waves in precordial leads

Causes of a prolonged Q-T$_c$ (and/or torsades)*‡
1 Ischemic heart disease
2 Hypocalcemia
3 Subarachnoid hemorrhage
4 Anorexia nervosa
5 Severe bradycardia (e.g. complete heart block)
6 Rheumatic carditis
7 Heredofamilial long Q-T syndrome¶
8 Drugs: quinidine; tricyclics, phenothiazines (e.g. pimozide), amiodarone, terfenadine, astemizole, erythromycin, ketoconazole

* In general, normal Q-T interval < 50% R-R interval. Non-specific causes of bradycardia (myxedema, hypothermia, raised intracranial pressure) may increase Q-T interval, but not when *corrected* (Q-T$_c$) for rate
‡ Sudden death in chronic CCF is commoner in patients with higher inter-lead Q-T variability ('Q-T dispersion')
¶ Left stellectomy (surgical denervation of left cardiac sympathetic supply) may help prevent arrhythmias in patients resistant to β-blockers

Absent 'p' waves: differential diagnosis
1 Atrial fibrillation
2 Nodal rhythm; sinoatrial block
3 Severe hyperkalemia

Inverted 'p' waves in standard lead I
1 Nodal rhythm
2 Dextrocardia
3 Reversed limb leads

ECG manifestations of digoxin therapy
1 Prolonged P-R interval
2 Shortened Q-T$_c$
3 S–T depression ('reverse-tick'); T-wave flattening

ECG manifestations of quinidine therapy
1 Increased QRS width (25% increase may denote toxicity)
2 Prolonged Q-T$_c$; prolonged P-R interval; low wide T-wave
3 Torsades de pointes*
   — Polymorphous, twisting VT with prolonged Q-T$_c$
   — Indicates toxicity

* May also complicate idiopathic long Q-T syndrome or perhexiline therapy

ECG manifestations of hyperkalemia
1 Peaked ('tent-shaped') T waves
2 P wave flattening
3 Broad QRS
4 Non-specific ST–T wave abnormalities
5 Asystole

ECG localization of acute myocardial infarction
1 Anterior
   — Q waves/ST elevation V_{2-4}
2 Extensive anterior
   — Q waves/ST elevation I, aVL, V_{1-6}
3 Anteroseptal
   — Q waves/ST elevation V_{1-3}
4 Anterolateral
   — Q waves/ST elevation V_{4-6}
5 Inferior
   — Q waves/ST elevation II, III, aVF
6 True posterior
   — Abnormalities in V_{1-2} (see below)
7 Right ventricular
   — ST elevation in V_{4R}

ECG in true posterior infarction
1 Dominant widened 'R' (V_{1-2}): no RBBB/RVH/WPW
2 Tall widened 'T' (V_{1-2})
3 Concave-up ST depression (V_{1-2})
4 Usually associated with signs of inferior infarction

ECG in cor pulmonale
1 P pulmonale
2 Right axis deviation
3 RBBB
4 Dominant R wave in V_1 and aVR
   Dominant S wave in V_6
5 Inferior leads: ST depression, T wave inversion

ECG in rheumatic fever
1 Tachycardia: sinus or idionodal
2 Heart block: first degree ($\uparrow$ P-R)
3 Prolonged Q-T_c

ECG with reversed limb leads
1 Lead I appears to have reversed polarity
2 Leads II and III appear interchanged
3 aVr and aVl appear interchanged; aVf is normal

ECG in myotonic dystrophy
1 Sinus bradycardia
2 First-degree heart block (± higher-grade heart block)
3 Left axis deviation (± LAHB, LBBB)
4 Sporadic ventricular or re-entrant arrhythmias

MANAGING CARDIOVASCULAR DISEASE

SURGERY AND THE HEART

Cardiovascular risk factors for general surgery
1 Poor left ventricular function
   — Myocardial infarction in last 6 months
   — Third heart sound
   — Elevated jugular venous pressure
   — Ejection fraction < 30% on echo
2 ECG
   — Not sinus rhythm, *or*
   — Sinus rhythm *plus* 5 VEBs/min.
   — Ischemic S–T segment changes
3 General
   — Thoracic or upper abdominal surgery
   — *Severe* aortic stenosis or hypertension

Morbidity of open-heart surgery
1 LV dysfunction ± perioperative myocardial infarction
2 Cerebral sequelae
   — Stroke (mechanism unclear)
   — Personality change, confusion
   — Depression; sleep disturbance
3 Bleeding tendency
   — Post-pump syndrome (see below)
4 Exacerbation of peptic ulcer disease
5 Delayed complications
   — Post-cardiotomy syndrome
   — Endocarditis (after valve surgery)
   — CMV viremia; hepatitis
   — Wound infection

Coronary artery bypass grafting: rationâle
1 Operate for pain, not for dyspnea
2 Improved LV function *only* → hibernating myocardium

Coronary artery bypass grafting: survival benefit*
1 Accepted
   — Left main coronary artery disease
   — Triple-vessel disease
     • Symptomatic
     • Asymptomatic + poor LV function
2 Probable
   — Double-vessel disease + $\downarrow$ LV function
   — Double-vessel disease + high-grade proximal stenosis of left anterior descending branch of left coronary

* cf. low-risk patients: early CABG is associated with $\uparrow$ mortality

Factors influencing surgical evaluation of coronary disease
1 Severity of symptoms uncontrolled by medical therapy
   — i.e. Unstable angina
2 Size of left anterior descending branch of left coronary artery
   — Determines amount of myocardium jeopardized
3 Suitability for percutaneous angioplasty (PTCA)
   — Age, prior surgery, other disease

Contraindications to coronary artery grafting
1 Absolute
   — Technically ungraftable vessels
2 Relative
   — Lack of symptoms*
   — Inadequate trial of medical therapy
   — Severe left ventricular dysfunction

* Exceptions: (1) left main disease, and (2) triple vessel disease with positive exercise test (silent ischemia) – though aspirin may have a role in the latter

Operability criteria in coronary artery grafting
1 Satisfactory general medical condition
2 Adequate left ventricular function
3 Discrete proximal stenoses with good distal run-off

The 'post-pump' (cardiopulmonary bypass) syndrome
1 Coagulopathy (may respond to dextran or DDAVP)
   — Heparin effect
   — Thrombocytopenia
   — Massive transfusion
   — Coagulation factor depletion
2 Anemia, leucopenia
   — Mechanical intravascular hemolysis
3 Systemic inflammatory reactions
   — e.g. 'Shock lung' (due to complement activation)
4 Pancreatitis
   — Associated with perioperative $CaCl_2$ administration
5 Central nervous system dysfunction: stroke, amnesia, dementia
   — Very common if sufficient filtering precautions not taken
   — Due to microinfarcts from 'spray' of cardiac microemboli

Post-cardiotomy (Dressler's) syndrome: clinical features
1 Acute febrile illness within 6 months of heart surgery/infarct

2 Chest pain: pleuritic or pericarditic
3 CXR may show effusion(s), cardiomegaly; ECG often normal
4 Self-limiting; may need NSAIDs, aspirin, steroids, aspiration
5 Diagnosis of exclusion (DD$_x$: acute myocardial infarction)

PACEMAKING

Indications for permanent pacing
1 Major indication
  — Symptomatic bradyarrhythmias
2 Relative indications
  — Complete heart block (if symptomatic)
  — 'At-risk' for complete heart block
    • Intermittent Möbitz type II AV block (wide QRS)
    • Bi-/trifascicular block + ↑ H-V interval on EPS
    • Alternating RBBB and LBBB
  — Drug-resistant tachyarrhythmias (incl. sick sinus)

Indications for transvenous pacing in anterior infarcts
1 Second- or third-degree AV block
2 Relative
  — New RBBB with old 1° HB/LAHB/LPHB
  — New LBBB with pre-existing 1° HB
  — Alternating RBBB and LBBB

Sources of interference
1 Arc welding
2 Intraoperative unipolar diathermy
3 Pectoralis overactivity (myoinhibition)
4 NMR scanners

Reasons for failure of pacemaker to prevent syncope
1 Failure of stimulus artefact
2 Failure of ventricular capture
3 Failure of demand function
  — Oversensing (will not 'fire')
4 Symptoms not due to cardiac arrhythmia

Features of the pacemaker syndrome
1 Definition
  — Retrograde ventriculoatrial conduction (despite blockade of anterograde conduction)
2 Mechanism
  — Ventricular pacemaker induces atrial contraction, increasing atrial pressure + reducing cardiac output
3 Presentations
  — Dizziness, episodic dyspnea

PROSTHETIC HEART VALVES

General considerations influencing valve selection
1 Topographic considerations
  — Problems commoner in mitral/tricuspid position
    • Thromboembolism
    • Acute obstruction
  — Problems commoner in aortic position
    • Intravascular hemolysis
    • Infection
    • Valve dysfunction
2 Mechanical valves (see below)
  — Main advantage: durability
  — Main disadvantage: anticoagulant requirement‡ (hence, bleeding complications)
3 Tissue valves (e.g. Hancock, Carpentier–Edwards)
  — Main advantage: no anticoagulant requirement*
  — Main disadvantage: not durable‡, prone to calcify

* Esp. in aortic position
‡ 50% need redo by 8 years

Specific factors influencing mechanical valve selection
1 Ball-in-cage (Starr–Edwards)
  — Disadvantages
    • Flow impediment (esp. with exercise)
    • Thrombogenicity (need to keep INR > 3.5)
  — Advantage
    • Durability
2 Tilting disc (e.g. Björk-Shiley, single-leaflet; St Jude, bileaflet)
  — Disadvantages
    • Prone to massive valve thrombosis
    • Significant incidence of strut fracture
  — Advantage
    • Excellent hemodynamics
    • Less peripheral thromboembolism

Features of valvar hemolysis
1 Diagnosis
  — Normochromic (rarely, hypochromic) anemia
  — Blood film: schistocytes, no spherocytes
  — Haptoglobin with negative Coombs'/Ham's tests
  — Hemosiderinuria (implies long-standing hemolysis)
2 Significance
  — Suspect valve dysfunction (e.g. regurgitation)
  — *Actively* exclude valve infection
3 Management
  — Transfuse
  — Treat infection
  — Valve repair or replacement

Tissue valves: relative indications for use*
1 Elderly patient requiring aortic valve replacement
2 Elderly patient in sinus rhythm with normal size left atrium requiring mitral valve prosthesis
3 Young woman in sinus rhythm desiring pregnancy
4 Any absolute contraindication to anticoagulation‡

* NB: Durability is usually the most important consideration; homografts tend to be superior to heterografts (Carpentier–Edwards, Hancock) in this regard
‡ Use homograft if so; heterografts still require 3 months' initial warfarinization, followed by aspirin therapy

Anticoagulant management of the pregnant patient
1 Use subcutaneous heparin prophylaxis (10 000 U b.d.) throughout first trimester to avoid warfarin embryopathy
2 Switch to warfarin at start of second trimester, and maintain until halfway through third trimester

(prolonged use of heparin prophylaxis may result in severe osteoporosis)

3 Change back to heparin (subcutaneous at home, infusion in hospital) and monitor closely using protamine sulfate neutralization and platelet count, esp. prior to delivery (neonatal intraventricular hemorrhage is a major risk)
4 Avoid epidural anesthesia throughout confinement. At delivery, reverse heparin with protamine sulfate
5 Recommence SC heparin immediately following delivery
6 Recommence warfarin 1 week after delivery (not contraindicated in lactation; cf. phenindione)

HEART TRANSPLANTS

Contraindications to transplantation
1 Satisfactory quality of life
2 Active infection (incl. HIV) or peptic ulcer
3 Severe pulmonary hypertension ($\geq$ 5 Wood units)
4 Past history of thromboembolism or CVA
5 Insulin-dependent diabetes
6 Renal or hepatic insufficiency; chronic hepatitis B/C
7 Major systemic/psychiatric illness (e.g. alcoholism)
8 Positive cytotoxic crossmatch with donor organ
9 Prior thoracotomy
10 Advanced age

Signs of rejection
1 Fever (early sign)
2 CXR: cardiomegaly
3 ECG: conduction disturbances, reduced QRS voltage
4 Cardiac failure (late sign)

Indications for heart–lung transplantation
1 Pulmonary hypertension
 — Primary (advanced)
2 Pulmonary hypertension
 — Congenital heart disease (Eisenmenger's)
3 Pulmonary hypertension
 — Secondary to cystic fibrosis

CORONARY ANGIOPLASTY/ATHERECTOMY

Percutaneous transluminal coronary angioplasty (PTCA)
1 All angiographic lesions are suitable for attempted PTCA
 Ischemia and angina commonly occur during PTCA
2 Commonest lesion (80%) is a proximal concentric non-calcified stenosis in a patient with single-vessel disease
3 80–90% of such lesions are successfully dilated*
 30% of dilated lesions re-occlude within 6 months‡
 (stent placement may be more durable than PTCA)
4 2% require urgent thoracotomy post-PTCA (acute occlusion)
 2% incidence of non-Q-wave myocardial infarction

1% mortality from elective PTCA for single-vessel disease
5 Similar success (~ 80%) in restenosis and graft occlusion
 Efficacy approximates that of CABG

* i.e. 10–20% failure rate
‡ Risk increases with prior CMV infection

Potential indications for PTCA
1 Angina
2 After thrombolysis for acute myocardial infarction

DRUG THERAPY

Elimination pathways of cardioactive drugs
1 Initial hepatic metabolism
 — Quinidine
 — Lidocaine (lignocaine)
 — Antianginals
 • Nitrates
 • β-blockers (e.g. propranolol)
 • Verapamil
2 Initial renal excretion
 — Digoxin
 — Disopyramide
 — Procainamide

Popular drug combinations in cardiological practice
1 ACE inhibitor + diuretic
 — Chronic left ventricular dysfunction
2 Nitrates + dopamine/dobutamine
 — Acute left ventricular dysfunction
3 β-blocker + isosorbide mononitrate
 — Angina

Cardiovascular effects of tricyclic antidepressants
1 Tachycardia (anticholinergic effect)
2 Hypotension (esp. postural)
3 Prolonged Q-T$_c$ (quinidine-like effect)
4 Prolonged P-R interval
5 Antagonism of guanethidine and methyldopa
6 Precipitation of ventricular arrhythmias (esp. in overdose)

CALCIUM ANTAGONISTS

Calcium blocker indications and contraindications
1 Main indication: angina
2 Main contraindication: congestive cardiac failure

Verapamil: absolute contraindications
1 High-degree AV block
2 Sick sinus syndrome*
3 Wolff–Parkinson–White syndrome with anterograde conduction causing recurrent atrial fibrillation/flutter
4 Digoxin toxicity
5 Heart failure, hypotension (incl. post-infarct)
6 Simultaneous IV use with β-blockers

* Unless manifests as atrial fibrillation

Calcium antagonists: which one?
1 Verapamil ($\to$ greatest AV nodal block)
   — Supraventricular tachycardia
   — Hypertrophic cardiomyopathy
   — Do not prescribe with β-blockers
2 Slow-release nifedipine ($\to$ greatest drop in peripheral resistance)
   — Angina (with β-blockers)
   — Left ventricular dysfunction/cardiac failure
   — Hypertension: systemic or pulmonary
   — Sinus bradycardia; impaired AV conduction
   — Coronary artery spasm
   — Peripheral vasospasm (Raynaud's)
   — Peripheral vascular disease
3 Diltiazem (intermediate in both respects)
   — Less negative ionotropy/chronotropy than verapamil
   — Permits increased heart rate with exercise
   — May be used for angina with (oral) β-blockers
4 Amlodipine, felodipine
   — New-generation dihydropyridines
   — Safe in cardiac failure; appear preferable to older calcium blockers for treating cardiac failure due to non-coronary disease

ANTIARRHYTHMIC THERAPY

Practical classification of antiarrhythmic drugs
1 'AV node' drugs
   — Digoxin
   — Verapamil
   — β-blockers
2 'Ventricle' drugs
   — Lidocaine (lignocaine)
   — Mexiletine, tocainide
3 'Whole-heart' (incl. bundle of Kent) drugs
   — Amiodarone
   — Disopyramide
   — Quinidine, procainamide

Electrophysiological classification* of antiarrhythmic drugs
1 #I
   — Block membrane Na^+ transport
   — ↓ Rate of action potential rise (phase O depolarization)
   — e.g. Quinidine, procainamide, disopyramide; lidocaine (lignocaine)
2 # II
   — Sympathetic nervous system blockers
   — Reduce phase 4 depolarization
   — e.g. β-blockers
3 # III
   — Prolong duration of action potential/refractory period
   — No effect on phase 0 depolarization
   — e.g. Amiodarone, bretylium
4 #IV
   — Calcium blockers
   — e.g. Verapamil (cf. nifedipine: *not* antiarrhythmic)

* Vaughan-Williams classification

Drugs reducing ventricular rate in atrial fibrillation*
1 Digoxin
2 Adenosine
3 Verapamil
4 Amiodarone
5 β-blockers

* i.e. AV blockers

Quinidine: contraindications to use
1 Single agent use in atrial flutter/fibrillation
2 Prolonged $Q-T_c$
3 Hypotension
4 Sick sinus syndrome
5 Myasthenia gravis

Quinidine: toxicity
1 Diarrhea
2 Nausea, vomiting, abdominal pain, fever
3 Thrombocytopenia, agranulocytosis
4 Cinchonism
   — Tinnitus, deafness, vertigo, amblyopia
   — Sweats, flushing, urticaria
5 Potentiation of digoxin and warfarin toxicity

Disopyramide: toxicity
1 Anticholinergic, esp. urinary retention in males
2 Negative inotropy, esp. when given by IV bolus
3 Ventricular tachyarrhythmias (usually preceded by ↑ $Q-T_c$)

Amiodarone: toxicity
1 Pneumonitis (10% incidence, 0.5% mortality)
2 Thyroid dysfunction*
   — Hypothyroidism (6–10% within 3 years)
   — Hyperthyroidism (< 3% within 3 years)
   — Euthyroid hyperthyroxinemia‡
3 Corneal microdeposits (reversible)
4 Peripheral neuropathy (irreversible)
5 Liver damage (irreversible)
6 Photosensitivity
7 Bradycardia, idioventricular rhythm
   Hypotension if rapidly infused
8 Nightmares, sleep disturbance

* Thyroid toxicity reflects high (37%) iodine content
‡ Due to impaired deiodination of T_4 to T_3

Antiarrhythmic efficacy of magnesium
1 Torsades de pointes
2 Digoxin-dependent arrhythmias
3 Multifocal or re-entrant supraventricular arrhythmias

DIGOXIN THERAPY

Side-effects of digoxin
1 Gastrointestinal
   — Diarrhea, abdominal pain, ulceration (local effect)
   — Nausea, vomiting (central effect)
2 Central
   — Confusion, convulsions, depression
   — Commoner in elderly patients

3 Visual (dose-related)
— Xanthopsia, haloes, blurring
4 Rare
— Facial pain; gynecomastia; hyperkalemia
— Muscle necrosis

Contraindications to digoxin therapy
1 Wolff–Parkinson–White syndrome*
2 AV block
3 HOCM (or severe aortic stenosis) in sinus rhythm
4 Constrictive pericarditis; acute myocarditis
5 Prior to elective cardioversion (relative‡)

* Antidromic (with tachycardias)
‡ cf. do *not* cardiovert in digoxin toxicity

Metabolic predispositions to digoxin toxicity
1 General
— Old age, low body weight
— Pre-existing myocardial disease
2 Renal impairment
3 Metabolic abnormality
— Hypoxia (esp. cor pulmonale)
— Hypokalemia
— Hypomagnesemia
— Hypercalcemia
— Hypothyroidism
4 Cardiac amyloidosis

Arrhythmias in digoxin toxicity
1 'Classical'
— AV block plus junctional/ventricular arrhythmia
2 Common in elderly patients: ↑ automaticity
— Frequent ventricular ectopic beats (in 50%)
— Ventricular bigeminy
— Ventricular tachycardia (in 5%); VF
3 Common in young patients (esp. overdoses): ↑ AV block
— Junctional rhythm (seen in 20%)
— Atrial tachycardia + varying block ('SVT with block')
— Sinus bradycardia, sinoatrial nodal block, sinus arrest

Management of digoxin toxicity*
1 Cease digoxin administration
2 Correct electrolyte imbalance
— Aim to maintain serum K^+ at 4.5–5.5 mmol/L
— Do *not* administer KCI in presence of AV block
— Infuse potassium in saline (not in dextrose)
3 AV block
— Atropine, phenytoin
— Temporary pacing
4 Supraventricular tachycardia
— Propranolol
5 Ventricular arrhythmias
— Phenytoin
— Temporary pacing
— (Emergency) cardioversion
6 Rarely needed therapies
— Antidigoxin antibodies (Fab fragments)
— Dialysis

* *Most* patients can be managed with the first two measures alone

SYMPATHOLYTIC AND SYMPATHOMIMETIC THERAPY

Physiological manifestations of adrenergic stimulation
1 α_1 (post-synaptic) stimulation
— Peripheral vasoconstriction, pressor effects
— Catecholamine agonists
• Dopamine, (nor)adrenaline ((nor)epinephrine)
— Peripheral α_1 antagonist
• Prazosin
2 α_2 (presynaptic) stimulation
— Sympathetic inhibition
— Central α_{2a} receptor agonist
• Clonidine
3 β_1 (predominantly cardiac) stimulation
— Tachycardia, positive inotropy
— Increased AV conduction
— Catecholamine agonists
• (Nor)adrenaline ((nor)epinephrine), isoprenaline
• Dopamine, dobutamine
— Cardioselective blockers
• Metoprolol, bisoprolol, atenolol; acebutolol*
4 β_2 (predominantly peripheral) stimulation
— Peripheral vasodilatation
— Bronchodilatation
— Catecholamine agonists
• Adrenaline (epinephrine), isoprenaline
• Dopexamine, dobutamine
5 Dopaminergic
— Low-dose: coronary/cerebral/renal *vasodilatation*
— Moderate-dose: mainly β_1 effects
— High-dose: mainly α_1-mediated *vasoconstriction*

* Also has some α-blocking activity

Hazards of combining β-blockers with other therapy
1 Verapamil*
— Depression of myocardial contractility and conduction
2 Ergotamine, dopamine
— Non-selective block of β_1-mediated vasodilatation (→ severe vasoconstriction and necrosis)
3 Prazosin
— Accentuation of 'first-dose' hypotension
4 Adrenaline (epinephrine)
— Immediate severe hypertension
5 Indometacin
— Antagonism of therapeutic hypotensive effect
6 Cimetidine
— Potentiation of therapeutic hypotensive effect
7 Antianginal therapy of coronary artery spasm
— Antagonism by β-blockade

* Esp. parenteral administration

Rationâle of β-blockade in myocardial infarction
1 IV (within 4 h of infarct ± streptokinase/angioplasty)
— May reduce chest pain
— May reduce infarct size (and ? cardiogenic shock)
— May prevent some arrhythmias (incl. SVT, VF)

2 Oral (post-infarct maintenance)
— Reduced mortality/reinfarction rate, esp. if
• Modest LV dysfunction
• Positive exercise test prior to discharge (may indicate need for catheterization ± CABG)

β-blockers used to slow ventricular rate in cardiac failure*
1 Carvedilol‡
2 Metoprolol¶; atenolol
3 Bisoprolol

* IV β-blockers may also be combined with thrombolytic therapy in acute myocardial infarction to reduce the risk of cardiac rupture
‡ Also has α-blocking activity causing vasodilatation
¶ Metabolism varies widely due to genetic polymorphisms

ANGIOTENSIN-CONVERTING ENZYME (ACE) INHIBITORS

Distinguishing features of ACE inhibitors
1 Captopril
— Rapid onset of action, short half-life
— Requires b.d./t.d.s. dosage regimen (on empty stomach)
2 Enalapril
— Hepatically bioactivated to enalaprilat
— Slower onset of action; once-daily dosage
3 Lisinopril
— Substitution of lysine for proline in enalaprilat
— 24-h duration of action; once-daily dosage
4 Others
— Alecapril (prodrug for captopril)
— Pentopril, ramipril (long duration of action)

Proposed mechanisms of action of ACE inhibitors
1 Reduction of angiotensin II levels
— Vasodilatation
— ↓ Renin release
— ↓ Aldosterone secretion
2 Increased bradykinin, prostacyclin, prostaglandin E_2 levels
— Vasodilatation

Indications for ACE inhibitors in hypertension management
1 Refractory heart failure with left ventricular dysfunction
2 Severe high-renin hypertension in scleroderma
3 Left ventricular hypertrophy
4 Diabetic nephropathy*
5 Cardioprotection in acute myocardial infarction
6 Stroke prevention

* Note that polycystic nephropathy does not appear to benefit

Therapeutic benefits of ACE inhibitors in hypertension
1 Peripheral vascular resistance is reduced
2 Renal, cardiac, and cerebral perfusion is maintained or increased due to selective vasodilating activity
3 No effect on myocardial conductivity or contractility
4 No effect on metabolism of glucose, urate, lipids or electrolytes; safe to use in diabetes and gout

5 Reduce proteinuria, nephropathy in hypertensive diabetics*
6 Safe to use in asthma and depression
7 Do not cause fatigue or impotence; hence, high compliance

* But benefit reduced if ACE genotype is *DD*

Benefits of ACE inhibitors in refractory heart failure
1 Improved hemodynamics
— No reflex tachycardia (reflecting ↓ preload)
2 Improved exercise tolerance and angina threshold
— ↓ Myocardial oxygen use despite ↑ cardiac output
3 Improved renal function and electrolyte balance
— No secondary hyperaldosteronism
4 Regression of LV hypertrophy
5 Improved survival

Side-effects of ACE inhibitors
1 Sulfhydryl moiety-related (i.e. seen with captopril/alecapril)
— Rash (dose-related; commoner in renal failure)
— Taste disturbance
— Mouth ulcers
— Neutropenia/agranulocytosis ⎫ Unusual at
— Proteinuria/nephrosis ⎬ doses now used
— Euphoria ⎭
2 'Class' effects (→ longer-acting ACE inhibitors)
— Hypotension (see below) and dizziness
— Hyperkalemia* (esp. in renal failure); hypoglycemia
— Cough (see below)
— Angioedema (in 0.1%; may be fatal)
— Renal insufficiency (esp. in bilateral renal artery stenosis or concurrent loop diuretic therapy)

* Hence, discontinue potassium supplements or potassium-sparing diuretics before initiation

Cough associated with ACE inhibition
1 Affects 10–20% patients
Causes change of therapy in up to 5%
Lower incidence with fosinopril than with enalapril
2 Affects mainly female non-smokers
3 Probably rises due to potentiation of ACE substrates such as bradykinin, substance P, neurokinin A, or prostaglandins
4 Diagnosis
— Stops within 4 days of ceasing medication
— Recommences within a week (usually within hours) of restarting same or different ACE inhibitor
5 May respond to cromoglycate (vagolytic) prophylaxis
6 Currently represents the main indication for commencing angiotensin II receptor antagonist therapy (losartan, valsartan, irbesartan, candesartan) in patients with known high-renin hypertension

Risk factors for 'first-dose' hypotension with ACE inihitors
1 Advanced cardiac failure, esp. if
— Hyponatremia (± salt restriction)
— Diuretic therapy

2 High-renin hypertension
3 Hemodialysis

VASODILATOR THERAPY

Indications for vasodilator therapy
1 Cardiac failure*
— Cardiogenic shock, cardiomyopathy
— Acute valvular incompetence; septal rupture
— Hypertensive heart failure
2 Hypertension
— Crisis (incl. encephalopathy)
— Refractory hypertension
3 Angina‡

* Hypotension and/or reflex tachycardia do not usually occur when vasodilators are used appropriately for CCF
‡ Best vasodilator in this context: glyceryl trinitrate

Predominant preload reducers
1 Nitrates*
2 Furosemide (frusemide)
3 Morphine (in pulmonary edema)

NB: Furosemide (frusemide) causes initial rapid venodilatation, followed by slower off-loading effect due to diuresis
* Including high-dose isosorbide dinitrate (for pulmonary edema), given as repeated IV bolus

Predominant afterload reducers
1 Hydralazine
2 Nifedipine
3 Nitroprusside
4 Prostacyclin (PGI_2)*

* Particularly useful as a vasodilator in Buerger's disease

Pre- and afterload reducers
1 Prazosin
2 ACE inhibitors (e.g. captopril)
3 Sodium nitroprusside ('SNIP')
4 Atrial natriuretic peptide (ANP)

NB: Nitroprusside best for 'forward failure', e.g. in septal/chordal rupture, acute mitral/aortic incompetence due to endocarditis

Toxicity of prolonged (> 48 h) nitroprusside infusions
1 Cyanide intoxication*
2 Lactic acidosis
3 Hypothyroidism

* Plasma CN^- levels can be monitored

THROMBOLYTIC THERAPY

Potential indications for thrombolytic therapy
1 Hyperacute phase (< 6 h) myocardial infarction*
2 *Massive* pulmonary embolism (> 40% vascular bed)‡, or
Any life-threatening pulmonary embolism
— i.e. Patient is hypotensive and sick
3 Massive iliofemoral thrombosis¶

* Thrombolytic therapy is coadministered with heparin in this context

‡ e.g. alteplase (tissue plasminogen activator, tPA) 100 mg over 2 h is one recommended regimen, notwithstanding the hazards
¶ Thrombolytic therapy reduces incidence of post-phlebitic syndrome

Contraindications to thrombolytic therapy
1 Absolute
— Recent prolonged or traumatic cardiac resuscitation
— Active bleeding (e.g from peptic ulcer)
— Increased risk of hemorrhagic stroke
• Any history of cerebral hemorrhage
• Recent skull trauma
• Brain tumor
— Retinal hemorrhages (e.g. diabetic*, hypertensive)
— Blood pressure > 200/120 mmHg
— Surgery within the last 3 weeks
— Pregnancy/puerperium
— Previous allergic reaction to SK or APSAC‡
2 Relative
— History of CVA, peptic ulcer or severe hypertension
— Recent surgery or trauma (but > 3 weeks ago)
— Suspected intracardiac thrombus (e.g. MS with AF)
— Coagulopathy, or severe chronic liver disease
— Prior thrombolytic treatment with SK or APSAC‡

* Controversial
‡ In this situation, treat instead with urokinase or tPA

Monitors of thrombolytic therapy
1 PTTK/APTT, (pro)thrombin time, euglobulin lysis time
2 Resolution of condition requiring treatment
— As determined by lung scan, blood gases, etc.
3 Overdosage may be corrected by aprotinin or FFP

CORONARY THROMBOLYSIS

Considerations favoring post-infarct thrombolytic therapy
1 No known contraindication to thrombolysis (see above)
2 Symptom duration < 6 h (preferably < 1 h)
3 Anterior or posterior (i.e. > inferior) infarct
4 Patient younger than 75

ECG criteria influencing thrombolysis outcomes
1 Features favoring utility of thrombolysis
— ST elevation (esp. anterior)
— Bundle branch block
2 Features opposing utility of thrombolysis
— Lone ST segment depression
— Normal ECG

Coronary recanalization efficiency
1 Intravenous streptokinase   — 50%
2 Intracoronary streptokinase   — 70%
3 Intravenous tPA   — 70%

tPA or streptokinase? Points to consider

1 tPA is a recombinant human protein which binds fibrin in clots then activates (cleaves) plasminogen to plasmin, causing localized thrombolysis. Streptokinase (or urokinase) also binds fibrin in clots, but degrades fibrinogen as well, leading to generalized fibrinolysis

2 Despite the apparently greater specificity of tPA, neither its efficacy nor its safety record has been proven superior to that of streptokinase; both are complicated by cerebral hemorrhage in 0.5–1.0% of cases

3 Clinical trials of tPA have shown 50% (the TIMI-1 study) and 26% (the ASSET study) reductions in death from myocardial infarction

4 Clinical trials of streptokinase have shown 25% (the ISIS-2 study) and 18% (the GISSI study) reductions in death from myocardial infarction, the latter increasing to 50% if given in the first hour of symptoms

5 tPA is far more expensive than streptokinase

UNDERSTANDING CARDIOVASCULAR DISEASE

TACHYARRHYTHMIAS

Management of atrial flutter

1 Slow ventricular rate
   — Digoxin (*if* digoxin toxicity excluded)
2 If *tachycardia* persists despite digitalization, consider
   — Adenosine, *or*
   — β-blocker, *or*
   — Verapamil
3 If *sinus rhythm* does not occur despite digitalization, add
   — Quinidine (in CCU)*, *or*
   — Disopyramide
4 If above measures fail
   — Prepare for elective synchronized cardioversion
   — Commence heparin infusion 48 h before
   — Cease digoxin 24 h prior to version
   — Commence quinidine after; maintain for 3 months
5 For long-term control of recurrent atrial flutter
   — Radiofrequency ablation

* If quinidine is commenced, the maintenance dose of digoxin should be reduced by 50% pending attainment of a new steady state

Cardioversion: indications and contraindications

1 Indications
   — Coarse ventricular fibrillation
   — Ventricular tachycardia or rapid atrial fibrillation of recent onset with hemodynamic deterioration
   — Atrial flutter or paroxysmal atrial tachycardia resistant to medical therapy
2 Relative contraindications
   — Suspected intracardiac thrombus
   — Digoxin toxicity and/or hypokalemia
   — Low anticipated success rate
     • Long-standing atrial fibrillation, *or*

   • AF with thyrotoxicosis*, *or*
   • AF with left atrial diameter > 50 mm on echo

* Best treated with β-blocker

Rapid atrial fibrillation resistant to digoxin?

1 Inadequately treated CCF + myocardial infarction
2 Thyrotoxicosis*
3 Wolff–Parkinson–White syndrome
4 Mitral stenosis
5 Pulmonary embolism
6 Myocarditis, congestive cardiomyopathy
7 Intracardiac (or pericardial) metastases

NB: Digoxin toxicity *rarely* causes lone atrial fibrillation
* Even in the absence of overt hyperthyroidism, low or undetectable TSH levels can indicate patients at risk of atrial fibrillation

High-risk atrial fibrillation: indications for warfarin*

1 Previous TIA or stroke
2 Paroxysmal AF alternating with sick sinus syndrome
3 Stroke risk factors from echocardiogram
   — Left atrial enlargement (± thrombus), *or*
   — Mitral annulus calcification, *or*
   — LV dysfunction
4 Prior to elective cardioversion

* Fibrillators *not* meeting these criteria should receive *aspirin* 150 mg/day

ECG clues to the diagnosis of recurrent palpitations

1 Long Q-T
   — Ventricular tachycardia
2 Short P-R
   — Re-entrant supraventricular tachycardia
3 P mitrale
   — Atrial fibrillation
4 Ventricular premature depolarizations, Q waves or complete heart block
   — Ventricular tachycardia
5 Inverted T in V_2 with epsilon wave
   — Right ventricular dysplasia giving rise to arrhythmias

Electrophysiologic clues to the diagnosis of recurrent palpitations

1 Normal electrophysiologic study
   — Idiopathic
   — Anxiety
   — Thyrotoxicosis
   — Pheochromocytoma
2 Abnormal electrophysiologic study
   — Intranodal bypass tract (commonest*)
   — Wolff–Parkinson–White syndrome
   — Atrio-His bypass (Lown–Ganong–Levine syndrome)
   — Intra-atrial/sinus node re-entry

* Palpitations distinctively associated with sensation of pounding in neck

Indications for electrophysiologic study in tachyarrythmias

1 Wide-complex tachycardias indistinguishable from ventricular tachycardia
2 Ventricular tachycardia

3 Recurrent symptomatic supraventricular tachycardia with
— Hemodynamic compromise ('presyncope')
— Syncopal episodes
— Wolff–Parkinson–White syndrome on resting ECG

Complications of radiofrequency ablation for tachyarrythmias
1 Femoral arterial hematoma, thrombosis or fistula
2 Coronary artery spasm or thrombosis
3 Mitral or aortic regurgitation
4 Cardiac tamponade
5 AV block
6 Death (< 0.1%)

Differential diagnosis of wide-complex tachycardia
1 Ventricular tachycardia (VT)
— Usually regular
— No effect of adenosine
2 Wolff–Parkinson–White with anterograde conduction
— May be regular or irregular
— Slowing of ventricular response by adenosine
3 Torsades de pointes (p. 40)
— Irregular
— Terminated by $MgSO_4$ (2 g IV over 3 min)
4 Supraventricular tachycardia (SVT) with aberrant conduction
— Termination by adenosine (unless WPW or asthma)

ECG characteristics of common paroxysmal SVTs
1 Atrioventricular nodal re-entrant SVT
— Hidden P waves, pseudo-R (V_1), pseudo-S (II or III)
2 Orthodromic* atrioventricular re-entrant SVT
— Inverted P waves; QRS alternans
3 WPW with atrial fibrillation
— Irregular rhythm, variable QRS conformation
4 Multifocal atrial tachycardia
— Variable P, P-R, and rate

* i.e. accessory pathway-mediated, not antidromic conduction

VT or SVT with aberrancy? Factors favoring VT*
1 Past history of ventricular disease (e.g. aneurysm)
2 Heart rate < 170/min; no effect of carotid sinus massage
3 Clinical evidence of AV dissociation
— Cannon waves in JVP; 'a' waves slower than
— Beat-to-beat variation in systolic blood pressure
— Varying intensity of S_1
4 ECG evidence of AV dissociation
— Dissociated 'P' waves
— Fusion beats, capture beats
— Left axis deviation
— QRS duration > 140 ms
— QRS morphology different to previous tracings
5 No benefit from adenosine

* NB: Do not give verapamil (dangerous in VT) to any patient with broad-complex tachycardia of unknown cause; try adenosine, procainamide or (if urgent) cardiovert

Antiarrhythmic role of IV adenosine
1 Action
— A purine nucleoside which slows AV nodal conduction by activating adenosine (A_1) receptors
— Half-life of only a few seconds ($\rightarrow \downarrow\downarrow$ adverse effects); hence, administered as a rapid IV bolus
2 Diagnostic use
— Differentiates SVT from VT safely
• Arrhythmia terminated? Junctional origin
• Transient AV block induced? Atrial origin
• No effect? Ventricular origin or WPW
3 Therapeutic use
— Paroxysmal junctional tachycardia (drug of choice)
4 Side-effects and interactions
— Transient chest discomfort, flushing, headache
5 Contraindications
— Asthma
— 2nd/3rd degree heart block
— Concurrent R_x (may potentiate adenosine)
• Dipyridamole, disopyramide

WOLFF–PARKINSON–WHITE SYNDROME (WPW)

Associations of WPW
1 Mitral valve prolapse
2 Hypertrophic cardiomyopathy (uncommonly)
3 Ebstein's anomaly; secundum ASD

Arrhythmias encountered in WPW
1 Paroxysmal atrial tachycardia (in 70%)
2 Atrial fibrillation (in 10–15%)
3 Atrial flutter (in 5%)*

* Development of one-to-one conduction is highly suggestive of the diagnosis

Subtypes of WPW
1 Type A (left-sided)
— QRS above the isoelectric line in V_1
— Simulates posterior or inferior infarction
— Accessory pathway connects left atrium and ventricle
2 Type B (right-sided)
— QRS below isoelectric line in V_1
— Simulates anterior or inferior infarction
— Pathway connects right atrium and ventricle (e.g. in Ebstein's anomaly)

Management of WPW
1 Observe if asymptomatic
2 Refer for electrophysiologic study at first suspicion of symptoms
3 Medical therapy
— Amiodarone
— Disopyramide
— β-blockers/verapamil
Avoid
— Digoxin
— Carotid sinus massage (if high risk of AF)
4 Radiofrequency ablation of accessory AV pathways

5 Implantable defibrillator
6 Surgical division of bundle of Kent (following His-bundle studies) if refractory to medical measures

BRADYARRHYTHMIAS

Causes of bradyarrhythmias
1 Primary (e.g. ischemic) heart disease:
   — Sinoatrial dysfunction ('sick sinus')
   — Nodal rhythm
   — Complete heart block
2 β-blockade
3 Increased intracranial pressure
4 Metabolic
   — Hypothyroidism
   — Hypothermia
   — Hyperbilirubinemia (profound)

ECG manifestations of sick sinus syndrome
1 Prolonged episodes of sinus bradycardia
   — Absolute (< 40/min)
   — Relative (e.g. < 50/min going up stairs)
2 Marked sinus arrhythmia with symptoms of hypoperfusion
3 Periods of sinus arrest (> 2 sec)
4 Junctional escape rhythms
5 'Brady-tachy' syndrome: background bradycardia punctuated by paroxysmal bursts of rapid atrial flutter/fibrillation
6 Chronic atrial fibrillation (end-stage sinus node dysfunction)

Diagnosis and management of sick sinus syndrome
1 Resting ECG
   — Slow AF
   — Marked, atropine-resistant bradycardia (following β-blockade or digoxin therapy esp.)
2 Holter study (see above)
3 Stress test
   — Excessive tachycardia at submaximal load
4 Management
   — Atrial fibrillation
     • Warfarinization (INR ~ 1.5)
   — Syncope associated with bradycardias
     • Atrial demand pacing

AORTIC DISSECTION

Predispositions to aortic dissection
1 Ageing
2 Hypertension
3 Coarctation or bicuspid aortic valve
4 Marfan's syndrome
5 Pregnancy
6 Iatrogenic (post-cardiotomy or post-catheter)

Acute severe chest pain: is it thoracic aortic dissection?
1 Ascending aorta dissection
   — Marfanoid habitus
   — Continuous severe tearing chest pain radiating to back
   — New aortic incompetent murmur
   — Signs of cardiac tamponade
   — ECG: acute infarct (right coronary occlusion) in 1–2%*
2 Aortic arch dissection
   — Reduced pulse in left arm
   — Asymmetric blood pressure readings
   — Carotid occlusion, esp. left
3 Descending aortic dissection
   — Reduced femoral pulse, esp. on left
   — Microhematuria (renal infarction)
   — Left basal dullness (hemothorax)

* NB: The ECG may be normal in aortic dissection

Diagnostic modalities in suspected aortic dissection
1 Transesophageal echocardiography
   — Advantages: rapid, sensitive (95–100%), detects pericardial effusion
   — Disadvantages: misses distal ascending aorta; requires expertise
2 Ultrafast CT
   — Advantages: specific (95–100%)
   — Disadvantages: misses aortic branches
3 MRI
   — Advantages: highly sensitive and specific (95–100%), no contrast needed
   — Disadvantages: availability and high cost
4 Angiography
   — advantages: shows aortic entry site and aortic branches
   — disadvantages: availability and morbidity (e.g. nephrotoxicity)

Management priorities in thoracic aortic dissection
1 Ascending (type 1 dissection)
   — Reduce aortic filling pressure
     • Glyceryl trinitrate
     • IV propranolol ± nitroprusside infusion
     • Nifedipine ± nitroprusside infusion
   — Urgent thoracotomy to prevent
     • Intrapericardial rupture
     • Aortic incompetence
     • Carotid artery involvement
   — Vascular graft ± aortic valve replacement
2 Descending (type II) dissection
   — Urgent treatment of hypertension + negative inotrope
   — Non-operative management unless
     • Major arterial involvement (e.g. renal)
     • Uncontrolled hypertension
     • Continued pain
   — Long-term β-blockade

AORTIC COARCTATION

Congenital associations of coarctation
1 Bicuspid aortic valve (→ ~ 90%)
2 Congenital aortic valvular stenosis
3 Ventricular septal defect
4 Patent ductus arteriosus (differential cyanosis)
5 Male sex (M:F = 2:1); Turner's syndrome

Radiological features of aortic coarctation

1 Rib notching affecting inferior aspects of posterior ribs (3–8) due to collateralizing anastomoses between internal mammary and inferior epigastric arteries (Dock's sign); not usually present until adolescence
2 Rib notching confined to right hemithorax indicates coarctation proximal to left subclavian
3 Dilatation of ascending aorta and left subclavian artery visible at the left mediastinal border
4 Post-stenotic aortic dilatation ('reverse-3' sign)

Complications of coarctation

1 Intracranial hemorrhage (subarachnoid or intracerebral)*
2 Refractory hypertension (normoreninemic) ± IHD
3 Aortic dissection/rupture (esp. during pregnancy)
4 Infective endarteritis (rare)
5 Perioperative catastrophes
   — Mesenteric infarction
   — Renal ischemia
   — Paraplegia (due to anterior spinal artery occlusion); more likely if absent collaterals on angiography

* Due to associated berry aneurysms

ATRIAL SEPTAL DEFECT (ASD)

Murmurs encountered in ASD

1 Pulmonary flow murmur
2 Tricuspid flow murmur (usually implies large shunt)
3 Pulmonary incompetent (Graham Steell) murmur of pulmonary hypertension
4 Associated lesions
   — Late systolic murmur (MVP + secundum ASD)
   — Mitral incompetence (primum lesion: cleft valve)
   — Mitral stenosis (Lutembacher's syndrome)
   — Tricuspid incompetence (pulmonary hypertension)
     • Primum defect
     • Ebstein's anomaly (with secundum defect)

NB: Auscultatory hallmark of ASD is fixed splitting of the second sound, though slight respiratory variation can occur

Diagnostic work-up of suspected ASD

1 CXR
   — Pulmonary plethora
   — Right ventricular/pulmonary artery enlargement
   — 'Hilar dance' on fluoroscopy
2 ECG
   — Right axis deviation + incomplete RBBB (secundum)
   — Left axis deviation + complete RBBB (primum)
   — First-degree heart block (sinus venosus type)
3 Echo
   — Paradoxical septal motion
   — Right ventricular enlargement
   — Shunt visualization using bubble contrast
4 'First-pass' nuclear scan → shunt quantification
5 Cardiac catheterization
   — Shunt size (oximetry, dye dilution curve)
   — Pulmonary hypertension
   — Associated lesions

Indications for surgery in ASD

1 Pulmonary:systemic blood flow > 1.5:1.0
2 Pulmonary:systemic vascular resistance < 0.7:1.0

Determinants of shunt magnitude in ASD

1 Relative ventricular compliance
   — ↑ LV dysfunction may *increase* shunt
2 Relative resistance of pulmonary and systemic vasculature
   — ↑ Pulmonary hypertension may *decrease* shunt

COMPLICATIONS OF CONGENITAL HEART DISEASE

Common left-to-right shunts

1 VSD (30%)
2 ASD (10%)
3 PDA (10%)

Indications for surgery in ventricular septal defect

1 Pulmonary:systemic blood flow > 1.5:1.0
2 Pulmonary:systemic vascular resistance < 0.5:1.0

Signs of a developing Eisenmenger complex

1 Decreasing intensity of pulmonary/tricuspid flow murmurs
2 Increasing intensity of P_2 (palpable)
3 Development of right parasternal heave
4 Development of single S_2
5 Appearance of Graham Steell murmur
6 Development of central cyanosis; clubbing (late)

Eisenmenger's syndrome: precipitants of death

1 Right ventricular failure
2 Massive hemoptysis
3 Cerebral embolism/abscess
4 Pregnancy
5 Anesthesia

NB: Infective endocarditis *rarely* occurs in patients with Eisenmenger's

Congenital causes of left axis deviation on ECG

1 Ostium primum atrial septal defect
2 Tricuspid atresia
3 AV communis (endocardial cushion defect)
4 Myotonic dystrophy
5 VSD, PDA

Congenital lesions prone to endocarditis

1 Bicuspid aortic valve, esp.
   — With significant stenosis or regurgitation
   — Post-surgery
2 Patent ductus arteriosus
3 *Small* VSD (*maladie de Roger*)*
4 Ostium primum ASD
5 Cyanotic congenital heart disease
   — e.g. Tetralogy of Fallot
6 Hypertrophic cardiomyopathy with mitral regurgitation
7 Aortic coarctation

* 'Jet lesion': jet damages RV wall → prone to endocarditis

Congenital lesions at negligible risk of endocarditis
1 Mitral valve prolapse without murmur
2 Isolated secundum ASD

INFECTIVE ENDOCARDITIS

High-risk scenarios for infective endocarditis
1 Rheumatic valve damage
2 Congenital heart disease
3 Prosthetic valve
4 Intravenous narcotic abusers

Features of endocarditis in IV drug abusers
1 Predominant valve involvement
   — Tricuspid
   — Valve damaged initially by starch/lactose contaminants
   — Subsequently colonized by needle-borne bacteria/fungi
2 Predominant micro-organisms
   — *Staphylococcus aureus*
   — Enterococci (group D streptococci, e.g. *Streptococcus fecalis*)
   — *Pseudomonas* spp. (e.g. *Ps. cepacia, Ps. aeruginosa*)
   — *Candida parapsilosis, Bacillus cereus, Serratia marcescens*

Predispositions to various organisms
1 Normal valve (+ bedsores, IV drug abuse)
   — *S. aureus*
   — Poor oral hygiene/dentition
2 Rheumatic heart disease (+ dental surgery)
   — *St. viridans* (α-hemolytic)
3 Sigmoidoscopy/cystoscopy/intrauterine device
   — *St. fecalis*
4 Cardiac surgery, valve prosthesis
   — *S. albus* (> 50%)*
   — Fungi, esp. *Candida* spp.
   — *Pseudomonas* spp.
   — JK organism
5 Colonic carcinoma
   — *St. bovis* (classically)
6 Homelessness, alcoholism
   — *Bartonella* spp.

* 80% penicillin-resistant; R_x vancomycin + rifampicin ± gentamicin

Streptococcal endocarditis: organisms implicated
1 Viridans streptococci, esp. *St. mitior, St. sanguis*
   — Account for 50% of strep endocarditis
2 *St. mutans, St. bovis* (GI tract commensals)
   — Account for 30% of strep endocarditis
3 *St. milleri* (anerobic strep), enterococci
   — Account for 15% of strep endocarditis
4 Group A, group B, pneumococci
   — Account for < 1% each

Factors worsening prognosis of infective endocarditis
1 Prosthetic valve as nidus
2 Cultures negative (40% mortality)
3 *S. aureus* isolated from blood cultures

Negative blood cultures? Some considerations
1 Prior antibiotic therapy
2 Fastidious organism or inappropriate culture medium:
   — HACEK organisms*
   — *Brucella* spp., *Legionella* spp., *Neisseria* spp.
   — *Chlamydia psittaci*
   — Rickettsiae, esp. Q fever (*Coxiella burnetii*)
   — Pyridoxine-dependent streptococci
   — L-forms, anaerobes, fungi, acid-fast organisms
3 Right-sided endocarditis
4 Sampling error (cultures taken in abacteremic phase)
5 Misdiagnosis
   — Atrial myxoma
   — Non-bacterial thrombotic endocarditis‡

* *Hemophilus-actinobacterium-cardiobacterium-eikenella-kingella*
‡ Associated with mucinous adenocarcinomas (esp. lung, stomach, ovary)

Reasons for fever recrudescence in treated endocarditis
1 Antibiotic inappropriate
   Antibiotic levels subtherapeutic
   Antibiotic resistance
   Antibiotic allergy
   Antibiotic use complicated by superinfection (e.g. fungal)
2 Extensive valve ring infection
3 Metastatic abscesses (splenic, cerebral, myocardial)
4 Pulmonary emboli (septic or bland)
5 Phlebitis, esp. infected central line

Indications for surgery in infective endocarditis
1 Suspected extensive valve ring infection
2 Refractory heart failure, esp. with aortic incompetence
3 Repeated septic emboli. e.g. due to *Haemophilus parainfluenzae*
4 Persistent bacteremias/fevers despite optimal therapy
5 Prosthetic valve involvement (esp. fungal or early post-op)

Monitors of established endocarditis
1 Symptoms
2 Temperature
3 Daily physical examination
4 Urinalysis
5 White cell count, hemoglobin, ESR
6 Blood cultures during antibiotic therapy and on cessation
7 Weekly estimations of minimum bactericidal concentration (MBC) of antibiotic (see below); *Staph* titers (etc.)
8 Neutrophil alkaline phosphatase if abscess suspected

Mechanical complications of endocarditis
1 Obstruction by vegetations
2 Myocardial abscess
3 Fistula
4 Aneurysm (e.g. affecting sinus of Valsalva)
5 Valvar destruction

Determination of antibiotic dosage in infective endocarditis*

1 Streptococcal endocarditis
  — Maintain peak antibiotic level > 8 × MBC
2 Neutropenic patients
  — Maintain peak antibiotic level > 16 × MBC
3 Staphylococcal or pseudomonal endocarditis
  — Maintain trough antibiotic level > 16 × MBC
  — Maintain peak antibiotic level > 32 × MBC

* In practice, consult the microbiologists

Presumptive antibiotic therapy if organism unknown*

1 'Community-acquired' endocarditis
  — Ampicillin + gentamicin
2 Prosthetic valve or drug addict
  — Ciprofloxacin + rifampicin, or
  — Ampicillin + gentamicin + flucloxacillin
3 Elderly patient and/or renal failure
  — Ampicillin + netilmicin
4 Major penicillin allergy
  — Vancomycin‡

* In practice, consult the microbiologists
‡ cf. prophylaxis: clindamycin may be better tolerated

Patients requiring procedural antibiotic prophylaxis

1 Past medical history of infective endocarditis
2 Prosthetic heart valves
3 Rheumatic heart disease
4 Most congenital heart disease (exception: secundum ASD)
5 Mitral valve prolapse with incompetence (i.e. with murmur)
6 Hypertrophic cardiomyopathy

Procedures for which prophylaxis recommended*

1 Dental surgery with expected gingival bleeding
2 Tonsillectomy, adenoidectomy, cholecystectomy
3 Rigid bronchoscopy or esophagoscopy
4 Esophageal dilatation
5 Variceal sclerotherapy
6 Cystoscopy, and most genitourinary surgery (incl. TURP)
7 Colonoscopy, and most lower gastrointestinal surgery
8 Any surgery involving incision of septic tissue

* For examples of antibiotic scheduling, see p. 212

Procedures for which prophylaxis may be unnecessary*

1 Dental fillings above the gingival margin ± intraoral injection of local anesthetic
2 Flexible bronchoscopy ± biopsy
3 Endoscopy ± biopsy (i.e. fiberoptic gastroduodenoscopy)
4 Cardiac catheterization
5 Cesarean or vaginal delivery
6 Laparoscopy, D&C, abortion, IUD insertion/removal

* Unless (i) patients are 'high-risk' (p. 52) for endocarditis, or (ii) sepsis is anticipated

CARDIAC FAILURE

Concepts and definitions

1 Cardiac failure
  — A condition in which adequate cardiac output can only be maintained by elevated venous filling pressure
2 Preload
  — Left ventricular end-diastolic pressure
3 Afterload
  — Left ventricular systolic wall tension

Cardiac syndromes of systolic or diastolic dysfunction

1 Predominant diastolic dysfunction ('stiff heart')
  — Mitral or tricuspid stenosis
  — Cardiomyopathy
    • Hypertrophic
    • Restrictive
  — Pericardial disease
    • Constriction
    • Tamponade
2 Predominant systolic dysfunction ('weak heart')
  — Ischemic heart disease
  — Congestive cardiomyopathy
3 Combined systolic/diastolic dysfunction
  — Valvular heart disease (except MS/TS)
  — Hypertensive heart disease

Clinical implications of systolic vs diastolic dysfunction

1 Diastolic dysfunction
  — Clinical course
    • Onset typically sudden, deterioration rapid
    • Edema and/or cardiomegaly are unusual
  — Drugs used
    • Nifedipine, β-blockers, ACE inhibitors
2 Systolic dysfunction
  — Clinical course
    • Onset and decline typically gradual
    • Edema and/or cardiomegaly are common
  — Drugs used
    • Diuretics (e.g. spironolactone), digitalis

Radiological signs associated with cardiac failure

1 Dilated upper lobe veins
2 Kerley B lines
3 Perihilar alveolar opacities
4 Cardiomegaly
5 Effusion(s), esp. on right

Very high JVP plus a 'normal' chest X-ray?

1 Constrictive pericarditis
2 Tricuspid stenosis
3 Pulmonary embolism
4 Restrictive cardiomyopathy
5 Right ventricular infarction

Pulmonary edema with normal cardiac size on CXR

1 Myocardial infarction
2 Mitral stenosis
3 Constrictive pericarditis
4 Toxic
  — Chlorine inhalation
  — Heroin use
  — Oxygen toxicity

5 Intracranial catastrophe
6 Pneumonia; aspiration; septicemia; fat emboli

Precipitants of cardiac failure in valvular disease
1 Onset of atrial fibrillation
2 Infective endocarditis
3 Recrudescence of rheumatic fever
4 Acute myocardial infarction
5 Pregnancy; anemia; lack of compliance with medication

Diagnostic considerations in refractory heart failure
1 Silent myocardial infarction
2 Pulmonary emboli
3 High-output failure in elderly: thyrotoxicosis, Paget's disease
4 Left ventricular aneurysm
5 Silent valvular stenosis
6 Thiamine deficiency
7 Anemia
8 Myocarditis
9 Cardiac tamponade; constrictive pericarditis
10 Iatrogenic
 — Overvigorous diuresis
 — Tachyarrhythmia due to digoxin toxicity

Diagnosis of cor pulmonale
1 Cyanosis
2 Elevated JVP
3 Loud P_2 *or* tricuspid or pulmonary incompetent murmur
4 Congestive hepatomegaly
5 ECG changes (p. 41)
6 ↓ PaO_2 *and* ↑ $PaCO_2$

NB: Ankle edema is *not* a reliable pointer to the diagnosis

CXR correlation with pulmonary capillary wedge pressure (PCWP)
1 CXR → Dilated upper lobe veins
 — PCWP = 15 mmHg
2 CXR → Kerley B lines
 — PCWP = 20 mmHg
3 CXR → Pulmonary edema
 — PCWP ≥ 25 mmHg

NB: Therapeutic changes of PCWP precedes CXR changes by up to 48 h

Therapy according to PCWP
1 Elevated PCWP + normal cardiac output
 — Preload reduction
 Elevated PCWP + *low* output
 — Pre- *and* afterload reduction
2 Optimal PCWP (18–20 mmHg) + low output
 — Afterload reduction, positive inotropes
3 Low PCWP + low output*
 — Intravenous fluids + positive inotropes

* e.g. in right ventricular infarction or overvigorous diuresis

An outpatient approach to treating heart failure
1 Begin with a diuretic, e.g. furosemide (frusemide)*
2 If still symptomatic, add an ACE inhibitor

3 If still symptomatic, add digoxin‡ (even if sinus rhythm)
4 Symptomatic arrhythmia? Consider amiodarone

* Assuming here that the diagnosis is clear and that conservative measures have not helped
‡ Note that digoxin is the only inotrope recognized to be safe in heart failure (with the possible exception of growth hormone)

Differential diagnosis of low central venous pressure (< –3 cm)
1 Warm extremities
 — Drug overdose
 — Brainstem lesion
 — Septic shock
2 Cool extremities, low hemoglobin
 — Hemorrhage
3 Cool extremities, normal/high hemoglobin
 — Gastrointestinal fluid losses (diarrhea, vomiting)
 — Renal fluid loss (e.g. diabetic ketoacidosis)
 — Third spacing (e.g. rapid accumulation of ascites)

NB: CVP is *not* accurate in determining LV filling pressure (and hence guiding treatment), e.g. in cardiogenic shock

Differential diagnosis of nocturnal dyspnea
1 Cardiac
 — Left ventricular failure
 — Coronary spasm
2 Pulmonary
 — Asthma
 — Extrinsic allergic alveolitis; emboli
3 CNS/pharyngeal
 — Sleep apnea
4 Anxiety

NATRIURETIC PEPTIDES

Natriuretic peptides (ANP, BNP) in cardiac failure
1 Compensatory ↑ ANP/BNP seen in heart failure and edema states
2 Increased atrial filling pressure → ↑ ANP/BNP secretion
3 ANP/BNP levels are inversely proportional to left ventricular function; LV deterioration → further ANP/BNP elevation
4 Reduction in ANP/BNP follows successful treatment of failure
5 BNP is more sensitive (and hence useful) than ANP for the diagnosis of heart failure and/or left ventricular hypertrophy*
6 High ANP/BNP levels following myocardial infarction predict high mortality

* But confirm with echo

Functions of natriuretic peptides
1 Diuretic function
 — Inhibit distal tubular reabsorption of sodium
 — Promote excretion of sodium and water (not K^+)
 — May also increase GFR (see below)
2 Vasodilator function
 — Inhibits vasoconstriction mediated by angiotensin II and noradrenaline (norepinephrine)

— Secondarily inhibits renin–aldosterone axis and ADH

— Does *not* lead to reflex tachycardia despite lowering BP

CARDIOMYOPATHY

Restrictive cardiomyopathy > constrictive pericarditis?
1 Pulse
— No paradox
2 Jugular venous pulse
— Normal 'y' descent, no Kussmaul's sign
3 Apical impulse
— Prominent
4 Auscultation
— Associated AV valvular incompetence (often)
5 Extra sounds
— S_3 (low-pitched)
6 CXR
— No pericardial calcification; cardiomegaly
7 ECG
— LVH, 'Q' waves, ventricular conduction disturbances
8 Echo
— No pericardial thickening/effusion; LV and/or valvar thickening
9 Catheter
— LV end-diastolic pressure > RV end-diastolic pressure (often by > 5 mmHg)
— RV systolic pressure > 60 mmHg
10 Endomyocardial biopsy
— Abnormal

Hypertrophic cardiomyopathy > aortic valvular stenosis?
1 Family history
— Premature sudden death
2 Pulse
— Jerky (steeply rising)
3 Apex beat
— Double impulse (due to S_4)
4 A_2
— Normal intensity and splitting
5 Murmur
— Late systolic (ejection) ± mitral regurgitation
— Maximal at sternal edge, inaudible in carotids
— ↑: Valsalva/standing/nitrates; ↓: squatting/isometrics
6 CXR
— No valvular calcification or post-stenotic dilatation
7 ECG
— Septal 'Q' waves; WPW (rarely)
8 Echo

Features favoring myocarditis over cardiomyopathy*
1 Young patient
2 Recent history of fevers/myalgias prior to cardiac symptoms
3 Minor cardiomegaly only

* i.e. acute myocarditis vs chronic congestive (dilated) cardiomyopathy

Reversible causes of dilated cardiomyopathy
1 Ischemic heart disease
— 'Hibernating' myocardium (p. 59)
Valvular heart disease
— Aortic stenosis
2 Infiltration by systemic disease
— Sarcoidosis
— Amyloidosis
— Lymphoma
3 Infectious
— Viral (e.g. CMV*)
— Bacterial, esp. *Corynebacterium diphtheriae*
— Parasitic, e.g. *Toxoplasma gondii* ‡
4 Poisoning
— Alcohol (± thiamine deficiency)
— Lead, mercury
— Cocaine
— Antiretroviral drugs (e.g. AZT)
5 Nutritional
— Thiamine deficiency (± alcohol): beri-beri
— Selenium deficiency (Keshan disease)
6 Endocrinopathy
— Thyrocardiac disease (hypo- or hyper-)
— Acromegaly, pheochromocytoma
— Peripartum

* cf. Coxsackie: commoner but not reversible
‡ cf. Chagas', trichinosis: probably irreversible

HYPERTROPHIC CARDIOMYOPATHY (HOCM)

Associations of hypertrophic cardiomyopathy
1 Familial (↑ penetrance in males)
2 Friedreich's ataxia
3 Pompe's disease
4 Familial lentiginosis

Echocardiography of hypertrophic cardiomyopathy
1 Asymmetric septal hypertrophy (septum > 12 mm thick *and* > 130% posterior wall thickness)
2 Systolic anterior motion of anterior leaflet of mitral valve
3 Premature closure of the aortic valve
4 Reduced EF slope due to reduced ventricular compliance

Features of catheterization in hypertrophic cardiomyopathy
1 Distorted left ventricular cavity with systolic obliteration
2 Elevated left ventricular end-diastolic pressure
3 Associated thickening of papillary muscles
4 Post-ectopic reduction in intra-aortic pressure
5 Systolic compression of the left anterior descending coronary artery (myocardial bridging) is predictive of early mortality

Drugs contraindicated in hypertrophic cardiomyopathy
1 Digoxin (unless in atrial fibrillation) and other positive inotropes
2 Atropine and other positive chronotropes
3 Nitrates and other vasodilators
4 Diuretics (*unless* in cardiac failure)

5 Alcohol (ingestion increases left ventricular outflow gradient)

Principles of management in hypertrophic cardiomyopathy

1 Echocardiographic screening of all family < 18 years
2 Arrhythmia detection (Holter) and therapy (amiodarone or sotalol*)
3 Minimization of strenuous activity
4 Prophylaxis against infective endocarditis
5 Symptoms: β-blockers (do *not* reduce risk of sudden death)
6 Symptoms refractory to medical therapy: septal myomectomy

* Reduce morbidity if VT has occurred

ISCHEMIC HEART DISEASE

Reversible independent risk factors for premature heart disease

1 LDL-hypercholesterolemia (± low HDL-cholesterol)
2 Hypertension
3 Smoking
4 Uncontrolled diabetes
5 Estrogen deficiency

Irreversible risk factors for ischemic heart disease

1 Age
2 Male sex
3 Positive family history
4 Elevated lipoprotein(a) level
5 Abnormal T wave axis on ECG

Other plasma levels correlating with ischemic heart disease

1 Homocysteine
2 C-reactive protein
3 Fibrinogen, factor VII
4 tPA and/or PAI-1
5 D-dimer

Gene mutations predisposing to cardiovascular disease*

1 Dyslipoproteinemias
   — LDL receptor (familial hypercholesterolemia)
   — Apo-B (apo-B100): hypertriglyceridemia
   — HDL deficiency: ApoA I–IV/CIII, ABC1 transporter, lipoprotein lipase, hepatic lipase, cholesteryl ester transfer protein
   — Lipoprotein(a)
2 Hyperhomocystinemia
   — Methylene tetrahydrofolate reductase
3 Hypercoagulability
   — Factor VII
   — Prothrombin
   — Fibrinogen B
   — Plasminogen activator inhibitor type 1
4 Atherosclerosis
   — Angiotensin-converting enzyme
   — Paraoxonase
   — Factor XIII
   — Endothelial nitric oxide synthase

* See also, Genetic causes of hypertension, p. 63

Unstable angina: definition(s)

1 Recent symptomatic progression
   — Increasing frequency and/or duration of angina
   — Development of pain at rest/at night/after meals
   — Development of nitrate-resistant angina
2 Recurrent angina despite maximal medical therapy
3 Clinically suspected infarct with negative ECG and enzymes

Features of coronary artery spasm (variant angina, syndrome X)

1 Symptoms (e.g. dizziness)
   — Often occur at rest or at night
2 ECG (classically)
   — ST elevation before and during pain
3 Stress ECG
   — Typically negative if no associated coronary disease
4 Angiography
   — Absent collateralization, varying stenotic sites
   — Spasm may be microvascular
5 ^{31}P-NMR spectroscopy
   — May confirm large metabolic perturbations in the left ventricle

Drugs of choice for treating angina

1 Nitrates
2 β-blockers
3 Calcium antagonists

Primary prevention of cardiovascular morbidity

1 Aspirin 75 mg/day
   — for well-controlled 'at-risk' hypertensives older than 50
2 Statin therapy (e.g. pravastatin, simvastatin)
   — for patients with cholesterol > 5.5 mmol/L and estimated risk of coronary event > 3% per year (e.g. angina patients, or those with peripheral vascular disease, including carotid disease, or individuals with diabetes or hypertension)

SMOKING

Plasma and urinary markers of cigarette smoke exposure

1 Cotinine (and/or nicotine)
2 Carbon monoxide
3 Thiocyanate
4 Urinary mutagenesis assays

Physiological sequelae of cigarette smoking

1 ↑ Platelet adhesion/aggregation/whole blood viscosity
2 ↑ Heart rate; ↑ catecholamine sensitivity/release
3 ↑ Carboxyhemoglobin level, ↑ hematocrit
4 ↓ HDL-cholesterol/vascular compliance
5 ↓ Threshold to ventricular fibrillation

Cardiovascular sequelae of cigarette smoking

1 Increased incidence of
   — Sudden death*
   — Coronary artery disease

— Malignant hypertension
— Subarachnoid hemorrhage
— Ischemic stroke
2 Increased mortality due to aortic aneurysm
3 Increased morbidity from peripheral vascular disease
4 Increased thromboembolism if taking oral contraceptives

* Note that using 'low-tar' cigarettes does *not* substantively reduce the incidence of cigarette-related myocardial infarction

PASSIVE SMOKING

Passive smoking: characteristics of sidestream smoke
1 Contributes 85% of cigarette smoke in an average 'smoking' room (cf. 15% from exhaled 'mainstream' smoke)
2 Exposure of non-smoking individual living or working with smokers averages 1–2 cigarettes/day
3 Sidestream smoke is of higher pH and contains smaller particles than does mainstream smoke
4 Sidestream smoke contains higher carbon monoxide concentrations than does mainstream smoke

Childhood disease associations of passive (parental) smoking
1 Exacerbation of asthma
2 Impairment of lung function
— ↓ FEV_I and forced midexpiratory flow rate
3 ↑ Bronchitis/glue ears/tonsillectomy/adenoidectomy

CARDIAC ARREST

Cardiac arrest: emergency intervention
1 Precordial 'thump' *if* definitely pulseless
— May revert asystole or VT (but only 2% of VF)
2 Crash cart arrives: → 'blind' cardioversion
— May revert VF (but not asystole)
3 Get ECG trace
— If VF, defibrillate again
— Intubate and ventilate with 100% O_2
— Get IV line in
— If still in VF, shock again @ 360 J
4 Commence CPR
— 10 cycles of 5:1 compression:ventilation
5 Repeat cardioversion cycle (see below)

ECG concomitants of cardiac arrest
1 Asystole
2 Ventricular fibrillation
3 Pulseless sinus rhythm (electromechanical dissociation)

ECG-guided management of cardiac arrest
1 Asystole
— Check leads
— Give IV adrenaline (epinephrine) 1 mg IVI (10 mL 1:10 000)
— Can't exclude VF? Shock @ 200 J

— Definitely no VF? Atropine 2 mg IV*
— Consider transvenous pacing *if* electrical activity‡
2 Ventricular fibrillation
— Shock @ 200 J
— Still fibrillating? Repeat shock @ 200–300 J ± @ 360 J
— Fine VF can be 'coarsened' with IV adrenaline (epinephrine)*
— Still fibrillating? Lidocaine (lignocaine) 100 mg (1.5 mg/kg) IV*
— Shock again, and give (say) bretylium 5 mg/kg‡
— Continued resuscitation
• CPR for 1–2 min between each drug
• Repeat adrenaline (epinephrine) every 5 min
• Bicarbonate (50 mL 8.4%) every 20 min
3 Documented hyperkalemia? (rare)
— Calcium chloride IV
— More frequent (incl. initial) bicarbonate

NB: Effective chest compression and hyperventilation between countershocks is *vital* to prospects of success
* Things are fairly desperate at this point
‡ *Very* desperate

Positive prognostic associations of cardiac arrest*
1 Presence of a witness
2 Ventricular fibrillation on initial ECG

* cf. asystole or electromechanical dissociation: < 5% survival

Guidelines for judging when to terminate resuscitation
1 Once commenced, 10 min is usual minimum*
— Usually continue while VF remains recognizable
— Persistent asystole usually indicates failure
2 Should mentally exclude important contingencies
— Defibrillator malfunction
— Electromechanical dissociation
3 Prolonged (> 60 min) resuscitation justified in
— Hypothermia or drowning (esp. children)
— Drug overdose

* Assuming that patient's overall condition is not already recognized to make resuscitation inappropriate

Indications for bicarbonate administration
1 Severe acidosis refractory to ventilation
2 Significant hyperkalemia
3 Concomitant overdosage with aspirin

Hazards of indiscriminate bicarbonate administration
1 Pulmonary edema
2 Paradoxical worsening of intracellular acidosis*

* Acidosis is best managed with hyperventilation alone; bicarbonate is only routinely indicated in prolonged resuscitation

Drugs used in cardiac arrest
1 VF, pulseless VT, or asystole: adrenaline (epinephrine)
2 Refractory VF or pulseless VT: amiodarone, lidocaine (lignocaine), procainamide, magnesium
3 Stable VT: lidocaine (lignocaine), amiodarone
4 Symptomatic bradycardia or heart block: atropine
5 Supraventricular tachyarrhythmia: amiodarone*
6 Shock: dopamine, noradrenaline (norepinephrine)

* May try carotid sinus massage and IV adenosine first, followed by cardioversion

MYOCARDIAL INFARCTION

Preventive initiatives relevant to myocardial infarction*
1 Smoking cessation
  — 50% ↓ risk within 5 years of stopping
2 Reduction of hypertension
  — 2% ↓ risk for each 1 mmHg ↓ diastolic BP
3 Reduction of hyperlipidemia
  — 2% ↓ risk for each 1% ↓ plasma cholesterol
4 Exercise
  — 40% ↓ risk for active vs sedentary lifestyle
5 Ideal body weight
  — 30% ↓ risk for ideal weight vs obese
6 Estrogen replacement therapy (in menopause)
  — 40% ↓ risk compared to unreplaced women
7 Low-dose aspirin prophylaxis
  — 30% ↓ risk compared with non-users
8 Mild alcohol consumption
  — 25% ↓ risk compared to teetotallers

* Risk reductions are not additive, and do not imply reductions in overall (non-disease-specific) mortality; moreover, associations may not be causal

Clinical spectrum of acute coronary syndromes
1 Unstable angina
2 Non-Q-wave myocardial infarction
3 Transmural myocardial infarction

Features of non-Q-wave (nontransmural) myocardial infarction
1 Fewer acute occlusions demonstrable, but overall extent of (chronic) coronary disease similar to transmural infarcts
2 Less myocardial necrosis
  Less marked enzyme elevations
3 Fewer acute complications
  Lower short-term mortality
4 *Higher* incidence of reinfarction
  Long-term prognosis equivalent or worse
5 Aspirin (and perhaps diltiazem) improves outlook

Myocardial infarction without coronary artery block?
1 Coronary microvascular disease
  Coronary artery spasm
  Coronary angiography-induced
2 Acute plaque rupture
3 Recanalized coronary thrombosis (endogenous thrombolysis)
4 Aortic stenosis
  Ascending aortic dissection (very rare)
  Arteritis: Takayasu's, PAN

Acute myocardial infarction: early diagnosis
1 Myoglobin
  — Levels rise within 2 h post-infarct
  — Low specificity*
2 Cardiac troponin I and troponin T
  — Levels rise within 4 h post-infarct
  — High specificity‡
3 CK-MB (total creatine kinase)
  — Levels rise within 6 h post-infarct
  — Moderate specificity

4 $CK-MB_2$ (isoform of CK-MB)
  — Levels rise within 6 h post-infarct
  — High specificity
5 ^{99m}Tc-labeled sestamibi myocardial scanning
  — Uptake reflects myocardial perfusion
  — Does not wash out quickly (cf. thallium)
  — Sensitive and specific; 95% negative predictive value

* Specificity can be improved by combining with measurement of carbonic anhydrase III, elevations of which indicate non-cardiac muscle injury
‡ Cardiac troponin T may also be raised in myocardial contusion, and correlates with poor outlook in patients with ischemic stroke. A normal level > 6 h after chest pain onset usually permits discharge of patients with normal ECGs from the ER

Bad prognostic indicators in acute myocardial infarction
1 Advanced age, previous infarct, female sex
2 Prolonged, relentless crushing substernal chest pain ('time is muscle')
3 Heart rate > 100, systolic BP < 100
4 Associated S_3 *or* new mitral regurgitant murmur
5 CK-MB > 2000 IU/mL, very high troponin T
6 ECG
  — Heart block
  — ST segment changes > T wave changes alone
  — New conduction defects, complex arrhythmias
7 Poor left ventricular function
  — Pulmonary edema on CXR

Myocardial infarction: pathogenesis and extent
1 Anterior infarct
  — Due to occlusion of left anterior descending coronary
  — Extent of jeopardized myocardium indicated by
    • Number of 'acute' precordial leads
    • Degree of ST elevation
    • RBBB*
2 Inferior infarct
  — Caused by occlusion of right coronary or left circumflex
  — ↓↓ Jeopardized myocardium; hence, ↓ CCF (see below)

* Signifies LAD occlusion proximal to first septal branch

Myocardial infarction: complications by site
1 Anterior infarct
  — Ventricular arrhythmias (incl. late-onset VF)
  — Left ventricular aneurysm or thrombus formation
  — Cardiac rupture/VSD
2 Inferior infarct
  — Atrial/junctional arrhythmias
    • Bradycardia
    • High-degree AV block
    • Complete heart block
  — Papillary muscle dysfunction
  — Associated right ventricular infarction (in 40%)

Diagnosis of right ventricular infarction
1 Clinical suspicion: 'inferior' infarct + arrhythmias
  — Absent preinfarction angina

— High-degree AV block (indicates need for RV pacing)
— Atrial fibrillation: may require cardioversion
— Ventricular arrhythmias → ? complete heart block
2 Signs/CXR
— Elevated JVP *but* clear lung fields
3 ECG
— 1 mm ST elevation in *right* precordial lead V_{4R}*
4 Hemodynamic monitoring
— Low/normal PCWP despite low output failure
— Right atrial pressure: PCWP > 0.86
5 Therapeutic response
— Improve with preload enhancement
• IV saline
• Dobutamine (if no response to saline)
— Deteriorate with preload reduction
• Nitrates
• Diuretics
• Morphine

NB: Such patients have a high mortality (30% vs 5% for uncomplicated inferior infarct) and should receive thrombolysis or angioplasty
* i.e. this lead should be recorded in patients presenting with classical 'inferior' infarcts (ST elevation in II, III, aVF)

'Cardiogenic shock': could it be anything else?
1 Hypovolemia
— Overvigorous diuresis
— Third-spacing
— Hemorrhage
2 Electromechanical dissociation
— Cardiac tamponade*
— Cardiac rupture‡
— Massive pulmonary embolism
— Tension pneumothorax
3 Other causes of shock
— High output failure
— Adrenal failure
— Septic shock
— Anaphylaxis

* NB: Tamponade may be associated with ↑ BP due to increased peripheral vascular resistance; may fall after pericardiocentesis
‡ Ruptured interventricular septum or papillary muscle

Therapeutic modalities in acute coronary syndromes
1 Antiplatelet modalities: aspirin, clopidogrel*, abciximab‡
2 Antithrombotic modalities: thrombolytic drugs, heparin
3 Anti-ischemic modalities: β-blockers, nitrates
4 Mechanical modalities: angioplasty, coronary bypass

* Inhibits ADP-dependent platelet aggregation
‡ An antibody which inhibits the platelet integrin GP IIb/IIIa

Drugs reducing mortality after myocardial infarction*
1 Proven benefit:
— β-blockers‡
• IV (acute): Mortality reduction 0.5%
• Oral (long-term): Mortality reduction 1.5%
— Aspirin¶
• Acute (150 mg/day for 1 month): Mortality reduction 2%
• Long-term (75 mg/day): Mortality reduction 1.5%

— Thrombolytic therapy
• Preadmission: Mortality reduction 3%
• Inpatient: Mortality reduction 2%
— ACE inhibitor§ (begin after nitrates ceased)
• AMI → LV failure: Mortality reduction 4%
• AMI → LV dysfunction: Mortality reduction 1%
— Statin
• If total cholesterol > 4.8 mmol/L, *or*
• If LDL-cholesterol > 3.2 mmol/L
2 Precise benefit uncertain
— Nitrates§ (use in first 24 h)
— Heparin (IV *or* low molecular weight)
• Net value uncertain (i.e. if given with tPA, aspirin)
• Consider in large anterior infarcts
— Amiodarone

* i.e. secondary prevention of AMI
‡ Excluding those partial agonists with intrinsic sympathomimetic activity, e.g. pindolol, acebutolol, oxprenolol
¶ Also maintains patency of CABG
§ Limit infarct size

Treatments of no value in acute myocardial infarction
1 Prolonged bedrest
2 Magnesium sulfate*
3 Calcium antagonists (may be detrimental)
4 Class I antiarrhythmics

* Hitherto believed to prevent reperfusion injury of 'stunned' myocardium (see below)

Common mechanisms of death following myocardial infarction
1 First few hours — Ventricular fibrillation
2 First few days — Pump failure
3 First few months — Reinfarction

REPERFUSION INJURY

Myocardial definitions in acute infarction
1 'Jeopardized' myocardium
— Myocardium 'at-risk' of infarction during early (reversible) period of coronary occlusion
— Extent of jeopardized myocardium represents potential benefit of thrombolytic intervention
2 'Hibernating' myocardium
— Myocardium which is persistently (but reversibly) impaired in function by reduced oxygenation due to coronary artery disease; an autoregulatory mechanism of myocardial self-preservation
3 'Stunned' myocardium
— Myocardium which requires a time lag (often several weeks) to improve functionally following revascularization; a retrospective characterization

Pathophysiology of post-infarction reperfusion injury
1 Intracellular calcium overload*
2 Osmotic myocyte swelling
3 Free radical-induced microvascular damage

* May be prophylactically reduced by pharmacologic inhibitors of the sodium–hydrogen exchanger (e.g. the amiloride derivative cariporide) which will minimize intracellular acidosis

Clinical manifestations of reperfusion injury

1 Reperfusion arrhythmias
   — Common after intracoronary thrombolysis or PTCA
   — Include ventricular fibrillation ($\to$ 6–7% post-PTCA)
   — Early reperfusion (< 30 min) potently causes VF
2 Myocardial stunning
   — Reversible ventricular dysfunction
   — Systolic performance may improve up to 6 months
3 Lethal myocyte injury
   — Contraction band necrosis may lead to cardiac rupture
   — Rupture commoner following thrombolysis

Therapeutic prevention of reinfarction

1 Stop smoking
2 β-blockade
3 Aspirin
4 Coronary artery bypass grafting for patients found to have left main disease following positive convalescent stress ECG
5 Angioplasty

HYPERLIPIDEMIA

Macroscopic appearance of hyperlipidemic serum

1 Chylomicronemia   — Lipemic supernatant
2 Increased VLDL/IDL — Diffusely lipemic
3 Increased LDL   — Clear

Individuals worth screening routinely for hyperlipidemia

1 Known (cardio)vascular disease
2 Diabetes mellitus
3 Xanthoma or xanthelasma (any age); arcus senilis (if younger than 50)
4 Hypertension (if younger than 60)
5 Any individual younger than 60 who requests screening, esp. if positive family history of vascular disease

Incidence and genetics of primary hyperlipidemias

1 Common hyperlipidemias
   — Autosomal dominant transmission (familial)
   — WHO types IIa, IIb, IV
   — Major excesses of *cholesterol* and *triglycerides*
      • IIa: cholesterol ($\uparrow$ LDL)
      • IIb: cholesterol ($\uparrow$ LDL) + triglyceride ($\uparrow$ VLDL)
      • IV: triglycerides ($\uparrow$ VLDL) + cholesterol
2 Uncommon hyperlipidemias
   — Autosomal recessive transmission
   — WHO types I, III, V
   — Major (primary) excesses of *lipoproteins*
      • I: chylomicrons ($\uparrow$ triglycerides, cholesterol)
      • III: IDL 'remnants' ($\uparrow$ cholesterol, triglycerides)
      • V: VLDL ($\uparrow$ triglycerides/cholesterol/chylomicra)

Clinical characterization of hyperlipidemias

1 Fasting hypertriglyceridemia
   — Chylomicronemia (I, V) due to:

• Lipoprotein lipase deficiency
• Apo C-II deficiency
   — Excess VLDL (IIb, IV, V)
   — *Not* associated with accelerated atherosclerosis
   — Symptoms and signs of hypertriglyceridemia
      • Eruptive xanthomata (usually *resolve* with R_x)
      • Abdominal pain ± pancreatitis
      • Hepatosplenomegaly
      • Lipemia retinalis (whitish arterioles)
2 Hypercholesterolemia with excess LDL (IIa, IIb)
   — Due to 1° LDL receptor defect or LDL overproduction
   — Strongly associated with accelerated atherosclerosis
   — Symptoms and signs of hypercholesterolemia
      • Tendinitis, polyarthritis
      • Tendon xanthomata (usually *persist* despite R_x)
      • Planar xanthomata (in homozygotes only)
      • Arcus senilis: pathological *if* younger than 40
      • Xanthelasma
3 Broad-beta 'remnant' hyperlipidemia with excess IDL (III)
   — Strongly associated with accelerated atherosclerosis
   — Responds well to fibrates (xanthomata regress)
   — Symptoms and signs of excess IDL
      • Tuberous xanthomata (esp. elbows, knees)
      • Linear palmar-crease (planar) xanthomata
      • Peripheral vascular disease

Atherogenicity of lipoproteins

1 Highly atherogenic
   — LDL, IDL
2 Moderately atherogenic
   — VLDL
3 Minimally atherogenic
   — Chylomicra*
4 Anti-atherogenic
   — HDL

* *Unless* associated with lipoprotein lipase (*LPL*) gene mutations (or mutations affecting the LPL cofactor apo C-II)

Secondary hyperlipidemias

1 Predominantly increased cholesterol
   — Hypothyroidism
   — Cholestasis (esp. PBC)
   — Anorexia nervosa
2 Predominantly increased triglycerides
   — Alcohol abuse
   — Diabetes mellitus
   — Chronic renal failure
3 Increased cholesterol and triglycerides
   — Nephrotic syndrome
   — Paraproteinemic states (rarely)
   — High-dose steroid therapy

Drugs adversely affecting blood lipids*

1 Thiazides‡
2 β-blockers*‡
3 Isotretinoin (for acne)
4 Levonorgestrel-containing oral contraceptives

* Increased triglycerides and/or reduced HDL-cholesterol
‡ Clinical significance is probably nil: favorable hemodynamic effects outweigh the adverse biochemical correlates

Factors affecting HDL-cholesterol levels

1 Factors associated with low levels
   — Obesity, dietary sugar, diabetes
   — Progestogens, androgens, male sex
   — Cigarette smoking
   — Nephrotic syndrome
   — Drugs (see above), incl. probucol
   — Tangier disease, familial LCAT deficiency
2 Factors associated with high levels
   — Regular exercise ($\uparrow$ HDL-2)
   — Estrogens, female sex
   — Moderate alcohol intake ($\uparrow$ HDL-3)
   — Increasing age/education status
   — Phenytoin use
   — Fish oil (e.g. cod liver oil; see below)

Hypolipidemic states in clinical medicine

1 Bassen–Kornzweig syndrome
   — $\downarrow$ Apolipoprotein B and all lipid fractions except HDL
   — Characterized by acanthocytosis, ataxia, retinopathy, steatorrhea and death before mid-life
   — R_x: vitamin E (A, D, K) + medium-chain triglycerides
2 Tangier disease
   — $\downarrow$ HDL but *no* cardiovascular disease; no treatment
   — Manifests with orange tonsils, neuropathy, splenomegaly and corneal opacities
3 LCAT deficiency
   — $\downarrow$ HDL, $\uparrow$ VLDL
   — Manifests with atheroma, uremia, hemolysis

Lipid profiles predictive of maximal benefit from hypolipidemic therapy

1 LDL:HDL ratio > 5:1
2 Fasting serum triglycerides > 2.3 mmol/L

APOLIPOPROTEINS

Apolipoproteins in cardiovascular disease

1 Apolipoproteins are the polypeptide components that make up lipoproteins; these apolipoproteins include A-I, A-II, A-IV; B48, B100; C-I, C-II, C-III; D, E, F
2 Lipoproteins are water-soluble protein complexes which transport lipids (cholesterol and triglycerides) in plasma; they comprise LDL, VLDL, HDL, IDL and chylomicrons
3 Lipoprotein(a) antigen [Lp(a)] is a variant LDL which is associated with coronary artery disease*
4 Apolipoprotein B is the main lipid transport protein
   — Apo B100 is the sole protein constituent of LDL and the major protein constituent of VLDL
   — Apo B48 is the major protein of chylomicrons
   — $\uparrow$ Apo B $\rightarrow$ coronary artery disease
   — $\downarrow$ Apo B $\rightarrow$ Bassen–Kornzweig syndrome
5 Apo A-I is the major protein constituent of HDL
   — $\downarrow$ Apo A-I $\rightarrow$ hypertriglyceridemia (#IV, V)
   — $\downarrow$ Apo A-I, apo B $\rightarrow$ coronary artery disease
6 Apo C-II is an activator of lipoprotein lipase
   — $\downarrow$ Apo C-II $\rightarrow$ fasting chylomicronemia (#I, V)

7 Apo E consists of three isoforms: E3, E4, E2
   — Apo E3 is the commonest allele
     • An abnormal apo E3 $\rightarrow$ IDL 'remnants' (#III)
   — $\uparrow$ Apo E4 $\rightarrow$ high LDL and cholesterol
   — $\uparrow$ Apo E2 (uncommon) $\rightarrow$ low LDL and cholesterol

* Despite its strong association with atherogenesis, reduction of Lp(a) levels by apheresis does *not* correlate well with regression of atheroma

HYPOLIPIDEMIC DRUGS

Mechanisms underlying hypolipidemic therapy

1 Statins: lovastatin, simvastatin, pravastatin
   — HMG CoA reductase (cholesterol synthesis) inhibitors
   — Cause 30% $\downarrow$ plasma LDL levels
   — Also enhance LDL receptor expression
   — Very well tolerated (occasional myalgias, $\uparrow$ CK)
   — Use in hypercholesterolemia
2 Fibrates: bezafibrate, gemfibrozil (± clofibrate)
   — Isobutyric acid derivatives activating lipoprotein lipase
   — Reduce VLDL (± LDL, fibrinogen, urate); $\uparrow$ HDL
   — Clofibrate also reduces IDL but *increases* LDL
   — Use in type III (esp.) or mixed hyperlipidemias
3 Colestyramine, colestipol
   — Non-absorbable anion-exchange resins; bind bile acids
   — Reduce LDL (but *increase* VLDL/triglycerides)
   — Use in familial hypercholesterolemia
4 Acipimox, nicofuranose
   — Nicotinic acid derivatives inhibiting lipolysis
   — Reduce VLDL mainly, but also reduce LDL and IDL
   — Use in hypertriglyceridemia or as adjunctive therapy
5 Probucol (an antioxidant)
   — Lowers LDL cholesterol (but may also lower HDL)
   — May lower LDL levels by 30% when used with resin
   — Also an antioxidant, but therapeutic value unclear
6 Fish oils (omega-3 fatty acids), e.g. eicosapentanoic acid
   — Substitute for essential fatty acids in cell membranes
   — Metabolized by cyclo-oxygenase to prostaglandins
   — Reduce platelet aggregation, triglycerides (see below)

Side-effects of hypolipidemic therapy

1 Statins
   — Gastrointestinal upset
   — Liver dysfunction (asymptomatic transaminitis)
   — Myositis (esp. in patients who exercise heavily)
   — Rhabdomyolysis, esp. if also receiving
     • Ciclosporin A ($\rightarrow$ 5-fold $\uparrow$ plasma level)
     • Gemfibrozil, nicotinic acid
2 Fibrates
   — Nausea, abdominal discomfort

— Gallstones, cholecystitis; also transaminitis
— Loss of libido, alopecia, weight gain
— Myopathy (esp. if hypoalbuminemic or azotemic)
— Potentiation of warfarin (cf. colestyramine)
  • Displacement from plasma protein (transient)
  • Inhibits hepatic metabolism
3 Resins
— Constipation (usual), abdominal distension (common); steatorrhea (only with large doses)
— Nausea, vomiting
— Reduced absorption of digoxin, thyroxine, warfarin, folate and fat-soluble vitamins (A,D,E,K)
4 Nicotinates
— Flushing; headaches
— Nausea, abdominal pain, diarrhea
— Hepatotoxicity; gout; glucose intolerance

NB: Aggressive hypocholesterolemic therapy has been associated with an increased risk of *hemorrhagic stroke*

Rhabdomyolysis due to hypolipidemic drugs
1 Fibrates
— Clofibrate
— Bezafibrate
— Gemfibrozil
2 Statins
— Simvastatin
— Pravastatin

Which hypolipidemic – statin, fibrate or resin?*
1 Predominant hypercholesterolemia
— Start with a statin ($\rightarrow \uparrow$ HDL, $\downarrow$ TGs; $\downarrow$ LDL-chol.)
— Maximum statin dose *not tolerated*? Substitute
  • A resin (e.g. colestipol; less well tolerated)
  • A fibrate (e.g. gemfibrozil)
  • Nicotinic acid
— Maximum statin dose *ineffective*? Add
  • A resin
2 Predominant hypertriglyceridemia
— Start with a fibrate ($\downarrow$ TGs by 30%), esp. if overweight and $\downarrow$ HDL
— Alternatives
  • Nicotinic acid (less well tolerated)
  • Fish oil (see below)
3 Mixed hyperlipidemia
— Start with a fibrate
— Second-line
  • Nicotinic acid, *or*
  • A statin‡

* i.e. assuming dietary measures (e.g. stopping alcohol) and appropriate patient selection
‡ Try not to combine fibrates and statins (increased risk of myopathy)

Therapeutic targets in treating hyperlipidemic patients
1 Aim to keep *total cholesterol* < 5.0 mmol/L*
2 Aim to keep *LDL-cholesterol* < 3.0 mmol/L‡
3 Aim to keep *total:HDL cholesterol ratio* < 5
4 Aim to keep triglycerides < 2 mmol/L

* Every 2 mmol/L reduction yields a risk reduction of 65%
‡ Or, failing that, cut level by at least one-third

FISH OILS

Observations suggesting cardiovascular benefits of fish oils
1 Fish oils, esp. those containing the *n*-3 (ω-3) polyunsaturated acids eicosapentanoic acid (EPA; C20:5) and docosahexanoic acid (DHA; C22:6) are abundant in the diet of populations with little coronary disease, e.g. Eskimos, Japanese, Greenland Inuits
2 High membrane *n*-3:*n*-6 fatty acid ratios are associated with reduced incidence of coronary disease
3 Dietary *n*-3-polyunsaturated fatty acids are associated with the following alterations in atherogenic risk factors
— $\downarrow$ Plasma cholesterol/triglycerides, $\downarrow$ VLDL/LDL
— $\uparrow$ HDL$_2$
— $\downarrow$ Blood pressure
4 Dietary *n*-3 polyunsaturated fatty acids are associated with the following alterations in thrombogenic risk factors
— $\uparrow$ Bleeding time (reduced platelet aggregation)
— $\downarrow$ Platelet thromboxane A$_2$
— $\uparrow$ Vascular prostacyclin
— $\downarrow$ Platelet reactivity to ADP/epinephrine/thrombin

Fish oil: putative mechanisms of action
1 Antiatherogenic action ($\downarrow$ coronary artery disease*)
— $\downarrow$ Triglycerides (plus $\downarrow$ cholesterol/LDL/VLDL, $\uparrow$ HDL)
2 Antithrombotic action ($\downarrow$ incidence of vascular 'events')
— Competitive inhibition of arachidonic acid
— Cyclo-oxygenase inhibition
— $\downarrow$ Thromboxane A$_2$-mediated platelet aggregation
3 Anti-inflammatory action (?$\downarrow$ severity of arthritis, migraine)
— Competitive inhibition of arachidonic acid
— $\downarrow$ lipo-oxygenase inhibition; $\downarrow$ IL-I
— $\downarrow$ TNF/leukotriene B$_4$-induced neutrophil chemotaxis

* But only applicable to males without overt cardiovascular disease *if* severely hypertriglyceridemic

HYPERTENSION

Differential diagnosis of hypertension
'RECAP'
1 'R'— **R**enal
  • Renal artery stenosis
  • Chronic renal failure with fluid overload
  • Unilateral parenchymal renal disease
  • Polycystic kidneys
2 'E' — **E**ssential
— **E**ndocrine
  • Pheochromocytoma
  • Primary hyperaldosteronism
  • Cushing's syndrome

- Thyrotoxicosis
- Acromegaly
- Hyperparathyroidism

3 'C' — **C**ollagen-vascular diseases (e.g. polyarteritis nodosa)
  — **C**erebral (e.g. raised intracranial pressure)
  — **C**ontraceptive pill
  — **C**lonidine withdrawal
4 'A' — **A**lcohol
  — **A**ortic coarctation
  — **A**cute intermittent porphyria
5 'P' — **P**regnancy-associated hypertension
  — **P**olycythemia rubra vera

Hypertension in children

1 Aortic coarctation
2 Congenital or acquired renal arterial disease
3 Parenchymal renal disease
4 Hormonal anomalies (e.g. congenital adrenal hyperplasia)

Causes of malignant phase

1 Essential hypertension
2 Rapidly progressive glomerulonephritis
3 Pregnancy-associated hypertension
4 Renovascular*
5 Polyarteritis; scleroderma
6 Pheochromocytoma
7 Iatrogenic
  — Interaction with MAO inhibitor
  — Clonidine withdrawal

* Onset may be *acute* if hemorrhage occurs into atheromatous plaque, or if aortic aneurysm expands over renal artery origin

Genetic syndromes of hypertension in childhood

1 Liddle's syndrome (mutations of epithelial sodium channel, causing amiloride-sensitive hyporeninemic hypoaldosteronism)
2 Gitelman's syndrome (mutations of Na^+/Cl^- cotransporter)
3 Congenital adrenal hyperplasia (11β- or 17α-hydroxylase deficiency)
4 Apparent mineralocorticoid excess (11α-hydroxysteroid dehydrogenase deficiency associated with high cortisol levels that activate mineralocorticoid receptors)
5 Glucocorticoid-suppressible aldosteronism (stroke-prone hyperaldosteronism syndrome due to fusion of aldosterone synthase and 11β-hydroxylase genes)

Alternating hypotension and hypertension: differential diagnosis

1 Iatrogenic
  — e.g. Diuretics, methyldopa
  — Hemodialysis
2 Pheochromocytoma, esp. if secreting adrenaline (epinephrine)
3 Hyponatremic hypertensive syndrome
  — Seen in renovascular hypertension of recent origin
4 Syndrome of baroreflex failure*
  — Hypertensive attacks prevented by clonidine

* cf. syndrome of baroreflex failure: labile hypertension but *little* orthostasis

Non-pharmacological management of mild hypertension

1 Stop smoking (reduces morbidity; does not reduce BP)
2 Ideal body weight
3 Low salt diet
4 Alcohol restriction
5 Biofeedback/relaxation/hypnotherapy
6 Regular exercise

Efficacy of antihypertensive treatment

1 Therapy reduces mortality in *moderate/severe* hypertension*
2 Less effective in *mild* hypertension‡ or in elderly patients
3 Reduces risk of *stroke* (>> myocardial infarction)
4 Does not *reverse* ischemic heart/peripheral vascular disease
5 Smoking may negate benefits of antihypertensive therapy
6 Clinical efficacy depends critically on patient *compliance*

* Diastolic BP > 100 mmHg
‡ Diastolic BP < 95 mmHg

Indications for treatment of 'mild' hypertension* in elderly

1 History of coronary or cerebrovascular disease
2 Development of fourth heart sound
3 Retinopathy (grade III or IV)
4 Elevated serum creatinine.
   Elevated urinary microalbumin excretion.
5 ECG: left ventricular hypertrophy/strain
6 CXR: cardiomegaly

* BP < 180/95

An approach to antihypertensive prescribing

1 Commence with a β-blocker or diuretic
2 If still uncontrolled, combine the two
3 If still uncontrolled, increase the dose of β-blocker, pending side-effects
4 If still uncontrolled, consider adding or substituting a calcium blocker (e.g. slow-release nifedipine, or amlodipine)
5 If still uncontrolled, substitute or add an ACE inhibitor (± diuretic)
6 If still uncontrolled, investigate the hypertension

Classical indications for antihypertensive drug treatment

1 Pheochromocytoma — combined α-/β-blockade
2 Hyperaldosteronism — spironolactone
3 Liddle's syndrome — amiloride
4 Glucocorticoid-suppressible hyperaldosteronism, *or* apparent mineralocorticoid excess — dexamethasone

Important contraindications for antihypertensive drug prescribing

1 α-blockers — pre-existing orthostasis
   — urinary incontinence

2 β-blockers — asthma, chronic obstructive airways disease
— peripheral vascular disease
— heart failure (possibly) or heart block
3 Verapamil — heart failure or heart block
— concomitant β-blocker treatment
4 Nifedipine — risk of myocardial infarction, esp. if diabetic
— hypertensive emergencies (don't use sublingual short-acting version)
5 Thiazides — gout
6 ACE inhibitors — renovascular disease*, renal impairment‡
Ang IIR blockers — pregnancy

* Suspect in the presence of peripheral vascular disease
‡ Serum creatinine > 150 mmol/L. Functional deterioration may occur on starting ACE inhibitor in patient receiving allopurinol, NSAIDs or potassium-sparing diuretics

Prerequisites for discontinuation of antihypertensive therapy
1 Persistently well-controlled blood pressure (in the normal range) on low-dose monotherapy
2 No left ventricular hypertrophy, retinopathy, renal impairment, diabetes, hypercholesterolemia, or active cardiovascular disease
3 Normal ECG and echocardiogram

Drug therapy of orthostatic hypotension
1 Fludrocortisone + pindolol
2 Octreotide

RENOVASCULAR HYPERTENSION

Hypertension: indications for further investigation*
1 Age < 35
2 Associated postural hypotension
3 Hypertensive retinopathy
4 Abnormal urinalysis (proteinuria/hematuria/glycosuria)
5 Hypokalemia without diuretic therapy, esp. if marked
6 Azotemia (esp. if recent onset)
7 Severe hypertension poorly controlled by multiple drugs

* NB: Experienced radiologists and vascular surgeons are a prerequisite

Investigational modalities in renovascular hypertension
1 Plasma renin activity ± captopril 'challenge'
2 Pre- and post-captopril renal isotopic uptake of ^{99m}Tc-DTPA*
3 Rapid-sequence intravenous pyelography
4 Venous digital subtraction angiography
5 Selective venous sampling for renal vein renins*
6 Renal arteriography ± immediate angioplasty (best approach)

* ↓ In stenosed kidney, ↓ post-captopril; *lateralization* indicates improved chance of successful BP control following revascularization

Varieties of renovascular disease
1 Fibromuscular dysplasia (age < 30 years)
— More common* in females (no family history)
— Rarely associated with renal impairment
— Presents with refractory hypertension de novo
— Responds to angioplasty
2 Atheromatous (age > 60 years)
— More common in males (esp. smokers)
— Often associated with renal impairment (minimal proteinuria)
— Presents with worsening control of long-standing hypertension
— Responds to stenting (i.e. better than to balloon angioplasty)

* But much *less common* than atheromatous renal artery stenosis

Diagnostic potential of arteriography in hypertension
1 Renal artery stenosis
2 Aortic coarctation
3 Polyarteritis nodosa
4 Pheochromocytoma

NB: Severe uncontrolled hypertension contraindicates elective angiography

Abnormal plasma renin activity: differential diagnosis
1 Elevated, no hypertension
— Addison's disease
— Hemorrhage
— Liver disease
— Pregnancy
— Bartter's syndrome
— Drugs
• Diuretics, vasodilators
• Estrogens
• Sympathomimetics; lithium
2 Elevated, hypertensive
— Malignant hypertension
— 'Essential' hypertension (in 15% of cases)
— Renovascular disease or end-stage renal failure
— Hemangiopericytoma (reninoma)
3 Low, no hypertension
— Old age
— Drugs
• β-blockers
• Clonidine, methyldopa; guanethidine
4 Low, hypertensive
— Essential hypertension (85%, esp. if elderly)
— Conn's/Cushing's syndromes
— Congenital adrenal hyperplasia
• 17-hydroxylase deficiency
— Drugs
• Corticosteroids

Therapeutic options in 'renal' hypertension
1 Salt and fluid restriction
2 Drug therapy
— ACE inhibitors* (e.g. captopril)
— β-blockers (e.g. metoprolol)
— Vasodilators (e.g. prazosin)
3 If refractory, treat 'operable' renovascular disease by
— Percutaneous angioplasty
— Vascular surgery

4 If refractory and *no* operable extrarenal vascular lesion:
  — Consider bilateral nephrectomy (a desperation move)

* *Unless* bilateral renal artery stenosis

Surgical intervention in renovascular hypertension: indications
1 Percutaneous transluminal angioplasty
  — Fibromuscular dysplasia
  — Single atheromatous plaque in arterial midportion
  — Intrarenal arterial stenosis inaccessible to surgery
  — Transplant artery stenosis
  — Contraindication to surgery
2 Surgical revascularization
  — Ostial lesions
  — Extensive atheromatous plaques

Renovascular hypertension: predictors of surgical cure
1 Young patient
2 Recent onset of hypertension
3 Normal serum creatinine
4 Homolateral:contralateral renal vein renin ratio > 1.5
5 Captopril challenge → ↓ BP, ↑ plasma renin activity

Indications for emergency drug therapy of severe hypertension
1 Sodium nitroprusside infusion + arterial monitor (urgent)
  — Hypertensive encephalopathy (MRI diagnosis)
    • Avoid β-blockers, methyldopa
  — ↑ BP + myocardial infarct and/or pulmonary edema
    • Avoid hydralazine
  — Dissecting aortic aneurysm (plus β-blocker)
    • Avoid hydralazine
  — Contraindicated in uremia, raised intracranial pressure
2 Captopril 25 mg
  — Hypertensive retinopathy without encephalopathy
    • Avoid β-blockers, methyldopa
  — Severe hypertension + acute renal failure*
    • Avoid β-blockers
3 Phentolamine or labetalol infusion
  — Clonidine withdrawal (rare now)
  — Pheochromocytoma
  — MAOI interaction (e.g. with dietary tyramine)
    • Avoid β-blockers
  — Labetalol contraindicated in acute LVF
4 Hydralazine
  — Eclampsia
    • Avoid diuretics, ACE inhibitors, β-blockers
    • Use magnesium
  — Contraindicated in angina
5 Enalapril
  — Acute LVF
6 Fenoldopam mesylate
  — A dopamine-1-receptor agonist

NB: Diazoxide is now obsolete. Clonidine should be avoided in this setting due to its CNS depressant effects

* *Unless* bilateral renal artery stenoses, stenosis in a solitary functioning kidney, or severe renal failure, in which cases avoid captopril

ESTROGENIC STATES AND CARDIAC DISEASE

Dangerous cardiac conditions in pregnancy
1 Stenoses
  — Tight mitral stenosis
  — Severe aortic stenosis
  — Aortic coarctation
2 Pulmonary hypertension
  — Primary
  — Eisenmenger's syndrome with reversed shunt
3 Marfan's syndrome
  — With aortic root dilatation

Treatment options in pregnancy-associated hypertension*
1 Oral treatment‡
  — Hydralazine
  — Methyldopa
2 Emergency treatment (e.g. for eclampsia)
  — Diazoxide
  — Labetalol, nifedipine
3 Prophylaxis during third trimester
  — Low-dose aspirin

* Linked to an activating mutation affecting the mineralocorticoid receptor
‡ β-blockers may also be used, but beware of fetal bradycardia/hypoglycemia

Metabolic alterations in oral contraceptive users
1 ↑ Fibrinogen/plasminogen/FDPs/factors VII, VIII, X
2 ↓ Antithrombin III; ↓ albumin, haptoglobin
3 ↑ Transferrin, ceruloplasmin (↑ total serum iron, copper)
4 ↑ Triglycerides (VLDL), insulin, aldosterone, cortisol
5 ↓ Renin, ACTH

Clinical concomitants of estrogen replacement therapy
1 Reduced incidence of coronary artery disease
2 Reduced mortality from coronary artery disease
3 No change in stroke risk

PULMONARY HYPERTENSION

Mechanisms of pulmonary hypertension
1 Increased pulmonary blood flow
  — Left-to-right shunt
2 Elevated pulmonary venous pressure
  — Mitral stenosis
3 Obliteration of vascular bed
  — Pulmonary emboli
  — Emphysema
  — Primary pulmonary hypertension
  — Collagen-vascular diseases

Diseases involving pulmonary arteries
1 Primary pulmonary hypertension
2 Churg–Strauss syndrome (cf. PAN)

3 Wegener's granulomatosis
4 Takayasu's arteritis
5 Systemic sclerosis

Associations of primary pulmonary hypertension
1 Raynaud's phenomenon, SLE*, scleroderma
2 Familial
3 Pregnancy
4 Iatrogenic: oral contraceptives, metformin, anorectic drugs (aminorex, dexfenfluramine, fenfluramine) or crotolaria alkaloids

* Esp. if anticardiolipin antibody positive

Diagnosis of primary pulmonary hypertension
1 CXR
   — Peripheral oligemia ('pruned' peripheral vasculature)
   — Proximal-dilated pulmonary arteries ('deer's antlers')
   — Pulmonary arterial calcification if long-standing
2 Pulmonary angiography*
   — No emboli
   — No peripheral arterial stenosis
   — No intracardiac shunt
   — Normal PCWP (excludes mitral stenosis, cor triatriatum)

* Note that choriocarcinoma growing down the pulmonary arteries is a rare, curable cause of 'primary' pulmonary hypertension; diagnose by plasma β-HCG

Drugs used to treat primary pulmonary hypertension
1 Prostacyclin (e.g. IV epoprostenol, oral beraprost, inhaled iloprost) drugs
2 Intravenous adenosine
3 Inhaled nitric oxide
4 Calcium blockers (nifedipine, diltiazem)
5 Other vasodilators (e.g. tolazoline)
6 Warfarin

VENOUS THROMBOSIS

Differential diagnosis of the swollen calf
1 Deep venous thrombosis
2 Cellulitis
3 Ruptured plantaris
4 Ruptured Baker's cyst
5 Popliteal artery aneurysm (incl. mycotic)
6 Hematoma (esp. in patient on anticoagulants)

'Post-phlebitic syndrome': pathogenesis, features and diagnosis
1 Previous venous thrombosis irreversibly damages venous valves (esp. in perforators) and distorts drainage
2 Gradual onset of symptoms worsened by upright posture
   — Tense ankle edema (implies deep vein incompetence)
   — Calf pain, esp. on exercise ('venous claudication')
   — Cyanosis, pigmentation, induration and ulceration

3 Essentially a diagnosis of exclusion
   — Negative venogram*
   — Negative impedance plethysmography
   — Negative radiofibrinogen scan
   — Doppler → deep venous reflux

* Misleading if thrombus has organized

ETIOLOGY OF VENOUS THROMBOSIS

Classical predispositions to thrombosis: Virchow's triad
1 Abnormal blood flow
   — e.g. Intrapelvic obstruction
2 Abnormal blood
   — e.g. Polycythemia vera, factor V mutation
3 Abnormal vessel wall
   — e.g. Coronary atherosclerosis

Non-specific predispositions to venous thrombosis
1 **H**istory
   — Previous thrombosis or embolism
2 **H**ypomobility
   — Cerebrovascular accident
   — Myocardial infarction, cardiac failure
   — Post-operative, esp. hip/pelvic/abdominal surgery
3 **H**ypovolemia
   — Nephrotic syndrome
   — Dehydration, esp. in elderly
4 **H**ypercoagulability
   — Malignancy*, esp. disseminated
   — Cigarette smoking
5 **H**ormones
   — Estrogens
   — Puerperium

* Cytotoxic chemotherapy per se may cause *additional* hypercoagulability

Specific conditions associated with thromboembolism
1 Hereditary causes of thrombophilia*
   — Common
      • Factor V Leiden mutation‡
      • Hyperhomocysteinemia¶
      • Elevated Lp(a)
   — Uncommon
      • Antithrombin III deficiency (1/2000)
      • Protein C (or S) deficiency
      • Heparin cofactor II deficiency
2 Specific diseases causing acquired hypercoagulability
   — SLE and/or lupus anticoagulant (anticardiolipin; p. 185)
   — Paroxysmal nocturnal hemoglobinuria
   — Polycythemia vera, essential thrombocythemia
   — 'Warm' autoimmune hemolytic anemia
   — Sickle-C disease
3 Drugs
   — e.g. Rifampicin

* Most DVT patients do *not* have any identifiable coagulation abnormality
‡ Mutation → resistance to activated protein C; occurs in up to 7% of population
¶ Important diagnosis since condition responds to vitamins (folate, pyridoxine, hydroxocobalamin)

Clinical sequelae of resistance to activated protein C*
1 Increased thrombosis, esp.
 — When taking oral contraceptives
 — When pregnant
2 Increased incidence of myocardial infarction
 — esp. In homozygotes

* i.e. due to factor V Leiden

ANTICOAGULANT THERAPY

Approximate duration of anticoagulation for thrombosis
1 Post-operative
 — 1 month
2 Uncomplicated sporadic DVT or pulmonary embolus
 — 3 months
3 Major pulmonary embolism or ileofemoral thrombosis*
 — 6 months

* NB: Initial (10-day) treatment with full-dose heparin (either subcutaneous or IV) appears essential in proximal venous thrombosis

Approximate extent of anticoagulation for thrombosis
1 Prophylaxis for cardiogenic emboli in chronic AF
 — Aim for INR > 2
2 DVT prophylaxis (incl. perioperative)
 — Aim for INR 2–2.5
3 Active treatment of DVT, pulmonary embolism, TIAs
 — Aim for INR 2.5–3
4 Treatment of recurrent DVT/pulmonary embolism, mechanical valve prostheses, myocardial infarction
 — Aim for INR 3–3.5

Distinguishing unfractionated and low-molecular-weight heparin
1 Intravenous (unfractionated)
 — Blocks factor Xa and circulating thrombin to a similar extent, thus prolongs APTT/PTTK
 — Neutralized by platelet factor IV in activated platelets
 — Side-effect: thrombocytopenia in 3%
2 Subcutaneous (low molecular weight), e.g. enoxaparin, dalteparin
 — Blocks factor Xa more potently than thrombin; does not prolong APTT/PTTK, and does not require monitoring
 — More bioavailable, durable, and predictable in its actions; not neutralized by platelet factor IV
 — Advantage: outpatient/home administration

Efficacy of GPIIb/IIIa inhibitors*
1 Unstable angina prior to PTCA, esp. if troponin T > 0.1 ng/mL
2 As adjunct to PTCA (reduces restenosis rate‡)

* Include abciximab (antibody), tirofiban and lamifiban (small-molecule inhibitors), eptifibatide (peptide antagonist), oral antagonists (sibrafiban, xemilofiban) and natural disintegrin antagonists (barbourin, trigramin)
‡ As does catheter-based intracoronary [192]iridium radiotherapy
Note that GPIIb/IIIa antagonists are associated with an increased risk of bleeding

INVESTIGATING THROMBOSIS

Indications for investigating thrombotic tendency
1 Venous or arterial thrombosis in young patient (< 40 years)
2 Recurrent thromboembolic events and/or family history
3 Recurrent abortion
4 Skin necrosis while taking warfarin*

* Affects individuals with protein C or S deficiency

Diagnostic imaging of suspected pulmonary embolism
1 Spiral CT
2 Ventilation/perfusion lung scan
3 Pulmonary arteriogram (esp. if embolectomy is entertained)

Techniques for detecting peripheral thrombi
1 Duplex B-mode ultrasound/color Doppler
 — Advantages
 • Quick, painless, non-invasive and cheap
 • Sensitive/specific for proximal thrombi
 • Currently the most popular approach
 — Disadvantages
 • Insensitive for distal (calf) thrombi
 • False-negative: non-occlusive proximal thrombi
 • False-positives possible in CCF
2 Venography
 — Advantages
 • Quick, accurate ('gold standard')
 — Disadvantages
 • May be painful and/or cause phlebitis
 • Risk of contrast hypersensitivity
 • Radioactivity exposure
 • False-negative: recanalized thrombus
3 ^{125}I-labelled fibrinogen scanning
 — Advantages
 • Non-invasive, painless
 • Accurate for actively extending calf thrombi
 — Disadvantages
 • Slow (results take 24–72 h) and expensive
 • Radioactivity exposure
 • Insensitive for iliofemoral thrombus
 • False-negative: non-extending thrombus
 • False-positives: hematoma or inflammation
4 Impedance plethysmography
 — Advantages
 • Non-invasive, painless, no radioactivity
 • Sensitive for proximal occlusive thrombi
 • Good when combined with ^{125}I-fibrinogen
 — Disadvantages
 • May require serial studies
 • Insensitive for calf thrombi
 • False-negative: non-occlusive proximal thrombi
 • False-positive: cardiac failure
5 Miscellaneous
 — D-dimer
 • Absence in plasma may *exclude* fresh thrombus
 — Edema fluid protein concentration
 • Levels > 10 g/L suggest cellulitis > thrombosis

— Thermography
  • False-positives with any inflammation

PERIPHERAL ARTERIAL DISEASE

Cardiogenic sources of systemic emboli
1 Mitral stenosis
2 Post-infarct
3 Atrial fibrillation
4 Prosthetic valve
   — Mitral > aortic
   — Mechanical > biological
5 Other
   — Sick sinus syndrome
   — Infective endocarditis
   — Left atrial myxoma

Digital gangrene with normal pulses
1 Diabetes mellitus
2 Vasculitis; cold agglutinins
3 Thromboembolism
4 Hyperviscosity
5 Iatrogenic
   — Excess ergot or dopamine
   — Intra-arterial thiopental or adrenaline (epinephrine)

Claudication of the upper limb
1 Atheroma
2 Buerger's disease
3 Takayasu's arteritis
4 Proximal coarctation
5 Thoracic outlet syndrome
6 Polymyalgia rheumatica

REVIEWING THE LITERATURE: CARDIOLOGY

2.1 Stelfox HT et al (1998) Conflict of interest in the debate over calcium channel antagonists. N Engl J Med 338: 101–106

Retrospective analysis of journal articles in the field of calcium channel antagonist safety, in which the relationship between the articles' conclusions and the authors' conflict of interest (or otherwise) was examined. A strong association (p < 0.01) was found between supportive articles and financial ties with related drug companies. This article preceded a belated acknowledgement by the Journal of Positive Results that an embarrassing number of recently published studies had failed to disclose financial conflicts of interest.

2.2 Hakim AA et al (1998) Effects of walking on mortality among nonsmoking retired men. N Engl J Med 338: 94–99

Erikssen G et al (1998) Changes in fitness and changes in mortality. Lancet 352: 759–762

Manson JE et al (1999) A prospective study of walking as compared with vigorous exercise in the prevention of coronary heart disease in women. N Engl J Med 341: 650–658

Boreham CA et al (2000) Training effects of accumulated daily stair-climbing exercise in previously sedentary young women. Prev Med 30: 277–281

Striking congruence between these four studies as to the benefits of exercise – notwithstanding the confounding possibilities of covert covariables and publication bias. The first showed a halving of mortality for elderly male non-smokers who walked more than 2 miles per day relative to those who walked less than a mile a day. The second showed that even a small increase in fitness in middle-aged men is associated with a significant mortality reduction, irrespective of the original level of fitness. The third showed that habitual brisk walking is associated with reduced incidence of coronary events in middle-aged females. The last, a small (n = 22) randomized study of a graded increase in daily stair-climbing over 7 weeks in young sedentary females, showed a significant (p < 0.05) rise in HDL-cholesterol associated with reduced exertional blood lactate, oxygen consumption and heart rate in the cohort randomized to exercise.

2.3 Tarnow-Mordi WO et al (2000) Hospital mortality in relation to staff workload: a 4–year study in an adult intensive care unit. Lancet 356: 185–189

Canto JG et al (2000) The volume of primary angioplasty procedures and survival after acute myocardial infarction. N Engl J Med 342: 1573–1580

Two studies supporting a relationship between manpower logistics and therapeutic outcomes. The first found a consistent four-fold increased risk of patient death at times of peak occupancy in an intensive-care unit relative to times of low occupancy. The second documented a 28% lower inpatient mortality for myocardial infarction patients undergoing coronary angioplasty for reperfusion in hospitals undertaking the top quartile of such procedures compared with hospitals undertaking the lowest quartile; in contrast, the outcomes for non-operative intervention (thrombolytic therapy) were identical.

2.4 Schwartz PJ et al (1998) Prolongation of the QT interval and the sudden infant death syndrome. N Engl J Med 338: 1709–1714

One-year follow-up study of 33 034 newborns who had routine ECGs done in the first week of life. Those who had a prolonged Q-T interval (long Q-T syndrome) were found to have a 40–fold increased risk of sudden infant death over the ensuing 12 months; moreover, in this series, half of all SIDS cases were associated with a long Q-Tc. Sudden arrhythmic death (reflecting the onset of ventricular fibrillation) during competitive sports in young adulthood has also been associated with this ECG diagnosis.

2.5 Newman MF et al (2001) Longitudinal assessment of neurocognitive function after coronary artery bypass surgery. N Engl J Med 344: 395–402

Study of 261 CABG patients of whom 53% had incurred deterioration of cognitive function at discharge (due to ministrokes) – 24% at 6 months and 42% at 5 years – thus confirming the predictive significance of perioperative cognitive decline for long-term mental functioning. A further 2–5% of CABG patients stroke out. Use of the heart–lung pump and aortic clamping are implicated in the pathogenesis.

2.6 Decousus H et al (1998) A clinical trial of vena caval filters in the prevention of pulmonary embolism in patients with proximal deep-vein thrombosis. N Engl J Med 338: 409–415

Patients managed with filters had fewer emboli but more DVTs than patients managed without, with no difference in mortality between the two groups. Moreover, patients managed with low-molecular-weight (subcutaneous) heparin had fewer emboli than those treated with unfractionated (intravenous) heparin.

2.7 Conolly HM et al (1997) Valvular heart disease associated with fenfluramine-phentermine. N Engl J Med 337: 581–588

Khan MA et al (1998) The prevalence of cardiac valvular insufficiency assessed by transthoracic echocardiography in obese patients treated with appetite-suppressant drugs. N Engl J Med 339: 713–718

Jick H et al (1998) A population-based study of appetite-suppressant drugs and the risk of cardiac-valve regurgitation. N Engl J Med 339: 719–724

Weissman NJ et al (1998) An assessment of heart-valve abnormalities in obese patients taking dexenfluramine, sustained-release dexenfluramine, or placebo. N Engl J Med 339: 725–732

Bad cardiovascular news for amphetamine-based appetite suppressants from these studies. Both right- and left-sided valvopathies (esp. aortic regurgitation), with or without pulmonary hypertension, were demonstrable, particularly in patients on combined-drug treatment.

2.8   Sacks FM et al (1996) The effect of pravastatin on coronary events after myocardial infarction in patients with average cholesterol levels. N Engl J Med 335: 1001–1009

Weverling-Rijnsburger A et al (1997) Total cholesterol and risk of mortality in the oldest old. Lancet 350: 1119–1123

The first of these studies was a 5–year double-blind outcome analysis of non-hypercholesterolemic myocardial infarction patients receiving either placebo or pravastatin; an approximate 25% reduction of coronary events and stroke was confirmed in the treatment group. The second observational study of 724 patients older than 84 years showed that hypercholesterolemic patients of this age live longer (15% better for each 1 mmol/L increase in total cholesterol): cardiovascular mortality was similar in each cholesterol range, but lower mortality for cancer and infection was associated with higher cholesterol. The speculation is made that hypolipidemic treatment may not confer the same mortality benefits in this aged cohort.

2.9   Appel LJ et al (1997) A clinical trial of the effects of dietary patterns on blood pressure. N Engl J Med 336: 1117–1124

Hu FB et al (1997) Dietary fat intake and the risk of coronary heart disease in women. N Engl J Med 337: 1491–1499

The first of these studies was a controlled analysis of dietary manipulation on blood pressure in 459 mildly hypertensive individuals. Use of a diet rich in fruits and vegetables, and low in saturated fats, reduced systolic blood pressure by 10 mmHg more than the control diet. In the second study, ingestion of a diet low in saturated fats was prospectively associated with a lower risk of coronary events: a 5% increase in energy intake from saturated fats was associated with a 17% increased risk in coronary events.

2.10   Burke AP et al (1997) Coronary risk factors and plaque morphology in men with coronary disease who died suddenly. N Engl J Med 336: 1276–1282

Gaeta G et al (2000) Arterial abnormalities in the offspring of patients with premature myocardial infarction. N Engl J Med 343: 840–846

In the first study – a post-mortem examination of 113 sudden coronary death cases – two correlations of coronary pathology with risk factors were discerned: acute thrombosis in smokers, and plaque rupture in individuals with high total:HDL cholesterol ratios. In the second study, 40 healthy children aged 6–30 of parents with early onset myocardial infarction underwent ultrasonic evaluation of brachial and carotid artery structure and function, revealing detectable abnormalities despite their young age.

2.11   Bernardi L et al (1998) Effect of breathing rate on oxygen saturation and exercise performance in chronic heart failure. Lancet 351: 1308–1311

Patients with chronic heart failure underwent respiratory training to reduce their respiratory rate to 6/min. This maneuver increased gas exchange, oxyhemoglobin saturation and exercise performance, while reducing dyspnea.

CHAPTER 3

Endocrinology

Physical examination protocol 3.1 You are asked to assess a patient for clinical evidence of hypopituitarism

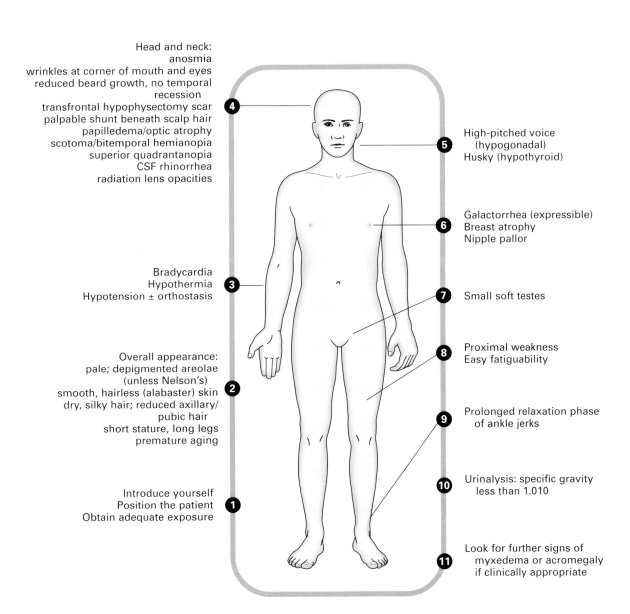

Head and neck:
anosmia
wrinkles at corner of mouth and eyes
reduced beard growth, no temporal
recession
transfrontal hypophysectomy scar
palpable shunt beneath scalp hair
papilledema/optic atrophy
scotoma/bitemporal hemianopia
superior quadrantanopia
CSF rhinorrhea
radiation lens opacities

High-pitched voice
(hypogonadal)
Husky (hypothyroid)

Galactorrhea (expressible)
Breast atrophy
Nipple pallor

Bradycardia
Hypothermia
Hypotension ± orthostasis

Small soft testes

Overall appearance:
pale; depigmented areolae
(unless Nelson's)
smooth, hairless (alabaster) skin
dry, silky hair; reduced axillary/
pubic hair
short stature, long legs
premature aging

Proximal weakness
Easy fatiguability

Prolonged relaxation phase
of ankle jerks

Urinalysis: specific gravity
less than 1.010

Introduce yourself
Position the patient
Obtain adequate exposure

Look for further signs of
myxedema or acromegaly
if clinically appropriate

Physical examination protocol 3.2 You are asked to examine a patient who has recently noticed increasing hat size

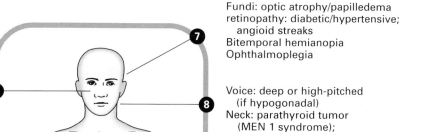

Face: hypophysectomy scar
Thick lips, prominent
nasolabial folds
Seborrhea, acne, hirsuties
Prominent brow
Underbite
Wide-spaced teeth
Macroglossia

Proximal weakness
Axilla:
fibromata mollusca
± acanthosis
nigricans

Hypertension
Palpable ulnar nerve,
supraclavicular nerve

Hands:
spadelike
spatulate fingers
positive Tinel's sign
thenar wasting
weak opponens
sweaty palms

Overall appearance:
? acromegaly

Introduce yourself
Position the patient
Obtain adequate exposure

Fundi: optic atrophy/papilledema
retinopathy: diabetic/hypertensive;
angioid streaks
Bitemporal hemianopia
Ophthalmoplegia

Voice: deep or high-pitched
(if hypogonadal)
Neck: parathyroid tumor
(MEN 1 syndrome);
goiter

Gynecomastia
Galactorrhea
Cardiomegaly, S_3, S_4
Kyphosis

Hepatosplenomegaly
Palpable kidneys

Testicular atrophy

Proximal weakness
Palpable peroneal nerve ± footdrop
Osteoarthritis: knee, hip

'Hung-up' ankle jerks
Large feet, thick heels

Glycosuria

Emotional lability

Physical examination protocol 3.3   You are asked to examine a patient with recent onset of lethargy and cold intolerance

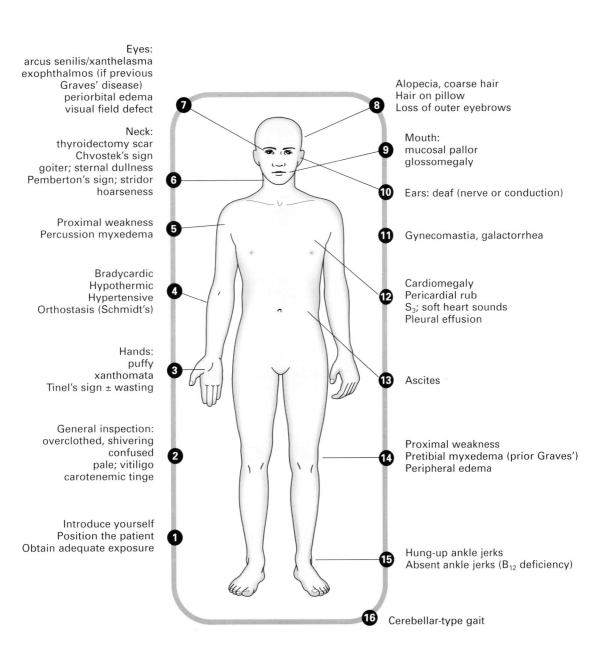

Eyes:
arcus senilis/xanthelasma
exophthalmos (if previous
Graves' disease)
periorbital edema
visual field defect

Neck:
thyroidectomy scar
Chvostek's sign
goiter; sternal dullness
Pemberton's sign; stridor
hoarseness

Proximal weakness
Percussion myxedema

Bradycardic
Hypothermic
Hypertensive
Orthostasis (Schmidt's)

Hands:
puffy
xanthomata
Tinel's sign ± wasting

General inspection:
overclothed, shivering
confused
pale; vitiligo
carotenemic tinge

Introduce yourself
Position the patient
Obtain adequate exposure

Alopecia, coarse hair
Hair on pillow
Loss of outer eyebrows

Mouth:
mucosal pallor
glossomegaly

Ears: deaf (nerve or conduction)

Gynecomastia, galactorrhea

Cardiomegaly
Pericardial rub
S_3; soft heart sounds
Pleural effusion

Ascites

Proximal weakness
Pretibial myxedema (prior Graves')
Peripheral edema

Hung-up ankle jerks
Absent ankle jerks (B_{12} deficiency)

Cerebellar-type gait

Physical examination protocol 3.4 You are asked to begin by examining the neck of a patient who looks possibly thyrotoxic

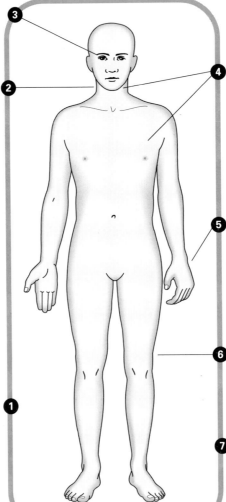

Eyes: stare; can they be closed?
exophthalmos (look from above
and from side)
lid lag/lid retraction; chemosis
diplopia/ophthalmoplegia
impaired convergence/acuity
corneal/fundal examination

Neck: is there a goiter?
Inspect:
nodularity
motion on swallowing

Palpation:
consistency
tenderness
discrete cyst(s)
fixation
adenopathy (regional)
Pemberton's sign, Berry's sign
Sternal percussion

Auscultate:
bruit
venous hum

Voice:
stridor
hoarseness

Introduce yourself
Position the patient
Obtain adequate exposure

Prominent jowls
Lymphadenopathy (generalized)
Gynecomastia
Cardiomegaly, S_3
Loud S_1, systolic flow murmur
Lerman–Means scratch
Systolic hypertension
Irregular large-volume pulse
Splenomegaly
Tender spine (osteoporosis)

Hands:
fine tremor
sweaty palms
acropachy
capillary pulsations
onycholysis
palmar erythema

Legs:
proximal weakness
pretibial myxedema
fasciculations
edema
brisk reflexes

Temperature

Physical examination protocol 3.5 You are asked to examine a patient who is known to have diabetes mellitus

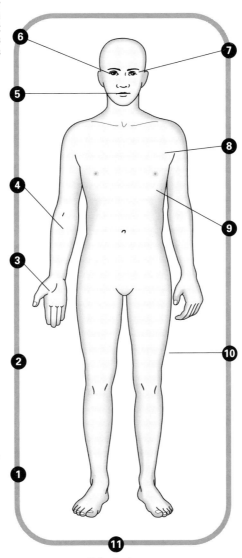

Eyes:
visual acuity
iridial rubeosis/hyphema
visual field defect
ocular movements
pupillary reactions

Oral thrush
Dental hygiene

Eruptive xanthomata
Peripheral pulses
Fistula (for dialysis)
Waxy skin
Fungal nail infections
Fingers: flexion deformities

Blood pressure
Orthostasis

General appearance:
Cushingoid
pigmented (bronzed)
uremic
balding/thick glasses (myotonic
dystrophy)
obese; wasted; lipodystrophy

Introduce yourself
Position the patient
Obtain adequate exposure

Ophthalmoscopy:
cataract ('snowflake'/senile);
  aphakia
background retinopathy
new vessel formation
hemorrhages
macular edema (retinal glistening)
photocoagulation scars
hypertensive changes

Carotid bruit
Cardiomegaly, S_3
Thoracotomy (CABG) scar

Abdomen:
hepatomegaly (fat, iron)
palpable kidneys
enlarged (atonic) bladder
injection sites/lipoatrophy
sympathectomy scar
femoral bruit; renal bruit

Legs:
amputations
proximal wasting (amyotrophy)
hemiparesis (CVA)
Skin:
  warmth
  anhidrosis
  color
  ulcers, foot sepsis
  hair distribution
popliteal and distal pulses
elevation pallor
dependency rubor
painless, deformed ankle
  (Charcot's)
absent deep tendon reflexes
absent vibration/light touch
reduced pinprick/deep pain/heat
claw toes, toenail deformity
ankle edema
sensory (pseudotabetic) ataxia

Urinalysis:
glycosuria
ketonuria
proteinuria
Perineal moniliasis

Physical examination protocol 3.6 You are asked to examine a patient suspected of having Cushing's syndrome

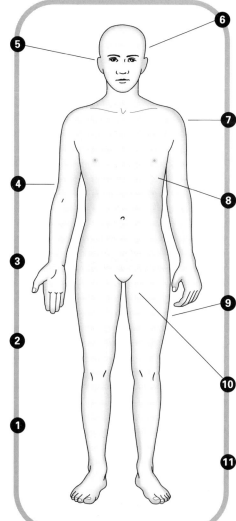

Face:
hypophysectomy scar
moon shape
plethora
acne
hirsuties
telangiectasia

Mouth:
thrush
deep voice (if virilized)

Skin:
fine, fragile
purpura, esp. forearm
± pigmentation (esp. in scars)
puffy hands

Hypertension

General:
degree of obesity (% > ideal weight)
truncal obesity
Affect:
depressed/euphoric

Introduce yourself
Position the patient
Obtain adequate exposure

Fundoscopy:
cataract (posterior subcapsular)
hypertensive changes
diabetic retinopathy
Rarely:
visual field defect
optic atrophy
papilledema

Buffalo hump
Supraclavicular fat pads
Vertebral tenderness
Kyphosis
Sacral edema

Abdomen:
pink striae
ballottable mass (adrenal)
hepatomegaly (fatty)
adrenalectomy scar

Legs:
proximal wasting/weakness
purpura
hirsute
tibial tenderness
ankle edema

Urinalysis: glycosuria
Clitoromegaly

Stigmata of underlying steroid-
dependent disease, e.g. asthma,
SLE, RA, skin disease

Diagnostic pathway 3.1   This patient has a goiter. What is the differential diagnosis?

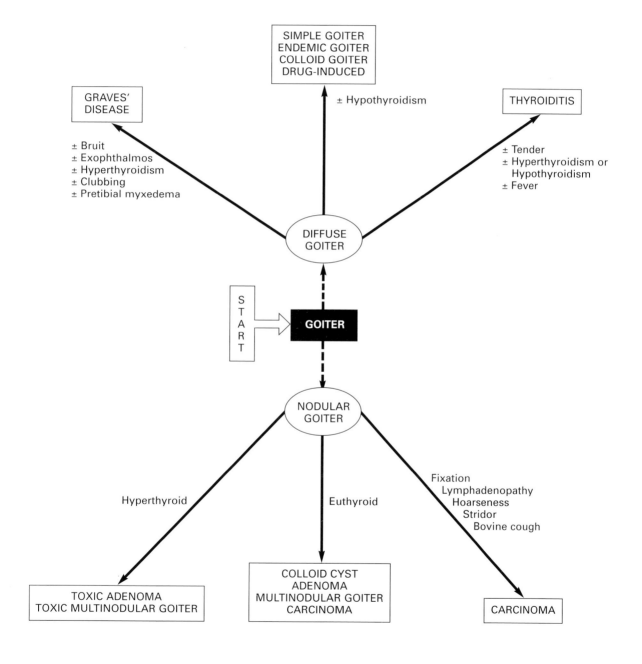

COMMON AND CLASSIC ENDOCRINE PROBLEMS

Common endocrine problems in clinical practice
1 Diabetic vascular, renal or neuropathic disease
2 Hypothyroidism following treatment of hyperthyroidism
3 Hirsutism

Classic endocrine problems in clinical exams
1 Diabetic retinopathy
2 Graves' disease/goiter
3 Acromegaly

ENDOCRINE EMERGENCIES

Thyroid storm: approach to management
1 Prevention
   — Treat possible precipitating factors (e.g. sepsis)
   — Render euthyroid prior to elective surgery
2 IV fluids as required to maintain BP; tepid sponge
3 Propylthiouracil (PTU) 200 mg p.o. q 6 h
4 Potassium iodide 200 mg IV over 15 min (give 1 h post-PTU)
5 Propranolol 1 mg IV, then 2 mg IV q 4 h p.r.n.*
6 Dexamethasone in supraphysiological ('shock') dosage

* NB: Beta-blockers may *not* be contraindicated in rate-dependent thyrocardiac failure; use short-acting IV esmolol, or combine propranolol with digoxin

Potential hazards in ketoacidosis
1 Insulin-induced *hypophosphatemia* may enhance oxygen-hemoglobin affinity and thus aggravate tissue hypoxia; phosphate supplementation is not routine, however
2 Severe *acidemia* may
   — Impair cardiac and respiratory (@ pH < 6.9) function
   — Reduce ventricular threshold to fibrillation
   — Increase ventilatory work
   — Lead to insulin resistance
3 *Rapid* correction of acidemia with intravenous *bicarbonate* may be associated with the following hazards
   — Alkalemia, as correction of CSF acidosis (which controls ventilatory rate) lags behind periphery
   — Paradoxical worsening of CSF acidosis as CO_2 (but not HCO_3) equilibrates across the blood–brain barrier*
   — CSF hyperosmolality leading to cerebral edema
   — Exacerbation of tissue hypoxia due to Bohr effect
4 Intracellular potassium depletion may result if supplements not prescribed when K^+ falls below 5.0 mmol/L

* i.e. rapid correction of acidosis enhances oxyhemoglobin affinity, accompanied by a slower increase in red cell 2,3-DPG

An approach to managing diabetic ketoacidosis (DKA)
1 Insulin
   — Administer via pump at 0.1 U/kg/h initially
   — Aim to lower blood glucose by 3 mmol/L/h
   — Increase rate by 2 U/h if no improvement after 2 h
2 Potassium
   — Give about 20 mmol/h if K^+ < 6 mmol/L
   — Withhold if anuric *or* K^+ > 6 mmol/L *or* ECG → ↑ K^+
   — If serum K^+ < 3 mmol/L, give 30–40 mmol/h
   — Aim to maintain K^+ > 4 mmol/L during insulin infusion
3 Fluids
   — Must be clinically assessed
   — A typical regimen in a dehydrated DKA patient might be: normal saline 1 L IV stat, 1 L over 1 h, 1 L over 2 h, then 1 L q 4 h as needed*
4 Bicarbonate
   — Consider giving 50 mmol $NaHCO_3$ *if* pH < 7.0
5 Tapering off
   — When blood glucose < 10 mmol/L, change saline to 5% dextrose; monitor glucose and potassium hourly

* cf. hyperosmolar coma: fluids and insulin are more conservatively administered; aim for complete rehydration and normoglycemia only after 36–72 h

Managing the acutely ill diabetic: a few tips
1 An acutely ill insulin-dependent diabetic may need to increase (rather than reduce) insulin dose
2 Even if meals have been missed due to illness, elevated blood or urine glucose indicates an increase in insulin dosage
3 Vomiting may indicate severe ketosis, therefore requiring urgent insulin supplementation
4 Heavy ketonuria and/or severe vomiting constitute indications for hospitalization in any ill diabetic patient

CLINICAL ASSESSMENT OF ENDOCRINE DISEASE

PITUITARY DISORDERS

Distinguishing features of hypopituitarism
1 Hypothyroidism (without goiter)
2 Hypoadrenalism (with pallor: 'alabaster skin')
3 Hypogonadism (with fine wrinkled skin: 'crows feet')
4 Hyposthenuria* (diabetes insipidus)

* Note that *serum* osmolality or sodium concentration may be normal (i.e. not increased) if water intake has been adequate

Acromegaly: indicators of disease activity
1 Severity of
   — Seborrhea, sweating, skin tags*
   — Hypertension, edema
   — Glucose intolerance
2 Serial measures of
   — Visual fields
   — Visual acuity

3 Plasma insulin-like growth factor-1 (IGF-I) level

* Fibromata mollusca

Common causes of morbidity/mortality in acromegaly
1 Diabetes
2 Sleep apnea
3 Hypertension
4 Cardiomyopathy
5 Cerebrovascular disease
6 Colonic polyps and carcinoma

Mechanisms of polydipsia in acromegaly
1 Dehydration secondary to hyperhidrosis
2 Osmotic diuresis (in 10%) due to glucose intolerance (in 50%)
3 Diabetes insipidus

Mechanisms of galactorrhea in acromegaly
1 Concomitant adenomatous secretion of prolactin (in 30%)
2 Compression of posterior pituitary stalk by adenoma, causing reduced ingress of prolactin-inhibitory factor (PIF)
3 Reduced pituitary TSH secretion → compensatory elevation of hypothalamic TRH secretion → prolactin release

HYPERTHYROIDISM

Pointers to the diagnosis of Graves' disease*
1 Smooth diffuse goiter
  — Esp. with bruit
2 Ophthalmopathy (see below)
  — Clinically apparent in 40%
3 Classical but rare
  — Localized mucinous edema (pretibial myxedema)
  — 'Acropachy'‡
4 Non-specific
  — Splenomegaly
  — Lymphadenopathy
5 Laboratory
  — Thyroid-stimulating immunoglobulin (TSI)
  — Low or undetectable TSH (i.e. hyperthyroidism)

* Note that incidence of both Graves' and ophthalmopathy is higher in smokers who, if so diagnosed, should be advised to stop smoking
‡ = Clubbing + subcutaneous fibrosis + phalangeal periosteal proliferation

Clinical manifestations of Graves' ophthalmopathy
1 Primary (autoimmune) manifestations
  — Proptosis, exophthalmos
  — Ophthalmoplegia
    • Lymphocytic infiltration of external eye muscles
    • Inferior recti most affected → vertical diplopia
2 Secondary (mechanical) complications
  — Optic nerve compression
    • Often occurs insidiously with *mild* proptosis
    • ↓ Acuity, central scotoma
    • ↓ Color vision; Marcus Gunn pupil
    • Variable disc appearance on fundoscopy
  — Impaired convergence
  — Corneal ulceration (exposure keratitis)
    • Occurs with *marked* proptosis of acute onset
  — Glaucoma
3 Sympathetic manifestations (*if* thyrotoxic*)
  — Lid-lag
  — Lid retraction ('stare')
    • Sclera visible above and below iris
    • Due to overactivity of Müller's muscle

* These signs also occur in non-autoimmune hyperthyroidism

Graves' ophthalmopathy: indicators of activity*
1 Retrobulbar pain (at rest and/or on movement)
2 Eyelid edema or swelling
3 Conjunctival injection or chemosis

* Severity of ophthalmopathy is exacerbated by smoking

Graves' ophthalmopathy: classification of severity*
1 Class 0 *N*o signs
2 Class 1 *O*nly signs (no symptoms)
3 Class 2 *S*oft tissue symptoms and/or signs
4 Class 3 *P*roptosis
5 Class 4 *E*xtraocular muscle involvement (ophthalmoplegia)
6 Class 5 *C*orneal involvement (exposure keratitis)
7 Class 6 *S*ight impairment (optic nerve compression)

* 'NO SPECS' classification of American Thyroid Association

Bilateral exophthalmos: differential diagnosis
1 Graves' disease
2 Uremia
3 Alcoholism
4 Malignant hypertension
5 Carcinomatosis
6 SVC obstruction

Unilateral exophthalmos: differential diagnosis
1 Graves' disease (commonest cause)
2 Contralateral Horner's syndrome (i.e. misdiagnosis)
3 Cavernous sinus pathology
  — Cavernous sinus thrombosis
  — Caroticocavernous fistula (pulsating)
  — Rhinocerebral mucormycosis
4 Intraorbital pathology
  — Histiocytosis X
  — Wegener's granulomatosis
  — Riedel's thyroiditis with pseudotumor oculi
  — Tumor (e.g. optic nerve glioma)

Neuromyopathies in thyroid disease
1 Proximal myopathy
  — Seen in thyrotoxicosis, less in hypothyroidism
  — Affects mainly upper limbs; reverts when euthyroid
2 Hypokalemic periodic paralysis
  — Seen in association with toxic multinodular goiter
  — Commonest in Asian males, esp. in hot season
  — Linked to hyperinsulinemia; treated with propranolol

3 Myasthenia gravis
— Affects 5% Graves' patients; suspect if bulbar weakness
— Exacerbated by thyrotoxicosis or hypothyroidism
4 Graves' ophthalmoplegia
— Seen also in euthyroid patients
— Predominant weakness of upward and lateral gaze
5 Hoffmann's syndrome
— Pseudomyotonia of myxedematous muscles
— Manifests with muscle aching following exertion

Endocrine causes of proximal weakness: differential diagnosis
1 Thyroid dysfunction
— Thyrotoxicosis (myopathy or periodic paralysis)
— Hypothyroidism
2 Adrenal dysfunction
— Cushing's disease
— Corticosteroid therapy (esp. triamcinolone)
— Nelson's syndrome
— Addison's disease
3 Acromegaly
4 Primary hyperparathyroidism
5 Primary hyperaldosteronism
6 Vitamin D deficiency (osteomalacia)

HYPOTHYROIDISM

Signs suggesting severe hypothyroidism
1 Hoarseness
2 Profound bradycardia or hypothermia
3 Mental confusion or coma
4 Markedly prolonged relaxation phase of deep tendon reflexes

Differential diagnosis of 'hung-up' tendon jerks
1 Myxedema
2 Other (rare) causes
— Diabetes mellitus
— Sarcoidosis
— Syphilis
— Profound hypothermia
— Post-partum
— Anorexia nervosa
— β-blockade

Factors favoring secondary (pituitary) hypothyroidism
1 No goiter
2 No soft-tissue (myx)edema
3 Stigmata of hypopituitarism (pale areolae, hyposthenuria)
4 Normal plasma cholesterol
5 Enlargement of sella turcica
6 TSH not elevated despite low free T_4

Pathogenetic mechanisms of thyroid enlargement
1 **T**hyroiditis (Hashimoto's)
2 **T**SI (thyroid stimulating immunoglobulin; → Graves')
3 **T**SH (multinodular goiter)
4 **T**umor

Clinical varieties of thyroiditis
1 Chronic lymphocytic (Hashimoto's) thyroiditis
— Common
— Female:male = 20:1
— Onset: gradual, painless
— Transient 'Hashitoxicosis' unusual
— Signs: diffuse painless goiter, no bruit
— Biopsy: lymphocytic infiltrate, Askanazy cells
— Associations: thyroid autoantibodies, HLA DR5
— Sequelae: persistent hypothyroidism in 80%
2 Subacute granulomatous (de Quervain's) thyroiditis
— Uncommon
— Female:male = 2:1
— Onset: acute, painful, transient thyrotoxicosis usual
— Signs: small goiter, extremely tender
— Biopsy: giant cell infiltrate, granulomata
— Associations: viral infection
— Sequelae: transient hypothyroidism in 10%
3 Subacute lymphocytic ('silent') thyroiditis
— Common
— Female:male = 5:1
— Onset: acute (often peripartum), painless
— Transient thyrotoxicosis usual
— Signs: goiter usually absent
— Biopsy: similar to Hashimoto's
— Associations: thyroid autoantibodies, HLA DR5
— Sequelae: transient hypothyroidism in 25%
4 Chronic fibrosing (Riedel's) thyroiditis
— Rare
— Onset: gradual
— Signs: woody (ligneous) indurated thyroid
— Biopsy: widespread fibrosis
— Associations: retroperitoneal fibrosis, sclerosing cholangitis, Peyronie's disease
— Sequelae: persistent hypothyroidism in 50%

Cardiac manifestations of thyroid disease
1 Hypothyroidism
— Hypercholesterolemia, ischemic heart disease
— Pericarditis, pericardial effusion
— Cardiomyopathy, cardiac failure
— Hypotension or hypertension
— Bradycardia; low-voltage ECG
2 Thyrotoxicosis
— Sinus tachycardia; AF ± thromboembolism
— Bounding pulse, widened pulse pressure
— Angina, myocardial infarction
— High-output CCF; cardiomyopathy, focal myocarditis
— Sudden death (presumed VF)

DIABETES MELLITUS

Abdominal pain in diabetic patients: differential diagnosis
1 Gastric dilatation
— Acute (ketoacidosis)
— Chronic (autonomic neuropathy)
2 Pancreatitis
— Acute (a complication of type IV hyperlipidemia)
— Chronic (precedes development of diabetes)

3 Infarction
— Mesenteric
— Myocardial (painless in autonomic neuropathy)
4 Genitourinary
— Urinary tract infection
— Bladder retention (painless in early stages)
5 Hepatobiliary
— Cholecystitis
— Hepatic capsular distension due to steatosis, esp. in poorly controlled patients receiving high insulin
6 Thoracolumbar radiculopathy (amyotrophy)
— Due to nerve root ischemia

Clinical features of diabetic amyotrophy
1 Presents acutely in a poorly-controlled type 2 diabetic with ↑↑ HbA_{1c} but no known microvascular disease
2 Initially manifests with asymmetric weakness of hip/knee
3 Radicular pain and/or other sensory symptoms may be associated; almost always accompanied by hyporeflexia
4 Often complicated by contralateral pelvic girdle weakness, wasting, weight loss, incontinence and impotence
5 Occasionally associated with extensor plantar response and/or ↑ CSF protein
6 Excellent long-term prognosis: partial recovery usual within 1–2 years, though recurrence not uncommon

Clinical anomalies of diabetic adiposities
1 Lipodystrophy
— Associated with insulin-resistant diabetes, i.e. type A insulin receptor abnormality (see above)
2 Lipoatrophy
— Occurs at sites of porcine insulin injection; responds to injection of monocomponent insulin
3 Lipohypertrophy
— Commoner with monocomponent insulin use, esp. if injection sites not rotated

Clinical and biochemical features of syndrome X*
1 Insulin resistance with central obesity, hyperinsulinemia and glucose intolerance (but clinical diabetes is unusual)
2 Hypertension
— Severity proportional to hyperinsulinemia
3 Hyperuricemia
4 Hyperlipidemia
— ↑ VLDL‡ (esp. males)
— ↓ HDL (esp. females)
5 Increased PAI-1

* a.k.a. Reaven's syndrome; associated with polycystic ovaries
‡ cf. LDL: usually *normal*, but small dense LDL-cholesterol particles are increased

DIABETIC EYE DISEASE

Differential diagnosis of ocular pain in diabetic patients
1 Third nerve palsy
2 Iridial rubeosis
3 Mucormycosis
4 Secondary glaucoma
5 Poor visual acuity → eyestrain

Characteristics of a diabetic third nerve palsy
1 Sudden onset
2 Painful
3 Pupillary sparing
4 Probably reflects microvascular disease of vasa nervorum
5 Diplopia usually improves within 12 months

Common causes of impaired visual acuity in diabetic patients
1 Macular edema in acute hyperglycemia
2 Retinopathy impinging on macula
3 Retinal detachment or vitreous hemorrhage
4 Hyphema secondary to iridial rubeosis
5 Cataract (classical, rare 'snowflake' type in type 1 diabetes)
6 Cerebrovascular accident

Diabetic retinopathy: characterizing the lesions
1 Maculopathy (commonest cause of diabetic blindness)
— Macular edema
— Macular exudates
— Macular ischemia
2 'Background' retinopathy (i.e. acuity unimpaired)
— Microaneurysms
— Hemorrhages (dot and blot)
— Hard exudates (lipid deposits)
— Soft exudates ('cotton wool' spots = infarcts)
— Venous calibre changes: beading, looping, dilatation
— Arteriolar changes: narrowing, tortuosity, a–v nipping
3 Proliferative retinopathy (→ type 1 diabetes)
— New vessels (arising from disc or periphery)
— Fibrous patches
— Vitreous hemorrhage
— Retinal detachment
— Rubeosis iridis

COMPLICATIONS OF DIABETES

Key prognostic variables influencing diabetic complications
1 Major predictive factors in *macrovascular* complications
— Age
— Duration of diabetes
— Hypercholesterolemia
2 Major predictive factors in *microvascular* complications
— Hyperglycemia (correlates with HbA_{1c} level)
— Hypertension
3 Retinopathy
— Smoking
— Hyperglycemia (4-fold greater risk for HbA_{1c} > 11.7% than < 8.5%)

— Hypercholesterolemia (4-fold greater risk for cholesterol > 7 vs < 5.3 mmol/L)
— Hypertension (2-fold risk of visual acuity decline for BP > 154/87 vs < 144/82)
4 Nephropathy
— Hypertension
— Family history of cardiovascular disease*
— Hyperglycemia
5 Neuropathy/amyotrophy
— Hyperglycemia

* Serum Lp(a) concentrations correlate with occurrence of proteinuria

Patterns of fetal morbidity in gestational diabetes
1 Mild (newly dignosed) diabetes
— Macrosomia (→ dystocia)
2 Severe (known microvascular disease)
— Small-for-dates
3 Spontaneous abortions*
— Intrauterine fetal death
4 Malformations (esp. anencephaly)
— Increased with maternal ketosis
5 Neonatal morbidity
— Jaundice, respiratory distress
— Hypoglycemia (maternal hyperglycemia → ↑ insulin)
6 Reduced childhood intelligence
— IQ inversely proportional to third-trimester ketosis

* Incidence reduced if blood glucose levels tightly controlled in first trimester

Pathogenetic phases of diabetic nephropathy
1 Preclinical phase
— GFR normal or high
— Blood pressure normal
— Urinary albumin excretion elevated but undetectable by routine tests (i.e. microalbuminuria*)
2 Clinically overt nephropathy
— Declining GFR
— Hypertension
— Frank proteinuria

* Microalbuminuria = 20–200 μg urinary protein/min, urinary albumin concentration > 30 mg/L; often apparent in the first 10–15 years of type I diabetes, and predictive of cardiovascular complications. In contrast, overt proteinuria = > 200 μg/min proteinuria, tends to supervene after 15 years type I diabetes

Clinical presentations of nephropathy
1 Worsening of hypertension
2 Development of nocturia
3 Unexplained ↓ glycosuria (i.e. 'threshold' elevation)
4 Increase in microalbuminuria
5 Decrease in insulin requirement
6 Increase in hypoglycemic frequency

Causes of premature death in insulin-dependent diabetes
1 Macrovascular disease
— Ischemic heart disease (35%)
— Cerebrovascular disease (15%)
2 Microvascular disease
— Renal failure (25%)

3 Ketoacidosis (20%)
4 Hypoglycemia (15%)

Infections increased in poorly controlled diabetics
1 Rhinocerebral mucormycosis
2 Emphysematous cholecystitis (*Clostridia* spp.)
3 Necrotizing cellulitis/fasciitis (mixed aerobes and anaerobes)
4 Malignant otitis externa (*Ps. aeruginosa*)
5 Oral or vulvovaginal candidiasis
6 Furunculosis (staphylococcal)
7 Abscesses (e.g. perinephric)
8 Influenza/*Staph.* pneumonia
9 Tuberculosis

NB: infection may either complicate or precipitate ketoacidosis

THE FOOT IN DIABETES

The diabetic foot: factors contributing to morbidity
1 Ischemia
— Microvascular disease (esp.)
— Macrovascular disease (atheroma) ± thrombosis
2 Infection (incl. osteomyelitis)
— Stiff (glycosylated) collagen
  • → Ulcers (cellulitis)
— Hyperglycemic leukocyte dysfunction
  • → Poor wound healing
3 Neuropathy (in 80%)
— Sensory loss (incl. Charcot joint development)
  • → Trauma, burns
— Motor loss
  • Weak intrinsics → 'claw toe' → plantar ulcers
— Visual loss
  • Reduced visual acuity (→ poor foot care)
4 Deformity
— Callus, bunion, hammer-toe → ↑ trauma

Ischemic or neuropathic feet in diabetes?
1 The ischemic foot
— painful
— cold; reduced pulses
— ulcers at extremities
2 The neuropathic foot
— painless
— warm; normal pulses
— ulcers at pressure points

The infected diabetic foot: bacteriology and therapy
1 Mild infections (tend to be Gram-positive)
— *Staph. aureus*
— Streptococci
2 Serious infections
— Gram-negative aerobes
— Anaerobes
3 Empirical (preculture) treatment options:
— Non-limb-threatening infection
  • Oral flucloxacillin *or* IV cefazolin
— Limb-threatening infection
  • Ciprofloxacin + clindamycin (oral/IV)
— Life-threatening infection
  • Vancomycin + metronidazole (IV)

CLINICAL DIAGNOSIS OF ADRENAL DISORDERS

Pathophysiologic prevalence in Cushing's syndrome
1 Cushing's disease   — 70%
2 Ectopic ACTH   — 10%
   Adrenal adenoma   — 10%
3 Adrenal carcinoma   — 5%
4 Adrenal hyperplasia   — 1%
   Depression, alcohol   — 1%

Cushing's syndrome: features of discriminative value
1 Cushing's (benign ACTH-dependent) disease
   — Atrophic livid striae (skin atrophy)
   — Proximal myopathy   } → 'lemon-on-sticks'
   — *Truncal* obesity   }   habitus
   — Spontaneous purpura
   — Osteoporosis (esp. males, premenopausal females)
2 Adrenal carcinoma
   — Childhood onset
   — Hirsutism/virilism/acne
   — Abdominal mass
3 Ectopic ACTH (paraneoplastic)
   — Hypokalemia → weakness
   — Pigmentation *if* survival sufficient (e.g. thymoma)
4 Iatrogenic
   — Posterior subcapsular cataracts
   — Aseptic necrosis of bone
   — Glaucoma; papilledema (pseudotumor)
5 Simple obesity*/polycystic ovaries
   — Pale striae
   — Generalized (may be massive) > truncal
   — 'Buffalo hump'
   — Oligomenorrhea
   — Hypertension, glucose intolerance

* i.e. these features are of *poor* diagnostic value

Hypoadrenalism: primary or secondary?
1 Primary (adrenal failure)
   — Pigmentation
   — Hyperkalemia
   — Metabolic acidosis
2 Secondary (pituitary failure)
   — Depigmented areolae
   — Despite normal aldosterone secretion, symptomatic hypovolemia *may* still occur due to vomiting/diarrhea or diabetes insipidus
   — Similarly, hyponatremia *may* still occur due to concomitant hypothyroidism or SIADH
3 The above may be distinguished by
   — Plasma ACTH assay
   — Tetracosactrin (Synacthen) test*

* Unless *long-term* pituitary failure → adrenal atrophy → false-positive

Differential diagnosis of grossly elevated plasma ACTH
1 Addison's disease
2 Nelson's syndrome
3 Ectopic (neoplastic) ACTH production

PHEOCHROMOCYTOMA

Common sites of extra-adrenal pheochromocytoma
1 Organ of Zuckerkandl (aortic bifurcation)
2 Paraspinal sympathetic ganglia
3 Bladder wall (symptoms on micturition)
4 Spermatic cord
5 Glomus jugulare (usually non-secreting tumors)

Clinical aspects of pheochromocytoma
1 **H**eadache
   Hypertension
   — Non-paroxysmal in 50%
   — May paradoxically *worsen* following β-blockade
   Hypotension (orthostatic in 50%)
   Heartbeat awareness (palpitations)
   Hyperhidrosis (sweating)
2 10% are malignant (histology not predictive)
   10% are extra-adrenal (greater risk of malignancy)
   10% are familial (often bilateral): usually non-secretory
   10% are multiple (30% in children)
3 Noradrenaline-secreting type
   — May mimic essential hypertension
   — Absent tachycardia
   — Pallor
   — *Angor animi*
4 Adrenaline-secreting type
   — May mimic acute anxiety attacks
   — Orthostasis
   — Flushing *may* follow initial upper body pallor
5 Aspects distinguishing diagnosis from carcinoid syndrome
   — Pallor > flushing
   — Hypertension > hypotension
   — Constipation > diarrhea
   — Cardiomyopathy > valve defects
6 **C**omplications
   — **C**onstipation
   — **C**ardiomyopathy
   — **C**erebral hemorrhage
   — **C**holelithiasis
   — **C**hronic renal failure
   — **C**arcinoma (medullary) of thyroid (MEN2; p. 7)
   — **C**ushing's syndrome (ACTH secretion by tumor)

DISORDERS OF GROWTH AND DEVELOPMENT

Presentations of congenital adrenal hyperplasia
1 21-hydroxylase deficiency (*CYP21* gene mutation)
   — Commonest (90%) subtype; allele → 1:50*
   — ↓ Aldosterone/cortisol → hypotension, salt-wasting
   — *Secondary* ↑ ACTH → ↑ androgens (incl. testosterone)
     • Precocious puberty in males (but *atrophic* testes)
     • Virilization in females ('ambiguous genitalia')
   — ↑ Urinary 17-hydroxysteroids (e.g. 17-hydroxyprogesterone)
   — ↓ Plasma renin activity

2 3-β-hydroxysteroid dehydrogenase‡ deficiency
— ↓ Cortisol/aldosterone → Hypotension, salt-wasting
— ↓ Testosterone (primary) → sexual infantilism
• Male pseudohermaphroditism
— Secondary ↑ ACTH → ↑ DHEA (weak androgen) →
• Female virilization
— ↑ Urinary 17-ketosteroids
3 11-β-hydroxylase deficiency (apparent mineralocorticoid excess)
— ↓ Cortisol/aldosterone → ↑ 11-desoxycorticosterone
• Hypertension (in 70%)
— ↑ ACTH → ↑ androgens (like 21-hydroxylase deficiency)
• Precocious puberty, virilization
— ↑ Urinary 17-hydroxy- *and* 17-ketosteroids
4 17-α-hydroxylase deficiency
— ↓ Cortisol → 2° ↑ aldosterone → hypertension, ↓ K+
— ↓ Testosterone → sexual infantilism
• Male pseudohermaphroditism
• Primary amenorrhea in females
— Urinary 17-hydroxysteroids and 17-ketosteroids
5 18-hydroxylase deficiency (very rare)
— ↓ Aldosterone → salt-wasting
— Normal cortisol/ACTH/androgens; no genital defects
— Normal 17-hydroxysteroids and 17-ketosteroids
— ↑ Plasma renin activity

* Heterozygotes detectable by post-ACTH ratio of 17-hydroxyprogesterone to 11-desoxycorticosterone (< 12 in normals, > 12 in heterozygotes)
‡ Inhibited by licorice ingestion (causes transient hypertension)

Differential diagnosis of dwarfism
1 Dwarfism with normal limb proportions
— Growth hormone deficiency (e.g. hypopituitarism)
— Severe systemic disease
2 Dwarfism with disproportionately short limbs
— Achondroplasia
— Ellis van Creveld syndrome
— Hereditary hypophosphatasia

Symptoms and signs of adult growth hormone deficiency
1 Muscle wasting and weakness
2 Reduced energy, well-being and mood
3 Increased body fat
4 Decreased sweating
5 Increased anxiety

Physiologic concomitants of adult growth hormone deficiency
1 Decreased cardiac muscle and function
2 Decreased bone density
3 Decreased insulin sensitivity
4 Increased atherogenesis
5 Increased LDL-cholesterol, apo B, fibrinogen, PAI-1

Aging-related endocrine changes
1 Menopause
— Caused by low estradiol levels
2 Andropause
— Caused by low free testosterone levels
3 Adrenopause
— Caused by low DHEA (sulfate) levels
4 Somatopause
— Caused by low IGF-1 (or growth hormone) levels

INVESTIGATING ENDOCRINE DISEASE

THE PITUITARY AND HYPOTHALAMUS

Tests of hypothalamic integrity
1 Insulin tolerance (stress, hypoglycemia) test →
— ↑ Cortisol (i.e. implies ↑ CRH → ↑ ACTH*)
— ↑ Growth hormone (GH; due to ↑ GHRH)‡
— ↑ Somatostatin, dopamine
2 Clomifene stimulation →
— ↑ LH, FSH (GnRH)
3 Metyrapone (11-β-hydroxylase inhibitor) test →
— ↑ ACTH (CRH)
— ↑ Urinary 17-hydroxysteroids
— *Exaggerated* response in (pituitary) Cushing's disease
4 Water deprivation test¶ →
— ↑ ADH (synthesized in hypothalamus)

* In *long-standing* hypoadrenalism, give tetracosactide (synthetic ACTH, Synacthen) for 2 weeks to prevent false-positives due to adrenal atrophy
‡ Note that direct GHRH stimulation testing may be an alternative to ITT for detecting GH deficiency in adults
¶ *Inappropriate* (dangerous) for diagnosis of *acute* diabetes insipidus, e.g. post-microadenomectomy

Contraindications to insulin tolerance testing*
1 Hypoadrenalism (unless pretreated with dexamethasone)
2 Ischemic heart disease
3 Epilepsy

* Note that for assessing HPA axis integrity following long-term steroids, a CRH stimulation test (or short Synacthen test) is almost as good as ITT

Tests of pituitary reserve post-hypophysectomy
1 TRH stimulation
→ ↑ TSH, ↑ prolactin
2 GnRH stimulation
→ ↑ LH, ↑ FSH
3 Arginine vasopressin stimulation
→ ↑ GH (in children)
4 Tetracosactide/ACTH stimulation
→ ↑ Cortisol*

* Indirectly confirming normal *long-term* ACTH release. Value at 30 min correlates with insulin stress test (i.e. with HPA axis function)

Investigating pituitary function*
1 Screening: serum levels of *target* hormones
— e.g. T4, cortisol
2 Serum levels of *pituitary* hormones
— e.g. TSH, prolactin
3 Pituitary hormone suppression (if *excess* suspected), e.g.

— Dexamethasone suppression (↑ ACTH: Cushing's)
— Glucose tolerance test (fail to suppress GH: acromegaly)

4 Pituitary hormone stimulation (if *deficiency* suspected), e.g.
   — Synacthen test
   — GnRH stimulation (see below)

* NB: So-called 'non-functioning' (clinically silent) pituitary tumors may be detectable by measuring the α-subunit of glycoprotein hormones (FSH, LH, TSH) in peripheral blood

Common endocrine deficiencies post-hypophysectomy
1 ↓ GH increment on stimulation (80%)
2 ↓ FSH/LH (75%)
3 ↓ ACTH/TSH (40%)
   — *Always* signifies need for replacement

Imaging the pituitary gland
1 Lateral skull X-ray with coned views of the pituitary fossa
   — Sellar enlargement (pituitary tumor, empty sella)
   — Double floor of dorsum sellae (may be normal variant)
   — Erosion of posterior clinoid processes
   — Suprasellar calcification (craniopharyngioma)
2 High-resolution coronal-plane CT with contrast
   — Obviates need for pneumoencephalography to demonstrate suprasellar tumor extension
   — Metrizamide cisternography excludes empty sella
3 Magnetic resonance imaging (MRI)
   — Investigation of choice for suspected pituitary disease
   — More sensitive than CT for microadenomas
   — Clearly localizes tumor microanatomy
   — Reliably excludes giant aneurysm

Differential diagnosis of an enlarged sella turcica
1 Pituitary tumor
2 Primary hypothyroidism (hyperplasia of TSH-secreting cells)
3 Pregnancy
4 Empty sella syndrome

Features of empty sella syndrome
1 Reflects arachnoid herniation via sellar diaphragm Pituitary is flattened against sellar floor; pituitary stalk may be laterally deviated
2 May be primary (congenital), or secondary to
   — Surgery, radiotherapy
   — Tumor infarction; classically affects obese hypertensive multipara
3 Most have normal pituitary function 15% have mild hyperprolactinemia
4 Degree of sellar enlargement correlates with probability of pituitary dysfunction
5 Factors making the diagnosis unlikely
   — Visual field defect
   — Erosion of posterior clinoids/dorsum sellae on SXR

Laboratory diagnosis of acromegaly
1 Diagnostic serology
   — Failure to suppress plasma GH with oral glucose load*
   — ↑ Plasma IGF-1 level‡

2 Supportive serology
   — ↑↑ Fasting morning GH (10% false-negative rate)
   — Paradoxical GH elevation following TRH, GnRH
   — Loss of GH circadian rhythm
   — ↑ Prolactin (in 30%)
3 Supportive radiology
   — Enlarged sella turcica (in 90%)
   — Enlarged frontal sinuses; increased skull thickness
   — Macrognathia, underbite, wide-spaced teeth
   — 'Arrowhead' tufting of fingertips; ↑ joint space
   — Heelpads > 22 mm thick (female), > 25 mm thick (male)
4 Confirmatory (post-operative) histology
   — Eosinophilic pituitary adenoma

* Currently the best test; normally suppresses to < 4 mU/L. *Random* level < 1 mU/L effectively excludes acromegaly. Levels < 5 mU/L throughout GTT, or on multiple random samples, indicate satisfactory treatment of acromegaly
‡ Reduced by effective treatment, e.g. with the growth hormone receptor antagonist pegvisomant (a peptide blocker)

Screening tests for growth hormone deficiency
1 Overnight urinary GH levels
2 Plasma levels of IGFBP-3*
3 Combined IGF-1 and IGF-2 plasma levels

* The main IGF-binding protein in serum

Diagnostic confirmation of growth hormone deficiency
1 Failure of GH rise following insulin hypoglycemia*
2 Failure of GH rise following physiologic stimuli
   — Exercise
   — Sleep
3 Failure of GH rise following pharmacologic stimuli
   — Arginine infusion
   — Clonidine

* Glucose < 2.2 mmol/L plus sweating, tachycardia; associated with significant mortality and long-term neurologic damage

Diagnostic pointers in diabetes insipidus (DI)
1 Definition: daily passage of more than 3 L of dilute urine
2 The water-deprivation/desmopressin sensitivity test may not distinguish pituitary DI (ADH deficiency) from primary polydipsia or partial nephrogenic DI*
3 T1-weighted MRI scanning reveals loss of the normal posterior pituitary hyperintense signal in most pituitary DI patients
4 The definitive diagnosis of pituitary DI is made by infusing hypertonic saline and then measuring the plasma ADH response

* Only diagnostic of pituitary DI if urine osmolality is < 300 mosmol/kg after fluid deprivation *and* > 800 mosmol/kg after desmopressin (cf. primary polydipsia, both > 800 mosmol/kg; 'full' nephrogenic DI, both < 300 mosmol/kg)

THYROID FUNCTION TESTS

A quick approach to excluding thyroid dysfunction
1 Suspected thyrotoxicosis? Order
   — TSH, *plus*

— Free T_4, *plus*
— Free T_3 (*if* free T_4 normal)
2 Suspected hypothyroidism? Order
— TSH* (if *primary* hypothyroidism suspected)
— Free T_4

* cf. plasma ACTH in Addison's disease – *no* use in monitoring cortisol replacement (*unless* elevation occurs during post-adrenalectomy cortisol replacement, indicating development of Nelson's syndrome)

Monitoring the TSH level: clinical significance

1 Elevated TSH in patient receiving T_4 replacement may indicate *non-compliance* (esp. if TSH fluctuates from test to test) rather than underreplacement. For this reason alone, it is reasonable to check the TSH and T_4 levels annually, even in stabilized patients who appear clinically euthyroid
2 Patients on T_4 suppression to inhibit regrowth of differentiated thyroid carcinoma should maintain the TSH level below the lower limit of normal (if not undetectable)
3 Asymptomatic patients with mild TSH elevations (< 10 mU/L) without microsomal (thyroid peroxidase) antibodies may be observed in preference to immediate thyroxine replacement. Note, however, that chronic underreplacement accelerates atherogenesis
4 Long-term suppression of TSH to below-normal levels (subclinical hyperthyroidism) may increase the risk of atrial fibrillation in those older than 60. Evidence that osteoporosis is also increased in this cohort, however, is inconclusive
5 T_4 suppression may be useful in reducing the size of small functioning multinodular goiters, but is contraindicated if the TSH level is already suppressed

Specific indications for T_3 radioimmunoassay

1 Suspected hyperthyroidism (T_3 toxicosis), esp. in elderly
2 Monitoring of thyroid status following discontinuation of antithyroid drugs
3 Diagnosis of amiodarone-induced thyrotoxicosis
— To exclude euthyroid hyperthyroxinemia

NB: T_3 is produced by TSH-stimulated thyroid gland; hence, typically *not* elevated in (say) factitious T_4 toxicosis

Clinical and biochemical spectrum of thyroid dysfunction

1 T_3 toxicosis
— Clinically toxic
— $\uparrow T_3$, normal free T_4
— Commoner
• In iodine-deficient communities
• In toxic adenomas
• Following ablative therapy for toxicosis
2 T_3 euthyroidism
— Clinically euthyroid
— $\downarrow T_4$, normal/$\uparrow T_3$
— Occurs in
• Compensated (early) hypothyroidism
• Ophthalmic Graves'
• Functioning adenoma

3 T_4 toxicosis
— Clinically toxic in 50% ('sick hyperthyroid')
— $\uparrow T_4$, $\downarrow T_3$
4 Sick euthyroid
— Clinically euthyroid (but sick)
— $\downarrow T_3$, $\uparrow rT_3$ (reverse T_3); $\uparrow T_3$ receptors
— $\downarrow T_4$ (often), normal TSH
5 Euthyroid hyperthyroxinemia
— Clinically euthyroid
— T_4 (total or free): variable TBG and total T_3
— *Normal* TSH rise in response to TRH stimulation
6 Pituitary hyperthyroidism
— $\uparrow T_4$, $\uparrow T_3$, $\uparrow$ TSH

Elevated T_3/T_4 with detectable TSH?

1 Euthyroid hyperthyroxinemia (see below)
— T_3, T_4 *normal* by equilibrium dialysis assay
2 TSH-secreting pituitary tumor
— Associated with $\uparrow\uparrow$ SHBG (± abnormal CT)
3 Thyroid hormone resistance syndrome*
— $\uparrow\uparrow$ Free α-subunit:total TSH ratio

* Usually due to mutant ligand-binding domain of thyroid hormone receptor

Differential diagnosis of euthyroid hyperthyroxinemia

1 Elevated thyroid-binding globulin (any cause, e.g. estrogens, heroin)
2 Familial dysalbuminemic hyperthyroxinemia
3 Hyperemesis gravidarum
4 Iatrogenic
— Iodine-rich drugs (e.g amiodarone)
— High-dose propranolol (blocks $T_4 \rightarrow T_3$)

Thyrotoxicosis with low radioactive iodine uptake

1 Thyroiditis (see p. 80)
— Subacute granulomatous (de Quervain's) thyroiditis
— Subacute lymphocytic ('silent') thyroiditis
• Post-partum painless thyroiditis
• Spontaneously resolving hyperthyroidism
— Chronic lymphocytic thyroiditis ('Hashitoxicosis')
2 Iatrogenic
— Recent iodine exposure (Jod–Basedow phenomenon)
— Incompletely radioiodine-treated Graves' disease
— Thyrotoxicosis factitia* (self-administration of T_4)
3 Neoplastic
— *Struma ovarii*
— Functioning metastases from follicular thyroid Ca‡
— Extrinsic compression of normal gland by tumor mass

* Characterized by low thyroglobulin levels
‡ cf. functioning primary thyroid cancer, molar hyperthyroidism or pituitary hyperthyroidism: uptake *increased* (as with Graves', toxic adenoma, etc.)

Indications for a TRH stimulation test*

1 Investigation of symptomatic patients with inappropriately normal (or elevated) plasma TSH
— TSH-induced hyperthyroidism (pituitary adenoma)
— Thyroid hormone resistance syndromes

2 Assessment following pituitary surgery or irradiation
   — Documentation of adequate thyrotropin (TSH) reserve following pituitary irradiation and/or surgery
   — Documentation of adequate treatment of acromegaly; i.e. TRH does *not* cause ↑ GH
   — Documentation of adequate excision of prolactinoma; i.e. TRH → *no change* in serum prolactin
3 Evaluation of hypogonadism with borderline LH/FSH
   — Delayed puberty (TRH → ↑ prolactin) vs
   — Hypogonadotropic hypogonadism (TRH → *no change* in prolactin)
4 Characterization of 'non-functioning' pituitary adenomas
   — LH/FSH (or β-subunit) rise indicates cell of origin

* NB: The advent of highly sensitive TSH assays has now almost eliminated this test

Abnormalities of the TRH stimulation test
1 'Flat' TSH response
   — Thyrotoxicosis (primary)
   — 'Euthyroid' patients with
     • Ophthalmic Graves' disease
     • Functioning adenoma
     • Recently treated toxicosis
     • Multinodular goiter
   — Other: acromegaly, Cushing's, L-DOPA use
2 Exaggerated or prolonged TSH rise
   — Primary hypothyroidism
   — Pregnancy

Common symptomatic indications for excluding hypothyroidism
1 Unexplained fatigue
2 Unexplained infertility
3 Unexplained depression or dementia
4 Unexplained dementia

Routine indications for screening to detect hypothyroidism
1 Neonates
2 Past history of
   — Pituitary surgery/irradiation
   — Neck irradiation (including for Hodgkin's disease)
   — Treatment of hyperthyroidism (e.g. radioiodine)
3 Addison's disease
4 Long-term treatment with lithium or amiodarone

INVESTIGATING THE DIABETIC PATIENT

Indications for a glucose tolerance test
1 Pregnancy
   — Glycosuria
   — Risk factors for diabetes mellitus
2 Non-diagnostic elevation of blood glucose *plus* glycosuria
3 Investigation of peripheral neuropathy

Abnormalities of the glucose tolerance test
1 Pronounced glycemia
   — Diabetes mellitus
2 'Flat' response
   — Malabsorption
   — Addison's disease
3 'Lag storage' curve
   — Post-gastrectomy
   — Thyrotoxicosis
   — Chronic liver disease

Indications for home blood glucose monitoring (HBGM)
1 Stabilization of any young or insulin-dependent diabetic
2 Gestational diabetes
3 Abnormal renal threshold for glucose (e.g. renal failure)
4 Impaired color vision (e.g. due to retinopathy + photocoagulation; hinders urinalysis interpretation)
5 Unexplained insomnia, anxiety attacks, angina or epilepsy

Factors elevating the glycosylated hemoglobin (HbA$_{1c}$) level
1 Hyperglycemia (in previous 8 weeks), esp. ketoacidosis
2 Hypertriglyceridemia
3 Pregnancy (first and second trimester)
4 Renal failure
5 Iron deficiency
   Hereditary spherocytosis (post-splenectomy)
   Elevated HbF (e.g. thalassemia: mimics HbA$_{1c}$)
6 Aspirin/alcohol ingestion

Factors depressing the HbA$_{1c}$ level
1 Reticulocytosis (e.g. hemolysis, hemorrhage) + anemia
2 Pregnancy (third trimester)
3 Assay performed in hot environment

Practical limitations of HbA$_{1c}$ measurement
1 Only reflects glycemic control over previous 8 weeks*
   Hence, *not* useful in monitoring short-term therapy; home blood glucose monitoring is essential for this
2 Fasting glucose measures may be more reliable in diagnosing and monitoring patients with type 2 diabetes

* cf. Serum *fructosamine*: reflects shorter-term glycemic control, thus may be useful during (say) pregnancy

Technical considerations in diabetic monitoring
1 *Arterial* glucose levels are higher than venous; capillary blood samples are intermediate
2 *Plasma* glucose is 10% higher than whole blood
3 Glucose metabolism continues (i.e. levels decline) in vitro at ~ 3–4% per hour (esp. in heparinized whole blood), making it imperative to use inhibitors (e.g. NaF, Li) and process samples promptly
4 Urine glucose monitoring is useless in patients with normal renal thresholds since good diabetic control should keep glucose below the glycosuric level

Urinary ketone detection and significance

1 Urinary dipstick tests detect reaction of only one ketone body (acetoacetate) with nitroprusside
2 Other ketones (acetone, -hydroxybutyrate) may predominate in hypoxic patients, yet be undetected by dipstick
3 Heavy ketonuria combined with glycosuria indicates developing ketoacidosis
4 Mild ketonuria can occur during fasting or pregnancy

HYPOGLYCEMIA

Predispositions to recurrent hypoglycemia

1 Inappropriate insulin regimen, e.g.
— 'Sliding scale' urinalysis with renal glycosuria
— Somogyi effect (see below)
— Inadvertent IM injections
— Low renal threshold, patient monitoring urinalysis*
2 Insulin sensitivity
— Renal failure
— Celiac disease; diabetic gastroparesis
— Hypothyroidism
3 Alcohol abuse
4 Absence of neuroglycopenic 'warning signs'
— Recurrent hypoglycemia (e.g. due to insulinoma)
— Coexisting hypoadrenalism ± hypopituitarism‡
— Autonomic neuropathy
— β-blockade (esp. non-selective)
5 Factitious hyperinsulinism or sulfonylurea ingestion Non-compliance, manipulative behavior (esp. adolescents)

* Largely a theoretical hazard these days
‡ e.g. post-hypophysectomy for retinopathy

Hypoglycemia without hyperinsulinemia?

1 Alcohol ingestion
— Inhibits hepatic gluconeogenesis (as does lactic acidosis)
— Usually presents as hypothermic coma in semi-starved alcoholics with depleted hepatic glycogen
2 Non-islet cell tumors (release IGF-2)
— Bulky mesenchymal tumors (e.g. fibrosarcoma)
— Hepatoma, adrenal carcinoma
3 Sepsis
— esp. *Plasmodium falciparum*
4 Physiologic
— Starvation
— Prolonged exercise
— Post-prandial (rare)
5 Iatrogenic
— Oral hypoglycemics
— Post-Polya gastrectomy (late dumping)
— Salicylism (in children)
— Propranolol (inhibits hepatic glycogenolysis)

Insulinoma: making the diagnosis

1 Clinical
— Symptoms (syncope, amnesia) on fasting or exercise
— Symptoms accompanied by low plasma glucose
— Symptoms relieved by glucose

2 Screening test: 3 overnight 16-hour fasts
— Blood sugar abnormally low in 90% of insulinomas
— Non-suppression of insulin (> 6 μU/mL) and C-peptide
— ↓ C-peptide/proinsulin? Factitious hypoglycemia
3 Supporting tests
— Elevated fasting insulin:glucose ratio
— High proinsulin (> 20% total insulin)
— Stimulation of insulin secretion by calcium infusion
4 Insulin (or tolbutamide) tolerance test
— Non-suppression of proinsulin and/or C-peptide
— Non-suppression excludes post-prandial hypoglycemia
5 Tumor localization and biopsy
— CT and/or angiography (initial work-up)
— Endoscopic or intraoperative ultrasonography

NB: Paradoxically, insulinoma may be associated with post-prandial hyperglycemia, since normal post-prandial ↑ insulin may be suppressed

Factitious hypoglycemia

1 Clinical: recurrent hypoglycemia in a (para)medically employed patient or member of diabetic patient's family
2 Grossly elevated plasma insulin during attacks
3 Low proinsulin and/or C-peptide levels (cf. insulinoma)
4 Insulin antibodies may be assayed if porcine insulin used
5 Sulfonylurea abuse may lead to elevated insulin and C-peptide levels, normal proinsulin levels and positive urine/serum drug screens

NB: Most iatrogenic hypoglycemia is *inadvertent*; cf. thyrotoxicosis factitia

NOCTURNAL HYPOGLYCEMIA

Nocturnal hypoglycemia: diagnostic considerations

1 Clinical
— Nocturnal distress, nightmares
— Mental dullness/depression
— Morning headaches and/or hypothermia
— Onset of idiopathic epilepsy
2 Overnight voided urine sample
— ↑ Cortisol:creatinine ratio
3 Confirm hypoglycemia
— 3 a.m. (inpatient) blood sugar

Nocturnal hypoglycemia: the Somogyi effect

1 Suggested by confirmation of nocturnal hypoglycemia associated with a.m. urinalysis → glucose + ketones
2 Pathogenesis: nocturnal hypoglycemia due to insulin overtreatment causes compensatory release of glucose-mobilizing hormones (e.g. cortisol, catecholamines) resulting in paradoxical waking hyperglycemia
3 For diagnosis, distinguish
— *Dawn effect* (greater endogenous a.m. insulin requirement) from

— *Somogyi effect* (where hyperglycemia occurs due to reactive, rather than circadian, excess of counter-regulatory hormones)

Nocturnal hypoglycemia: therapeutic approach
1 Supper late
  — Complex carbohydrate, protein
2 Extra supper if
  — Heavy evening exercise, *or*
  — Glucose < 6.5 mmol/L
3 Give intermediate-acting insulin
  — At bedtime instead of with the evening meal
  — In thigh, not in abdominal wall
4 Use longer-acting evening insulin
  — e.g. Isophane, ultralente

DIAGNOSING DIABETES AND ITS COMPLICATIONS

Rapid assessment of glucose tolerance using single plasma levels
1 Random (post-prandial) glucose < 8 mmol/L
  Fasting glucose < 6 mmol/L
  — Normal
2 Random glucose 8–11 mmol/L
  Fasting glucose 6–7 mmol/L
  — Impaired glucose tolerance
3 Random glucose > 11 mmol/L
  Fasting glucose > 7 mmol/L
  — Diabetes mellitus

Assessing diabetic treatment using glycosylated hemoglobin*
1 HbA_{1c} < 10%
  — Reasonable control
2 HbA_{1c} 10–14%
  — Control can be improved: ?compliance ?regimen
3 HbA_{1c} > 15%
  — Treatment plan needs major overhaul

* HbA_{1c} normal range = 5–8.5%

Hyperosmolar coma: making the diagnosis
1 Blood glucose level > 50 mmol/L
  Serum osmolality < 350 mosmol/L
2 Minimal or absent ketonuria and acidosis
3 Azotemia and/or hypernatremia (if severe or prolonged)
4 Plasma insulin usually detectable; lactate/alcohol usually not

Indications for renal biopsy in diabetes mellitus
1 Red cell casts or persistent (micro)hematuria (sterile urine)
2 Unusually early (e.g. no retinopathy) or rapid nephropathy

INVESTIGATING ADRENAL DISEASE

Diagnostic sequence in suspected Cushing's syndrome
1 Overnight dexamethasone (1–2 mg) suppression test
  — 10–30% false-positive results (see below)
2 Extended low-dose dexamethasone suppression
  — 0.5 mg q 6 h for 48 h; collect urine for free cortisol
  — Best single screening test
3 24-h urinary free cortisol
  — Unless renal impairment
4 Plasma ACTH
5 8 a.m. and midnight cortisol levels
6 CRH stimulation test
  — Establishes ACTH-dependency (see below)
  — Distinguishes pituitary and ectopic ACTH*
7 MRI of sella with gadolinium and T1-weighted images
  CT of adrenals (± thorax, abdomen if ectopic ACTH)

NB: No *single* test should be relied upon
* Distinguishes pituitary Cushing's from ectopic ACTH syndrome

False-positive 1 mg dexamethasone suppression tests*
1 Simple obesity (cf. false-negatives: rare)
2 Non-compliance (check dexamethasone level)
3 Depression
4 Alcoholism
5 Iatrogenic
  — Estrogens
  — Antiandrogens: spironolactone, cyproterone
  — Phenytoin, alcohol, other enzyme inducers

* Occur in up to 20% of tests

Features of alcohol-induced pseudo-Cushing's syndrome
1 Vaguely 'Cushingoid' appearance
  — Central adiposity
  — Bruising
  — Myopathy
  — Osteoporosis, rib fractures
  — Hypertension; impaired glucose tolerance
  — Depression, psychosis
2 Typical biochemical abnormalities
  — Increased free plasma or urinary cortisol*
  — Decreased circadian rhythm of plasma cortisol‡
  — Overnight (1 mg) dexamethasone → no suppression
3 Spironolactone treatment for ascites may underlie some false-positive tests
4 Distinguished from 'true' Cushing's by
  — Extended (2-day) dexamethasone suppression followed by CRH stimulation test
  — Naloxone stimulation test: detects pseudo-Cushing's CRH *hyper*secretion (cf. true Cushing's: ↓ CRH)

* Esp. following (1) ethanol withdrawal, or (2) liver damage leading to impaired production of cortisol-binding globulin (CBG)
‡ *Poor* sensitivity and specificity for diagnosis of Cushing's

Features of 'food-dependent' Cushing's syndrome
1 Arises due to aberrant adrenal *sensitivity* to GIP (glucose-dependent insulinotrophic polypeptide; p. 124), presumably reflecting 'illicit' adrenal gland expression of GIP receptors
2 GIP hypersensitivity leads to *ACTH-independent* bilateral adrenal hyperplasia (may be nodular)

3 Ingestion of meals leads to elevated cortisol levels paralleling rises in GIP; *no* abnormality of GIP regulation or secretion
4 Responsive to octreotide or lanreotide (pp. 91–2)

ACTH-dependence of Cushing's syndrome

1 ACTH-dependent
— ↑ ACTH on CRH stimulation
• Cushing's disease*
• Ectopic ACTH (or CRH) syndrome
2 ACTH-independent
— *No* ↑ ACTH on CRH stimulation
• Food-(GIP receptor)-dependent Cushing's
• Adrenocortical tumors (cortisol-secreting)

* NB: Peripheral plasma ACTH levels are often in the normal range – rather than elevated – in pituitary Cushing's. ACTH levels from the inferior petrosal sinus may be of greater sensitivity here (see below)

Etiological clues in established Cushing's syndrome

1 Pituitary Cushing's ('disease')
— High-dose (8 mg/day) dexamethasone → cortisol *suppression* (< 10% basal levels)
— CRH test → *normal* ↑ ACTH (in 90%)
— Inferior petrosal sinus ACTH at least double plasma ACTH (cf. in ectopic ACTH: < 1.8)
— Petrosal sinus sampling also *lateralizes* pituitary lesion following CRH stimulation
2 Primary adrenal adenoma
— Plasma ACTH undetectable; no rise with CRH
— ^{75}Se/NP59 scanning: lateralizes lesion (cf. hyperplasia)
3 Primary adrenal carcinoma
— Urinary cortisol excretion may exceed 5000 nmol/24 h
— Plasma ACTH undetectable
— ↑ DHEA/urinary 17-ketosteroids
— ↑ Testosterone in females
— ^{75}Selenium scanning if lesion not visible on CT*
4 Ectopic ACTH secretion
— Absolute plasma ACTH level may exceed 500 ng/L
— Urinary cortisol excretion may exceed 5000 nmol/24 h
— Metyrapone/CRH test → no (further) ↑ ACTH‡
5 Alcohol- or depression-induced pseudo-Cushing's syndrome
— Normal insulin hypoglycemia test (p. 84)

* Adrenal nodular hyperplasia may occur in pituitary Cushing's; hence, visualization of adrenal nodule is *not* diagnostic of primary adrenal tumor. Note also that NP59 scan is often *negative* in adrenal carcinoma
‡ Exception: ACTH-secreting bronchial carcinoids. Note also that tumors may secrete 'big ACTH' which can be missed by some ACTH assays

Diagnostic approach to the patient with an adrenal mass

1 Key symptoms and signs
— Hypertension
• Absent? Pheo-, Conn's, Cushing's *unlikely*
— Hirsuties, virilization
• Assay plasma androgens (DHEA, testosterone)
— Obesity
• Absence makes Cushing's unlikely

2 Key investigations
— Hypokalemia
• Absence virtually excludes Conn's
— CT mass > 6 cm diameter
• Favors carcinoma over other lesions
— Urinary VMA, metanephrines, catecholamines
• To exclude pheochromocytoma

Conn's syndrome (primary hyperaldosteronism): diagnosis

1 Suggestive presentations
— Unexpected occurrence of severe hypokalemia in a mild hypertensive on diuretic therapy
— *Untreated* hypertensive with hypokalemia and urinary postassium excretion > 30 mmol/24 h*
2 Proposed screening tests
— Lack of aldosterone suppressibility despite
• High-salt diet or IV sodium loading
• Oral fludrocortisone or captopril
— Aldosterone elevation following IV metoclopramide
— Plasma renin activity suppressed
— Plasma aldosterone:renin ratio > 30:1
— High-salt diet (→ *persistent* hypokalemia)
3 Dexamethasone suppression test *if* screening test positive
— Glucocorticoid-suppressible hyperaldosteronism (see below)
— Suppressibility contraindicates laparotomy
4 Tests distinguishing aldosterone-producing adenomas (70%) from bilateral adrenal hyperplasia (30%)
— Angiotensin II or postural test → *no* ↑ aldosterone if adenoma
— CT scan → unilateral adrenal enlargement
— Selenocholesterol (or NP59) scan
— Venous catheterization + effluent analysis
— Biopsy (cf. excision: *only* indicated for adenoma)

* NB: Untreated renovascular or 'malignant' hypertension may also be associated with hypokalemia due to secondary hyperaldosteronism

Features of glucocorticoid-suppressible aldosteronism

1 Associated with 8q22 genetic locus
2 Autosomal dominant disorder presenting in children and young adults
3 Often associated with family history of CVA or labile hypertension
4 Causes ACTH-driven hyperaldosteronism
5 Urinary 18-oxocortisol excretion is elevated (cf. adrenal hyperplasia)

Liddle's syndrome (pseudohyperaldosteronism): diagnosis

1 Hypertension
2 Low aldosterone levels
3 Responds to salt restriction or triamterene

Bartter's syndrome (primary hyperreninemia): diagnosis

1 Usually presents in childhood with failure to thrive, enuresis (due to potassium-depletion nephropathy) and weakness

2 Normotensive (intravascular hypovolemia); no edema
3 Low serum potassium, elevated urinary potassium Hypochloremic metabolic alkalosis
4 Elevated urinary chloride*
5 Insensitivity to IV angiotensin or vasopressin Hypersensitivity to IV saralasin‡ or captopril
6 Therapeutic response to indometacin

* cf. diuretic abuse, laxative abuse, surreptitious bulimic vomiting; p. 233
‡ An angiotensin II inhibitor

Pheochromocytoma: how to diagnose your first
1 24-h urinary free catecholamines/VMA
2 Plasma adrenaline/noradrenaline: sample taken at rest via an indwelling needle inserted 30 min previously
3 Pentolinium (or clonidine) catecholamine suppression test
4 Whole-body ^{131}I-MIBG scanning*
5 Abdominal CT scanning
6 Selective venous sampling, or angiography (premedicate with the β-blocker phenoxybenzamine for 3 days first)

NB: No *single* investigation excludes the diagnosis
* Esp. useful for extra-adrenal, multiple or metastatic pheo's

Secondary adrenal insufficiency after long-term steroids?
1 Short Synacthen (tetracosactide) test
2 CRH stimulation test
3 Insulin tolerance test (p. 84)

MANAGING ENDOCRINE DISEASE

Pituitary tumors: therapeutic considerations
1 Transsphenoidal microadenomectomy
   — Good results in Cushing's disease, esp. in children
   — Complications: CSF rhinorrhea, diabetes insipidus
   — 10 year recurrence rate averages 25%
2 Transfrontal hypophysectomy
   — Treatment of choice for patients with macroadenomas and/or visual symptoms or signs
   — Usual first-line treatment for craniopharyngioma
3 Radiotherapy (incl. ^{90}yttrium implantation)
   — Reduction of adenoma size/function may take *years**
   — High incidence of subsequent hypopituitarism
   — Occasionally complicated by (late) pituitary apoplexy
4 Medical management
   — Somatostatin analogs
     • Octreotide or lanreotide, esp. for acromegaly → tumor shrinkage in up to 50%
     • Add UDCA to prevent gallstones
   — D$_2$ receptor agonists‡
     • Cabergoline, lisuride, pergolide, quinagolide
     • Bromocriptine (less effective than cabergoline, quinagolide)

   — Metyrapone (11-β-hydroxylase inhibitor)
     • For Cushing's disease presurgery
5 Bilateral adrenalectomy
   — For Cushing's disease *not* cured by adenomectomy
   — Must also irradiate pituitary to prevent Nelson's

* Hence, *inappropriate* for patients with visual symptoms or infertility
‡ *First-line* therapy for prolactinomas or hyperprolactinemic hypogonadism

Replacement therapy in panhypopituitarism
1 Cortisone acetate 25 mg mane, 12.5 mg nocte*
2 Levothyroxine 100–150 μg/day
3 Intranasal dDAVP 2–6 times per day
4 Conception not desired
   — Females: daily combined oral contraceptive pill
   — Males: IM testosterone enantate every 2–3 weeks
5 Conception desired: short-term administration of
   — FSH, *or*
   — HCG, *or*
   — Low-dose pulsatile GnRH analogs

* May monitor adequacy of replacement with plasma renin activity

Metabolic effects of growth hormone replacement
1 Increased lean body mass (anabolic effect)*
2 Increased basal metabolic rate
3 Increased muscle strength, heart and exercise capacity
4 Increased bone mass, density (and turnover)
5 Increased GFR, renal plasma flow
6 Increased plasma glucose (catabolic effect)
7 Reduced plasma LDL-cholesterol‡8   Sodium retention, edema
9 Improved sleep, social functioning, well-being

* Note that in *adults* no change in *total* body weight usually occurs
‡ But ? also ↑ Lp(a)

SOMATOSTATIN ANALOGS

Main physiologic actions of somatostatin*
1 Effects on anterior pituitary
   — Inhibits GH secretion (and thus IGF-1)
   — Inhibits LH release
2 Effects on gut and peripheral hormones
   — Inhibits insulin release
   — Inhibits gastrin and CCK release
   — Inhibits secretin release
   — Inhibits motilin release
   — Inhibits pancreatic polypeptide release
   — Inhibits VIP release

* A hypothalamic tetradecapeptide also present in gut – gastric D cells and small intestine, by far the most abundant source – pancreatic islets, and in the nervous system (myenteric and submucosal neural plexuses)

Indications for octreotide/lanreotide therapy
1 Acromegaly
2 Other pituitary adenomas
   — ACTH-secreting tumors

— TSH-secreting tumors
— 'Non-secreting' pituitary adenomas*
3 Other hypersecreting endocrine tumors
— VIPoma
— Carcinoid syndrome
— Glucogonoma, insulinoma
4 GIP-receptor-dependent Cushing's
5 Variceal bleeding
— Safer and cheaper than vasopressin
6 Anecdotal indications
— Polycystic ovary syndrome
— Pancreatic pseudocysts
— Pancreatic and enterocutaneous fistulae
— Secretory diarrhea
— Dumping syndrome
— Psoriasis
— Intestinal pseudo-obstruction‡

* May relieve headache within minutes
‡ e.g. due to scleroderma; R_x may reduce bacterial overgrowth

Problems with octreotide/lanreotide therapy
1 Expense; need for parenteral administration
2 Impaired glucose tolerance
 Diabetics receiving insulin or oral hypoglycemics may require close monitoring (glucagon release also inhibited)
3 May precipitate cholelithiasis (reduced gallbladder motility)
 Biliary colic (rare)
4 Reduces gut absorption of cimetidine, ciclosporin
5 Thyroid function may be altered
6 Abdominal cramps, tenesmus, flatulence (common)
 Steatorrhea (rare)

GOITER

Non-toxic multinodular goiter: management considerations
1 Reduction of nodule size using T_4 suppression (150–200 μg/day)* of TSH may be *less* effective if
— Goiter is long-standing
— TRH-stimulation test is 'flat'‡
2 Antithyroid drugs (thionamides) confer no benefit
3 Biopsy and/or thyroidectomy should be undertaken if no shrinkage within 3 months of conservative therapy
4 Carcinoma occasionally complicates multinodular goiter

* First ensure that goiter is not *already* associated with TSH suppression
‡ i.e. subclinical autonomous T_4 production

Failure of TSH suppression by T_4: differential diagnosis
1 Non-compliance with T_4
2 TSH measured too early (wait 2 months)
3 Increased dose needed (e.g. pregnancy, obesity)
4 Malabsorption of T_4 (e.g. due to colestyramine, sucralfate, phenytoin)
5 TSH-secreting pituitary tumor
6 Thryoid hormone end-organ resistance syndrome

Approach to thyroid nodules
1 Clinical characterization
— Multiple nodules? fixed? nodes? bruit? euthyroid?
2 ^{99}Tc scan
— 'Hot' nodule (1% cancer risk; exclude thyrotoxicosis)
— 'Cold' nodule (20% cancer risk*)
3 Ultrasound
— Smooth thin-walled cyst‡ → lower cancer risk
4 T_4-suppression
— Therapeutic trial for up to 3 months¶
5 Fine needle aspiration (FNA) cytology
— Negative cytology does *not* exclude malignancy (up to 25% of FNA results are indeterminate)
6 Thyroidectomy: partial or total
— Pending frozen section and operative findings

* i.e. increased malignancy risk; but *most* are benign
‡ Note, however, that cystic nodules per se are often malignant; i.e. ultrasound examination provides strictly limited reassurance on this score
¶ In practice, most solitary thyroid nodules *rarely* shrink in response to TSH suppression

Cytological diagnoses possible with fine needle aspiration
1 Thyroid cancer, esp. papillary*
2 Colloid goiter
3 Hashimoto's thyroiditis

* cf. follicular or Hürthle cell tumors: often require large bore needle biopsy or excision for diagnosis

Complications of thyroidectomy
1 Short-term
— 'Thyroid storm' (if thyrotoxic pre-op)
— Hypocalcemia (hypoparathyroidism)
— Recurrent laryngeal nerve palsy; hemorrhage
2 Long-term
— Hypothyroidism (may be late or insidious)

THERAPY OF THYROTOXICOSIS

Rationâle of dexamethasone therapy in thyroid storm
1 Prevents Addisonian crisis in patients with associated (albeit unrecognized) autoimmune hypoadrenalism
2 Inhibits glandular release of T_4
3 Inhibits peripheral conversion (activation) of $T_4 \rightarrow T_3$

Drugs inhibiting glandular release of thyroxine
1 Dexamethasone
2 Lithium
3 Iodine*

* cf. the *Wolff-Chaikoff effect*, where iodine inhibits organification/coupling

Pharmacological actions of propylthiouracil
1 Inhibits organification of tyrosine
2 Inhibits coupling of MIT (monoiodotyrosine) and DIT
3 Inhibits peripheral conversion (activation) of $T_4 \rightarrow T_3$

Management of thyrotoxicosis

1 Antithyroid drugs (thionamides: carbimazole/methimazole, PTU)
   — Usually given for 12–18 month therapeutic trial
   — 60% patients relapse (99% of toxic adenoma patients)
   — Occasionally used long-term in elderly patients
   — Ineffective in thyroiditis-induced toxicosis*
   — Agranulocytosis is the most notorious toxicity
   — Carbimazole preferred over PTU due to once-daily dosing
2 Radioiodine (^{131}I)
   — Takes 2–3 months to achieve response
   — Teratogenic; contraindicated if pregnancy possible‡
   — *Not* carcinogenic (cf. external thyroid radiation)
   — 30% will still be thyrotoxic after a single treatment
   — 60% will be hypothyroid within 20 years of treatment
   — Risk of deteriorating ophthalmopathy may be greater than with other antithyroid therapies
3 Subtotal thyroidectomy
   — Undertaken after thyrotoxicosis controlled (e.g. after 6 weeks of carbimazole + 1 week's iodine ± propranolol)
   — 30% will be hypothyroid within 10 years of treatment
   — Losing popularity now to ^{131}I

* cf. β-blockers: often the only treatment needed
‡ No longer contraindicated in young patients per se

Clinical monitors of response to antithyroid therapy

1 Slowing of heart rate
2 Weight gain
3 Goiter shrinkage

Factors predictive of prolonged remission to thionamides*

1 Small goiter
2 Reduction in goiter size on treatment
3 Mild thyrotoxicosis
4 T_3-toxicosis
5 Low or absent TSI titre
6 HLA-DRw3 negative

* Methimazole/carbimazole, propylthiouracil; inhibit organification of iodide, and coupling of iodothyronine

Relative indications for PTU > methimazole/carbimazole*

1 Thyroid storm
2 Pregnancy
3 Puerperium

* NB: In other circumstances methimazole is to be preferred; longer plasma half-life, and lower risk of agranulocytosis

Potential indications for β-blockers

1 Rapid control of symptoms during initial treatment
2 Thionamide hypersensitivity or toxicity
3 Preparation for surgery

Factors contributing to high-output thyrotoxic heart failure

1 Factors contributing to volume overload
   — Reduced systemic vascular resistance
   — Increased blood volume*
   — Increased diastolic relaxation
2 Factors contributing to reduced diastolic filling
   — Increased heart rate
   — Increased myocardial contractility (stroke volume)
   — Atrial fibrillation‡

* Treat with diuretics
‡ Slow ventricular rate with digoxin ± propranolol; larger-than-usual doses may be needed

Relative indications for ablative therapy in Graves' disease

1 Elderly patient
2 Poor compliance
3 Large goiter
4 Nodular change in goiter
5 Recurrent disease despite conservative therapy

Prerequisites for radioiodine therapy

1 Patient is not pregnant
2 Patient has been *already* rendered *euthyroid*

Relative indications for radioiodine therapy

1 Thyrotoxic patient relapsing following thionamide therapy
2 Thyrotoxic patient relapsing following thyroidectomy
3 Thyrotoxic patient normally treatable with surgery (e.g. toxic adenoma) but unfit for anesthesia
4 Euthyroid patient with metastatic differentiated thyroid cancer (esp. lung metastases from follicular cancer)

Indications for total thyroidectomy

1 Medullary thyroid carcinoma (± MEN2; p. 7)
2 Anaplastic thyroid carcinoma
3 Differentiated thyroid carcinoma involving both lobes

Indications for subtotal thyroidectomy in thyrotoxicosis

1 Thyrotoxic patient with large symptomatic goiter
   — e.g. SVC obstruction, thoracic outlet syndrome
2 Young thyrotoxic patient unable to tolerate thionamides
3 Young thyrotoxic woman desiring pregnancy

Graves' disease in pregnancy: management considerations

1 The placenta is crossed by
   — TSI (but not T_4) → fetal goiter
   — Thionamides: → fetal goiter*; teratogenic (PTU least)
   — ^{131}I (→ cretinism; teratogenic)
   — Propranolol (→ fetal bradycardia)
2 *Neonatal* hyperthyroidism (suggested by persistent fetal tachycardia) may pose greater risks than hypothyroidism‡
   — Intrauterine hyperactivity
   — Growth retardation, craniosynostosis
   — Increased perinatal mortality

3 If ultrasound reveals fetal goiter, fetal hypothyroidism may be confirmed by percutaneous umbilical blood sampling and treated by amniotic fluid injection of T_4

4 Thyrotoxic maternal Graves' disease may be treated with the smallest possible dose of thionamide and/or propranolol

5 Neonates may require thionamides for up to 2 months even if maternal antithyroid treatment has ensured fetal euthyroidism at delivery (TSI may persist in the neonate)

* Due to fetal TSH; may obstruct labor
‡ In contrast, mild non-autoimmune *maternal* hyperthyroidism may be less hazardous in pregnancy (to mother and child) than hypothyroidism; elevated maternal and fetal TBG elevations may 'mop up' excess

Therapeutic approach to Graves' ophthalmopathy
1 Assess severity
   — Clinical examination (p. 79)
   — MRI (or CT) scanning; B-scan ultrasound
2 Conservative therapy
   — Lubricating eyedrops, for
     • Corneal protection
   — Fresnel prisms, for
     • Diplopia
3 Medical therapy
   — Oral/IV prednisone and/or ciclosporin
   — Retro-orbital steroids
   — Botulinum toxin injected into affected muscle(s)
4 Radiotherapy
   — 20 Gy to retro-ocular tissues in 10 fractions (for motility impairment only, e.g. diplopia)
5 Palliative surgical therapy
   — Lateral tarsorrhaphy, for:
     • Exposure keratopathy
   — Muscle transposition/recessing, for
     • Ophthalmoplegia
6 Definitive surgery
   — Orbital decompression, for
     • Rapidly progressive optic neuropathy/retinal impairment
     • Severe ocular pain or inflammation
     • Steroid dependence

HYPOTHYROIDISM

Treatment of myxedema associated with ischemic heart disease
1 Begin replacement with low-dose L-thyroxine (e.g. 25 μg/day: probably safer than T_3 in this context)
2 Increase to full dose by 25 μg/day every 2 weeks; monitor symptoms (of angina, arrhythmia or failure) and ECG
3 Reduce digoxin if toxicity suspected (despite plasma levels)
4 Avoid β-blockers if bradycardic or borderline CCF

Common perioperative complications in hypothyroid patients
1 Intraoperative
   — Hypotension
   — Cardiac failure (esp. during cardiac surgery)

2 Post-operative
   — Lack of fever despite documented infection
   — Constipation, ileus
   — Neuropsychiatric disorder, esp. confusion

Rationâle for monitoring thyroxine replacement
1 Clinical assessment correlates poorly with TFTs
2 Chronic underreplacement accelerates atherogenesis*

* But be careful not to acutely *overreplace* (or even rapidly replace) a patient who has long been hypothyroid, precipitating ischemia

INSULIN THERAPY

Insulin varieties
1 Conventional insulins
   — Short-acting (duration 6–8 h), e.g. Actrapid
   — Medium-acting (duration 18–24 h), e.g. Monotard
   — Long-acting (duration 24–36 h), e.g. Ultratard
2 'Designer' analogs
   — Rapid-acting (better meal matching; onset 15 min, duration 2–4 h)
     • insulin lispro (reversal of proline-28 and lysine-27 in insulin B chain*)
     • insulin aspart (substitution of aspartate for proline-28 in insulin B chain)
   — Longer-acting 'designer' analogs (reduced nocturnal hypoglycemia)
     • insulin glargine (glycine/di-arginine)

* Prevents insulin dimer formation; hence, insulin lispro is monomeric. Receptor affinity is similar to soluble insulin, absorption is quicker (must eat immediately after injection) and action shorter, and the frequency of insulin-dependent hypoglycemia is 10–15% lower

Tight blood glucose control: benefits and uncertainties
1 Measures of 'tight control'
   — Mean amplitude of glucose excursion
   — Mean plasma glucose < 8.5 mmol/L
   — HBA_{1c} 7%
2 Benefits
   — Prevention/regression of retinopathy
   — Reduced microalbuminuria, ↑ GFR
   — Improved neuropathy
3 Problems
   — Increased frequency of severe hypoglycemia
   — No proven reduction of ketoacidosis
   — Retinopathy may *initially* deteriorate

Indications for using recombinant human insulin
1 Newly diagnosed diabetes
2 Lipoatrophy at porcine insulin injection sites
3 Proven allergy to porcine insulin
4 Diabetic pregnancy (? prevents fetal pancreatic insulitis)
5 Insulin resistance due to antibody production (rare)

Indications for commencing insulin in type II diabetics
1 Planned pregnancy
2 Progressive weight loss

3 Development of hyperlipidemia or vascular complications
4 Non-obese patients with poor glycemic control
5 Diet-refractory obese patients with poor glycemic control

Causes of insulin resistance in treated diabetics
1 Common
   — Poor compliance with insulin regimen
   — Obesity ($\rightarrow$ downregulation of endogenous receptors)
2 Acute
   — Acidemia (e.g. in ketoacidosis)
   — Profound hypokalemia
3 Circulating antagonists
   — Acromegaly
   — Cushing's syndrome
   — Pregnancy
4 Rare
   — Insulin receptor abnormalities
   — Pathogenic insulin antibodies (*very* rare)
5 Iatrogenic, e.g.
   — Thiazide administration
   — Steroid therapy

MANAGEMENT OF RETINOPATHY

Diabetic retinopathy: indications for photocoagulation
1 Proliferative retinopathy*
   — New vessels within one disc diameter of optic disc
   — Fibrosis, retinal detachment
2 Fresh hemorrhages
   — Preretinal and/or vitreous hemorrhages, esp.
3 Maculopathy
   — *Focal* photocoagulation controls early exudative maculopathy
   — *Peripheral* ('panretinal') photocoagulation is needed to control maculopathy due to edema or ischemia

NB: Do *not* photocoagulate macula or optic disc
* May also be treated with vitrectomy if no severe macular ischemia

Efficacy of retinal laser photocoagulation
1 Renders hypoxic retina anoxic, thus preventing further secretion of putative neovascularizing factors
2 Central visual acuity remains normal if therapy undertaken early, but visual fields constrict and night vision worsens
3 New vessels atrophy within a month of treatment
4 In general, argon laser is better for focal photocoagulation, while xenon laser is better for peripheral lesions

Indications for fluorescein angiography
1 To evaluate and follow up patients with significant retinopathy evident on fundoscopy
2 To evaluate patients with known retinopathy in whom visual deterioration occurs
3 To evaluate major changes in fundoscopic signs

4 To direct laser treatment in patients with maculopathy or proliferative retinopathy

NB: Fluorescein angiography is *not* indicated in patients without fundoscopic abnormality

Potential indications for vitrectomy*
1 Retinitis proliferans
2 Removal of vitreous hemorrhages if
   — Bilateral
   — Causing visual acuity < 6/60
   — Threatened retinal detachment involving macula
3 Failure of laser photocoagulation to preserve visual acuity

* A risky procedure that may lead to iatrogenic retinal detachment or painful neovascular glaucoma necessitating enucleation

SURGERY IN THE DIABETIC PATIENT

Perioperative management of insulin-dependent diabetes
1 Admit at least 2 days pre-op to assess glycemic control
2 Cease long-acting insulin and stabilize on short-acting and intermediate-acting insulin
3 Schedule operation for first thing in the morning
4 On day of operation, commence infusion of dextrose, soluble insulin (1–2 U/h at first) and KCl at least 1 h pre-op
5 Measure blood glucose q 2 h initially; aim for 5–10 mmol/L level; measure serum potassium q 6 h
6 Post-op, continue insulin infusion until first meal, then recommence preprandial subcutaneous soluble insulin in lieu of infusion, and commence intermediate-acting insulin prior to evening meal

Perioperative management of sulfonylurea-treated diabetics
1 Omit tablets on morning of surgery
2 If preoperative blood glucose > 15 mmol/L, cancel surgery and reschedule while stabilization underway
3 If preoperative blood glucose > 12 mmol/L, commence 'sliding scale' insulin titrated against blood/urine glucose
4 If glucose drops below 10 mmol/L while receiving insulin, commence dextrose infusion
5 Cease insulin when euglycemic
6 Once eating, recommence tablets if hyperglycemia recurs

ORAL HYPOGLYCEMICS

Postulated mechanisms of action of oral hypoglycemic agents
1 Sulfonylureas
   — Cause pancreatic β-cell membrane depolarization by closing the potassium–ATP channel

— Stimulate pancreatic insulin release and reduce glucagon secretion
— May also increase number of insulin receptors
2 Metformin (a biguanide)
— Suppresses hepatic gluconeogenesis
— Increases peripheral glucose utilization
— Increases anerobic glycolysis (hence lactic acidosis risk)
— Induces anorexia (and hence weight loss); therefore prescribe with meals, for overweight patients (including polycystic ovary patients on clomiphene), or after failure of glycemic control with sulfonylureas
— Unlike sulfonylureas, does not cause weight gain or hypoglycemia
3 Meglitinides (repaglinide)
— Short-acting sulfonylurea analogs (take before meals)
4 Alpha-glucosidase inhibitors (acarbose, miglitol)
— Inhibit intestinal brush border enzymes which break down sugars
— Hence, reduce post-prandial gut sugar absorption
— Hypoglycemic effect enhanced by colestyramine coadministration
5 Lipase inhibitors (orlistat)
— Inhibit intestinal fat absorption; cause steatorrhea
6 Thiazolidinediones (glitazones: e.g. rosiglitazone, pioglitazone)
— Activate peroxisome proliferator-activated receptor (PPAR)-gamma
— Reduce abdominal fat but promote peripheral fat deposition*
— May cause liver toxicity; contraindicated in liver disease or cardiac failure
— Useful for treatment of syndrome X (p. 81)

* i.e. anabolic, reduces basal lipolysis; cf. metformin (catabolic, increases basal lipolysis). Both increase insulin sensitivity and glucose transport, however

Clinical problems with sulfonylurea therapy
1 High failure rate
— 80–90% overall
— 40% failure within first 3 months
— Of those 'successfully' controlled, 25% per annum will need to be changed to insulin
— Of those successfully controlled in the longer term, 50% can cease drug treatment if challenged
2 Hypoglycemia (cf. metformin), esp. with chlorpropamide
3 Leukopenia/thrombocytopenia
4 Cholestasis
5 Photosensitivity
6 Weight gain (increased insulin availability)

Metabolic associations of oral hypoglycemia therapy
1 Drugs undergoing predominant renal excretion
— Chlorpropamide
— Metformin
Drugs undergoing predominant hepatic metabolism
— Glibenclamide
— Tolbutamide*

2 Drugs with long half-life (once-daily administration)
— Chlorpropamide‡
— Glimepiride
Drugs with medium half-life (up to b.d. administration)
— Glibenclamide
Drugs with short half-life (up to three times daily)
— Metformin
— Tolbutamide*
3 Effects on water metabolism
— Chlorpropamide $\rightarrow \uparrow$ ADH sensitivity (mimics SIADH)
— Glibenclamide $\rightarrow$ diuretic effect
4 Chlorpropamide $\rightarrow$ alcohol-induced flushing, esp if
— Family history of non-insulin-dependent diabetes
— No microangiopathic complications

* Virtually superseded by glibenclamide now
‡ Drugs with long half-lives are most likely to cause hypoglycemia. Drugs with short half-lives are thus particularly suitable for elderly patients

Predispositions to metformin-induced lactic acidosis
1 Renal failure, cardiac failure, respiratory failure
2 Perioperative (or other cause of hypoxia)
3 Liver failure, alcohol abuse
4 Severe infection
5 Radiographic IV contrast agent usage
6 > 2 g/day dosage
7 Associated cimetidine therapy

OTHER MANAGEMENT MODALITIES IN DIABETES

Principles of dietary management
1 Non-insulin-dependent diabetes
— 2000 kcal/day
— Regular exercise
2 Insulin-dependent diabetes
— Caloric restriction as required for ideal body weight
— Balanced diet: a variety of foods enjoyed by the patient
— Protein intake averaging 1 g/kg/day
— Approximately 50% of total caloric intake should consist of complex carbohydrate (high fiber)
— Restrict alcohol, refined sugar, saturated fats, salt
— Regular exercise program

Pros and cons of antihypertensive prescribing in diabetes
1 ACE inhibitors
— Advantages
• No hyperglycemic/hyperlipidemic effects
• *Improve* proteinuria/nephropathy
— Disadvantages
• Hyperkalemia
• May *impair* renal function in renovascular hypertension (reversible)
2 β-blockers
— Advantages
• Cardioprotective

— Disadvantages
  • Impotence
  • Hypoglycemia ($\downarrow$ awareness; prolongation)
  • Worsening of peripheral vascular disease
  • $\uparrow$ Triglycerides, $\downarrow$ HDL
3 Thiazides
  — Advantages
    • Cheap
  — Disadvantages
    • Hyperglycemia, hypercholesterolemia
    • Impotence; postural hypotension
4 Calcium antagonists
  — Advantages
    • No hyperglycemic/hyperlipidemic effects
  — Disadvantages
    • Postural hypotension

Useful drugs in diabetic autonomic neuropathy
1 Gustatory facial sweating
  — Amitriptyline
2 Gastroparesis
  — Metoclopramide
  — Erythromycin
  — Cisapride*
  — sildenafil (Viagra)
3 Diarrhea
  — Tetracycline‡
4 Painful neuropathy
  — Amitriptyline
  — Topical capsaicin

* May cause cardiac arrhythmias
‡ Efficacy is probably *not* via its antibacterial action

Anticipated problems in uremic diabetics
1 If managed with hemodialysis
  — Vascular access
  — Worsening of retinopathy
2 If managed with peritoneal dialysis
  — Hyperglycemia
  — Recurrent peritonitis
3 If managed with transplantation
  — Steroid-induced worsening of diabetic control
  — Severe and/or recurrent infections

CUSHING'S DISEASE

Treatment modalities in Cushing's disease
1 For adults, transsphenoidal microadenomectomy is best
2 Best indicator of surgical cure is post-op hypocortisolism
3 Bilateral adrenalectomy now only for failed transsphenoidal microadenomectomy in women desiring pregnancy
4 Nelson's syndrome (ACTH-secreting pituitary tumor) occurs in 10% adults (30% children) after bilateral adrenalectomy
5 ^{60}Co (heavy-particle) pituitary irradiation is used primarily in children; ocular nerve palsies may result
6 Medical management alone (e.g. cyproheptadine) may suffice

UNDERSTANDING ENDOCRINE DISEASE

Characteristics of hormonal action
1 Steroid and thyroid hormones
  — Lipid soluble; require plasma carrier protein
  — Long plasma $t^{1/2}$; easily measured in serum
  — Actions are gradual in onset (hours to days)
  — Hormone binding induces conformational change in nuclear receptor which then binds DNA
2 Polypeptide hormones and catecholamines
  — Water soluble; circulate free, bind membrane receptors
  — Short plasma $t^{1/2}$; serum levels hard to interpret
  — Actions are rapid in onset (minutes to hours)
  — Binding to membrane receptor proteins activates cytoplasmic 'second messenger' (e.g. cAMP) which transduces signals to nucleus

Prohormones: hormones requiring activation for function
1 T_4
  — Prohormone for T_3
2 Testosterone
  — Prohormone for dihydrotestosterone (DHT)
3 (Dietary) vitamin D_2 = ergocalciferol
  (Skin-derived *or* dietary) vitamin D_3 = cholecalciferol
  — Prohormones for 1,25–dihydroxyvitamin D

Peptide hormones with structural similarities
1 Glycoproteins with identical β-subunits
  — LH, FSH
  — TSH
  — HCG*
2 Large single-chain polypeptides with amino acid homology
  — Growth hormone (GH)
  — Prolactin (PRL)
  — Human placental lactogen (HPL)
3 CNS neurotransmitters
  — Melatonin
  — Serotonin
4 Receptor tyrosine kinase ligands
  — Insulin
  — Insulin-like growth factors (IGF)-1 and -2
  — Relaxin
5 Serine/threonine kinase ligands
  — Inhibin
  — Activin
  — Transforming growth factor-β
  — Bone morphogenetic proteins

* NB: Weak TSH agonism may rarely cause thyrotoxicosis in choriocarcinoma patients with grossly elevated β-HCG

Stress-inducible peptide hormones
1 ACTH/cortisol
2 ADH*
3 Prolactin
4 Growth hormone (in lean patients)
5 Glucagon

* Potently induced by nausea

BIORHYTHMS

Circadian rhythmicity of hormone release
1 Late afternoon
   — Prolactin*
2 Early phase of sleep
   — Growth hormone
3 Late phase of sleep
   — ACTH/cortisol
   — TSH, LH

* Hence, to demonstrate hyperprolactinemia, test in morning

Melatonin secretion: regulation and function
1 Secreted by pineal gland* during the night (darkness)
   Inhibited by light (even in some consciously blind patients)
2 Influences circadian sleep–wake rhythms
3 Implicated in 'jet-lag' pathogenesis. Taking 5–10 mg oral melatonin beginning on the day of travel may have therapeutic value
4 High levels may cause hypogonadotropic hypogonadism‡
   Increased levels also seen in anorexia nervosa

* Pineal calcification may indicate secretory hyperfunction
‡ Suspected to be due to inhibition of hypothalamic gonadotrophin release

Clinical spectrum of sleep–wake disturbances
1 Sleep onset insomnia
   — late to sleep but normal wake time
2 Delayed sleep phase syndrome
   — late to sleep and wake
3 Advanced sleep phase syndrome
   — both fall asleep and wake early
4 Early morning waking
   — common in elderly and depressed
5 Non-24-h sleep–wake cycle
   — common in blind subjects
6 Gross arrhythmicity of the sleep–wake cycle
   — e.g. due to hypothalamic lesions or fatal familial insomnia

HORMONE RECEPTORS

Diseases caused by end-organ resistance to hormones*
1 Testicular feminization syndrome, Reifenstein's syndrome
   — Defective androgen receptors
   — Causes feminization or pseudohermaphroditism
   — Androgen resistance also due to 5-α-reductase defects
2 Albright's hereditary osteodystrophy
   — Associated with apparent resistance to PTH‡
   — Linked to constitutively activating mutations of adenyl cyclase-stimulatory G-protein subunit (G_s)
3 X-linked nephrogenic diabetes insipidus (XR)
   — Resistance of distal nephron to ADH
   — Due to mutated vasopressin V2-receptor

4 Type II vitamin D-dependent rickets
   — End-organ resistance to 1,25-dihydroxyvitamin D
5 Laron dwarfism (AR)
   — $\downarrow\downarrow$ GH receptors → $\downarrow\downarrow$ IGF-1 release
   — Treatable with IGF-1
   Pygmy dwarfism
   — $\downarrow\downarrow$ Plasma GH-binding protein (GHBP)
   — May reflect loss of GH receptors
6 Type A insulin receptor abnormality (AR)
   — Reduced number of insulin receptors
   — Linked with Stein–Leventhal (polycystic ovaries; p. 382)
7 Familial hypocalciuric hypercalcemia (AD; p. 235)
   — Failure of PTH suppression by calcium due to mutations affecting a calcium-sensing receptor
8 Familial thyroid hormone resistance (AD)
   — Due to dominant-negative mutant T_3 receptors
   — Most mutations affect T_3-binding domain of c-*erb*A
9 Familial male-limited precocious puberty (AD)
   — Null mutations affect the LH receptor¶
10 Familial isolated GH deficiency (AD)
   — Some cases due to GH receptor gene mutations

* i.e. all such diseases may be associated with *high* hormone levels
‡ (Pseudo)pseudohypoparathyroidism; some may respond to vitamin D
¶ cf. testotoxicosis: precocious puberty due to activating mutations affecting the same molecule; activating mutations affecting the stimulatory G-protein downstream of the LH receptor cause precocious puberty as part of McCune–Albright syndrome

Thyroidopathies associated with thyrotropin (TSH) receptor activation
1 Autosomal dominant non-autoimmune hyperthyroidism
2 Autonomously hyperfunctioning thyroid adenomas
3 Graves' disease (secondary to autoantibody production)
4 Differentiated thyroid cancers

Antibodies detectable in diabetes mellitus
1 Insulin antibodies
   — Usually seen in patients treated with porcine insulin
   — IgE type may mediate allergic reactions
   — Rarely associated with insulin resistance
2 Islet cell antibodies
   — May play a pathogenetic rôle in type 1 diabetes
   — Predicts young family members at high risk of IDDM
3 Islet cell insulin receptor-blocking antibodies
   — IgG-mediated reduction in receptor affinity for insulin
   — Associated with SLE-like phenotype
4 Islet cell insulin receptor-stimulating antibodies
   — May play a rôle in disturbed glucose homeostasis

Polyglandular endocrine syndromes
1 Schmidt's syndrome
   — Addison's + Hashimoto's
   — Hypoparathyroidism (±)

— Primary gonadal failure
— Diabetes mellitus
2 Candidiasis/endocrinopathy syndrome
— Hypoparathyroidism
— Addison's disease
— Pernicious anemia
3 Lipodystrophies
— Diabetes mellitus
— Stein–Leventhal syndrome
— Acromegaly, Cushing's
4 Albright's syndrome
— Precocious puberty in girls (predominantly)
— Cushing's syndrome, acromegaly (±)
5 Pinealoma
— Diabetes insipidus (ectopic location)
— Precocious puberty in boys (only about 10%)

DRUG INTERACTIONS IN ENDOCRINE DISORDERS

Alcohol abuse and glucose homeostasis
1 Hypoglycemia may occur due to
— Prolonged fasting
— Reduced hepatic glycogen storage capacity
— Impaired gluconeogenesis due to high NADH levels
— 'Reactive' to carbohydrate diet (i.e. ↑ insulin release)
— Acute potentiation of drug-induced hypoglycemia
2 Hyperglycemia may occur due to
— Obesity
— Chronic pancreatitis
— Insulin resistance due to elevated free fatty acid levels
— Induced hepatic metabolism of sulfonylureas with chronic ingestion (i.e. worsening of diabetic control)

β-blockers and glucose homeostasis
1 May predispose to hypoglycemia due to prevention of catecholamine-induced hepatic glycogenolysis
2 May lead to potentiation and prolongation of sulfonylurea-induced hypoglycemia due to lack of negative feedback on insulin release (esp. if α-agonism, e.g. labetalol)
3 Impair awareness of developing (systemic) hypoglycemia, with attendant risk of profound neuroglycopenia, esp. with non-selective β-blockade

REVIEWING THE LITERATURE: ENDOCRINOLOGY

3.1 Yaffe K et al (2000) Cognitive decline in women in relation to non-protein-bound oestradiol concentrations. Lancet 356: 708–712

High serum concentrations of free (bioavailable) estradiol were associated with a protective effect on cognition in this study of 425 women, suggesting that declining estrogen levels may contribute to cognitive impairment in a subset of ageing women.

3.2 Takala J et al (1999) Increased mortality associated with growth hormone treatment in critically ill adults. N Engl J Med 341: 785–792

Randomized double-blind studies of over 500 intensive care patients assessing the effects of high-dose growth hormone on survival; the unexpected result was that patients treated with growth hormone did worse.

3.3 Franklin JA et al (1998) Mortality after the treatment of hyperthyroidism with radioactive iodine. N Engl J Med 338: 712–718

Bartelena L et al (1998) Relation between therapy for hyperthyroidism and the course of Graves ophthalmopathy. N Engl J Med 338: 73–78

Two studies analysing outcomes of treatment for hyperthyroidism. The former is a retrospective population analysis of 7209 patients treated for hyperthyroidism, showing that radioiodine treatment was associated with increased incidence of vascular death, as well as of bone fracture. The latter is a randomized study of 443 Graves' disease patients with minimal ophthalmopathy, showing more frequent worsening of ophthalmopathy following radioiodine treatment compared with methimazole; this was transient, however, and could be prevented with steroids.

3.4 Bunevicius R et al (1999) Effects of thyroxine as compared with thyroxine plus triiodothyronine in patients with hypothyroidism. N Engl J Med 340: 424–429

Crossover study of 33 hypothyroid patients, showing that mood and neurocognitive function were improved in patients receiving T_3 in addition to T_4.

3.5 Adler AI et al (2000) Association of systolic blood pressure with macrovascular and microvascular complications of type 2 diabetes. Br Med J 321: 412–416

Gress TW et al (2000) Hypertension and antihypertensive therapy as risk factors for type 2 diabetes mellitus. N Engl J Med 342: 905–912

Two prospective studies documenting different correlations between diabetes and hypertension. In the British study of 4801 patients, all measured complications except for cataract extraction were significantly and directly associated with systolic blood pressure. In the US study of 12 550 non-diabetic patients, an increased incidence of diabetes developed in patients receiving β-blocker therapy, but not thiazide (or ACE inhibitor or calcium blocker) therapy.

3.6 Inzucchi SE et al (1998) Efficacy and metabolic effects of metformin and troglitazone in type II diabetes mellitus. N Engl J Med 338: 867–872

Schwartz S et al (1998) Effect of troglitazone in insulin-treated patients with type II diabetes mellitus. N Engl J Med 338: 861–866

Two of the first studies indicating a comparable antidiabetic benefit of thiazoledinediones (which increase the rate of peripheral glucose utilization via their effects on peroxisome proliferator-activated receptors) compared with biguanides (with metformin acting by decreasing gluconeogenesis) or insulin, respectively, in type 2 diabetes. Troglitazone has since been discontinued due to liver toxicity, but new drugs such as pioglitazone and rosiglitazone appear promising.

3.7 Chandalia M et al (2000) Beneficial effects of high dietary fiber intake in patients with type 2 diabetes mellitus. N Engl J Med 342: 1392–1398

In this randomized crossover study of 13 patients, glycemic control, hyperinsulinemia, and hyperlipidemia were improved by a diet highly enriched in soluble fiber.

3.8 UK Prospective Diabetes Study (UKPDS) Group (1998) Intensive blood-glucose control with sulphonylureas or insulin compared with conventional treatment and risk of complications in patients with type 2 diabetes (UKPDS 33). Lancet 352: 837–853

Meta-analysis of 3867 newly diagnosed type 2 diabetics, showing that tight glycemic control decreases the risk of microvascular but not macrovascular complications.

3.9 UK Prospective Diabetes Study Group (1998) Efficacy of atenolol and captopril in reducing risk of macrovascular and microvascular complications in type 2 diabetes (UKPDS 39). Br Med J 317: 6–11

Analysis of 1148 hypertensive diabetics suggesting that blood pressure reduction per se is the critical variable in preventing complications, not the class of antihypertensive agent.

3.10 Skyler JS et al (2001) Efficacy of inhaled human insulin in type 1 diabetes mellitus: a randomised proof-of-concept study. Lancet 357: 331–335

Open-label randomized study of 73 diabetic patients, showing no difference in efficacy or hypoglycemic frequency between the subcutaneous and inhaled insulin schedules.

CHAPTER 4

Gastroenterology

Physical examination protocol 4.1 You are asked to examine the gastrointestinal system

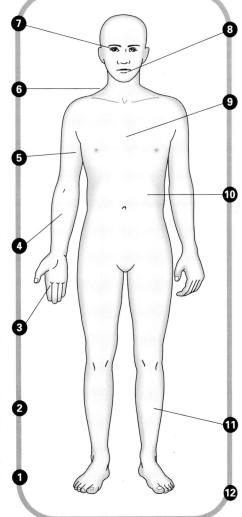

Eyes: xanthelasma, arcus (PBC)
scleral icterus
Kayser–Fleischer rings
nystagmus (Wernicke's)
uveitis (IBD)

Supraclavicular adenopathy
Parotidomegaly
Spider nevi

Proximal wasting/weakness
Absent axillary hair
Arthropathy (IHC)
Acute arthritis (IBD)

Skin:
scratch marks
pigmentation (IHC, Whipple's)
bullae, atrophic scars (PCT)
scleroderma
xanthomata

Hands: clubbing
leukonychia, koilonychia
palmar erythema
Dupuytren's contracture
flapping tremor

Overall appearance:
malnourished
unkempt
jaundiced

Introduce yourself
Position the patient
Obtain adequate exposure

Mouth and pharynx:
fetor
cheilitis, glossitis
aphthous ulcers
telangiectasia
xerostomia (PBC)
pigmentation (Peutz–Jeghers)

Gynecomastia

Abdomen:
operation scars
visible mass on respiration
flank distension; caput
palpate/percuss/measure liver
  and spleen
percuss ascitic level
roll patient to right, repeat
  ascitic percussion and
  splenic palpation
lie flat: ballotte kidneys
palpate inguinal nodes
check hernial orifices
examine perineum, genitalia
auscultate:
  bowel sounds
  venous hums
  bruits, rubs
  request PR examination,
  sigmoidoscopy

Edema (peripheral ± sacral)
Pyoderma, erythema nodosum
Peripheral neuropathy
Cerebellar examination

Urinalysis
Higher center examination

Diagnostic pathway 4.1   The patient is jaundiced. Why do you think this might be?

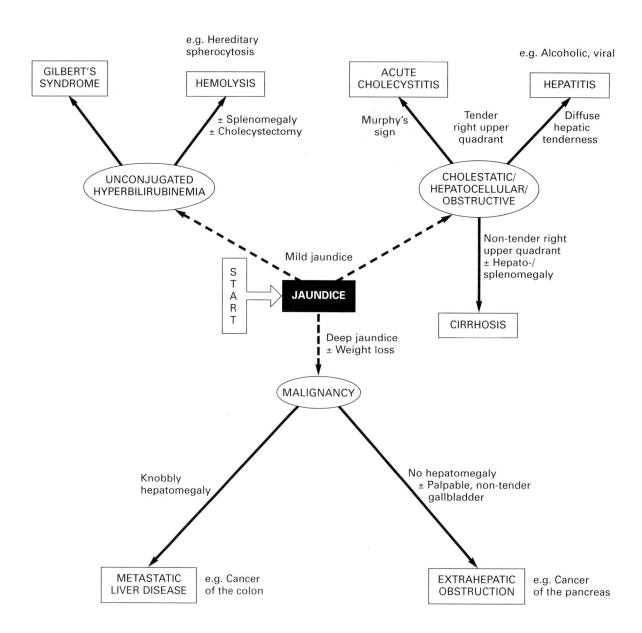

Diagnostic pathway 4.2   This patient is noted to have hepatomegaly. What is your provisional diagnosis?

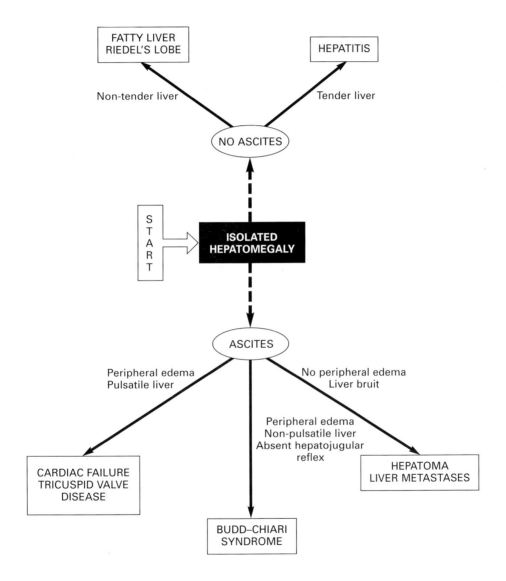

COMMON AND CLASSIC GASTROENTEROLOGIC PROBLEMS

Common gastrointestinal problems in clinical practice
1 Dyspepsia ± reflux
2 Irritable bowel syndrome
3 Chronic hepatitis

Classic gastrointestinal problems in clinical exams
1 Hepatosplenomegaly
2 Ascites
3 Jaundice

GASTROENTEROLOGIC EMERGENCIES

Acute management of upper gastrointestinal hemorrhage
1 Patients with known or suspected liver disease
  — Correction of coagulopathy and thrombocytopenia
  — Encephalopathy regimen (p. 118)
2 Hemodynamic homeostasis
  — Adequate transfusion (maintain Hb > 10 g/dL)
  — IV fluid and electrolyte balance (central line if needed)
3 Emergency surgery, e.g.
  — Oversewing of Mallory–Weiss tear
  — Partial gastrectomy ± vagotomy for bleeding ulcer
  — Total gastrectomy for erosive gastritis (last resort)

Effective drugs for gastrointestinal bleeding
1 Acute variceal bleeding
  — Octreotide (drug of choice), somatostatin
  — Vasopressin/terlipressin + nitroglycerine
2 Portal hypertensive bleeding prophylaxis (gastropathy, varices)
  — Propranolol, nadolol ± nitrates
3 Stress ulcer prophylaxis
  — High-dose intragastric antacids (in ICU)
  — Acid suppression with H_2-blockade, proton pump inhibitors (IV or oral)
4 Prevention of ulcer bleeding following initial healing
  — Acid suppression (e.g. maintenance ranitidine)

Endoscopic management of bleeding peptic ulcers
1 Injection of vasoconstrictors (e.g. adrenaline 1:20 000)
2 Direct injection of sclerosant*: ethanolamine 5%, or absolute alcohol
3 Uni- or multipolar electrocoagulation (diathermy), or thermocoagulation
4 Endoscopic hemoclipping
5 Nd-YAG laser photocoagulation
6 Band ligation

* NB: Risk of perforation

Bleeding esophageal varices: specific therapeutic options
1 Endoscopic variceal band ligation (most popular)
  Endoscopic injection sclerotherapy
  — Proven value in acute bleeding (not prophylaxis)
  — Potential complications: sepsis, esophageal ulceration

2 TIPS (transjugular intrahepatic portosystemic shunting): a radiologic approach
  — Used for failed banding or sclerotherapy
  — Hepatic and portal veins are joined by metallic transhepatic stent
  — Controls bleeding but risks encephalopathy
3 Other
  — Continuous infusion: somatostatin, (intermittent) octreotide, vasopressin
  — Staple-gun esophagogastric devascularization, or esophageal transection
  — Balloon tamponade (Sengstaken–Blakemore tube)*
  — Portocaval shunting‡

* Short-term measure, must remove within 24 h; justified only if varices will be ablated on removal
‡ Not of proven value in acute bleeding; 50% mortality in emergency shunting

CLINICAL ASSESSMENT OF THE GASTROENTEROLOGY PATIENT

Precipitants of morning vomiting
1 Pregnancy (rarely, trophoblastic tumors)
2 Alcoholic gastritis
3 Migraine
4 Intracranial space-occupying lesion

Diagnostic significance of macroglossia
1 In adults
  — Amyloidosis
  — Acromegaly
2 In children
  — Hypothyroidism
  — Down's syndrome

Recurrent alcohol-induced abdominal pain? Causes
1 Common
  — Alcoholic hepatitis
  — Alcoholic gastritis/peptic ulcer
  — Acute pancreatitis
2 Classical
  — Hodgkin's disease
  — Acute intermittent porphyria

Recurrent acute abdomen of obscure cause
1 Narcotic addiction (malingering)
2 Familial Mediterranean fever (± narcotic addiction)
3 Sickle-cell anemia
4 Acute intermittent (or variegate) porphyria
5 C_1-esterase inhibitor deficiency (p. 182)
6 Lead poisoning
7 Iatrogenic (digoxin, anticholinergics, erythromycin)

GASTROINTESTINAL BLEEDING

Common causes of recurrent gastrointestinal bleeding
1 Ulcerative colitis
2 Colorectal cancer
3 Hemorrhoids (diagnosis of exclusion)

Unusual local causes of recurrent gastrointestinal bleeding

1 Angiodysplasia (telangiectasia)
  — Often multiple
  — Tend to affect right colon
  — Higher incidence in elderly patients
  — Angiography may be required for visualization
2 Hemangioma
  — Tend to affect stomach, small bowel, or rectum
  — Typically gross (visible) lesions; cf. angiodysplasia
3 Telangiectasia
  — e.g. Hereditary hemorrhagic telangiectasia

Hematemesis in the alcoholic: pathogenetic considerations

1 Variceal hemorrhage
2 Peptic ulcer
3 Alcoholic gastritis (or esophagitis)
4 Mallory–Weiss syndrome
5 Coagulopathy

LIVER DISEASE

Clinical signs of portal venous hypertension

1 Specific signs
  — Caput medusae
  — Venous hum (rare)
  — Anorectal varices (*not* hemorrhoids)
2 Non-specific signs
  — Ascites
  — Splenomegaly*

* Insensitive sign; absent in 50%

Natural history of patients with symptomatic varices

1 One-third will die during the first bleed
2 One-third will rebleed within 6 weeks
3 One-third will remain alive after 12 months

Direction of abdominal venous flow: diagnostic significance

1 Outwards (i.e. from umbilicus)
  — Portal hypertension (caput medusae)
2 Upwards
  — Budd–Chiari syndrome or IVC thrombosis
3 Downwards
  — SVC obstruction

Clinical signs associated with alcohol abuse

1 Dupuytren's contracture
2 Parotidomegaly
3 Wernicke's syndrome

Differential diagnosis of palmar erythema/spider nevi

1 Fewer than five spider angiomata may be normal
2 Chronic liver disease
3 Pregnancy/oral contraceptive use
4 Thyrotoxicosis
5 Rheumatoid arthritis

Massive hepatomegaly: some causes

1 Fatty infiltration
2 Metastatic liver disease
3 Polycystic disease

Differential diagnosis of hepatomegaly and heart failure

1 Right ventricular failure ± tricuspid incompetence
2 Constrictive pericarditis
3 Alcoholic cardiomyopathy with fatty liver
4 Hemochromatosis
5 Amyloidosis
6 Carcinoid syndrome

Liver disease and splenomegaly without portal hypertension?

1 Chronic active hepatitis
2 Alcoholic hepatitis
3 Idiopathic hemochromatosis
4 Primary biliary cirrhosis
5 Infiltrations: sarcoid, amyloid

Helpful clinical features in characterizing chronic liver disease

1 Fever
  Ascites, edema
  Gynecomastia   } Alcoholic cirrhosis
  Dupuytren's
  Parotidomegaly

2 Pigmentation
  Hepatomegaly
  Testicular atrophy
    and hypogonadism
  Gynecomastia   } Hemochromatosis*
  MCP arthropathy
  Cardiac failure
  Glycosuria
  Usually male

3 Splenomegaly (often without
    portal hypertension)   } Autoimmune
  Prominent spider nevi   chronic active
  Often young (15–30) and   hepatitis‡
    female

4 Scratch marks
  Xanthelasma   } Primary biliary
  Pigmentation   cirrhosis
  Usually female

* Jaundice and ascites uncommon; in any case, most patients today are diagnosed very early on the basis of family studies and/or biochemical screening
‡ Pigmentation uncommon

Fever and abnormal liver function? Differential diagnosis

1 Acute viral hepatitis
2 Alcoholic hepatitis
3 Cholangitis
4 Liver abscess
5 Lymphoma

LIVER FAILURE

Features of hepatic encephalopathy

1 Grade I
  — Fluctuating confusion ± euphoria/depression
  — Inversion of sleep pattern
  — Slow, slurred speech

2 Grade II ('hepatic precoma')
 — Drowsiness, inappropriate behavior
 — Fetor hepaticus
 — Flapping tremor
 — Constructional apraxia
3 Grade III
 — Incoherent
 — Sleeps all day, but rousable
 — Hyperreflexia, myoclonus, extrapyramidal signs
4 Grade IV
 — Unrousable (comatose)
 — Extensor plantar responses

The flapping tremor: differential diagnosis
1 Hepatic precoma
2 Uremia
3 CO_2 narcosis

ASCITES

Ascites: sudden worsening in stable cirrhosis
1 Spontaneous bacterial peritonitis*
 — e.g. Coliforms (*Escherichia coli* 40%, *Klebsiella* 10%), *Streptococcus* (25%), *Flavobactenum* spp., TB
 — Predisposition: ascitic protein < 10 g/L
 — R_x Ceftriaxone, cefotaxime; prophylaxis with norfloxacin‡
2 Hepatic vein thrombosis
 — Budd–Chiari syndrome
3 Hepatoma
 — Associated with high AFP
4 Acute deterioration of hepatocellular function
 — e.g. Due to sepsis, alcoholic binge, gut hemorrhage
5 Rupture of dilated abdominal lymphatics
 — Causes chylous ascites

* Positive ascitic culture *and* WCC > 250/μL; cf. *bacterascites* (positive culture but WCC < 250/μL) and *culture-negative neutrocytic ascites* (WCC > 250/μL but negative culture)
‡ Not yet shown to reduce mortality

Differential diagnosis of chylous ascites
1 Intra-abdominal lymphoma or carcinoma
2 Hepatic cirrhosis
3 Nephrotic syndrome
4 Tuberculosis
5 Trauma (incl. surgery, e.g. distal splenorenal shunt)

Further examination of the patient with ascites
1 Abdominal signs suggesting primary liver disease
 — Ballottable spleen
 — Caput medusae, venous hum, testicular atrophy
2 Signs suggesting intra-abdominal malignancy
 — Absent ankle edema
 — Palpable supraclavicular nodes
 — Hepatic bruit
 — Palpable tumor (e.g. on rectal examination)
3 Signs suggesting cardiac etiology
 — Elevated jugular venous pressure ± 'v' waves
 — Pulsatile tender hepatomegaly

 — Cardiomegaly, S_3, tricuspid murmur
 — Pulsus paradoxus (constriction)
4 Signs suggesting hepatic vein/IVC thrombosis
 — Ascites > edema
 — Absent hepatojugular reflux (patient lying flat)
 — Upward-draining lower abdominal wall veins
 — Non-pulsatile tender hepatomegaly

Ascites: indications for diagnostic tap
1 First presentation with ascites (?infection, ?malignant)
2 Symptoms or signs suggesting sepsis
3 Hospitalization required for severe or refractory ascites
4 Unexplained worsening of ascites, or of overall clinical status

INTESTINAL DISEASES

Chronic diarrhea*: factors favoring organic bowel pathology
1 Nocturnal diarrhea (interrupting sleep)
2 Passage of blood per rectum
3 Steatorrhea
4 Weight loss; fever; anemia
5 Age at symptom onset > 50 years

* i.e. duration > 4 weeks

Differential diagnosis of chronic diarrhea
1 Inflammatory bowel disease
2 Malabsorption
3 Infection
 — Giardiasis
 — Amebiasis
 — *Clostridium difficile*
 — AIDS-associated gut infections
4 Endocrinopathy
 — Thyrotoxicosis*
 — Adrenal insufficiency
 — Diabetes mellitus
5 Spurious
 — Ca colon
 — Stricture
 — Ischemic colitis
 — Fecal incontinence
6 Iatrogenic, e.g.
 — SSRIs (e.g. sertraline)
 — Statins (e.g. atorvastatin, leflunomide)
 — Antibiotics, antacids
 — Post-gastrectomy
 — Radiation enteritis
 — Laxative abuse
7 Irritable bowel syndrome
 — Diagnosis of exclusion (but the commonest diagnosis)

* Also a rare cause of constipation

Diarrheal syndromes responsive to fasting
1 Osmotic diarrhea
 — Carbohydrate malabsorption
 — Laxative abuse

2 Non-osmotic malabsorption
— Steatorrhea
— Bile acid malabsorption
• After ileal resection
• After cholecystectomy
3 Incontinence

Inflammatory bowel disease (IBD): indicators of severity
1 Extent of colonic disease
— May not be ascertainable during exacerbation
2 Number of stools/day
— esp. If bloody; < 4 = mild, > 8 = severe
3 Constitutional
— Fever, tachycardia, pain, tenderness, distension
4 Weight loss
— esp. if > 5 kg
5 Blood count
— ↓ Hb, ↑ WCC/platelets/ESR
6 Biochemistry
— ↓ K$^+$/albumin
Acute phase reactants
— ↑ CRP
7 AXR
— Transverse colonic diameter (> 6.5 cm = severe)
— Subphrenic free gas (?asymptomatic if on steroids)
— Mucosal 'islands' (pseudopolyps)

Diagnostic clues in chronic diarrhea
1 Fever
— IBD, Whipple's
— TB, amoebiasis
2 Neuropathy
— Amyloidosis
— Diabetic diarrhea
3 Wasting
— Malabsorption
— Thyrotoxicosis
— Uncontrolled IBD
— Cancer
4 Lymphadenopathy
— Lymphoma, Whipple's
— HIV
5 Skin rash
— Celiac disease (dermatitis herpetiformis)
— Ulcerative colitis (pyoderma)
— Carcinoid syndrome (flushing)

Common sites of ischemic colitis
1 Splenic flexure
— Watershed of inferior/superior mesenteric arteries
2 Rectosigmoid junction
— Watershed of inferior mesenteric/internal iliac arteries

ENTERIC DYSMOTILITY SYNDROMES

Secondary causes of gut motility disorders
1 Diabetes mellitus*
2 Amyloidosis

3 Parkinson's disease
4 Myotonic dystrophy
5 Neurofibromatosis
6 Chagas' disease

* Gastroparesis may respond to sildenafil (Viagra) treatment or erythromycin (a motilin agonist)

Anatomic spectrum of gut motility disorders
1 Esophageal
— Achalasia
— Diffuse esophageal spasm
— Scleroderma
2 Delayed gastric emptying/gastric outlet obstruction
— Infantile hypertrophic pyloric stenosis*
— Scleroderma
3 Chronic intestinal pseudo-obstruction
— Autosomal dominant visceral neuropathy
— Acquired neuropathies
4 Megacolon
— Hirschsprung's disease (loss-of-function *Ret* gene mutation)
— Waardenburg's syndrome
5 Irritable bowel syndrome

* Associated with loss of nitric oxide synthase in pyloric sphincter neurons

Common presentations of irritable bowel syndrome*
1 Abdominal pain relieved by defecation
2 Chronic or recurrent abdominal distension
3 'Morning rush' (urgency, loose stools)
4 Sensation of incomplete evacuation
5 Passage of mucus in stool

* Diagnosis of exclusion, prob. pathologically heterogeneous

Differential diagnosis of irritable bowel syndrome
1 Psychological precipitant
— Depression
— Stress-related
— Laxative abuse
2 Inflammatory bowel disease
3 Colorectal cancer (if recent onset)
4 Endocrinopathy
— Thyrotoxicosis
— Hypothyroidism
— Addison's disease
5 Neuropathy
— Autonomic
— Lead poisoning
— Porphyria
6 Malabsorption, dietary intolerance
— Alactasia
— Gluten-induced enteropathy

Features favoring functional bowel disorders
1 Long-standing symptoms (years)
2 Vague or variable localization of discomfort
3 Symptomatic failure of all therapeutic measures
4 Non-specific accompaniments
— Tiredness, headache, insomnia
— Nausea, flatulence, easy satiety
5 Affective disturbance

INVESTIGATING GASTROINTESTINAL DISEASE

GASTROESOPHAGEAL DISORDERS

Investigation of dysphagia
1 Barium swallow*
— Good for confirming
  • Web
  • Pouch
  • Stricture
  • Achalasia
  • Spasm
— Reduces risk of endoscopic perforation in these disorders, esp. pouch
2 Endoscopy‡ ± biopsy
— Proceed to this even if swallow is negative

* Limited diagnostic utility for patients without dysphagia
‡ In general, this investigation is hard to beat

Investigation of non-dysphagic esophageal dysfunction
1 Is reflux present?
— Most precise test: 24-h esophageal pH monitoring
— Positive if pH < 4, esp. during sleep
2 Are symptoms due to reflux?
— Best test: therapeutic trial of proton pump inhibitor
3 Is there esophagitis/peptic stricture/erosion?
— Best test: endoscopy
4 Is a high lesion (e.g. pouch) suspected?
— Best test: barium swallow
5 Is mucosal disease (viral/fungal esophagitis, Barrett's esophagus) likely?
— Best test: endoscopic biopsy
6 Is there a dysmotility syndrome?
— Best test: esophageal manometry

Clinical varieties of esophageal dysmotility syndromes
1 Diffuse spasm
2 'Nutcracker' esophagus
3 Achalasia

Applications of radionuclide esophageal transit studies
1 May provide a non-invasive alternative to endoscopy in patients (esp. children) with suspected gastroesophageal reflux
2 Correlates well with manometry in assessment of dysmotility

ENDOSCOPY

Absolute indications for endoscopy
1 Gastrointestinal blood loss
— Hematemesis, hematochezia, melena
— Unexplained iron-deficiency anemia and/or positive fecal occult blood
2 Suspected esophageal disease without tissue diagnosis
— Progressive dysphagia or odynophagia
— Suspicious barium swallow
3 Suspected gastric pathology without tissue diagnosis
— Gastric ulcer on barium meal
— Follow-up of gastric ulcer
— Progressive weight loss, epigastric pain or vomiting

The dyspeptic patient: to endoscope or not to endoscope?
1 Endoscopy generally not indicated
— Self-limiting dyspepsia
— Known duodenal ulcer responding to therapy
— Typical symptoms of reflux or irritable bowel syndrome manageable with conservative measures
2 Endoscopy generally indicated
— Severe or persistent symptoms
— Refractory symptoms in a young (< 40 years) patient
— Recent onset of symptoms in patients > 40 years

HYPERGASTRINEMIA

Indications for fasting serum gastrin estimation
1 Family history of peptic ulceration
2 Multifocal peptic ulceration
  Peptic ulceration of distal duodenum or jejunum
  Recurrent post-operative peptic ulceration
3 Peptic ulceration with hypercalcemia (i.e. ?MEN1)
4 Intractable watery diarrhea or steatorrhea
5 Radiologic/endoscopic evidence of gastric rugal hypertrophy

Gastric hyperacidity without elevated gastrin?
1 Duodenal ulcer
2 Elevated plasma histamine
— Systemic mastocytosis
— Mast cell (basophilic) leukemia

Hypergastrinemia: differential diagnosis
1 *Gross* elevation (> 600 ng/L)
— Achlorhydria
— Gastrinoma
— Renal failure
2 Minor elevation
— Failure of patient to fast
— Antral G-cell hyperplasia/retained antrum
— Gastric outlet obstruction and/or gastric ulcer
— Small bowel resection and/or Crohn's disease
— Hepatic insufficiency
— Hypercalcemia
— Proton pump inhibitor or H_2-receptor antagonist therapy

Gastrinoma: diagnostic confirmation
1 Fasting hypergastrinemia (*plus* gastric acid output)
2 Tumor visualization by CT or angiography*
  (→ biopsy)
  Tumor localization by endoscopic ultrasonography
  Tumor localization by examination of proximal duodenum‡
3 Percutaneous transhepatic portal venous sampling

* Up to 50% failure rate
‡ Duodenal tumors may be ≤ 2 mm diameter

PEPTIC ULCER DISEASE

Pathogenesis of peptic ulcers
1 *Helicobacter pylori*
2 NSAIDs
3 Rare causes: Crohn's disease, herpes simplex, gastrinoma

Varieties of gastritis
1 Type A
   — Antrum not involved
   — Achlorhydria → hypergastrinemia
   — Associated with pernicious anemia and autoantibodies to gastric H^+/K^+-ATPase ('parietal cell antibodies'); hence, atrophic
   — Premalignant
2 Type B
   — Antrum involved
   — Hyperacidity → hypogastrinemia*
   — Associated with *H. pylori* infection
   — Premalignant‡

* But loss of antral gastrin-secreting cells is a more important cause of gastrin decline
‡ Predisposes to both cancer and MALT lymphoma; the latter may regress with *H. pylori* eradication alone

HELICOBACTER PYLORI INFECTIONS

Epidemiology of *H. pylori*
1 Progressively acquired from childhood at a rate ~ 1% per year
2 Higher prevalence in lower socioeconomic communities
3 ~ 30% adult prevalence in developed countries, ~ 70% in developing countries

Clinical manifestations of *H. pylori*
1 Non-ulcer dyspepsia
2 Atrophic gastritis and metaplasia
3 Non-malignant non-NSAID gastric ulcers
4 Duodenitis, leading to secondary acid release and duodenal ulceration
5 MALT (mucosa-associated lymphoid tissue) B cell lymphoma* or gastric cancer

* May regress following antibiotic eradication of *H. pylori*

Diagnosis of gastric *H. pylori* infection
1 Serology (IgG)
   — Useful for epidemiological studies of prevalence
   — *Not* useful for monitoring therapeutic response
2 ^{13}C-urea or ^{14}C-urea breath tests
   — Excellent for diagnosing active infection
   — Useful for monitoring therapeutic response

DIAGNOSTIC ASPECTS OF LIVER DISEASE

True liver 'function' (> damage) tests
1 Albumin
2 Prothrombin time

Elevated alkaline phosphatase: features favoring liver origin
1 Heat-stable isoenzyme ('bone burns')
2 ↑ GGT
3 ↑ Serum bile acids

Investigation of suspected alcoholic liver disease
1 ↑ Gamma-glutamyl transpeptidase (GGT)*
   — Induced by alcohol ingestion
   — May also reflect intrahepatic obstruction in cirrhosis
2 Blood film
   — Round macrocytes (*unless* coexisting folate deficiency)
   — Target cells (*non-specific* indicator of liver disease)
3 Biochemical profile
   — AST:ALT > 2:1, AST < 500 IU/L (cf. viral hepatitis)
   — ↑ Urate, ↑ triglycerides, ↓ Mg^{2+}, ↓ albumin (less specific)
4 ↑ Blood alcohol
   — If drinking within last 24 h suspected
5 ↑ Plasma AFP; abdominal ultrasound, gallium scan
   — If hepatoma suspected
6 Liver biopsy (see below)

* Alkaline phosphatase is also inducible, but less sensitive

Investigation of occult gastrointestinal blood loss
1 Fecal occult blood testing
   — For confirmation of bleeding
   — Negative testing does *not* reliably exclude bleeding
2 Endoscopy
   — Esophagogastroduodenoscopy and colonoscopy
3 Angiography
   — Detects angiodysplasias and small bowel bleeding
4 Small bowel series*
   Video capsule enteroscopy (if available)
5 Radionuclide studies
   — ^{59}Fe (oral) whole body counting
     • Good for assessing intermenstrual blood loss
   — ^{99m}Tc-labelled sulfur colloid (IV)
     • Detects *active* hemorrhage (> 0.5 mL/min)
   — ^{51}Cr-RBC or ^{99m}Tc-RBC labelling (IV 'blood pool scan')
     • May also be of value in intermittent bleeding
   — ^{99m}Tc pertechnate (IV)
     • → Ectopic gastric mucosa (Meckel's diverticulum)

* NB: Angiography *impossible* for days if barium studies performed first

Laboratory diagnosis of idiopathic hemochromatosis
1 Transferrin saturation
   — *Suspect* if > 55%
   — *Diagnostic* if > 80% (*plus* ↑ serum Fe, ↓ TIBC)
2 Serum ferritin > 1000 µg/L (best screening test)
   Serum ferritin increases following desferrioxamine
   Desferrioxamine-chelatable urinary Fe excretion > 7.5 mg/24 h
3 Mutation detected by PCR in *HLA-H* gene (Cys282Tyr is commonest)*

4 Liver biopsy: stainable Fe grade 3 or 4
Hepatic iron index‡
5 Quantitative phlebotomy > 7.5 g Fe

* Extremely important for diagnosis in Caucasians
‡ i.e. hepatic iron quantitation in μmol/g dry weight divided by the age; > 2.0 favors diagnosis

Distinction of hemochromatosis from alcoholic liver disease
1 Ferritin > 1000 μg/L (normal range < 300 μg/L)
— cf. Alcoholics: often 300–1000 μg/L
2 *Massive* iron overload on liver biopsy
— cf. Alcohol: moderate only
— Hepatic iron index > 2.0
3 Elevated ferritin levels
— In first-degree relatives as well as patient
4 HLA-A3 linkage
— An association only; *not* a diagnostic test

Diagnosis of hepatic vein thrombosis (Budd–Chiari)
1 Confirmatory investigations
— Doppler ultrasound of hepatic veins and IVC
— Contrast abdominal CT and MRI/MR angiography
— Hepatic venography
 • Thrombosis (± inferior vena caval thrombosis)
2 Supportive investigations
— Isotope liver scan
 • Selective caudate lobe uptake (hypertrophied)
— Liver biopsy
 • Centrizonal venous congestion

Biochemical characterization of jaundice
1 Conjugated hyperbilirubinemia
↑ GGT/alkaline phosphatase
Bilirubinuria, absent urobilinogen*
— Common bile duct obstruction‡
2 Conjugated (± unconjugated) hyperbilirubinemia
AST/ALT > 1000 IU/L
Bilirubinuria
— Acute hepatitis
3 Unconjugated hyperbilirubinemia
— Gilbert's, Crigler–Najjar
— Hemolysis

* NB: Urobilinogen *not* routinely measured now
‡ NB: Mixed patterns occur in early or partial obstructions

HEPATITIS

Differential diagnosis of chronic transaminitis
1 Hepatitis B or C
2 Alcoholism
3 Fatty liver (steatohepatitis)
4 Autoimmune hepatitis
5 Metabolic: Wilson's, hemochromatosis, α_1-antitrypsin deficiency
6 Drugs, esp.
— Statins
— Chinese herbs, shark cartilage, homeopathic remedies
— Illicit (e.g. Ecstasy (MDMA), phencyclidine, cocaine, glues)

Serologic investigation of acute hepatitis
1 IgM anti-HAV
2 HBsAg *and* IgM anti-HBc
3 Anti-HCV and hepatitis C RNA (PCR)
4 If above are *negative*, request
— IgM anti-HEV (or rising IgG anti-HEV)
— EB viral capsid antigen IgM
— CMV serology

Hepatitis B serology made easy
1 Presence of HBsAg implies active infection
Appearance of anti-HBs implies recovery and immunity
2 Presence of HBeAg implies patient is infective to others
Anti-HBe generally (not invariably) implies loss of infectivity
3 HBcAg (core antigen) cannot be detected in peripheral blood
High-titre IgM anti-HBc implies late, acute (usually severe) hepatitis B
4 Persistence of IgM anti-HBc or HbsAg implies chronic HBV (esp. CAH)
5 Presence of IgG anti-HBc indicates previous exposure to HBV

Mutant hepatitis B infections
1 Pre-core mutant
— Endemic in Mediterranean (e.g. 70% of all HBV in Italy)
— Negative HBeAg due to mutations of pre-core region
— Liver disease progresses despite anti-HBe, perhaps indicating cross-recognition of HBcAg by anti-HBe
— Positive HBV DNA
2 Surface gene 'escape mutants'
— Occurs post-vaccination, post-transplant
— Point mutation in 'a' determinant of surface gene leads to loss of immune recognition → reactivated HBV
3 Therapeutic significance
— Pre-core mutant: cannot monitor success of lamivudine therapy by reversion of HbeAg (ALT may rise during treatment)
— YMDD mutant may occur during lamivudine treatment
— Surface mutants: HBV vaccination may be less effective against HbsAg mutants

Diagnosis of hepatitis C
1 History of 'at-risk' behavior
— Injecting drug use, skin tattooing, ear piercing
— Blood transfusion, organ transplant
2 Anti-HCV serology
— Immunoenzymatic (ELISA-3) 99% specific
— May take up to 6 months to become positive (average 3 months)
— False-negatives in transplant patients; occasional false-positives in blood donors and in some individuals without risk factors but with cross-reactive antibodies
— ELISA results are confirmed by immunoblot (RIBA)

3 Plasma RNA PCR
— Sensitive, but some false-positives
— Mainly used for
• HCV diagnosis post-transplant
• Early diagnosis of acute hepatitis
• Perinatal transmission detection
• Monitoring of antiviral therapy
4 HBsAg and IgM anti-HAV negative
5 Abnormal liver function tests ± symptoms

Investigation of the patient with chronic hepatitis

1 If HBsAg and anti-HCV negative
— Request anti-HBc and anti-HBs
2 If HBsAg or anti-HBc positive > 6 months (chronic hepatitis)
— Request HBeAg and anti-HBe
3 If chronic HBsAg carrier deteriorates, request
— δ agent antibody
— IgM anti-HAV
— AFP
4 If patient is *not* proven to have hepatitis B or C, request
— Review history of medications, alcohol and illicit drug use
— Autoantibodies: smooth muscle/mitochondrial/ ANA
— Serum ceruloplasmin, 24-h urinary copper
— α_1AT level
— Iron studies
— Blood glucose and serum lipids

The stages of chronic hepatitis B infection

1 Replicative phase (→ acute, or chronic active, hepatitis)
— HBeAg+, anti-HBe
— HBV DNA+ (most sensitive marker)
— HBV DNA +++
— ↑ AST/ALT (T-cell-dependent liver necrosis)
2 Intermediate phase
— Cessation of HBV replication
— Acceleration of hepatocyte damage
3 Integrative phase (→ hepatoma; late complication)
— HbeAg–, anti-HBe+
— HBsAg remains + initially; then becomes negative as HbsAb becomes + (i.e. acquires immunity)
— HBV DNA becomes integrated into hepatocyte genome*
— AST/ALT normalizes

* i.e. HBV DNA becomes *negative* on *serum* testing

LIVER BIOPSY

Abnormal enzymes? Treatable diagnoses on liver biopsy

1 Chronic active hepatitis (esp. autoimmune)
2 Hemochromatosis
3 Wilson's disease
4 Granulomatous liver disease (esp. TB, sarcoidosis)

Provisional diagnoses contraindicating liver biopsy*

1 Hemangioma, angiosarcoma
2 Amyloidosis with prolonged bleeding time
3 Hydatid disease

4 Extrahepatic biliary obstruction‡
5 *Any* liver disease with uncorrected coagulopathy

* Associated with 0.01% mortality rate
‡ Predisposes to post-biopsy biliary leak

How to biopsy a chronically diseased liver

1 If prothrombin time, Hb and platelet count are normal, group and hold, then proceed with caution, including pre-biopsy ultrasound to image for liver abnormalities and to localize the liver (or, if available, real-time ultrasound-guided liver biopsy)
  If abnormal platelet function suspected, may be worthwhile to check bleeding time (debatable)
2 If prothrombin time abnormal and patient *not* jaundiced, give vitamin K 10 mg/day (IM, IV or SC for up to 3 days, or orally for 5 days) and repeat prothrombin time; if index < 1.3, proceed. If prothrombin time abnormal and patient jaundiced, give vitamin K (usually IM with anaphylactic kit ready) and check PT the next day; if normal, proceed
3 If prothrombin time remains > 4 sec prolonged after vitamin K (indicating major hepatic parenchymal damage), and if biopsy required urgently, cover with fresh frozen plasma (FFP). Check the prothrombin time following completion of FFP infusion, then biopsy. Further FFP may be needed post-biopsy.
4 If FFP ineffective, dispense with percutaneous biopsy altogether and opt for a transjugular biopsy catheter if histological diagnosis is still regarded as absolutely necessary

HEPATIC HISTOPATHOLOGY

Differential diagnosis of hepatic granulomata

1 Sarcoidosis
2 Berylliosis
3 Primary biliary cirrhosis
4 Infection: TB, syphilis, Q fever, brucellosis, histoplasmosis
5 Drug-induced: allopurinol, phenylbutazone, sulfonamIdes

Liver histology in selected disorders

1 Alcoholic liver disease
— Mallory's hyaline *(not* pathognomonic)
— Centrilobular necrosis
— Giant mitochondria
— Ballooning degeneration of hepatocytes
— Pericellular fibrosis → 'chicken wire' appearance
2 α_1AT deficiency
— PAS-positive globules within hepatocytes
3 'Chronic persistent' hepatitis
— Preserved lobular architecture (intact limiting plate)
— Minimal fibrosis
— Mononuclear infiltrate confined to portal tracts
4 'Chronic active' hepatitis
— Disruption of lobular architecture
• Piecemeal necrosis (erosion of limiting plate)
• Bridging necrosis
• 'Rosette' and pseudolobule formation
— Mononuclear infiltrate extends into lobules
— Councilman bodies, Kupffer cell hyperplasia

Differential diagnosis of 'disappearing bile-ducts' on biopsy

1 Primary biliary cirrhosis
   — Affects biliary ductules
2 Sclerosing cholangitis
   — Affects small and large bile ducts
3 Liver transplantation
   — Graft vs host disease
   — Chronic rejection

INVESTIGATING PANCREATIC DISEASE

Diagnostic confirmation of acute pancreatitis

1 ↑ Serum amylase
   — Good screening test, but frequent false-positives
   — False-negatives → hyperlipidemia-induced pancreatitis
2 ↑ Serum lipase
   — Most specific test
   — Equally sensitive as amylase
3 Urinary trypsinogen-2
   — Negative dipstick test reliably excludes diagnosis
   Urinary trypsinogen activation peptide (TAP)
   — Early positivity correlates with severity
4 CT
   — Detects necrosis, pseudocyst, etc.
5 ERCP
   — Not used just for diagnostic confirmation, as it may exacerbate acute pancreatitis
   — Used for removing bile duct stones in acute cholangitis associated with severe gallstone pancreatitis
   — Also used to sort out chronic pancreatitis (after MRCP)

Indicators of poor prognosis in acute pancreatitis

1 Clinical
   — Age > 60; first attack
   — Hypotension
   — Ascites (esp. with high protein level)
2 Hemorrhagic pancreatitis
   — Clinical signs
     • Grey Turner's sign (flank ecchymosis, esp. left)
     • Cullen's sign (periumbilical ecchymosis)
   — Methemalbuminemia
   — Low albumin; anemia; leukocytosis (WCC > 15 000)
   — Peritoneal lavage (confirms hemorrhagic ascites)
3 Reduced blood levels
   — ↓ Ca^{2+}*
   — ↓ PaO_2
4 Increased blood levels
   — ↑ Blood glucose
   — ↑ BUN, ↑ AST
   — ↑ Fibrinogen

* When corrected for albumin; cf. *elevated* calcium: exclude causative primary hyperparathyroidism

Pancreatic function tests

1 Plasma cholesterol, albumin, β-carotene*
   — Non-specific screens for fat malabsorption (if low)
   — 'False-positives' in liver disease
2 Imaging
   — CT
   — MRI/MRCP
3 3-day fecal fats
   — > 6 g/day confirms steatorrhea
   — Sudan III stool fat stain may suffice
4 Therapeutic trial of pancreatic enzyme supplements

* NB: *Folate* levels are normal in pure pancreatic insufficiency; hence, low folate plus steatorrhea suggests the need for jejunal biopsy

INVESTIGATING BILIARY DISEASE

Investigations of choice for gallbladder disease

1 Real-time ultrasonography
   — Quick, painless, non-invasive; difficult if obese
   — Risk-free: no radiation, no contrast hypersensitivity
   — High sensitivity for cholecystitis (incl. chronic)
   — Distinguishes obstructive from hepatocellular jaundice
   — May detect unsuspected non-biliary causes of pain
2 ERCP
   — Useful in post-cholecystectomy jaundice
   — Excludes false-negative ultrasound/cholecystography*
   — May be therapeutic (e.g. sphincterotomy, stenting)
   — Localizes obstruction in pancreatic/common bile duct
3 MRCP (magnetic resonance cholangiopancreatography)
   — Sensitivity for gallstone detection exceeds 90%
   — Technically superior to CT for bile duct examination; CT may be better for gallbladder visualization
   — As sensitive as ERCP for detection of pancreatic cancer
   — Non-invasive; hence, favored over ERCP for patients not suspected of requiring sphincterotomy or stenting (palliative drainage)
4 Percutaneous transhepatic cholangiogram (PTC)
   — Localizes obstruction when intrahepatic ducts dilated‡
   — Useful for draining bile in inoperable obstruction¶
   — Contraindicated in gross ascites or coagulopathy
   — Usually only done when ERCP fails (e.g. because of major risk of liver bleeding, or ongoing bile leak)
5 Cholecystokinin- (or fatty meal) enhanced ^{99m}Tc-HIDA hepatobiliary scintigraphy
   — Main indication: assessment of 'biliary' pain in patients without demonstrable gallstones
   — ↓ CCK-induced gallbladder ejection fraction in
     • Biliary dyskinesia
     • Sphincter of Oddi spasm
     • Chronic acalculous cholecystitis

— Ejection fraction < 30% may predict successful symptomatic response to cholecystectomy
— DISIDA preferred to HIDA in jaundiced patients

* For bile duct; reliability for gallbladder is less
‡ But ERCP better
¶ i.e. if stent placement proves impossible

Indications for ERCP
1 Suspected choledocholithiasis
2 Investigation and treatment of obstructive jaundice
3 Persistent symptoms following biliary surgery
4 Cholestasis without intrahepatic bile duct dilatation*
5 For diagnosis (or preoperative assessment) of chronic pancreatitis or pancreatic carcinoma
6 Stent insertion for acute post-laparoscopic cholecystectomy biliary leak

* i.e. cholestasis due to suspected biliary tract disease rather than due to medications or intrahepatic disease

INVESTIGATING INTESTINAL DISEASE

Indications for colonoscopy
1 Bleeding per rectum *or* occult blood loss
2 Persistent bowel symptoms with normal sigmoidoscopy
3 Dysplasia monitoring in long-standing ulcerative pancolitis
4 Surveillance for recurrence following surgery for Ca colon
5 Abnormal barium enema (e.g. stricture, polyp)
6 Diagnostic or therapeutic removal of colonic polyps

Contraindications to colonoscopy
1 Peritonism
2 Toxic megacolon
3 *Any* acute severe inflammatory colonic process
4 Pregnancy
5 Recent (< 6/12) history of myocardial infarction

Advantages of colonoscopy over barium enema
1 More sensitive for tumor/polyp detection
2 More accurate, esp. in sigmoid colon and cecum
3 May detect vascular lesions such as angiodysplasia
4 May be useful in emergency assessment of PR bleeding
5 Enables tissue diagnosis and polyp removal

Rectal biopsy: diagnostic value
1 Ulcerative proctitis
2 Amyloidosis
3 Amebiasis (and other infective proctocolitides)
4 Pseudomembranous colitis (though may spare rectum)
5 Solitary rectal ulcer syndrome (rectal prolapse)
6 Tay–Sachs disease, metachromatic leukodystrophy

GASTROINTESTINAL RADIOLOGY

Radiologic features of achalasia
1 Plain film
— Intrathoracic air-fluid level
— Absent gastric air bubble
— Lower zone lung fibrosis (bronchiectasis)
2 Barium swallow
— Tertiary contractions replacing peristaltic activity
— Dilated, tapering lower esophagus ('beaked', 'rattail')

Giant gastric rugae: differential diagnosis
1 Malignancy (e.g. lymphoma, leiomyoma)
2 Gastrinoma
3 Ménètrier's disease*

* Hypoproteinemic hypertrophic gastropathy

Jejunal ulcers: differential diagnosis
1 Ulcerative jejunitis (malignant histiocytosis)
2 Celiac disease, Crohn's disease
3 Gastrinoma
4 Meckel's diverticulitis (usually in boys; 5–10% bleed)
5 Mesenteric ischemia; polyarteritis
6 Lymphoma
7 Infection
— Typhoid, dysentery, syphilis, TB, actinomycosis, fungi
8 Iatrogenic
— Digoxin, potassium tablets

Multiple intestinal tumors? Differential diagnosis
1 Hereditary adenoma–carcinoma syndromes
— Familial adenomatous polyposis (FAP)
— Gardner's syndrome
— Turcot's syndrome
2 Hereditary non-polyposis colorectal cancer (HNPCC)
— DNA mismatch repair syndromes
— Muir–Torre syndrome
3 Hereditary hamartoma syndromes
— Peutz–Jeghers syndrome
— Cowden's disease
— Basal cell nevus syndrome
— Sotos' syndrome
4 Non-hereditary polyposis syndromes
— Cronkhite–Canada syndrome
— Pneumatosis cystoides intestinalis

Space-occupying lesions on liver scan: clinical significance
1 Thick-walled cavity on ultrasound
Gallium scan/^{111}In-WBC scan positive
— Pyogenic liver abscess
— R_x: Aspiration + antibiotics
2 Thick-walled cavity on ultrasound
Gallium negative; amebic serology positive (99%)
— Amebic liver abscess
— R_x: Metronidazole
3 Thin-walled cyst on ultrasound
'Daughter' cysts
— Hydatid disease*
— R_x: Open drainage (aspiration contraindicated)

4 Echodense lesion within cirrhotic parenchyma
AFP elevated
— Hepatoma‡
— R_x: Excision/transplant
5 Multiple echodense lesions
Biopsy positive for malignancy
— Metastatic liver disease
— R_x: Palliative chemotherapy
— Consider metastasectomy for resectable lesions
in one lobe (in colon cancer)

* Serology often inconclusive
‡ AFP > 1000 ng/mL obviates need for CT-guided biopsy

Abdominal imaging techniques: ultrasound or CT?

1 Ultrasound
— Advantages
• No radiation dose
• Quick and relatively cheap
• Good resolution of luminal structures (e.g.
biliary tree), cysts and abscesses
— Disadvantages
• Difficult in obese patients or if lots of bowel gas
• Less detail than CT
2 CT
— Advantages
• High quality images, esp. in obese patients
• Excellent delineation of retroperitoneal
structures (e.g. pancreas, psoas)
— Disadvantages
• Difficult if lots of bowel gas
• Not great for biliary tree (MRCP better if icteric)
• High radiation dose
• Time-consuming and expensive

MALABSORPTION

Diagnosis of bacterial overgrowth

1 High index of suspicion
— Crohn's
— Post-Polya
— Small bowel diverticulosis
— Hypomotility syndrome (e.g. scleroderma)
— Elderly
2 Low B_{12}
— Abnormal Schilling's test after intrinsic factor
3 ^{14}C-bile acid breath test (see below)
4 Duodenal aspiration and culture
— > 10^5 organisms/mL
5 Therapeutic trial of tetracycline

Diagnosis of lactose intolerance

1 History of milk-related diarrhea
2 Successful therapeutic trial of milk-free diet
3 Stool: pH < 6.5; Benedict's test positive
4 'Flat' lactose tolerance test (rarely used now)
5 Hydrogen breath test following oral lactose (best
screen)
6 Small bowel biopsy with lactase quantitation
(definitive)
— Primary alactasia: other disaccharidases normal
— Secondary lactose intolerance: all
disaccharidases ↓

Breath testing: diagnostic value in malabsorption

1 ^{14}C-glycocholate (bile acid) breath test*
— Bacterial overgrowth
• ↑ Deconjugation (small bowel) → ↑ Breath/
↓ fecal ^{14}C
— Ileal insufficiency
• ↑ Deconjugation (large bowel) → ↑ Breath/
↑ fecal ^{14}C
2 Hydrogen breath test (e.g. after oral glucose,
lactulose)
— Bacterial overgrowth
• Early H_2 peak (30 min; normally 2 h)
— Lactose intolerance (following oral lactose)
• 'Flat' H_2 response
— Indirect index of small intestinal transit time
• Early or late peak with ↑,↓ motility
3 ^{14}C-triolein breath test
— Steatorrhea ($→ ↓ ^{14}CO_2$ excretion)
4 ^{14}C-galactose breath test
— Galactosemia ($→ ↓ ^{14}CO_2$ excretion)
5 ^{13}C-urea breath test
— *Helicobacter pylori*‡
— Urea → ↑ NH_3 + $^{13}CO_2$

* Breath test now superseded by either (1) fecal bile acid
estimation for diagnosis of bile acid malabsorption; ^{75}SeHCAT is
used for this; or (2) therapeutic trial of colestyramine
‡ And other urease-positive gastric infections; not widely
available

Small bowel biopsy: diagnostic value

1 Celiac disease
— Villous atrophy, crypt hypertrophy,
mononuclears
2 Nodular lymphoid hyperplasia,
hypogammaglobulinemia
— Villous atrophy but *no* plasma cells
3 Abetalipoproteinemia
— Lipid infiltration
4 Infections
— Parasites (*Giardia, Strongyloides, Coccidia*)
— Fungal (*Candida, Histoplasma*) infections
— Whipple's disease (*Tropheryma whippelii*)
— Mycobacterium avium-intracellulare in AIDS
5 Other histopathologic diagnoses
— Crohn's disease
— Lymphoma, α heavy chain disease
— Intestinal lymphangiectasia

AN APPROACH TO DIARRHEA

Watery diarrhea: secretory or osmotic?

1 Withdraw medications
2 Stool examination
— Microscopy, culture and sensitivity
— Cysts, ova, parasites
— *Clostridium difficile* toxin
3 Therapeutic trial of metronidazole ± cipro
(erythromycin, amoxicillin)
4 If persistent proceed to investigate
— Colonoscopy
— Endoscopic duodenal biopsy
— Small bowel series

Diagnosing suspected laxative abuse
1 History
2 Colonoscopic appearance
   — Melanosis coli (if anthracene laxatives used)
   — Absent mucosal damage
3 Adjunctive/supportive investigations
   — Hypokalemia
   — Stool volumes/electrolytes/osmolality
   — Urinary phenolphthalein and/or fecal
     magnesium levels

Diagnosis of giardiasis
1 Stool examination
   — Trophozoites (in unformed stools)
   — Cysts (in formed stools)
2 Endoscopic sampling of duodenal/jejunal fluid
   Endoscopic deep duodenal/jejunal biopsy
3 Therapeutic trial of metronidazole/tinidazole*

* Commonest and most practical 'diagnostic' approach

Bloody diarrhea: microbiological differential diagnosis
1 *Shigella* spp.
2 Enteroinvasive *E. coli*
3 *Campylobacter jejuni*
4 *Salmonella* spp.
5 *Entameba histolytica* (esp. if recent travel)
6 *Yersinia enterocolitica*
7 *Cl. difficile* (if recent antibiotics)
8 Tuberculosis

Diarrhea with abundant fecal polymorphonuclear leukocytes?*
1 *Shigella* spp.
   — Classical cause of bacillary dysentery
2 Enteroinvasive *E. coli*
   — cf. Enterotoxigenic *E. coli* (few leukocytes)
3 *Campylobacter jejuni*
   — cf. *C. fetus* (mononuclears only)
4 *Salmonella enteritidis*
   — cf. *S. typhi* (mononuclears only)
5 Amebic dysentery, yersiniosis
   — cf. Giardiasis (few leukocytes)
6 *Vibrio parahemolyticus*
   — cf. *V. cholerae* (few leukocytes)
7 *Cl. difficile*

* i.e. *dysentery*; caused by *enteroinvasive* (not toxigenic) organisms

INFLAMMATORY BOWEL DISEASE

Histologic hallmarks of inflammatory bowel disease
1 Ulcerative colitis
   — Crypts reduced in number; irregular; branched
   — Cryptabscesses +++
   — Loss of goblet cells
   — Paneth cell metaplasia +++
   — Thickening of muscularis mucosae
   — Infiltrate: polymorphs, eosinophils, plasma cells
2 Crohn's disease
   — Transmural involvement, fissuring
   — Glandular pattern relatively undisturbed
   — Non-caseating granulomata
   — Focal inflammation
   — Goblet cell preservation
   — Infiltrate: lymphocytes, macrophages, histiocytes
   — Cryptabscesses infrequent
   — Paneth cell metaplasia rare

Radiologic hallmarks of inflammatory bowel disease
1 Ulcerative colitis
   — Indicators of disease diagnosis
     • Fine, spiculating superficial ulcers, fuzzy contour
     • 'Collarstud' ulcers
   — Indicators of disease *severity*
     • 'Pseudopolyps' (luminal mucosal filling defects = inflammatory polyps between ulcers)
   — Indicators of disease *chronicity*
     • Tubular 'hosepipe' colon (↓ haustration)
     • Shortened, narrowed colon
     • Retrorectal space > 2 cm
     • Barium reflux through patulous ileocecal valve
2 Crohn's disease
   — Early lesions
     • Thickening of valvulae coniventes
     • Aphthoid ulceration
   — Late lesions
     • 'Cobblestoning'
     • 'Rose-thorn' and 'collarstud' (deep) ulcers
     • Transmural fissuring
     • 'Skip lesions' (= involved segments)
   — Complications
     • Fistulae, sinuses, stenoses (on barium studies)
     • *Severe* colonic ulceration/edema may be evident on plain films
3 Ischemic colitis
   — Large asymmetric 'thumbprint' deformities (due to intramural edema), esp. at splenic flexure
   — Toxic dilatation

Radiographic stricture in Crohn's disease?
1 Transient bowel spasm
2 Inflammatory stenosis
3 Ischemic fibrosis
4 Pericolic abscess
5 Carcinoma

Diagnosis of Whipple's disease
1 Duodenal biopsy
   — PAS-positive staining of foamy macrophages in lamina propria
2 Polymerase chain reaction (PCR)
   — Primers specific for *Tropheryma whippelii* in infected tissues or peripheral blood
3 Electron microscopy
   — Whipple bacillus visible in infected tissues
4 Therapeutic trial
   — Penicillin/streptomycin; co-trimoxazole

ESOPHAGEAL DISEASE

Therapeutic measures in esophageal reflux
1 Minor disease
— Weight reduction, elevate bedhead
— Avoid alcohol/nicotine/caffeine/fat
— Post-prandial antacids
— Preprandial
  • Metoclopramide*
  • Domperidone‡
— Nocturnal H_2-receptor antagonists
2 Major disease (incl. CREST, scleroderma)
— Proton pump inhibitors (treatment of choice)
— Surgery (e.g. laparoscopic fundoplication¶)

* Enhances gastric emptying/lower esophageal sphincter tone
‡ Dopamine agonist
¶ Rarely used now, but good for controlling resistant regurgitative symptoms

Indications for surgery in esophageal reflux
1 Persistent, troublesome symptoms refractory to medical treatment
2 Penetrating ulcer unresponsive to medical treatment
3 Severe esophageal bleeding
4 Stricture requiring excessively frequent dilatation

Management of severe recurrent pain due to esophageal spasm
1 Endoscopy: exclude
— Intrinsic esophageal disease
— Peptic ulcer
2 Exclude non-gastroesophageal causes, e.g.
— Ischemic heart disease (ECG)
— Gallstones (OCG)
3 Nifedipine
4 Nitrates

MANAGEMENT OF PEPTIC ULCERATION

Factors to exclude in patients with ulcers
1 NSAID use
2 *H. pylori* infection
3 Smoking
4 Malignancy: carcinoma, lymphoma, MALToma, gastrinoma

Medical modalities available for peptic ulcer
1 Antisecretory agents
— H_2-receptor antagonists
  • Ranitidine, cimetidine, famotidine, nizatidine
— Proton pump (H^+/K^+-ATPase) inhibitors
  • Omeprazole, lansoprazole, pantoprazole
2 Antisecretory and cytoprotective agents
— Prostaglandin E_1/E_2 derivatives
  • Misoprostol
3 Other
— Antacids
  • Sodium bicarbonate (absorbed; may cause alkalosis, fluid overload)

• Magnesium salts, esp. trisilicate (tend to cause diarrhea)
• Aluminium salts, hydroxide/silicate (tend to constipate)
— Cytoprotective agents ('coat' mucosa; no antacid properties)
  • Colloidal bismuth (bactericidal to *H. pylori*)

Indications for proton pump inhibitor therapy
1 Gastrinoma (p. 108)
— 60 mg/day in divided doses initially
— Medical therapy of choice
2 Esophagitis (drug of choice) or troublesome reflux symptoms
— Endoscopy confirms severe esophagitis, *or*
— Failure of 8 weeks' H_2-blocker + antacids
3 Refractory duodenal ulceration
— *H. pylori* detected? Eradicated (but see below) with
  • Omeprazole + amoxicillin (80% success)
  • Omeprazole + amoxicillin/metronidazole + clarithromycin (90–95% success)
— *H. pylori* not detected, but ulcer persists after 8 weeks' H_2-blocker therapy (0.5% patients only)
  • Try omeprazole 20 mg b.d. for 4–8 weeks
4 NSAID-associated gastric ulcer, *if*
— NSAID must be continued, *and*
— Misoprostol ineffective or toxic (diarrhea)

NB: Proton pump inhibitor therapy may increase the risk of atrophic gastritis in patients with *H. pylori* infection, but significance of this is uncertain

Advantages of proton pump inhibitors over H_2-blockers
1 More prolonged action
— Once-daily dosage usually suffices
2 More potent acid inhibitor*; hence
— More rapid ulcer healing

* Omeprazole improves its own bioavailability by reducing gut acidity

Clinical use of misoprostol therapy
1 Action
— *Cytoprotective* oral analog of prostaglandin E_1
— *Antisecretory* effect (via histamine and prostaglandins)
2 Main indications
— Prophylaxis* or R_x of NSAID-induced gastric damage
— Permits ulcer healing in patients needing to continue NSAIDs; does not attenuate systemic NSAID effects
— Second-line or adjunctive therapy for peptic ulcers unassociated with NSAID therapy
3 Toxicity
— Diarrhea, cramps, flatulence (in 10%)
— Dysmenorrhea, menorrhagia (↑ uterine contractility)
4 Contraindications
— Pregnancy (promotes miscarriage)
5 Limitations
— *Not* shown to reduce incidence of complications from NSAID therapy (hemorrhage, perforation, death)
— Does *not* improve NSAID-induced dyspepsia

* In high-risk patients (e.g. past ulcer history) about to commence NSAIDs. Preferable, however, to prescribe COX2 inhibitors instead (e.g. celecoxib, rofecoxib)

Relative ulcerogenicity of NSAIDs
1 Least ulcerogenicity
   — Ibuprofen (< 1500 mg/day)
   — Diclofenac
2 Intermediate ulcerogenicity
   — Indometacin
   — Naproxen
3 Greatest ulcerogenicity
   — Azapropazone
   — Piroxicam

NB: Enteric-coated or buffered aspirin is not proven to be any less potent at causing upper gastrointestinal hemorrhage than normal aspirin

MANAGEMENT OF *H. PYLORI* INFECTIONS

Clinical scenarios for considering anti-*Helicobacter* therapy*
1 Duodenal ulcer
2 Gastric ulcer or chronic antral gastritis
3 MALT gastric lymphoma
4 Post-resection of early gastric cancer
5 Family history of gastric cancer
6 Troublesome non-ulcer dyspepsia or refractory esophagitis

* Assuming positive *H. pylori* screen

Some *H. pylori* eradication regimens
1 OCA: Omeprazole + clarithromycin + amoxicillin (1 week)
2 OCM: Omeprazole + clarithromycin + metronidazole (1–2 weeks)

Indications for endoscopy prior to *H. pylori* eradication
1 Sinister symptoms
   — Weight loss, anorexia, recurrent vomiting
   — Unusual, gnawing epigastric pain
2 Bleeding or anemia
3 Dysphagia or persistent vomiting
4 Epigastric mass or suspicious barium meal
5 Previous gastric ulcer or gastric surgery

A sequential approach to duodenal ulcer symptoms
1 Preliminary precautions
   — Confirm diagnosis; exclude gastric ulcer, esophagitis
   — Cease NSAIDs/cigarettes
   — Exclude anemia/iron deficiency
2 Treat initially with
   — Antacid + H_2-blocker for 6 weeks
3 No symptomatic improvement? Consider
   — Serology or breath testing for *H. pylori*
   Or switch medication empirically to
   — Proton pump inhibitor (4–8 weeks)
4 In the light of these outcomes, consider
   — *H. pylori* eradication (triple therapy; see above)

5 If *H. pylori* not suspected, consider
   — Fasting serum gastrin
   — Treating with proton pump inhibitor
   — Maintenance H_2-blockers following symptom control

POST-GASTRECTOMY SYNDROMES

Anemia following gastric surgery: mechanisms
1 Iron deficiency ($\rightarrow$ anemia in 50%)
   — Malabsorption due to duodenal bypass (Polya)
   — Hypochlorhydria (Fe^{2+} less soluble than Fe^{3+})
   — Recurrent bleeding (e.g. stomal ulcers, gastritis)
2 B_{12} deficiency ($\rightarrow$ anemia in 5%)
   — $\downarrow$ Parietal cell mass, esp. in total gastrectomy
   — Bacterial overgrowth due to
     • Blind loop (Polya): commonest cause
     • Reduced motility (vagotomy)
     • Hypochlorhydria
3 Folic acid deficiency ($\rightarrow$ anemia in 1%)

Mechanisms of post-Polya malabsorption
1 Inadequate luminal mixing of food and digestive secretions due to intestinal hurry (leading to steatorrhea)
2 Duodenal bypass $\rightarrow \downarrow$ biliary and pancreatic secretions
3 Stagnant loop syndrome
4 Inadvertent gastroileostomy
5 'Unmasking' gluten sensitivity/pancreatic insufficiency
6 Stomal ulceration leading to formation of gastrocolic fistula

Possible significance of stomal ulcer development
1 Inadequate vagotomy/gastrectomy ('retained antrum')
2 Inadvertent gastroileal (or gastrocolic) anastomosis
3 Gastrinoma

Other complications of gastric surgery
1 Dumping ('early', 'late'); R_x octreotide
2 Biliary vomiting, biliary gastritis; alkaline reflux esophagitis
3 Osteomalacia, osteoporosis
4 Protein-losing enteropathy (cause unknown); diarrhea
   Protein malnutrition (due to poor intake and absorption)
5 Reactivation of TB (cause unknown)
6 Development of malignancy in gastric remnant

HEMOCHROMATOSIS

Approach to presymptomatic hemochromatosis
1 Prevent complications by screening first-degree relatives
   — $\uparrow$ Serum ferritin
   — $\uparrow$ Transferrin saturation (> 55%)

2 Under certain circumstances, confirm suspected positives using
— Liver biopsy
— ± Quantitative phlebotomy, HLA-A3 phenotype
3 Venesection of affected patients
— Until Hb = 10 g/dL (i.e. not below; aim for ferritin 20–50)
4 Annual monitoring of these patients*
— Keep male ferritin levels < 350 µg/L
— Keep female ferritin levels < 200 µg/L

* Effectively prevents liver/cardiac disease and skin bronzing

Efficacy of therapy for established hemochromatosis
1 Benefits
— Prolongs life in symptomatic patients
2 Limitations
— *Arthropathy* fails to improve
— *Insulin requirement* in diabetics is rarely eliminated
— *Hypogonadotrophic hypogonadism* (impotence, premature menopause) seldom improves*
— *Risk of hepatoma* in cirrhotics is unaffected

* NB: Androgen therapy for impotence greatly increases hepatoma risk

MANAGEMENT OF ASCITES

Approach to managing ascites in chronic liver disease
1 Mild, minimally symptomatic ascites
— Spironolactone
— Low-salt diet
2 Tense, symptomatic ascites in patients with edema, normal renal function, and serum sodium > 130 mmol/L
— Hospital admission
— Large-volume controlled paracentesis
— Early discharge following stabilization on diuretics
3 Tense, symptomatic ascites in patients *without* edema, with renal impairment, or serum sodium < 130 mmol/L
— Hospital admission
— Large-volume paracentesis *plus* albumin infusion
— Early discharge following stabilization on diuretics
4 Recurrent ascites following paracentesis and diuretics
— Culture ascites (bacteria, AFB)
— Sudan III stain if fluid opalescent (chylous ascites)
— Cytology (malignant cells)
— Plasma AFP (hepatoma)
— Liver scan (hepatoma, hepatic vein thrombosis)
5 Intractable ascites
— TIPS*
• ↓ Portal pressure, ascites, variceal bleeding
• ↑ Risk of encephalopathy
— Rarely, peritoneovenous (LeVeen) shunt
6 Liver transplantation

* Transjugular intrahepatic portosystemic shunting

Complications of peritoneovenous shunting
1 Disseminated intravascular coagulation*
2 Sepsis
3 Shunt blockage (very frequent)
4 Intravascular fluid overload (→ pulmonary edema)
5 Peritoneal fibromatosis (foreign body reaction)

* May be clinical or subclinical

HEPATIC ENCEPHALOPATHY

Inpatient monitoring of the patient in hepatic precoma
1 Higher centers
— Regular close questioning by staff and relatives
2 Constructional apraxia
— Handwriting chart
— Five-pointed star chart
— Reitan trail test (consecutive number connection)
3 Investigations
— EEG (p. 269)
— CT (if *any* diagnostic doubt)
— Specific biochemistry (rarely done)
• Plasma ammonia (sampled without tourniquet)
• CSF glutamine

Hepatic encephalopathy: management of the 'at-risk' patient
1 Elimination of precipitants
— Detection and correction of hypoglycemia
— Correction of hypothermia, ↓ K$^+$, ↓ Mg^{2+}
— Withdrawal of loop diuretics, sedatives, alcohol
— Active exclusion of sepsis
— Treatment of gastrointestinal bleeding
— Avoidance of surgery and general anesthesia if possible
2 Diet
— High-calorie (incl. IV dextrose if necessary)
3 Bowel cleansing
— Magnesium sulfate enemas
— Lactulose (or lactilol)*
— Consider gut sterilization‡ with oral neomycin
4 *Consider* prophylactic broad-spectrum antibiotics (metronidazole) and antifungals
5 *Consider* steroids

* Acidifies gut lumen, thus converting liposoluble (absorbable) NH_3 to NH_4^+ (less absorbable) while promoting bowel washout. Can be used orally or as enema
‡ Promotes malabsorption of putative neurotoxin

PORTAL-SYSTEMIC SHUNTING

Relative contraindications to portal-systemic shunting
1 Age > 50 years
2 Previous episode(s) of encephalopathy
3 Jaundice
4 Ascites
5 Profound hypoalbuminemia
6 High IQ required for livelihood

Potential complications of portal-systemic shunting
1 Perioperative death ($\rightarrow$ 50% of 'poor-risk' patients)
2 Precipitation of hepatic encephalopathy
3 Development of hepatic nephropathy (hepatorenal failure)

DRUG-INDUCED LIVER DISEASE

Iatrogenic histopathologic mimics of primary liver disease
1 Viral hepatitis
   — Halothane, isoniazid, ketoconazole
2 Alcoholic hepatitis
   — Perhexiline maleate
3 Reye's syndrome
   — Aspirin, valproate
4 Acute fatty liver of pregnancy
   — Tetracycline
5 Cryptogenic cirrhosis/fibrosis
   — Long-term methotrexate ($\rightarrow$ fibrosis esp.)
   — Amiodarone
   — Vitamin A intoxication, vinyl chloride monomer
6 Primary biliary cirrhosis
   — Chlorpromazine
7 Chronic active hepatitis
   — Methyldopa, isoniazid, nitrofurantoin, dantrolene
8 Granulomatous (hypersensitivity) hepatitis
   — Allopurinol (+ many others)
9 Budd–Chiari syndrome
   — Synthetic estrogens
10 Veno-occlusive disease
   — 6-Thioguanine $\pm$ irradiation (for childhood tumors)
11 Cholestasis
   — (Flu)cloxacillin, amoxicillin–clavulanic acid
   — Estrogens, anabolic steroids

Halothane hepatitis: occurrence and outcome
1 Incidence
   — Clinically evident hepatitis: 1 in 10 000
   — Asymptomatic $\uparrow$ AST/ALT: 10–25%
2 Predisposition
   — 70% of affected patients are female
   — 50% of affected patients are obese
3 Exposure frequency
   — More than 80% patients have had at least 2 exposures
   — Initial exposure is often followed by unexplained fever
   — Toxic re-exposure usually occurs within 1 month
4 Associated features
   — Fever is seen in 75% of established hepatitis cases
   — Eosinophilia is seen in 30% of cases
5 Mortality of established halothane hepatitis is 50%

PRIMARY LIVER DISEASE

Autoimmune chronic active hepatitis: when to try steroids
1 Symptoms causing reduced quality of life, *plus*
2 Severe histologic abnormalities on biopsy, *plus*

3 HBsAg *and* anti-HBc negativity, *plus*
4 Exclusion of reversible etiology
   — Drug-induced chronic active hepatitis
   — Wilson's disease
   — α_1-antitrypsin deficiency

Therapeutic modalities in primary biliary cirrhosis
1 Ursodeoxycholic acid (UDCA)*
   — Improves LFTs and biopsy; doubtful mortality benefit
2 Debatable benefit
   — Colchicine; methotrexate
3 Liver transplantation‡

* cf. primary sclerosing cholangitis: UDCA *no* proven value
‡ If survival otherwise < 1 year, rising bilirubin/ascites

Treating the itch of primary biliary cirrhosis
1 Colestyramine (before and after breakfast)
2 Rifampicin
3 Ursodeoxycholic acid
4 Naloxone

THERAPY OF CHRONIC VIRAL HEPATITIS

Factors predicting good response to interferon in chronic hepatitis B
1 Short duration of disease
2 Low viral DNA levels
3 Active hepatitis on biopsy
4 HbeAg-positive (wild-type) virus
   Absence of δ virus coinfection
5 High AST/ALT levels

Factors predicting good response to interferon* in chronic hepatitis C
1 Short duration of disease
2 Low viral RNA levels
3 No fibrosis on biopsy‡
4 Young age, female sex
5 Normal bilirubin and GGT
6 Low hepatic iron/ferritin
7 Presence of cryoglobulinemia
8 HCV genotype 2 or 3

* Efficacy is greater with addition of oral ribavirin
‡ Though use of interferon-α in chronic HCV with cirrhosis reduces the incidence of hepatoma

Contraindications to interferon therapy of chronic hepatitis
1 Autoimmune etiology
2 Alcoholism or psychiatric disorder
3 Liver failure

Utility of lamivudine for chronic hepatitis B
1 Daily oral therapy produces > 50% rate of histological improvement within 1 year*
2 Efficacy greater if high ALT levels (cf. interferon: AST)
3 May cause sustained clearance of HbeAg

* cf. 35% for interferon-α and 25% for placebo

Problems with lamivudine treatment of chronic hepatitis B
1 YMDD mutant often appears during treatment
2 Viral flares following drug cessation are sometimes seen
3 Lactic acidosis, fatty liver, and fulminant liver failure may occur

LIVER TRANSPLANTATION

Varieties of liver transplantation
1 Orthotopic liver transplantation
2 Heterotopic auxiliary liver transplantation
   — For acute liver failure, or end-stage metabolic liver disorders

Principal indications for liver transplantation
1 Pediatric liver disease
   — Congenital biliary atresia with persistent cholestasis despite Kasai procedure (1-year survival > 90%)
   — Metabolic disease: α_1-antitrypsin deficiency, galactosemia, Crigler–Najjar syndrome, hypercholesterolemia
2 Wilson's disease with encephalopathy (consider all patients)
3 Acute liver failure due to paracetamol intoxication *and*
   — Arterial pH < 7.30, *or*
   — Severe encephalopathy *and* renal failure *and* coagulopathy
4 Fulminant liver failure due to other causes, including halothane, other drugs, or seronegative hepatitis *and*
   — Severe coagulopathy (PT > 100 sec), *or*
   — Jaundice precedes encephalopathy by > 1 week
5 End-stage (but stable) chronic liver disease
   — Alcoholic liver disease
   — Chronic hepatitis, esp. hepatitis C
   — Primary biliary cirrhosis; sclerosing cholangitis; Budd–Chiari; cryptogenic cirrhosis
6 Neoplasms*
   — *Small* hepatomas (< 5 cm) without grossly elevated AFP
   — Fibrolamellar tumors, hemangioendotheliomas
   — Carcinoid or APUDoma metastases (esp. if solitary)

* Disappointing results to date

Therapeutic outcome in liver transplantation

1 Overall 12-month survival	—	75%
2 Primary biliary cirrhosis	—	12-month survival 90%
3 Other causes of cirrhosis	—	12-month survival 60%
4 HBV-induced liver disease	—	12-month survival 50%
5 Hepatoma	—	12-month survival 30%
6 Patients alive at 12 months	—	80% 5-year survival

Contraindications to liver transplantation
1 Common
   — Irreversible symptomatic liver failure
   — Patient unfit for surgery
   — No suitable donor
2 Absolute
   — Active alcoholism*
   — Systemic or biliary infection (incl. HIV)
   — Extrahepatic malignancy
3 Relative
   — Age > 60 years
   — Portal vein thrombosis
   — Portocaval shunt ($\rightarrow$ uncontrollable surgical bleeding)
   — Intrapulmonary AV shunting (> 50%)
   — Multiple previous laparotomies
   — HBeAg/HBV DNA+; δ agent infection
   — Severe hepatic osteodystrophy

* Most centers require at least 6 months' abstinence; compliance can be assessed using carbohydrate-deficient transferrin. Similar post-graft prognosis

Complications of liver transplantation
1 Infection
   — esp. *Pseudomonas* spp., *Candida* spp., CMV
2 Hepatic artery thrombosis (in up to 20%)
   — May infarct graft $\rightarrow$ immediate retransplantation
   — May also cause biliary peritonitis (bile duct infarct)
3 Acute rejection
   — Almost invariable (day 4–10 post-transplant)
   — Treated with steroids, ciclosporin
4 Chronic rejection (in 10–20% patients)
   — Causes 'vanishing bile duct syndrome' (jaundice)
   — May respond to retransplantation
5 Ciclosporin toxicity
   — Nephrotoxicity, hypertension
   — CNS: confusion, cortical blindness, pyramidal lesions, headaches, tremulousness
6 Death
   — Affects up to 25% within 12 months of transplant

GALLSTONES: ALTERNATIVES TO CHOLECYSTECTOMY

Therapy of gallstones without open cholecystectomy
1 Oral dissolution using cheno- or ursodeoxycholic acid (CDCA, UDCA)
2 Laparoscopic cholecystectomy
   Minilaparotomy cholecystectomy
3 Endoscopic sphincterotomy* (during ERCP)
   — For common bile-duct stones
4 T-tube stone extraction using Dormia basket
5 Extracorporeal shock wave lithotripsy (ESWL)‡

* May delay, or even obviate, need for laparascopic cholecystectomy in frail or elderly
‡ May be combined with stone dissolution therapy

Indications for endoscopic sphincterotomy > cholecystectomy
1 Elderly patients, *plus*
2 Patent cystic duct, *plus*
3 Common duct stone(s)

Prerequisites for extracorporeal lithotripsy
1 History of biliary colic (i.e. patient must be symptomatic)
2 Solitary radiolucent gallstone < 3 cm diameter (or < 3 stones with equivalent combined mass)
3 Functioning gallbladder on oral cholecystography
4 No recent cholecystitis/cholangitis, clotting defect, pregnancy

GALLSTONE DISSOLUTION THERAPY

Potential indications for bile acid therapy
1 Gallstones (see below)
2 Primary biliary cirrhosis
3 Sclerosing cholangitis
4 Benign cholestasis of pregnancy

Prerequisites for dissolution therapy
1 Functioning gallbladder (patent cystic duct) on OCG
2 Radiolucent (cholesterol) stones*
3 Stone diameter(s) < 1.5 cm
4 No common bile duct stones
5 No history of liver or pancreatic dysfunction
6 Not pregnant or morbidly obese

* Success likely if OCG shows stones *floating* within gallbladder, since this implies hypodense stones with large surface area for dissolution

LAXATIVE THERAPY

Indications for laxatives
1 Short-term therapy of constipation/painful defecation
2 Long-term therapy in elderly or debilitated patients with chronic abdominal/perineal muscular weakness
3 Prevention of iatrogenic constipation (esp. opiates)
4 Bowel preparation prior to investigation or surgery

Classifying laxatives
1 Bulking agents
   — Bran, ispaghula husk, sterculia, methylcellulose
2 Fecal softeners
   — Paraffin, docusate sodium
3 Osmotic laxatives
   — Magnesium salts, lactulose, glycerol suppositories
4 Stimulant laxatives
   — Senna, bisacodyl, dantron, phenolphthalein

Individualizing laxative treatment
1 Rectal discomfort
   — Glycerol suppositories
   — Bisacodyl suppositories
2 Long-term therapy of constipation
   — Bran (esp. unprocessed)
   — Ispaghula husk
   — Sterculia
   — Methylcellulose
3 Short-term therapy of self-limiting constipation
   — Senna ± docusate sodium
4 Second-line therapy of constipation
   — Magnesium hydroxide
   — Lactulose (expensive)

5 Refractory constipation
   — Investigate to clarify cause

ANTIDIARRHEAL THERAPY

Infectious diarrhea: indications for antibiotics
1 Always
   — Giardiasis (metronidazole 2 g/day for 3 days; or tinidazole 2 g stat, possibly repeated)
   — Amebiasis *if* symptomatic
   — Severe bacillary (*Shigella*) dysentery
2 Usually
   — Pseudomembranous (antibiotic-associated) colitis*
3 Occasionally
   — Campylobacter enterocolitis
   — 'Traveller's diarrhea' (therapy or prophylaxis)

* Relapses may be due to loss of aerobic flora

Antibiotics relevant to pseudomembranous colitis
1 Frequent causes
   — Ampicillin/amoxicillin
   — Clindamycin
   — Cephalosporins
2 Therapy*
   — Oral metronidazole 250 mg q.i.d.
     • Cheap and effective first-line therapy
     • Some systemic absorption, hence side-effects (nausea, metallic taste) may occur
   — Oral vancomycin 125 mg q.i.d.
     • Expensive but effective
     • Minimal systemic absorption
   — Intravenous metronidazole
     • May be used in patients unable to tolerate oral therapy (e.g. post-operative, ileus)
     • Biliary excretion ensures effective luminal concentrations in bowel‡
   — Bacitracin (second-line therapy only)

* *Colestyramine* 4 g q.i.d. may also be used to bind clostridial toxin
‡ cf. IV vancomycin: *not* recommended

Specific remedies for noninfectious diarrhea
1 Carcinoid syndrome
   — Cyproheptadine
2 Gastrinoma
   — Ranitidine, omeprazole
3 Chologenic diarrhea (e.g. in ileal insufficiency)
   — Colestyramine
4 Radiation proctitis
   — Formalin application per rectum
   — Laser per rectum, or argon plasma coagulation
   — Butyrate enemas (NB: smell bad)

INFLAMMATORY BOWEL DISEASE

Indications for surgery
1 Crohn's disease
   — Chronic disabling symptoms
   — Persistent bowel obstruction

— Enteric fistulae with complications
— Perirectal suppuration
— Acute appendicitis; perforation
— Obstructive hydronephrosis
— Growth retardation (e.g. despite parenteral nutrition)
— Colonic cancer
2 Ulcerative colitis
— Chronic disabling symptoms
— Severe colitis with failure to stabilize on intensive medical therapy (e.g. 5 days of IV steroids, followed by trial of IV ciclosporin)
— Intractable pararectal or extraintestinal complications
— Acute complications (e.g. toxic megacolon, perforation)
— Severe dysplasia
— Carcinoma (colonic or cholangiocarcinoma)
— Unacceptable medical side-effects

Diagnosis of toxic megacolon
1 Colonic distension confirmed on X-ray, *and*
2 Tachycardia + fever + neutrophilia/anemia, *and*
3 Dehydration/hypotension *or* electrolyte disturbance *or* impaired consciousness

Colectomy: its effect on complications of ulcerative colitis
1 Complications responsive to colectomy
— Peripheral arthropathy
— Pyoderma gangrenosum
— Pararectal disease*
2 Complications resistant to colectomy
— Ankylosing spondylitis
— Sclerosing cholangitis

* NB: Uncommon in ulcerative colitis

Mechanisms of debility in inflammatory bowel disease
1 Anemia (normochromic *or* iron deficiency)
2 Portal pyemia
3 Liver disease
4 Fistulae (malabsorption)
5 Recurrent bowel obstruction (Crohn's)
6 Relapsing or refractory colitis

Therapeutic role of 5-aminosalicylic acid (5-ASA) formulations
1 Classification
— Prodrugs (act in colon): sulfasalazine*, olsalazine, balsalazide
— 5-ASA alone: mesalazine
— Delayed-release 5-ASA preparations (act in terminal ileum)
— Also available as suppositories, foams or enemas
2 Main value is in *maintaining* remission in ulcerative colitis
May also *induce* remission in active ulcerative colitis or Crohn's
3 Very little drug is absorbed in the small intestine
Unabsorbed 5-ASA exerts topical therapeutic effect in colon
Rectal aminosalicylates are more effective than rectal steroids

4 Dose-related toxicity is maximal in slow acetylators
Hypersensitivity is usually due to the sulfapyridine moiety

* = sulfapyridine (sulfonamide) and 5-ASA moieties joined by azo-bond (lysed in colon)

Side-effects of sulfasalazine
1 Headaches, fever
2 Gastrointestinal
— Anorexia, nausea, vomiting
3 Hematologic
— Hemolysis, methemoglobinemia, aplasia
— Agranulocytosis; folate deficiency
4 Male infertility
— Oligospermia, reduced sperm motility
5 Neurologic
— Peripheral neuropathy, tinnitus, vertigo
6 Other
— Hepatitis, nephrosis, orange urine; toxic epidermal necrolysis; depression

Crohn's disease: approach to management
1 Acute ileitis
— Steroids are effective in inducing remission
— Controlled-release oral budesonide is as effective as more traditional corticosteroids but less toxic (fewer side-effects due to rapid first-pass metabolism)
— Infliximab
— Azathioprine
2 Acute colitis
— Sulfasalazine + steroids induce remission
— Infliximab
3 Perianal disease or fistulae
— Metronidazole + ciprofloxacin (esp. perianal disease)
— Infliximab (enterocutaneous fistulae)
— Surgery
4 Cholorrheic enteropathy (= diarrhea due to ileal malabsorption of bile acids, leading to colonic irritation)
— Therapeutic trial of colestyramine
5 Extensive ileal resection (> 100 cm) with frank steatorrhea
— R_x: medium-chain triglycerides (MCT), low oxalate ± low lactose diet
— Vitamin (A, D, E, K, B_{12}) supplements, TPN
6 Bacterial overgrowth
— May underlie 'refractory' disease
— Treat with broad-spectrum antibiotics (e.g. tetracycline)
— May necessitate surgery
7 Post-surgical disease recurrence
— Typically occurs proximal to anastomoses
— Minimal surgical intervention is favored
8 Refractory disease (e.g. no response to budesonide)
— Consider high-dose mesalazine, azathioprine, or methotrexate
— Infliximab
— Thalidomide (investigational)
— Prolonged (1–2 years) antibiotics (e.g. rifabutin, clarithromycin + clofazimine)

9 Malignancy
— Affects surgically excluded segments, strictures, fistulae; anus (SCC)
— Routine colonoscopic surveillance not indicated
— Excess of right-sided colonic Ca occurs in Crohn's
10 Maintenance prophylaxis
— Stop smoking (most effective intervention)
— Post-operative azathioprine

Non-intestinal complications of Crohn's disease
1 Osteopenia
Growth retardation*
2 Gallstones
3 Renal (oxalate) stones
Ureteric obstruction
4 Psoas abscess
5 Amyloidosis
6 Thromboembolism

* May be *either* steroid-induced *or* disease-related

Use of continent ileoanal reservoirs* or ileostomy after proctocolectomy
1 Continence achievable in 80–95% patients
2 Anastomotic strictures occur in about 10%
3 Pouch failure occurs in 2–5%
4 Fecal stasis → anaerobic overgrowth → 'pouchitis' → diarrhea (responds to metronidazole)
5 'Primary' ileostomy diarrhea may respond to somatostatin analogs
6 If pouch requires dismantling, further bowel shortening may exacerbate pre-existing short bowel syndrome

* In ulcerative colitis

Therapeutic distinctions in inflammatory bowel disease
1 Surgical therapy
— Segmental resection may be useful in colonic Crohn's, not ulcerative colitis
— Proctocolectomy may be curative in ulcerative colitis, not Crohn's
2 Medical therapy
— Maintenance oral aminosalicylates are more useful in ulcerative colitis than in Crohn's
— Diet (e.g. low fiber diet) and metronidazole/ciprofloxacin (for colonic/perianal disease) are more useful in Crohn's than in ulcerative colitis
— Osteopenia and growth failure often require treatment in Crohn's, whereas autoimmune disorders (e.g. sclerosing cholangitis) often need treatment in ulcerative colitis.

UNDERSTANDING GASTROINTESTINAL DISEASE

GASTRIC ACID REGULATION

Anatomic localization of acid-regulatory cells
1 Body of stomach* (corpus/fundus; proximal two-thirds)
— Parietal (oxyntic) cells
• Secrete HCl, intrinsic factor into lumen
— Chief cells
• Secrete pepsinogen into lumen
2 Gastric antrum (pyloric region; distal third)
— G-cells (also found in proximal duodenum)
• Secrete gastrin/somatostatin into bloodstream

* Site of atrophic gastritis

Factors regulating parietal cell acid output
1 Increased by
— Vagal stimulation (e.g. food in stomach)
— Gastrin (via blood)
— Histamine
2 Reduced by
— Somatostatin
— Anticholinergics (block *vagal* activity)
— H_2-receptor antagonists (block parietal cell *activation*)
— Proton pump inhibitor (blocks acid *secretion*)

GUT HORMONES

Classification of regulatory peptides coexisting in gut and CNS
1 Paracrine (locally acting)
— Somatostatin
2 Neurotransmitters
— VIP, substance P, bombesin, endorphins
3 Endocrine (distantly acting)
— Cholecystokinin (CCK), neurotensin

NB: All other gut peptides mentioned below exhibit mainly *endocrine* action

Gut peptides exhibiting structural similarities
1 Gastrin, CCK
2 Secretin, (entero)glucagon, VIP, GIP
3 Bombesin, substance P

Physiology and clinical significance of gastrin
1 Location
— Gastric antrum (also jejunum)
2 Released by
— Vagal stimulation (esp. gastric distension)
— Protein meals; alcohol
— Bombesin
3 Effects
— Stimulates gastric acid and pepsin secretion
— Inhibits gastric emptying
— Trophic to gastric mucosa
— Increases lower esophageal sphincter tone
4 Clinical significance
— Zollinger–Ellison (gastrinoma) syndrome
— Achalasia (cholinergic denervation hypersensitivity to gastrin implicated in pathogenesis of ↑ LES tone)

Physiology of cholecystokinin ('hormone of satiety')
1 Location: duodenum and jejunum
2 Released by protein/fat ingestion
3 Effects
— Stimulates gallbladder contraction
— Relaxes sphincter of Oddi

— Releases pancreatic proteolytic enzymes
— Trophic to pancreas
4 Clinical significance
— Used to assess pancreatic/gallbladder function

Physiology of secretin ('physiological antacid')
1 Location: duodenum and jejunum
2 Released by entry of acid into duodenum
3 Effects
— Stimulates pancreatic bicarbonate secretion
4 Clinical significance
— ↓ Secretion in celiac disease

Physiology of vasoactive intestinal polypeptide (VIP)
1 Location: post-ganglionic gut nerve cells
2 Released by direct neural mediation (*not* by meals)
3 Effects
— Inhibits gastric acid secretion
— Stimulates pancreatic bicarbonate secretion
— Stimulates gut secretion and insulin release
— Induces vasodilatation and hypotension
4 Clinical significance
— VIPoma
— ↓ Secretion in Chagas' and Hirschsprung's
— ↑ Secretion in Crohn's disease
— Implicated in post-gastrectomy 'dumping' (p. 117)

Physiology of substance P
1 Location: gut nerve cells
2 Released by unknown stimuli
3 Effects
— Inhibits pancreatic bicarbonate/amylase release
— Inhibits biliary secretion
— Inhibits insulin, stimulates glucagon release
— Stimulates salivation, vasodilatation, natriuresis
4 Clinical significance
— Implicated in nociception, asthma

Physiology of bombesin (gastrin-releasing peptide)
1 Location: gut nerve cells
2 Released by unknown stimuli
3 Effects
— Stimulates gastrin/gastric acid secretion
— Stimulates pancreatic enzyme secretion
4 Clinical significance
— Secreted in SCLC but no recognized syndrome

Physiology of glucose-dependent insulinotrophic polypeptide*
1 Location: throughout gut, esp. duodenum/jejunum
2 Released by *oral* glucose
3 Effects
— Stimulates insulin release‡
— Inhibits gastric acid secretion
4 Clinical significance
— ↓ Secretion in celiac disease

* GIP; formerly, 'gastric inhibitory polypeptide'
‡ NB: Oral glucose induces greater insulin release than does parenteral glucose per unit glycemia, due to ?presence of 'incretin' hormone (see GLP-1; see below)

Physiology of motilin ('hormone of diarrhea')
1 Location: duodenum and jejunum
2 Released by meals (including drinking water; i.e. by vagally-mediated gastric distension; also by fat)
3 Effects
— Stimulates gastric emptying
— Stimulates small intestinal motility
— Mediates gastrocolic reflex
4 Clinical significance
— ↑ Secretion in infective diarrheas, inflammatory bowel disease, and carcinoid syndrome
— *Erythromycin* (IV or oral) activates motilin receptors, causing abdominal cramps (toxicity), but also enhances motility in patients with hypomotility syndromes such as diabetic gastroparesis

Physiology of neurotensin
1 Location: ileum
2 Released by entry of food (esp. fat) to ileum
3 Effects
— Inhibits gastric emptying and acid secretion
— Stimulates intestinal secretion
— Induces hypotension
4 Clinical significance
— Implicated in post-gastrectomy 'dumping'

Physiology of enteroglucagon
1 Location: ileum and colorectum
2 Released by: meals
3 Effects
— Trophic to small intestinal mucosa
— Inhibits gastric emptying and acid secretion
4 Clinical significance
— ↑ Secretion following bowel resection or bypass
— ↑ Secretion in celiac disease/cystic fibrosis
— Implicated in post-gastrectomy 'dumping'

Physiology of glucagon-like peptide 1 (GLP-1)
1 Location: terminal ileum and pancreatic α-cells
2 Released by oral glucose (gut), arginine (pancreas)
3 Effects
— Increases insulin secretion (? = 'incretin') if glucose is available
— Reduces plasma glucagon
4 Clinical significance
— Exaggerated post-prandial levels seen in post-gastrectomy dumping (together with excess insulin secretion)

Physiology of pancreatic polypeptide ('hormone of indigestion')
1 Location: pancreas
2 Released by vagal stimulation or (protein) meals
3 Effects
— Inhibits pancreatic and biliary secretion
4 Clinical significance
— Cosecreted in many gut endocrine tumor syndromes, esp. VIPoma (75%), glucagonoma (50%), gastrinoma (25%), carcinoid syndrome

Physiology of somatostatin (GH release inhibiting hormone)

1 Location: pancreas ('D' cells) and throughout gut
2 Released by diverse stimuli
3 Effects
   — Stimulates gastric emptying
   — *Inhibits* almost everything else
      • Gastric acid and pepsin secretion
      • Pancreatic/biliary secretion, celiac blood flow
      • Release of GH, TSH, insulin, glucagon, gastrin, secretin, PP, GIP, motilin, enteroglucagon
4 Clinical significance
   — Synthetic analogs successfully used in
      • VIPoma diarrhea control
      • Gastrinoma
      • Insulinoma, glucagonoma
      • Acromegaly (tumor sometimes reduces)
      • GI hemorrhage, pancreatitis

NB: *No* abnormality of gut hormones is linked to irritable bowel syndrome

GUT ENDOCRINE TUMOR SYNDROMES

General features of gut endocrine tumor syndromes*

1 *All* may be due to malignant tumors, and metastases are frequently evident at presentation (see below)
2 *Most* cause diarrhea
3 *Many* may be associated with secretion of other peptides (such as calcitonin, ACTH/CRH, PTH, adrenaline, noradrenaline, VMA), and clinical evolution from (say) VIPoma to insulinoma may occur
4 'Noisy' (clinically obvious) secreted hormones include
   — Insulin
   — Gastrin
   — VIP
   'Quiet' hormones include:
   — Glucagon
   — Somatostatin
   — Pancreatic polypeptide
5 *Any* may be associated with multiple endocrine neoplasia (MEN1); this possibility should be regularly excluded by measuring plasma Ca^{2+} (plus PTH if Ca^{2+} elevated), performing lateral SXR, and assaying pituitary hormones
6 Streptozotocin may be used to palliate unresectable disease, but response rates are modest (typically about 25%)

* Very rare

Gastrinoma: features

1 Primary G-cell tumors, usually found in pancreatic body/tail
2 50% develop parathyroid/pituitary adenoma (MEN1) Family history: renal stones, pituitary tumor, hypoglycemia
3 50% present with diarrhea or steatorrhea (see below)

4 95% present with duodenal ulceration, classically
   — Young patient without risk factors (unless MEN1)
   — Multiple large, deep ulcers
   — Ectopic position (post-bulbar, jejunal, esophageal)
   — Associated with pyloric stenosis or esophageal stricture
   — Prone to perforation or hemorrhage, esp. post-op
   — Healing resists normal-dose H_2-receptor antagonists
5 Management
   — Medical
      • Omeprazole (high-dose)
      • *High*-dose (5 × normal) H_2-receptor antagonists
      • Addition of anticholinergics (if needed)
      • Pancreatic enzyme supplements (for steatorrhea)*
      • Colestyramine (for diarrhea)
   — Surgical
      • If hypercalcemic: assess for parathyroidectomy
      • If no evidence of metastasis *or* MEN1: laparotomy
      • If primary tumor localizable: resection
      • If disease unresectable *and* preoperative ulceration controllable with drugs, close up
      • If disease unresectable *and* difficulties in ulcer control, consider highly selective vagotomy
      • If disease unresectable *and* symptoms resistant to drugs, consider total gastrectomy (last resort)

* Note that bowel strictures – fibrosing colonopathy – may develop as a side-effect (albeit more often in cystic fibrosis)

VIPoma: features

1 Primary tumors are usually pancreatic in adults Children may develop benign ganglioneuroblastomas
2 Pancreatic origin (in 80%) is confirmed by coexisting elevation of pancreatic polypeptide
3 Causes watery diarrhea, dehydration, ↓ K^+
4 Associated
   — Achlorhydria
   — Flushing, hypotension (esp. on tumor palpation)
   — Cholelithiasis and gallbladder dilatation
   — Hypercalcemia (with or without MEN1)
   — Glucose intolerance (usually subclinical)
5 Management
   — **S**urgery if feasible
   — **S**omatostatin analogs* (→ best symptom control)
   — **S**ymptomatic
      • Opiates (codeine, loperamide)
      • Metoclopramide; indometacin
      • Steroids
      • Fluid and electrolyte balance
   — **S**treptozotocin (cytotoxic) for metastases

* e.g. octreotide improves diarrhea by lowering VIP

Glucagonoma: features

1 Primary α-cell pancreatic tumors; commoner in females
2 Spontaneous symptomatic remissions characteristic

3 Sequelae
  — Diarrhea (see below); hypercatabolic weight loss
  — Stomatitis, glossitis, vulvovaginitis, nail dystrophy
  — Thromboembolism
  — Necrolytic migratory erythema (transient bullous or crusting rash, often involving perineum and leaving residual pigmentation)
  — Glucose intolerance (often symptomatic)
  — Hypocholesterolemia
4 Management
  — Somatostatin analogs (for diarrhea)
  — Insulin if required (for diabetes)
  — Oral zinc (for rash)
  — Anticoagulant prophylaxis (for thromboembolism)
  — Tumor resection (for operable disease)
  — Streptozotocin (for inoperable disease)

Other gut endocrine tumors: features
1 Somatostatinoma (D-cell tumor; rare)
  — Diarrhea, steatorrhea (see below)
  — Achlorhydria; dyspepsia
  — Cholelithiasis, dilated gallbladder
  — Glucose intolerance (usually subclinical)
2 Enteroglucagonoma (very rare)
  — Small intestinal hypomotility
  — Massive villous hypertrophy on jejunal biopsy
  — Edema due to protein loss (see below)
3 PPoma/neurotensinoma (very rare)
  — The only gut endocrine tumors which present with symptoms and signs of invasion or metastasis rather than of endocrine sequelae

Malignant potential of gut endocrine tumors
1 Insulinoma
  — 5–10% are metastatic at presentation
2 Gastrinoma
  — 30% are metastatic at presentation
3 Glucagonoma, VIPoma, somatostatinoma
  — 50% are metastatic at presentation
4 Carcinoid syndrome
  — > 98% are metastatic at presentation*

* cf. carcinoid tumors *without* syndrome: < 10% metastasize

CARCINOID SYNDROME

Symptoms and signs of carcinoid syndrome
1 *Acute* symptoms (induced by 5-HT, kinins, etc.)
  — Upper body flushing
  — Dependent edema
  — Pruritic wheals, serpentine flush (histamine-secreting)
  — Wheezing; hypotension; fever; tachycardia
  — Borborygmi, abdominal pain, diarrhea, vomiting
2 *Chronic* complications (indicative of disease duration)
  — Telangiectasia; pellagra-like rash; arthropathy
  — Hepatomegaly*; cirrhosis may also supervene
  — Mesenteric fibrosis ('sclerosing peritonitis')
  — Tricuspid incompetence (chordal fibrosis)
  — Pulmonic stenosis (valvular adhesions)

* *Rarely*, bronchial or ovarian primaries may cause the syndrome in the absence of liver metastases

Symptoms of atypical carcinoid syndrome (lung primary)
1 Lacrimation
2 Parotid enlargement, salivation
3 Facial (not dependent) edema
4 Left-sided cardiac valve lesions

Benefits of octreotide in carcinoid syndrome
1 Effective in reducing *diarrhea**
2 Best available treatment for *flushing* (effective in 90%)
3 Infusion valuable for treating 'carcinoid crisis'

* Octreotide slows colonic motility, thereby increasing colonic conversion of the bile acid cholate to deoxycholate; this raises hepatic saturation of recirculated bile-cholesterol, thus predisposing octreotide-treated acromegalics to gallstones

Other treatment modalities in carcinoid syndrome
1 Diarrhea (serotonin-induced)
  — Non-specific: codeine, loperamide
  — Serotonin blockers: cyproheptadine (cf. methysergide: *contraindicated* due to ↑ risk of fibrotic sequelae)
2 Flushing (due to kinins, substance P, serotonin)
  — Phenoxybenzamine, corticosteroids
  — Ketanserin (serotonin blocker)
3 *Serpentine* (histamine-induced) flushing of gastric carcinoids
  — H_1 and H_2 histamine receptor antagonists
4 Hepatic pain
  — Hepatic embolization
  — Surgical debulking
5 Carcinoid crisis (e.g. perioperative)
  — Corticosteroids
6 Pellagra
  — Nicotinamide supplements (see p. 229)
7 Metastases
  — Streptozotocin (limited efficacy)
  — Interferon-α

HUMORAL DIARRHEA

Characteristics of diarrhea due to gut endocrine tumors
1 Gastrinoma
  — Diarrhea not caused by ↑ gastrin but by ↓ intestinal pH
  — This denatures pancreatic enzymes and precipitates bile salts with consequent ileal bile salt malabsorption
    • Dietary fat malabsorption (steatorrhea)
    • Colonic irritation by bile salts (watery diarrhea)
2 VIPoma ('pancreatic cholera')
  — 'Rice-water' (secretory) diarrhea (1–20 L/day)
  — Frequently nocturnal or fasting diarrhea
  — ± Colicky abdominal pain, dehydration, azotemia
  — Hypokalemic *acidosis**
3 Glucagonoma
  — Diarrhea, no steatorrhea
  — May be associated with hypokalemic alkalosis

— Characteristic rash
— Normochromic anemia
4 Somatostatinoma
— Steatorrhea (↓ biliary secretion, intestinal absorption)
— Associated with achlorhydria (↓ gastric acidity)
5 Enteroglucagonoma
— Steatorrhea
— No diarrhea (gut hypomotility)
— Protein-losing enteropathy with edema (due to massive villous hypertrophy)
6 Carcinoid syndrome
— Profuse secretory diarrhea (5-HT-induced)
— Associated borborygmi, abdominal pain, nausea

* VIP-induced achlorhydria → life-threatening loss of *alkaline* secretions

THE UPPER GASTROINTESTINAL TRACT

Pathogenetic mechanisms contributing to reflux esophagitis
1 ↓ Lower esophageal sphincter (LES) tone*
— e.g. Scleroderma
2 ↓ Esophageal clearance of refluxed material
— e.g. Esophageal spasm, achalasia
3 ↑ Irritant content of refluxed material
— e.g. Post-gastrectomy biliary gastritis; gastrinoma
4 ↑ Volume of gastric contents
— e.g. Delayed gastric emptying, Ménètrier's disease
5 Irritant drug therapy (pill esophagitis)
— e.g. Alendronic acid, minocycline

* cf. achalasia: increased LES tone due to cholinergic denervation hypersensitivity to acetylcholine

Barrett's esophagus*: what is its clinical significance?
1 Commoner in males
2 Found in 10% of patients undergoing biopsy for esophagitis
3 Found in 40% of patients with chronic peptic strictures
4 Carcinoma risk
— Predisposes to about 5% of all esophageal cancer
— Lifetime risk in a given patient is about 5%
— This represents a 30-fold increase in relative risk
5 30% of patients presenting with carcinoma and Barrett's esophagus have *no* history of reflux symptoms

* Specialized intestinal metaplasia above gastric cardia

Approach to the patient with Barrett's esophagus
1 Antireflux therapy, including proton pump inhibition
2 Endoscopic surveillance for dysplasia
3 Multiple foci of high-grade dysplasia? Consider resection

Differential diagnosis of delayed gastric emptying
1 Pyloric stenosis (e.g. due to chronic duodenal ulceration)
2 Infiltration (amyloid, linitis plastica)
3 Scleroderma

4 Autonomic neuropathy (e.g. diabetes)
5 Iatrogenic (opiates, anticholinergics, antidepressants)

Clinical features of hypertrophic gastropathies
1 Ménètrier's disease
— Male predominance (3:1)
— Presents with epigastric pain and peripheral edema
— Barium meal/endoscopy: giant rugae, antral sparing
— Achlorhydria (5% develop carcinoma)
— Protein-losing enteropathy
2 Schindler's disease
— Giant gastric rugae
— Acid hypersecretion
— Normal protein balance

VIRAL HEPATITIS: PATHOPHYSIOLOGIC ASPECTS

Predominant modes of transmission
1 Fecal–oral route
— Hepatitis A virus (HAV)
— Hepatitis E virus (HEV)
2 Parenteral (esp. via blood)
— Hepatitis B virus (HBV)
— Hepatitis C virus (HCV)
— Hepatitis D virus (HDV)

Hepatitis A (HAV) pathophysiology
1 Picornavirus transmitted by fecal–oral route
2 Almost always self-limiting disease; most often subclinical
Adult-onset disease tends to be more severe
3 Onset abrupt, fever higher, transaminitis shorter; but may be clinically *indistinguishable* from other viral hepatitides
4 Prominent cholestasis later in the illness
5 IgM anti-HAV appears with symptoms, persists for 3–6 months

Hepatitis B (HBV) pathophysiology
1 Acute HBV (a hepadnavirus) usually subicteric, 'flu-like
10–20% get serum sickness prodrome due to HbsAg–HBsAb complexes depositing in skin and joints
2 Persistence of HBeAg beyond 12 weeks of symptom onset indicates possibility of disease chronicity. On the other hand, surgeons who are HbeAg-negative carriers can still transmit the disease
3 Antiviral efficacy
— Lamivudine
— Interferon-α
— Investigational: foscarnet/ganciclovir, adefovir
4 Interferon-α induces remission in 30% of those with chronic disease, esp. if:
— Female, heterosexual, non-Asian
— Short duration of infection
— Negative hepatitis D/HIV serology
— High pretreatment ALT (> 1.3 × normal)
— Low pretreatment serum HBV DNA

5 Remission marked by
  — Normalization of ALT
  — Conversion of HBeAg to HBeAb
  — Disappearance of serum HBV DNA
6 Vaccination with recombinant HBsAg induces HBsAb and immunity

Hepatitis C (HCV) pathophysiology

1 Non-A non-B hepatitis transmitted parenterally
  — Post-transfusion/-transplant (almost all cases), intraoperative
  — Injecting drug use, tattoos; needlestick (5–10% seroconvert); ear-piercing
  — Transplacental (vertical) transmission
  — Venereal transmission believed *rare*
2 Due to RNA flavivirus
  — Serologically detected; multiple serotypes
  — Multiple genotypes; HCV PCR is used to confirm infection
  — Incubation period intermediate between hepatitis A and hepatitis B (~ 60 days)
  Genotype variants (at least 6 major and 12 minor)
  — Genotype 1 (esp. 1b): more severe liver disease, poor response to interferon, compared to genotypes 2 and 3
3 Complicates << 1% of transfusions
  — Implicated in 95% of transfusional hepatitis
  — 90% of anti-HCV-positive donors are infectious
  — Some infectious donors are anti-HCV-negative
4 Manifests as
  — Mild anicteric infection* ± large ALT fluctuations
  — HCV infection *persists* long-term in 80%
  — Occult HBV infection may be masked by chronic HCV
  — *Chronic* hepatitis in 50% (after 10 years)
  — *Cirrhosis* in 15% (after 15 years)
  — *Hepatoma‡* in 5% (after 20 years)
5 Extrahepatic HCV complications (rare)
  — Membranoproliferative glomerulonephritis
  — Sjogren-like syndrome, thyroiditis
  — Essential mixed cryoglobulinemia (associated with positive serology)
  — Thrombocytopenic purpura
  — Porphyria cutanea tarda, lichen planus
  — Lymphoma
6 Management
  — Observation
  — α-Interferon (12-month course reduces viremia), *plus*
  — Ribavirin (oral guanosine analog)
  — Liver transplant (recurs, but OK in short term)

* NB: Chronic hepatitis may be confirmed on biopsy despite absent symptoms and persistently normal LFTs in patients who are anti-HCV-positive
‡ Synergistic tumorigenic effect of hepatitis B coinfection; hence, all anti-HCV patients should receive HBV vaccine

Hepatitis D (δ agent, HDV) pathophysiology

1 Defective RNA virus coated with HBsAg
  — Requires HBV to replicate but inhibits HBV replication
  — Mainly affects anti-HBe-positive patients
  — Minimally infective to HBsAg-negative individuals

2 Main reservoirs (incl. sexual partners of)
  — IV drug abusers
  — Polytransfused patients, esp. hemophiliacs
  — South Americans, Middle Easterns, Africans
3 Clinical scenarios
  — Co-primary infection with HBV (low morbidity)
  — Superinfection on chronic HBV (*high* morbidity)
  — May convert mild liver disease to severe (e.g. cirrhosis)
4 *Persistence* of anti-δ IgM usually signifies development of chronic active hepatitis or cirrhosis
5 *No* link with hepatoma

Hepatitis E (HEV) pathophysiology

1 Due to single-stranded RNA virus (?togavirus)
  — May mimic hepatitis A
2 Implicated in epidemic waterborne non-A hepatitis reported in India in association with high fetal wastage and mortality in pregnant women
3 Acute illness indistinguishable from other forms of hepatitis, but *no* chronic sequelae (i.e. in contrast to HCV)

'Hepatitis G' (GBV-C) pathophysiology

1 May not cause hepatitis (controversial)
2 Parenterally transmitted (e.g. during hemodialysis)
3 High active infection rate in general population (3–20% of blood donors)
4 Coinfection with this agent has been correlated with slower progression of AIDS

ACUTE AND CHRONIC HEPATITIS

Precipitants of fulminant hepatic failure*

1 Viral hepatitis (responsible for 50% of cases)
  — Acute hepatitis B (esp. pre-core mutants): commonest cause
  — Reactivation of hepatitis B (e.g. post-chemotherapy)
  — Chronic hepatitis B with δ agent superinfection
  — Acute hepatitis E, esp. in pregnant women in endemic areas
  — Acute hepatitis A superinfection of chronic hepatitis C
  — Hepatitis A or C: *rarely* causes fulminant hepatitis when occurring alone
2 Toxicity
  — Paracetamol overdose; responsible for 40% of cases
    • *N*-acetylcysteine is of benefit up to 36 h post-ingestion
  — Halothane hepatitis
  — Mushroom poisoning (*Anantis phylloides*)
3 Other
  — Leptospirosis (Weil's disease)
  — *Bacillus cereus* emetotoxic food poisoning
  — Wilson's disease (in children)
  — Acute fatty liver of pregnancy (AFLOP)
    • Best prognosis of all causes

* Defined as encephalopathy within 8 weeks of symptom onset; 80% mortality

Hepatitis in pregnancy
1 Most likely to transmit HBV if acquired in 3rd trimester
2 HBeAg-positive mothers have an 85% chance of transmission (cf. anti-HBe-positive: 25% chance)
3 δ Agent may also be transmitted at delivery
4 Cesarean section may reduce transmission (controversial)
5 Neonates at risk should be immunized (active and passive); 50% of infected male children die of cirrhosis or hepatoma
6 Hepatitis E infection may lead to fulminant hepatic failure

Chronic viral hepatitis: principal causes
1 Hepatitis B virus ± δ agent (HDV)
2 Hepatitis C

Antigens implicated in pathogenesis of chronic active hepatitis
1 Autoimmune type I ('lupoid') hepatitis
   — Actin
2 Autoimmune type II hepatitis
   — $P_{450}db1$ (a hepatic microsomal P_{450} isozyme)
3 Tienilic acid-induced hepatitis
   — P_{450} isozyme metabolizing tienilic acid

SECONDARY CAUSES OF LIVER DISEASE

Alcohol-induced liver disease
1 Steatosis (fatty infiltration)
   — Dose-dependent, reversible
2 Hepatic siderosis
3 Alcoholic hepatitis
   — 10–40% mortality
   — Precursor lesion for cirrhosis
4 Central hyaline sclerosis
   Pericellular fibrosis
5 Micronodular cirrhosis
6 Hepatocellular carcinoma

Hormone-induced liver disease
1 Pregnancy
   — Benign recurrent cholestasis (recurs with pregnancy or OC use)
   — Acute fatty liver of pregnancy (AFLOP; 75% mortality; rarely recurs in subsequent pregnancies): 3rd trimester
   — HELPP syndrome* (*h*emolysis, *e*levated LFTs, low *p*latelets, *p*re-eclampsia): 3rd trimester
   — Hepatic vein thrombosis (Budd–Chiari syndrome; 3rd trimester)
   — Hepatic rupture (follows pre-eclamptic liver disease; 3rd trimester)
2 Oral contraceptive (OC) use
   — Cholestasis (pruritus ± jaundice), cholelithiasis
   — Hepatic vein thrombosis
   — Adenoma(s) ± intraperitoneal rupture
   — Focal nodular hyperplasia
3 Androgens (C-17 alkyl-substituted testosterones)
   — Cholestasis
   — Peliosis hepatis
   — Hepatoma, angiosarcoma

* Risk increased if fetus is deficient in LCHAD (long chain 3-hydroxyacyl-coenzyme A dehydrogenase)

Cirrhosis: potential etiologies
1 Viruses
   — HBV, HCV
2 Alcohol
   — Chronic
3 Prolonged cholestasis
   — Intra- or extrahepatic
4 Prolonged venous obstruction
   — Budd–Chiari, constrictive pericarditis
5 Metabolic
   — Idiopathic hemochromatosis
   — Wilson's disease
   — $\alpha_1 AT$ deficiency
6 Drugs (long-term)
   — Methotrexate, INH, methyldopa, nitrofurantoin, vitamin A, dantrolene

LIVER DISEASE: CLINICAL BACKGROUND

Liver dysfunction in inflammatory bowel disease
1 **C**holangitis
   — Recurrent ascending cholangitis
   — Sclerosing cholangitis (in ulcerative colitis only)
     • No effective treatment, incl. colectomy
     • May mimic hepatitis, PBC, cholangiocarcinoma
     • May predispose to cholangiocarcinoma
   Cholangiocarcinoma
   Cholelithiasis (in Crohn's disease only)
2 **H**epatic vein thrombosis
   Hepatic infiltration (fat, amyloid)

Amebic liver abscesses
1 Right lobe affected in 90%
   Males affected in 80%
   Single abscess only in 70%
2 Liver function tests usually normal
3 Formed stools may contain cysts (DD$_x$: leukocytes) and vegetative forms (usually early stages)
4 Secondary bacterial infection in 20%
5 Past history of amebic dysentery *rare*
6 Amebic serology positive in virtually 100%

PREDISPOSITIONS TO LIVER DISEASE

Epidemiologic associations of hepatitis B surface antigenemia
1 Male homosexuality
2 Narcotic addiction
3 Hemophilia; hemodialysis; transplantation

Predispositions to hepatic vein thrombosis (Budd–Chiari)
1 Severe dehydration, esp. in early life
2 Post-partum; oral contraceptive use
3 Paroxysmal nocturnal hemoglobinuria
4 Malignancies
   — Myeloproliferative disease (commonest cause)
   — Hepatoma, renal cell carcinoma

5 Inflammatory bowel disease
6 Hepatic vein (or caval) webs*

* Esp. in Orientals

Fatty liver? Differential diagnosis
1 Alcohol ingestion*
2 Diabetes mellitus
 — esp. High-dose insulin patients
3 Pregnancy
 — Acute (fulminating) type
 — High-dose intravenous tetracycline therapy‡
4 Thyrotoxicosis; Cushing's syndrome
5 Inflammatory bowel disease
6 Obesity, hyperlipidemia
7 Protein-calorie malnutrition; ileal bypass
8 Hepatitis C

* 50% proceed to cirrhosis if drinking continues
‡ Should never be used in pregnancy in any case

ALCOHOLIC LIVER DISEASE

Factors contributing to ethanolic hepatotoxicity
1 Increased oxidative stress
 — ↑ NADH:NAD ratio
 — ↑ Lactate:pyruvate ratio
2 Formation of acetaldehyde adducts
 — Inhibition of enzyme activity
 — Cytoskeletal dysfunction*
 — Glutathione depletion
3 Free radical generation
 — Lipid peroxidation
4 Immune system activation
 — ↑ Interleukin-8 levels
5 Other effects
 — Nutritional deficiencies
 — Increased portal blood flow

* e.g. *Mallory bodies* are aggregated intermediate filaments

Management of alcoholic hepatitis
1 Abstention from alcohol
2 Nutritional support (does *not* prevent ethanolic damage)
 — Folate, B_{12}, B_6, thiamine
3 Adequate oxygenation and transfusion

HEPATIC ENCEPHALOPATHY

Pathogenesis of hepatic encephalopathy: general mechanisms
1 Hepatic insufficiency
 — Circulation of undetoxified metabolites (e.g. ammonia, aromatic amino acids) due to urea cycle breakdown
 — Abnormal cerebral metabolism
2 Urea cycle breakdown
 — ↓ Hepatic gluconeogenesis and insulin release
 — ↓ Uptake of branched-chain amino acids by muscle
3 Increased permeability of blood–brain barrier

4 Disturbed neurotransmitter balance
5 Impairment of cerebral Na^+/K^+-ATPase activity
6 Shunting via varices

Pathogenesis of hepatic encephalopathy: specific mechanisms
1 ↑ Blood ammonia → ↑ CNS ammonia
2 ↑ CNS ammonia → ↑ CNS (CSF) glutamine
3 CNS ammonia → abnormal α-ketoglutarate metabolism
4 ↑ Blood tryptophan (an aromatic amino acid) → ↑ CNS 5-HT (serotonin)
5 ↑ Methionine → ↑ mercaptan (→ fetor)
6 ↓ CNS dopamine/noradrenaline
7 ↑ CNS octopamine (a 'false' neurotransmitter)
8 ↑ GABA (an inhibitory CNS neurotransmitter) activation
9 ?Endogenous benzodiazepine-like activity

PATHOPHYSIOLOGY OF INTESTINAL DISORDERS

Predispositions to giardiasis
1 Hypogammaglobulinemia, selective IgA deficiency
2 Celiac disease
3 Achlorhydria; post-gastrectomy
4 Chronic pancreatitis
5 Homosexuality
6 Institutionalized children
7 Travel/residence in developing countries

Relationship of smoking to inflammatory bowel diseases
1 Ulcerative colitis occurs less often in smokers
2 Crohn's disease occurs (and relapses) more often in smokers

Malabsorptive mechanisms in bacterial overgrowth
1 Invasive mucosal damage (villous atrophy)
2 Mechanical barrier to absorption
3 Nutrient consumption by organisms (incl. B_{12} catabolism)
4 Production of abnormal gut motility
5 Deconjugation of bile acids leading to
 — Steatorrhea (jejunoileal malabsorption)
 — Colonic irritation → diarrhea

Mechanisms of diarrhea following ileal resection
1 Short bowel syndrome
 — Rapid transit → sodium/water malabsorption
2 Limited or recent resection
 — Cholorrheic diarrhea due to colonic irritation
3 Extensive resection
 — Frank steatorrhea due to bile salt insufficiency
4 Loss of ileocecal valve
5 Gastric hypersecretion
 — Due to impaired gastrin inactivation

Gastrointestinal concomitants of panhypogammaglobulinemia
1 Infections
 — Giardiasis
 — Bacterial overgrowth
 — Viral and bacterial enteritides

2 Celiac disease
3 Nodular lymphoid hyperplasia
4 Pancreatic insufficiency
5 Pernicious anemia, gastric carcinoma

GLUTEN-INDUCED ENTEROPATHY (CELIAC DISEASE)

Clinical presentations of gluten-induced enteropathy
1 Common
   — Persistent non-specific gastrointestinal upset
   — Constitutional symptoms; symptomatic anemia
   — Minor abnormality detected on full blood count (e.g. mild macrocytic anemia, hyposplenism)
2 Classical
   — Steatorrhea
   — Growth retardation
   — Osteomalacia
   — Dermatitis herpetiformis
3 Unusual
   — Amenorrhea, hypogonadism, infertility
   — Clubbing, bone pain, tetany, neuropathy
   — Edema, nocturia
   — Aphthous stomatitis
4 Rare
   — Fever of unknown origin
   — Lymphadenopathy; thrombocytosis
   — Recurrent pericarditis
   — Proctalgia fugax
   — Gastrointestinal lymphoma or adenocarcinoma

Diagnostic criteria in gluten-induced enteropathy
1 Best screening tests
   — Microcytic anemia (in a young non-menstruating person)
   — Red cell folate (↓ in 70%)
   — Howell–Jolly bodies on film*
2 Serology
   — Antigliadin antibodies (IgG and IgA)
   — Antiendomysial antibodies (produced after gliadin challenge/exposure; IgA)
   — Antitransglutaminase antibody is negative in IgA deficiency
3 Definitive diagnosis (to justify lifelong dietary switch)
   — Subtotal villous atrophy on small bowel biopsy, *plus*
   — Symptomatic ± histologic resolution on diet

NB: Often *poor* correlation between symptomatic, biochemical and histologic improvement following gluten-free diet (biopsy may take *months* to improve)
* Highly specific finding in appropriate symptomatic context

Composition of the gluten-free diet
1 Excluded
   — Wheat
   — Rye
   — Barley
   — Malt
2 Moderate amounts OK for adult celiacs
   — Oats *if* not contaminated by wheat

3 Not excluded
   — Rice
   — Corn
   — Soybean

Efficacy of the gluten-free diet
1 90% patients → clinical (symptomatic) remission
2 70% → 'biochemical' remission (e.g. normal red cell folate)
3 50% → 'mucosal' remission on re-biopsy (but the other 50% also improve)

Failure of clinical remission with gluten-free diet
1 Inadequate dietary compliance
2 Undiagnosed complication or misdiagnosis
   — Lactose intolerance
   — Hypogammaglobulinemia
   — Bacterial overgrowth
   — Pancreatic insufficiency
   — Tropical sprue
3 Development of collagenous sprue (treatable with steroids)
4 Development of small bowel lymphoma

INTESTINAL PSEUDO-OBSTRUCTION

Chronic intestinal pseudo-obstruction: etiopathogenesis
1 Familial neuromyopathies
   — Familial myenteric plexus degeneration
   — Familial dysautonomia (Riley–Day syndrome)
   — Familial amyloidosis with autonomic neuropathy
   — Myotonic dystrophy
   — Acute intermittent porphyria
2 Acquired neuromyopathies
   — Systemic sclerosis (smooth muscle replaced by fibrosis)
   — Polymyositis
   — Parkinson's disease
   — Lead poisoning
   — Pelvic irradiation
3 Endocrinopathies
   — Diabetes mellitus (delayed gastric emptying)
   — Myxedema
   — Pheochromocytoma (long-standing)
   — Congenital hypoparathyroidism
4 Anticholinergic drugs
   — Phenothiazines
   — Tricyclics
   — Antiparkinsonian medication

Management modalities in pseudo-obstruction
1 Cisapride
   — Prokinetic drug which promotes release of acetylcholine in the myenteric plexus
   — No longer used routinely (e.g. for reflux esophagitis) due to risk of arrhythmias
2 Erythromycin
   — Macrolide antibiotic which binds and activates motilin receptors in the proximal GI tract
3 Guanethidine plus neostigmine
   — For acute colonic pseudo-obstruction

4 Colonoscopic decompression
— Success rate of 75%, morbidity 3%, mortality 1%, in acute colonic pseudo-obstruction
5 Conservative management (drip and suck)
6 Long-term total parenteral nutrition

INTESTINAL NEOPLASIA

Histopathologic classification of polyps
1 Hyperplastic
— No malignant potential
2 Juvenile
— May be familial
3 Villous
— Larger; hence, high neoplastic potential
4 Hamartomatous
— e.g. Peutz–Jeghers
5 Inflammatory ('pseudopolyps')
— True, non-neoplastic polyps occurring as post-inflammatory sequelae
— Must be distinguished from carcinoma

Molecular events in the polyp–cancer sequence
1 Loss of heterozygosity on chromosome 5q*
2 DNA hypomethylation ($\to$ chromatin activation)
3 Mutation on chromosome 17 (MCC)
4 *Ras* and *p53* mutations
5 Deletion on chromosome 18 (DCC: adhesion molecule)
6 Mutation on chromosome 2 in hereditary non-polyposis colon cancer (DNA mismatch repair gene)

* Locus for adenomatous polyposis coli (*APC*) gene

MECHANISMS OF CIRRHOTIC SEQUELAE

Gynecomastia in alcoholic cirrhosis
1 $\uparrow$ Sex-hormone binding globulin (SHBG) levels
— $\downarrow$ Free testosterone levels
2 Hypothalamopituitary axis suppression
— $\downarrow$ Total testosterone levels
3 $\uparrow$ Estrogen production from precursors (e.g. DHEA)

Anemia in alcoholic liver disease
1 Hepatic insufficiency per se depresses erythropoiesis
2 Alcohol per se depresses erythropoiesis
3 Folate deficiency
4 Hypersplenism
5 Bleeding (see below)

Bleeding tendency in alcoholic cirrhosis
1 Reduced synthesis of coagulation factors
Reduced activation of coagulation factors
2 Platelet function defect
— Cirrhosis-induced von Willebrand's-type defect
— Separate alcohol-induced platelet function defect
3 Thrombocytopenia
— Hypersplenism
— Marrow suppression

4 Local factors
— Varices
— Peptic ulceration
— Gastritis
— Mallory–Weiss

Coagulopathy in cirrhosis
1 Synthesis of all clotting factors except VIII may be reduced
2 Jaundiced patients may malabsorb vitamin K
— $\downarrow$ activation of factors II, VII, IX, X, and proteins C and S
3 Prolongation of prothrombin time reflects reduced levels of factors II, V, VII, and X (cf. vitamin K dependence)
4 Since the half-life of factor VII is only 6 h, the prothrombin time is a sensitive index of hepatic function
5 Marked prolongation of both thrombin time and reptilase clotting time despite normal levels of fibrinogen antigen may reflect presence of abnormal fibrinogen*

* Dysfibrinogenemia; also associated with hepatoma

Ascitic tendency in cirrhosis
1 Activation of renin–angiotensin–aldosterone axis due to decreased effective central blood volume
— Vasodilatation of splanchnic vascular bed
— Peripheral vasodilatation (due to A–V shunting)
— High portal venous pressure
— Low serum albumin
2 Perivenular hepatic fibrosis
— Hepatic venous outflow obstruction
— $\uparrow$ Sinusoidal pressure (intrahepatic hypertension) $\to$ fluid transudation
3 Other factors
— $\uparrow$ Renal sympathetic tone/sodium retention
— Reduced hepatic degradation of aldosterone
— Excess thoracic duct lymph drainage

NB: Onset of refractory ascites signals 1-year mortality of 50%

BILE METABOLISM

Hepatobiliary defects predisposing to gallstone formation
1 Cholesterol-supersaturated bile
2 Increased tendency to cholesterol crystal nucleation
3 Impaired gallbladder contractility

Physiologic regulation of bilirubin metabolism
1 Bilirubin arises by cleavage of heme ring of hemoglobin, myoglobin, cytochromes. 70% of bilirubin originates from senescent RBC breakdown
2 Bilirubin binds tightly to albumin, and may be displaced by drugs such as sulfonamides (leading to elevation of potentially neurotoxic free bilirubin $\to$ kernicterus)
3 Albumin-bound bilirubin is not renally filtered, but rather is exclusively metabolized by the liver and excreted in bile

4 On entering the hepatocyte, bilirubin is transported to the endoplasmic reticulum where it undergoes conjugation to the sugar molecule glucuronide. The enzyme regulating conjugation is called UDP-glucuronyltransferase. Hence, deficiencies of UDP-glucuronyltransferase cause unconjugated hyperbilirubinemia

5 Conjugated bilirubin is transferred to the canalicular membrane where it undergoes transport into the bile canalicular space. This is the rate-limiting step of bilirubin metabolism

6 Hepatocellular disease prevents canalicular transport of bilirubin into the bile, causing reflux of conjugated bilirubin back into the bloodstream

Familial 'non-hemolytic'* hyperbilirubinemias

1 Gilbert's syndrome (autosomal dominant)
— Affects 2–5% of the population, esp. slow acetylators
— Mild unconjugated hyperbilirubinemia due to *minor* deficiency of UDP-glucuronyltransferase (promoter polymorphism) → ↓ conjugation/uptake (± ↓ RBC survival)
— Jaundice precipitated by
   • Fasting (e.g. GTT)
   • Illness (e.g. 'flu)
   • Stress (e.g. surgery)
   • Alcohol ingestion
— Liver function and histology *normal*
— Phenobarbital or rifampicin offer effective prophylaxis; but usually unnecessary

2 Crigler–Najjar syndrome type II (type I usually lethal)
— Rare, relatively benign autosomal dominant condition
— Unconjugated hyperbilirubinemia due to *major* deficiency of UDP-glucuronyltransferase
— Phenobarbital useful in management

3 Dubin–Johnson syndrome
— Conjugated hyperbilirubinemia due to defective canalicular excretion; failure of OCG
— Exacerbated by pregnancy, oral estrogens
— BSP elimination: biphasic (late 2° rise)
— Abnormal urinary coproporphyrin excretion
— Biopsy: black centrilobular pigment

4 Rotor's syndrome
— Conjugated hyperbilirubinemia due to defect in canalicular bilirubin excretion
— *Normal* cholecystogram, biopsy, BSP test
— Abnormal urinary coproporphyrin excretion

* Note that some patients with Gilbert's have associated mild hemolysis. In particular, neonatal hyperbilirubinemia due to ABO incompatibility (mother group O, baby group A or B) is increased in Gilbert's babies

Protein malfunctions predisposing to cholestasis

1 Inherited gene mutations
— P-type ATPase (18q21–22): benign recurrent cholestasis
— Multidrug resistance-3 transporter (7q21): progressive familial cholestasis

2 Acquired changes of expression
— ↑ Organic anion-transporting polypeptide: primary sclerosing cholangitis

— ↓ Chloride-bicarbonate anion exchanger: primary biliary cirrhosis
— ↓ Sodium-taurocholate cotransporter: biliary atresia

REVIEWING THE LITERATURE: GASTROENTEROLOGY

4.1 Rao M et al (1998) Effect of computed tomography of the appendix on treatment of patients and use of hospital resources. N Engl J Med 338: 141–146

Consecutive study of 100 appendiceal CT scans in patients hospitalized for observation of suspected appendicitis. The accuracy of CT was 98%, led to changes of management in 59%, and prevented unnecessary surgery in 13%. CT was thus deemed cost-effective in this setting.

4.2 Rossle M et al (2000) A comparison of paracentesis and transjugular intrahepatic portosytemic shunting in patients with ascites. N Engl J Med 342: 1701–1707

Randomized study of 60 German patients with cirrhosis and refractory ascites, showing that transjugular shunting improves survival without the need for liver transplantation. The incidence of hepatic encephalopathy was similar in the two groups.

4.3 Feagan BG et al (2000) A comparison of methotrexate with placebo for the maintenance of remission in Crohn's disease. N Engl J Med 342: 1627–1632

Randomized double-blind study of 76 patients with active Crohn's disease who had entered remission after weekly IM injections of methotrexate 25 mg/week. Those patients who received low-dose (15 mg/week IM) methotrexate for the next 40 weeks maintained their remissions for longer.

4.4 Moayyedi P et al (2000) Effect of population screening and treatment for *Helicobacter pylori* on dyspepsia and quality of life in the community: a randomised controlled trial. Lancet 355: 1665–1669

[13]C-urea breath testing was used in this Swiss study to screen 8455 community patients. Of the 30% who were positive, those randomized to receive antibiotic treatment were (only) 5% less likely to report dyspeptic symptoms 2 years later. The authors conclude that routine community screening is unlikely to prove cost-effective based on symptoms alone.

4.5 Hildebrand P et al (2000) Risk among gastroenterologists of acquiring *Helicobacter pylori* infection: case-control study. Br Med J 321: 149

Swiss study of 92 gastroenterologists and 168 adult control subjects. The annual rate of conversion to *H. pylori* positivity was 2.6%, compared with only 0.14% in controls, suggesting that endoscopies can transmit the infectious agent.

4.6 Jaakkimainen RL et al (1999) Is *Helicobacter pylori* associated with non-ulcer dyspepsia and will eradication improve symptoms? A meta-analysis. Br Med J 319: 1040–1044

McColl K et al (1998) Symptomatic benefit from eradicating *Helicobacter pylori* infection in patients with nonulcer dyspepsia. N Engl J Med 339: 1869–1874

The former review of 28 studies found an odds ratio of 1.6 for *H. pylori* infection in patients with non-ulcer dyspepsia, and confirmed an improvement in dyspeptic symptoms following eradication therapy. The latter randomized study of over 300 patients documented symptomatic benefit in the eradication (antibiotic) group which was 15% greater than in the controls.

4.7 Lau J et al (2000) Effect of intravenous omeprazole on recurrent bleeding after endoscopic treatment of bleeding peptic ulcers. N Engl J Med 343: 310–316

Randomized comparison of 240 patients, in which one half received a 72-hour infusion of omeprazole following achievement of endoscopic hemostasis; both groups subsequently received daily omeprazole 20 mg p.o. for 8 weeks. However, the omeprazole infusion patients bled less during the period of infusion, and consequently had less than half the mortality of the placebo group.

4.8 Yeomans ND et al (1998) A comparison of omeprazole with ranitidine for ulcers associated with nonsteroidal antiinflammatory drugs. N Engl J Med 338: 719–726

Hawkey CJ et al (1998) Omeprazole compared with misoprostol for ulcers associated with nonsteroidal antiinflammatory drugs. N Engl J Med 338: 727–734

Two studies examining the gastric chemoprophylactic effects of anti-ulcer treatment in patients treated with NSAIDs. The former study of 541 patients showed superior healing with omeprazole than with ranitidine, whereas the latter study showed similar healing efficacy but better remissions and tolerability associated with omeprazole, compared with misoprostol (which caused abdominal pain and diarrhea).

4.9 Abajo F et al (1999) Association between selective serotonin uptake inhibitors and upper gastrointestinal bleeding: population based case-control study. Br Med J 319: 1106–1109

Lanas A et al (2000) Nitrovasodilators, low-dose aspirin, other nonsteroidal antiinflammatory drugs, and the risk of upper gastrointestinal bleeding. N Engl J Med 343: 834–839

Two studies examining the effects of 'non-gastrointestinal' drugs on NSAID gastrotoxicity. In the former population-based case-control study of 1651 cases and 10 000 controls, a modest risk of bleeding (risk ratio of 3.0) was associated with use of SSRIs alone, whereas concurrent use of SSRIs and NSAIDs/aspirin was associated with a synergistic increase in gastrotoxicity (risk ratio 15.6). The second case-control study of 1122 cases and 2231 controls showed that nitric oxide-releasing drugs (such as glyceryl trinitrate) protected against NSAID-induced bleeding to an extent similar to that of anti-ulcer drugs (risk ratio 0.6).

4.10 Leitzmann MF et al (1999) Recreational physical activity and the risk of cholecystectomy in women. N Engl J Med 341: 777–784

Ten-year follow-up of 60 290 participants in the Nurses' Health Study, showing that the frequency of regular exercise was inversely related to the incidence of cholecystectomy. This relationship was independent of obesity and recent weight loss.

4.11 Schwizer W et al (2001) *Helicobacter pylori* and symptomatic relapse of gastro-oesophageal reflux disease. Lancet 357: 1738–1742

Randomized controlled trial of 70 reflux patients, showing that eradication of *H. pylori* helped to alleviate the reflux symptoms.

CHAPTER 5

Hematologic disease

Physical examination protocol 5.1   You are asked to examine the patient for signs of hematological disease

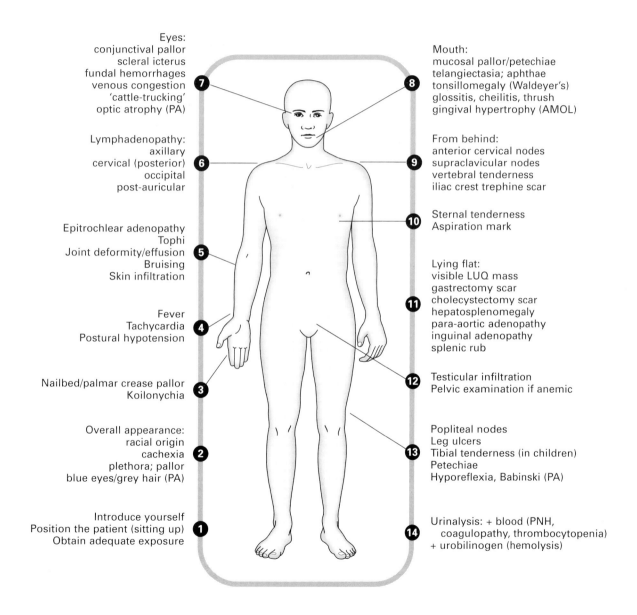

Eyes:
conjunctival pallor
scleral icterus
fundal hemorrhages
venous congestion
'cattle-trucking'
optic atrophy (PA)
7

8
Mouth:
mucosal pallor/petechiae
telangiectasia; aphthae
tonsillomegaly (Waldeyer's)
glossitis, cheilitis, thrush
gingival hypertrophy (AMOL)

Lymphadenopathy:
axillary
cervical (posterior)
occipital
post-auricular
6

9
From behind:
anterior cervical nodes
supraclavicular nodes
vertebral tenderness
iliac crest trephine scar

Epitrochlear adenopathy
Tophi
Joint deformity/effusion
Bruising
Skin infiltration
5

10
Sternal tenderness
Aspiration mark

Fever
Tachycardia
Postural hypotension
4

11
Lying flat:
visible LUQ mass
gastrectomy scar
cholecystectomy scar
hepatosplenomegaly
para-aortic adenopathy
inguinal adenopathy
splenic rub

Nailbed/palmar crease pallor
Koilonychia
3

12
Testicular infiltration
Pelvic examination if anemic

Overall appearance:
racial origin
cachexia
plethora; pallor
blue eyes/grey hair (PA)
2

13
Popliteal nodes
Leg ulcers
Tibial tenderness (in children)
Petechiae
Hyporeflexia, Babinski (PA)

Introduce yourself
Position the patient (sitting up)
Obtain adequate exposure
1

14
Urinalysis: + blood (PNH,
coagulopathy, thrombocytopenia)
+ urobilinogen (hemolysis)

Physical examination protocol 5.2   You are asked to examine a patient who has presented with bruising

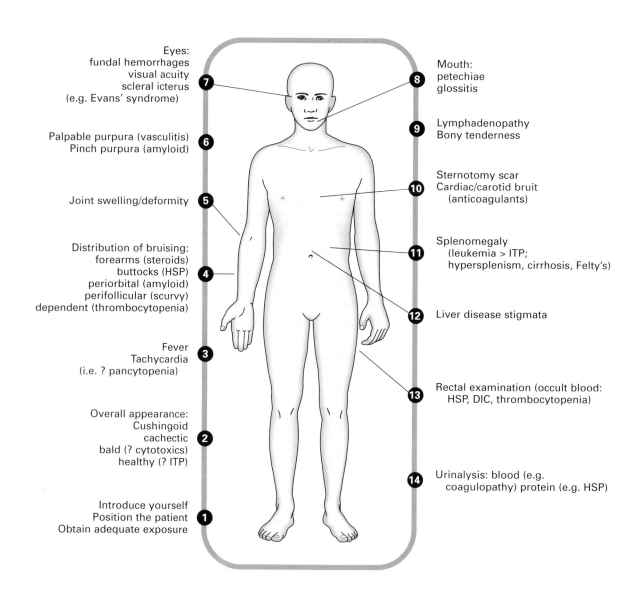

Eyes:
fundal hemorrhages
visual acuity
scleral icterus
(e.g. Evans' syndrome)   **7**

Palpable purpura (vasculitis)   **6**
Pinch purpura (amyloid)

Joint swelling/deformity   **5**

Distribution of bruising:
forearms (steroids)
buttocks (HSP)   **4**
periorbital (amyloid)
perifollicular (scurvy)
dependent (thrombocytopenia)

Fever   **3**
Tachycardia
(i.e. ? pancytopenia)

Overall appearance:
Cushingoid
cachectic   **2**
bald (? cytotoxics)
healthy (? ITP)

Introduce yourself   **1**
Position the patient
Obtain adequate exposure

8   Mouth:
petechiae
glossitis

9   Lymphadenopathy
Bony tenderness

10   Sternotomy scar
Cardiac/carotid bruit
(anticoagulants)

11   Splenomegaly
(leukemia > ITP;
hypersplenism, cirrhosis, Felty's)

12   Liver disease stigmata

13   Rectal examination (occult blood:
HSP, DIC, thrombocytopenia)

14   Urinalysis: blood (e.g.
coagulopathy) protein (e.g. HSP)

Physical examination protocol 5.3   You are asked to examine a patient who has been found to have an enlarged spleen

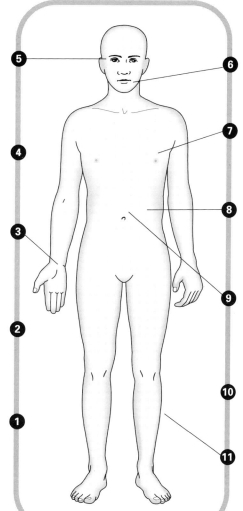

Eyes:
scleral icterus (HS, AIHA)
pingueculae (Gaucher's)
fundal hemorrhages (leukemia,
macroglobulinemia)
thyroid eye disease

Mouth: stomatitis; palatine
petechiae (mononucleosis)
macroglossia (amyloid)
xerostomia (Sjögren's)

Sternal tenderness
Cardiac bruit

Generalized lymphadenopathy
(CLL, lymphoma,
mononucleosis) –
tender/rubbery

Visibly massive spleen
(CML, MF, HCL, thalassemia)
Cholecystectomy scar (HS)
Tender (favors infection)
Rub (CML/SCA)

Pulse rate
Fever (leukemia/lymphoma;
infection: TB, SBE, brucellosis,
mononucleosis)
Hypertension (PRV)

Coexisting hepatomegaly
(primary liver disease, MF,
lymphoma, amyloid)
Para-aortic adenopathy
Liver disease stigmata
(e.g. ascites)

Overall appearance:
pallor (leukemia, thalassemia,
AIHA)
plethora
bruising
debility

Iliac crest trephine scar
(absence excludes diagnosed
myelofibrosis)

Introduce yourself
Position the patient
Obtain adequate exposure

Leg ulcers (congenital hemolytic
anemias, Felty's)

Diagnostic pathway 5.1 This patient has presented with hepatosplenomegaly. What underlying disorders might be responsible?

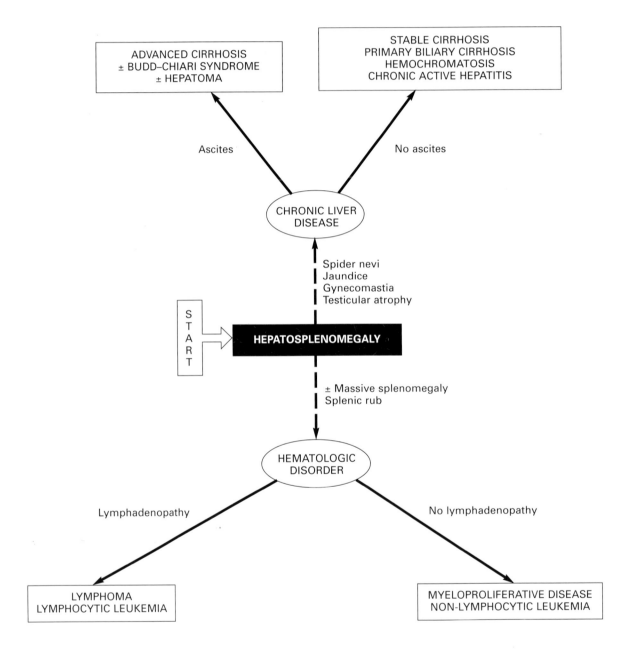

COMMON AND CLASSIC HEMATOLOGIC PROBLEMS

Common hematologic problems in clinical practice
1 Anemia
2 Bruising or bleeding tendency
3 Neutropenic fever in chemotherapy patients

Classic hematologic problems in clinical exams
1 Splenomegaly and/or lymphadenopathy
2 Venous thrombosis
3 Chronic joint ankylosis or deformity due to hemophilia

HEMATOLOGIC EMERGENCIES

Treatment modalities in bleeding cancer patients
1 Iatrogenic (cytotoxic-induced) thrombocytopenia
   — Platelet transfusion
2 Leukoerythroblastic thrombocytopenia (e.g. in lymphoma)
   — Cytotoxic therapy with transfusion cover
3 Autoimmune thrombocytopenia (e.g. in CLL)
   — Steroids
4 Hypersplenic thrombocytopenia (e.g. in hairy cell leukemia)
   — Splenectomy, splenic irradiation
5 Hyperviscosity
   — Plasmapheresis
6 Obstructive jaundice
   — Parenteral vitamin K
7 Uncontrolled neoplastic hemorrhage
   — Radiotherapy
8 Disseminated intravascular coagulation
   — Fresh frozen plasma (6 units; no heparin)
   — Platelet transfusion if count < 80×10^9/L
   — Cytotoxic therapy of underlying malignancy

Neutropenic fever: recognizing the high-risk patient
1 Very low absolute neutrophil count (< 100 mm^3)
2 Clinically apparent sepsis *and/or* positive blood cultures
3 Poor performance status
4 Severe comorbid condition
5 Onset within 1 week of chemotherapy initiation
6 Tachycardia or hypotension at presentation

Approach to the patient with disseminated intravascular coagulation
1 Treat underlying condition
2 Prevention (e.g. heparin prophylaxis in APL)
3 Treatment of symptomatic bleeding
   — Platelets
   — Transfusion
   — Fresh frozen plasma
   — Heparin (controversial): monitor AT III levels

Approach to the patient with tumor lysis syndrome
1 Prevention
   — Pretreatment allopurinol
   — Forced alkaline diuresis, or oral acetazolamide
2 Treatment of established syndrome
   — Hemodialysis

Clinical sequelae of hyperviscosity
1 CNS effects
   — Lassitude, headache, deafness, nystagmus, convulsions
2 Visual loss
   — Fundal hemorrhages, 'cattle-trucking', papilledema
3 Increased plasma volume
   — Dilutional anemia, hypertension, heart failure
4 Platelet dysfunction*
   — Bleeding, thrombosis, difficult venepuncture
5 Leukocyte dysfunction
   — Sepsis, difficult crossmatch
6 Renal failure
   — Plasmapheresis may minimize permanent damage

* esp. IgA myeloma

Clinical varieties of sickle cell crises
1 Painful (vaso-occlusive, thrombotic) crises
   — Commonest; often affects adults
   — Generalized bone pain
   — Infarcts (abdomen, brain, lung) precipitated by tissue hypoxia
   — May be accompanied by fever, fits, dyspnea
   — α-HBD may be elevated
   — Complications include
     • Autosplenectomy (hyposplenism)
     • Aseptic necrosis of bone
     • Permanent brain damage (stroke)
     • Renal failure
2 Acute chest syndrome (pulmonary infiltrates)
   — Fever, pleuritic pain, pulmonary infiltrates, cough, wheeze (mimics pneumonia)
   — May be triggered or exacerbated by fat embolism (secondary to bone marrow infarction) or community-acquired pneumonia (*Chlamydia, Mycoplasma*, viral)
   — Lung infarcts and becomes 'spleen-like'; older patients enter respiratory failure
   — Treat urgently with exchange transfusion to reduce HbS
3 Hand–foot syndrome
   — Affects infants → painful finger swelling
4 Splenic sequestration crises
   — Usually affects infants (may be triggered by hypovolemia)
   — Presents with rapid-onset hepato/splenomegaly and plummeting Hb
5 Hemolytic crises
   — May signify sepsis or associated G6PD deficiency
   — High reticulocyte count
   — Transfusion not routinely indicated
6 Aplastic crises
   — May signify parvovirus B19 infection or folate deficiency
   — Low reticulocyte count (cf. hemolytic crisis)

Prevention and management of sickle crises
1 Maintain Hb levels at 7–10 g/dL*
   — Transfusion (including exchange transfusion)
   — Hydroxyurea (→ ↑ HbF levels)‡

2 Active management
— Hydration, oxygenation, bronchodilators, antibiotics, analgesia

* Since HbS has a relatively low oxygen affinity, this may suffice to prevent vaso-occlusive crises (e.g. stroke). Note that erythropoietin is *useless* in this context
‡ Hydroxyurea may also inhibit sickling by reducing erythrocyte expression of the adhesion molecule VCAM-1

CLINICAL ASSESSMENT OF THE HEMATOLOGIC PATIENT

PRESENTATIONS OF HEMATOLOGIC DISEASE

Abdominal pain in the hematologic patient
1 Biliary colic (e.g. hereditary spherocytosis)
2 Splenic infarct (e.g. chronic myeloid leukemia)
3 Vaso-occlusive crisis (sickle-cell anemia)
4 Acute intermittent porphyria
5 Paroxysmal nocturnal hemoglobinuria
6 Hodgkin's disease (alcohol-induced pain)

History of the patient presenting with anemia
1 Duration of symptoms
2 Past history (e.g. ulcer, prosthetic valve, alcoholism)
3 Recent medications (e.g. NSAIDs, warfarin, steroids)
4 Operations (e.g. gastrectomy, ileal resection)
5 Menstrual history (esp. menorrhagia)
6 Diet (green vegetables, special restrictions)
7 Family history and racial background
8 Recent travel (e.g. to hookworm-endemic areas)
9 Toxic exposures (e.g. benzene, radiation)

Pathologic causes of epistaxis
1 Idiopathic thrombocytopenic purpura
2 Von Willebrand's disease
3 Hereditary hemorrhagic telangiectasia
4 Severe hypertension
5 Pertussis infection

Clinical manifestations of iron deficiency
1 Anemia
2 Koilonychia
3 Post-cricoid web (premalignant)
4 Atrophic glossitis
5 Angular stomatitis
6 Pica
7 Candidiasis
8 Impaired verbal learning and memory*

* May be improved by supplementation, even in the absence of anemia

Infections in the leukemic host: clinical pitfalls
1 Fevers may arise due to non-infectious causes (e.g. drugs, transfusion reactions, graft-versus-host disease)
2 Fevers may arise due to infection with multiple organisms, some of which may be difficult to identify
3 Fever may persist for the duration of neutropenia despite optimal antibiotic therapy

4 Fever may not occur at all in elderly or immunosuppressed patients with sepsis (± false-negative serologic responses)
5 Immunosuppressed febrile patients may fail to localize portal of sepsis due to poor inflammatory response

Complications of arteriovenous malformations
1 Spontaneous hemothorax
2 Cerebrovascular accident
3 Polycythemia, cyanosis

CLINICAL SIGNS OF HEMATOLOGIC DISEASE

Why do you think it's a spleen?
1 Can't get above it
2 Descends prominently on inspiration
3 Distinct edge ± medial notch
4 Not ballottable
5 Percussion dullness over spleen/Traube's space
6 ± Audible rub

Differential diagnosis of epitrochlear lymphadenopathy
1 Non-Hodgkin's lymphoma, chronic lymphocytic leukemia
2 Infectious mononucleosis; secondary syphilis
3 Sarcoidosis
4 Intravenous drug abuse

Widespread retinal hemorrhages: differential diagnosis
1 Malignant hypertension
2 Diabetes mellitus
3 Hyperviscosity syndrome
4 Severe anemia, severe thrombocytopenia
5 Hb SC (sickle-C) disease

Clinical evaluation of bleeding tendency
1 Skin petechiae, epistaxes, purpura after minor trauma
   Mucosal bleeding; menorrhagia
   Immediate bleeding after lacerations
   — Thrombocytopenia, or platelet function defect*
   — ↑ Bleeding time‡
2 Widespread intramuscular hematomas
   Spontaneous hemarthroses
   Delayed bleeding after lacerations
   — Coagulation factor deficiency (90% in males)
   — ↑ PTTK

* Incl. heterozygous von Willebrand's disease, even though platelets themselves are normal
‡ Clinical utility doubtful

POLYCYTHEMIA

Features common to primary and secondary polycythemia
1 Thrombotic tendency (esp. cerebral)
2 Hypertension
3 Headaches

4 Visual disturbances
5 Engorged retinal veins

Clinical features suggestive of polycythemia vera
1 Splenomegaly
2 Aquagenic pruritus
3 Bleeding (esp. gastrointestinal)
4 Gout
5 Peptic ulcer
6 Disease termination in myelofibrosis or leukemia (10%)

HODGKIN'S DISEASE

Clinical presentations of Hodgkin's disease
1 'B' symptoms (p. 149)
2 Pruritus (not a 'B' symptom)
3 Pel–Ebstein (cyclical) fever (p. 199): classical but rare
4 Alcohol-induced pain at sites of disease (incl. abdomen)
5 Infection (see p. 193)

Classical features of specific histologic subtypes
1 Lymphocyte predominant
   — Best prognosis
   — Usually early-stage (I, II) disease
2 Nodular sclerosing
   — Indolent chemosensitive but relapsing disease
   — Tends to affect young women
   — May cause bulky mediastinal adenopathy
   — Spreads by contiguity
   — Good prognosis unless bulky mediastinal disease
3 Mixed cellularity
   — Often associated with occult splenic involvement
   — Intermediate prognosis
4 Lymphocyte depletion
   — 'B' symptoms (e.g. fever of unknown origin)
   — Adenopathy more widespread than other subtypes
   — May present with visceral involvement, e.g. marrow fibrosis, osteoblastic bony disease ('ivory vertebrae')
   — Spreads by dissemination to distant sites
   — Worst prognosis

INVESTIGATING HEMATOLOGIC DISEASE

THE PERIPHERAL BLOOD FILM

Diagnosis suggested by blood film alone*
1 'Aleukemic' leukemia
   — Circulating blasts, leukoerythroblastic precursors
2 Compensated 'warm' autoimmune hemolysis
   — Spherocytes, polychromasia, reticulocytosis
   Hereditary spherocytosis
   — (Micro)spherocytes, ↑ MCHC
3 Dysproteinemias

   — Rouleaux, bluish background
4 Disseminated intravascular coagulation Microangiopathic hemolysis
   — Red cell fragments
5 Infection
   — Infectious mononucleosis (atypical lymphocytes)
   — Mycoplasma pneumoniae (autoagglutination)
   — Malaria (Plasmodium vivax/ovale → Schühffner's dots), babesiosis
   — Relapsing fever (Borrelia spirochetes visible on film)
6 Thalassemia trait‡
   — Microcytosis, teardrops, targets
   Hb C disease
   — Target cells in abundance
7 Pyruvate kinase deficiency (→ ATP deficiency)
   — Xerocytes (dehydrated RBCs)

* i.e. ± normal blood count
‡ cf. sickle cell trait: diagnosed by Hb electrophoresis (i.e. film normal)

Features of the postsplenectomy blood film
1 Howell-Jolly bodies
2 Pappenheimer bodies
3 Target cells
4 Spur cells, spherocytes
5 Thrombocytosis ± leukocytosis

Leukoerythroblastic blood film: diagnostic significance
1 **M**yelofibrosis
2 **M**arrow infiltration
   — Common causes
      • **M**etastatic cancer (e.g. breast, prostate)*
      • **M**yeloma
      • **M**alignant lymphoma
   — Uncommon causes
      • **M**arble bone disease (osteopetrosis)
      • **M**etabolic: Gaucher's disease

* Bone scan usually positive; cf. myeloma, lymphoma

Infectious diseases mimicking leukemic blood films
1 Infectious mononucleosis
   — May mimic ALL
2 Pertussis, mycoplasma
   — May mimic CLL

Differential diagnosis of eosinophilia
1 Allergy/atopy: asthma, eczema, urticaria, rhinitis
2 Parasitic infestations
3 Drug reactions
4 Rare neoplastic*, dermatologic or autoimmune associations

* e.g. hypereosinophilic syndrome

Clues to underlying sepsis on the peripheral blood film
1 Neutrophilia
2 'Left shift': bandforms, (meta)myelocytes
3 Toxic granulation
4 Döhle bodies

Differential diagnosis of the dimorphic blood film
1 Sideroblastosis
2 Post-splenectomy

3 Post-transfusion
4 Iron loss combined with B_{12}/folate malabsorption
   — Post-gastrectomy
   — Pernicious anemia with gastric cancer
   — Celiac disease and/or intestinal lymphoma
   — Crohn's disease, Whipple's disease
5 Iron loss combined with hyposplenism
   — Celiac disease
   — Radical gastrectomy (incorporates splenectomy)

Pathologic significance of red cell inclusions
1 Howell–Jolly bodies
  Cabot's rings
   — Nuclear remnants seen in hyposplenic states
2 Heinz bodies*
   — Denatured globin chains in RBC periphery seen in unstable Hb (e.g. Hb Zürich/Köln, G6PD deficiency)
   — Often associated with 'bite cells' on film
3 Pappenheimer bodies: iron granules in siderocytes
   — Positive Prussian blue reaction
   — Seen post-splenectomy and in lead poisoning
4 Basophilic stippling: implies dyserythropoiesis
   — Seen in lead poisoning (coarse stippling)
   — Also seen in thalassemia, 5'-nucleotidase deficiency

* Demonstrated using supravital stains, e.g. cresyl violet

Abnormal erythrocyte morphology: etiologic significance
1 Target cells
   — Chronic liver disease
   — Thalassemia; Hb C; Hb E*
   — Hyposplenism
   — Iron deficiency
2 Teardrop poikilocytes
   — Myelofibrosis
   — Dyserythropoiesis (e.g. thalassemia, megaloblastosis)
3 Schistocytes
   — Microangiopathic hemolytic anemia (e.g. TTP)
   — Disseminated intravascular coagulation
4 Spur cells (acanthocytes)
   — Chronic liver disease (esp. Zieve's syndrome)
   — Abetalipoproteinemia
   — Renal failure, hyposplenism

* Asymptomatic condition (Hb $\alpha_2\beta_2^{26Glu\rightarrow Lys}$) even when homozygous; but yields thalassemia major when crossed with β-thal trait. Very common in Thailand, Cambodia, Laos

Red cell distribution width (RDW) in anemia*
1 Normal RDW, ↑ reticulocyte count
   — α/β Thalassemia minor
   — Hereditary spherocytosis
   — Severe hemolysis (> 10% reticulocytes)
2 Normal RDW, ↓ reticulocyte count
   — Anemia of chronic disease
   — Aplastic anemia
   — Myelodysplastic syndromes
3 ↑ RDW, ↑ reticulocyte count
   — Microangiopathic hemolytic anemia
   — Immune hemolysis; cold agglutinin disease
   — Sickle-cell anemia; sickle-β-thal, sickle-C

   — Hb H disease
   — G6PD deficiency
4 ↑ RDW, ↓ reticulocyte count
   — Myelofibrosis
   — Sideroblastosis
   — Iron deficiency
* A quantitative measure of anisocytosis

IRON-DEFICIENCY ANEMIA

Abnormalities of plasma iron studies in hematologic disease
1 ↓ Fe, ↑ TIBC, ↓ ferritin   — Iron deficiency
2 ↓ Fe, ↓ TIBC, ↑ ferritin   — Chronic disease
3 ↑ Fe, ↓ TIBC, ↑ ferritin   — Chronic hemolysis
4 Normal Fe and TIBC, ↑ ferritin — β-thalassemia

Temporal sequence of iron deficiency
1 Iron depletion
   — ↓ Marrow stainable iron
   — ↓ Stainable sideroblast ferritin
   — ↑ Red cell protoporphyrin
2 Iron deficiency
   — Absent marrow stainable iron
   — ↓ Fe, ↑ TIBC
   — Transferrin saturation < 15%
3 Iron deficiency anemia
   — Hypochromic microcytic film
   — ↑ RDW*
   — ↓ Hb

* cf. chronic disease: RDW (red cell distribution width) normal

Differential diagnosis of microcytic anemia
1 Iron deficiency
   — Serum iron and ferritin ↓
2 Thalassemia trait
   — Serum iron normal; ferritin ↑
3 Sideroblastic anemia
   — Serum iron and ferritin ↑

Microcytosis disproportionate to anemia?
1 Thalassemia trait
2 Venesected polycythemia vera

Investigation of unexplained hypochromic microcytic anemia
1 Blood film
   — Red cell morphology
   — Reticulocyte count
2 Iron studies
   — Serum iron, TIBC, transferrin saturation
   — Serum ferritin
3 Exclusion of gastrointestinal (or uterine) bleeding
   — Fecal occult blood testing and/or endoscopy
   — Angiography; ^{99m}Tc-labelled red cells
4 Marrow aspiration
   — Stainable iron stores
   — Ring sideroblasts
5 Urinary hemosiderin
   — ↑ In chronic intravascular hemolysis (e.g. PNH)
6 Hb EPG
   — HbA$_2$ level (↑ in thalassemia trait)

Failure of microcytic anemia to respond to iron supplements
1 Wrong diagnosis
   — Thalassemia trait
   — Sideroblastosis (congenital)
2 Persistent bleeding
3 Malabsorption
   — Blind loop
   — Gastrectomy
4 Non-compliance

MEGALOBLASTIC ANEMIAS

Macrocytosis: clues to underlying megaloblastosis on blood film
1 Oval (not round) macrocytes (esp. if > 3%)
2 Markedly elevated MCV (> 115 fL)
3 Hypersegmented (> 5 lobes) neutrophils
4 Marked poikilo-/anisocytosis; mild basophilic stippling
5 No target/spur cells, round macrocytes (cf. liver disease)
   No polychromatophilic macrocytes (cf. hemolysis)

Clinicopathologic correlations in folate metabolism
1 Red cell folate is more informative than serum levels
2 Partial hematologic responses may be seen in (pure) B_{12} deficiency treated inadvertently with pharmacologic (5–15 mg/day) doses of folate*
3 Catastrophic progression of *neurologic* deficit may be seen in B_{12}-deficient patients treated inadvertently with folate. Hence, if in doubt, give both B_{12} and folate

* cf. primary folate deficiency, where maximal reticulocytosis follows physiologic – 200 μg/day – doses of folate

Clinicopathologic correlations in B_{12} deficiency
1 The microbiologic assay remains the 'gold standard' in determining B_{12} levels. Radioimmunoassay, though cheaper and more widely used, has a higher false-negative and (occasionally) false-positive rate with respect to B_{12} deficiency (e.g. due to R-protein (see below) errors)
2 In B_{12} deficient patients, serum folate (and iron) levels are often elevated ('normal' levels may indicate coexisting folate, or iron, deficiency), while red cell folate levels may be reduced due to the 'folate trap' mechanism
3 Neurologic degeneration may occur without anemia
4 Transient ileal mucosal changes (analogous to macrocytosis) may, misleadingly, lead to failure of normalization of the Schilling test following oral intrinsic factor in patients with pernicious anemia treated for less than (say) 6 weeks
5 Mean corpuscular volume may be normal in patients with coexisting iron deficiency (e.g. Crohn's, celiac disease, pernicious anemia with gastric cancer) or thalassemia trait
6 Blood transfusion is best avoided in initial management of severe megaloblastic anemia (risk of fluid overload)

Investigations distinguishing primary B_{12} from folate deficiency*
1 Deoxyuridine suppression test
   — Deoxyuridine and tritiated thymidine added to patient's bone marrow in vitro
   — Megaloblastic marrow takes up ↑↑ thymidine
   — Corrects upon adding B_{12} (in B_{12} deficiency) or methyltetrahydrofolate (in folate deficiency)
2 24-h urinary methylmalonic acid excretion
   — 10 g valine given as an initial loading dose
   — ↑ Methylmalonic acid excretion in B_{12} deficiency *only*

* i.e. if *both* B_{12} and folate levels low

Molecular regulation of B_{12} metabolism
1 Intrinsic factor (IF)
   — Synthesized by gastric parietal cells
   — Binds and transports dietary cobalamin (B_{12})*
   — B_{12}-IF complex attaches to specific ileal receptors
2 R-proteins
   — Incl. transcobalamin (TC) I, III; made by leukocytes
   — Compete with IF for intragastric binding of cobalamin
   — Bind B_{12} more avidly than IF at low gastric pH
   — Facilitate hepatic storage and excretion of cobalamin
   — Degraded in jejunum by pancreatic enzymes, whereas IF resists proteolysis and binds liberated B_{12}
3 TC-II
   — Plasma protein synthesized by liver
   — Binds newly absorbed B_{12} in portal blood
   — Transports B_{12} to target tissues

* Note however, that oral cobalamin in doses of 1000 μg/day may be effective in treating pernicious anemia, suggesting the presence of an alternative absorptive pathway

Abnormalities of transcobalamin metabolism
1 ↓ TC-II
   — Hereditary
   — Leads to ↓ B_{12} levels (with clinical deficiency)
2 ↑ TC-I
   — Occurs secondary to CML/polycythemia vera
   — May cause ↑ B_{12} levels
3 ↑ TC-III
   — Seen in benign leukocytosis (e.g. leukemoid reaction)
   — No change in B_{12} levels
4 ↑ TC-II
   — Seen with macrophage activation (e.g. SLE, sarcoid)
   — No change in B_{12} levels

Some causes of vitamin B_{12} deficiency
1 Pernicious anemia
2 Gastrectomy
3 Bacterial overgrowth (*Escherichia coli, Bacteroides fragilis*)
4 Ileal resection (usually > 1 meter)
5 Pancreatic exocrine insufficiency (↓ R-protein proteolysis)
   Gastrinoma (low pH inactivates pancreatic proteases)

6 Imerslund's disease; *Diphyllobothrium latum* infestation*

* Both conditions endemic in Finland

Significance of clinical B$_{12}$ deficiency in Crohn's disease
1 Bacterial overgrowth
2 Fistula
3 Ileal resection

NB: Major B$_{12}$ deficiency is *unusual* in uncomplicated Crohn's

Differential diagnosis of an abnormal Schilling* test
1 Corrects with addition of intrinsic factor
— Pernicious anemia
2 Does not correct with intrinsic factor
— Bacterial overgrowth ($\uparrow$ fecal bile acids)
— Ileal insufficiency, e.g. resection, severe Crohn's ($\downarrow$ fecal bile acids)
— Renal failure‡ (normal fecal bile acids)

* i.e. radioactive B$_{12}$ oral absorption; test will be *normal* in B$_{12}$ deficiency due to vegan diet
‡ i.e. renal failure *spuriously* reduces Schilling test yield; B$_{12}$ levels normal

Indicators of response following B$_{12}$ replenishment
1 Erythroblastosis (bone marrow) within 12 h
Reticulocytosis begins at 48 h, maximal after 1 week
2 $\uparrow$ Serum alkaline phosphatase
3 $\uparrow$ Urate
4 $\downarrow$ K$^+$ (may be profound)
5 $\downarrow$ Folate; $\downarrow$ iron (usually subclinical)

Megaloblastic anemias with normal B$_{12}$/folate levels
1 Antimetabolite therapy
2 Erythroleukemia
3 Hereditary orotic aciduria (uridine-responsive)
Lesch-Nyhan syndrome (adenine-responsive)

Etiology of non-megaloblastic macrocytosis
1 Alcohol ± liver disease
Liver disease ± alcohol
2 Hypothyroidism (exclude coexisting pernicious anemia)
3 Acquired sideroblastosis*
4 Reticulocytosis (any cause)
Autoagglutination ($\rightarrow$ *artefactual* $\uparrow$ MCV)‡
5 Aplastic anemia
6 Paroxysmal nocturnal hemoglobinuria

* cf. congenital sideroblastosis: usually microcytic
‡ e.g. in cold hemagglutinin disease (CHAD; pp. 154, 186)

AUTOIMMUNE HEMOLYTIC ANEMIA

Investigation of suspected hemolysis
1 Etiologic clues on blood film
— Spherocytes (hereditary, or autoimmune hemolysis)
— Schistocytes, helmet cells (microangiopathic hemolysis)
— Sickled cells

2 Signs of marrow compensation:
— Polychromatophilic macrocytes
— Reticulocytosis ('warm' > 'cold' hemolysis)
— Occasional nucleated red cells
3 Confirmation of red cell lysis:
— Mild unconjugated (direct) hyperbilirubinemia
— Urinalysis: urobilinogen+, bilirubin–
— $\downarrow$ Haptoglobin*
— $\downarrow$ Hemopexin
— $\downarrow$ Folate (secondary, esp. in pregnancy)
4 Confirmation of marrow compensation
— Erythroid hyperplasia on marrow aspirate
5 Signs of intravascular hemolysis
— Hemoglobinemia, hemoglobinuria‡
— Hemosiderinuria (implies chronicity; may $\rightarrow$ $\downarrow$ Fe^{2+})
— Methemalbuminemia (Schumm's+; implies severity)
6 Further diagnostic investigations
— Coombs' and Ham's tests
— Cold agglutinins, Donath–Landsteiner antibody
— Hb EPG; Heinz body prep; RBC G6PD levels
— ^{51}Cr-RBC survival and sequestration study

* NB: False-negatives in acute phase reactions, false-positives in liver disease
‡ Associated with pink serum; cf. myoglobinuria

Coombs' tests: what do they do?
1 Direct Coombs' antiglobulin test (DAT)
— Used to investigate *hemolysis*
— i.e. Do the *patient's red cells* have antibody/C$_3$?
2 Indirect Coombs' antiglobulin test (IAT)
— Used in blood *crossmatching*
— i.e. Does the intended *recipient's serum* contain antibodies to the planned red cell transfusion?

Autoimmune hemolysis: diagnostic aspects
1 'Warm' type
— IgG-mediated extravascular (intrasplenic) hemolysis: +DAT, +IgG
— Progressive anemia, mild jaundice, splenomegaly
— Blood film: spherocytes, marked reticulocytosis
— Often arises secondary to SLE, CLL, Hodgkin's, drugs
— Often responds to steroids/azathioprine, splenectomy
— Transfusion may be lifesaving
2 'Cold' type
— IgM-κ-mediated intravascular (intrahepatic) hemolysis: +DAT, +C$_3$
— Autoagglutination on blood film
— Symptom severity depends more on height of thermal amplitude than on absolute titre
— May signify lymphoma, macroglobulinemia, infection
— Treatment is best directed at the underlying condition
— Transfusion should be avoided if possible; if absolutely necessary, warm blood and transfuse slowly

Features of drug-induced autoimmune hemolysis
1 'Methyldopa' (autoimmune) type
   — Mild (rarely significant) extravascular hemolysis
   — +DAT, +IAT (i.e. Coombs+ without drug), $-C_3$
   — May remain Coombs+ for years after drug ceased
2 'Penicillin' (hapten) type
   — IgG directed against drug (a hapten)
   — IgG adsorbs to red cell after prolonged high-dose R_x
   — Causes extravascular hemolysis
   — +DAT, −IAT (i.e. Coombs+ *only* in presence of drug)
3 'Quinine' (immune complex) type
   — Intravascular hemolysis on second or subsequent exposures ('innocent bystander' mechanism)
   — IgM- (or IgG-) mediated complement activation
   — Drug–IgM complex dissociates from RBCs, leaving C_3
   — +DAT, $+C_3$

OTHER ANEMIAS

Significance of abnormal reticulocyte counts in anemia
1 Reticulocytosis
   — Blood loss/hemorrhage
     • Up to 15% reticulocytes
   — Hemolysis
     • Up to 30% reticulocytes
   — Response phase of iron/B_{12}/folate deficiency
     • Up to 50% reticulocytes
2 Reticulocytopenia (i.e. relative to degree of anemia)
   — Aplastic anemia
   — Chronic disease (e.g. uremia)

Hypersplenism: diagnostic criteria
1 Cytopenia
2 Splenomegaly
3 Marrow hypercellularity
4 Cytopenia corrected by splenectomy

Anemia of chronic disease: laboratory features
1 Blood film
   — Normocytic ± hypochromic; normal RDW
   — Reticulocytopenia (for degree of anemia)
2 Iron studies
   — ↓ Fe/TIBC/TF saturation
   — ↑ Ferritin
3 Special studies
   — ↓ Red cell survival
   — ↓ Erythropoietin activity
   — ↑ Red cell protoporphyrin
4 Bone marrow
   — Absent sideroblasts (RBC precursors)
   — ↑ Iron stores

Varieties of anemia in myxedema
1 Normochromic, normocytic
2 Macrocytic
   — Suggests associated pernicious anemia
3 Microcytic (in female)
   — Suggests menorrhagia

Diagnosis of hereditary spherocytosis
1 Family history (in 80%)
2 Clinical picture
   — Recurrent mild unconjugated jaundice (DD_x Gilbert's)
   — ± Splenomegaly, anemia, gallstones
3 Numerous microspherocytes on blood film
   Negative Coombs' test
4 ↑ MCHC (35–38 g%); normal MCV
5 Definitive diagnosis
   — ↑ RBC osmotic fragility (high-salt lysis)
   — Positive autohemolysis test*
6 Mutation in ankyrin/β-spectrin locus (not routine)
   — Genetic heterogeneity reflects clinical picture

* Corrects with glucose; cf. 'autoimmune' spherocytosis

Causes of a grossly abnormal ESR
1 > 100 mm/h
   — Malignancy
     • Myeloma
     • Hodgkin's
     • Carcinomatosis
   — Sepsis, esp. active TB
   — Active vasculitis, esp. giant-cell
   — Uremia; profound anemia
2 < 3 mm/h*
   — Polycythemia rubra vera
   — Sickle cell anemia
   — Massive leukocytosis (e.g. in CLL)
   — Hypofibrinogenemia (hereditary or DIC-induced)
   — High-dose steroids or salicylates

* NB: 95% of these will be *normal*

NORMAL AND ABNORMAL HEMOGLOBINS

Factors improving tissue oxygenation by red blood cells*
1 Acidosis, hypercapnia
   — Via Bohr effect
2 Hypoxia, anemia
   Thyrotoxicosis; pregnancy
   Renal failure
   — Via ↑ red cell 2,3-DPG
3 Increased blood temperature
4 Low-affinity Hb (see below)

* i.e. Reducing Hb affinity for oxygen; right shift of dissociation curve

Diagnostic value of hemoglobin electrophoresis
1 Hb S (sickle cell)
2 Hb A_2 (↑ in β-thal *trait* esp.)
3 Hb C, D, E

Hemoglobins with abnormal oxygen affinity
1 High-affinity hemoglobins
   — e.g. Hb F; Hb Chesapeake, Hb Rainier, Hb Köln
   — Detected as unexpected polycythemia on routine test
   — Cause left shift of oxyhemoglobin dissociation curve*
   — Usually asymptomatic with benign course

2 Low-affinity hemoglobins (rare)
— e.g. Hb Kansas, Hb Seattle, Hb Hammersmith
— Present with congenital cyanosis + 'pseudo-anemia'
— DD_x: genetic methemoglobinemia ('Hb M')
3 Unstable hemoglobins
— 'Heinz-body anemias' (p. 142)
— Abnormal isopropanol/heat stability test
— Usually autosomal dominant transmission
— Respond to splenectomy

* Also occurs in smokers due to binding of carbon monoxide to Hb

HEMATOLOGIC MALIGNANCIES

Diagnostic priorities in bone marrow biopsy
1 Aspiration more important
— Acute leukemias
— Chronic myeloid leukemia ($\rightarrow$ karyotyping)
— Myelodysplastic syndromes
— Megaloblastosis, sideroblastosis
— Thrombocytopenia, leukopenia
2 Trephine more important
— Chronic lymphocytic leukemia*
— Non-contributory aspirate: 'dry' or 'blood' tap

* NB: Can usually be diagnosed on blood film alone

Differential diagnosis of a dry tap
1 Operator inexperience
— Needle tip in wrong place
— Clot blocking needle lumen
2 Marrow fibrosis
— Myelofibrosis
— Myelodysplastic syndrome
— Hairy cell leukemia
— AIDS
3 Packed marrow
— Leukemia, lymphoma
— Metastatic carcinoma
— Osteopetrosis
4 Empty marrow
— Aplastic anemia
— Aleukemic leukemia
— Paroxysmal nocturnal hemoglobinuria (some)

Evaluation of the anemic patient with hypoplastic marrow
1 History
— Toxin exposure (incl. drugs)
— Previous transfusions*
2 Blood count: prognosis worse if
— WCC < 500/mL
— Platelets < 20 000/mL
— Reticulocyte count < 1%
3 Marrow aspiration and trephine
— Helps exclude
• Myelofibrosis
• Hypoplastic (aleukemic) leukemia
• Metastatic carcinomatosis
— Prognosis worse if cellularity < 25% normal

4 Ham's test
— Excludes paroxysmal nocturnal hemoglobinuria
— Prognosis better if positive
5 HLA-typing of siblings

* Higher success rate of marrow transplant if transfusions can be avoided altogether

Laboratory features of myelodysplastic syndromes
1 Film
— Hypersegmented neutrophils, *or*
— Hyposegmented neutrophils (Pelger–Huët-like)
2 NAP score
— Low
3 Hb electrophoresis
— Increased Hb F (often)
4 Marrow
— Hypercellular
— Scarcity of mature forms
— Slight excess of blasts

Common cytogenetic aberrations in hematologic malignancies
1 Ph^1
— Reciprocal 9:22 translocation of *Abl* and *Bcr* genes
2 Blastic transformation of CML
— Ph^2 (i.e. second Philadelphia chromosome)
— Aneuploidy
— Trisomy 8, isochromosome 17
3 8:14 translocation activating *Myc*
— Lymphomas, esp. Burkitt's
4 11:14 translocation activating cyclin D1
— Mantle cell lymphoma
5 15:17 translocation
— Acute promyelocytic leukemia (APL: $RAR\alpha/PML$ gene fusion)
6 8:21 translocation ($AML1–CBF\beta$ fusion gene)
— AML with maturation; good prognosis
Chromosome 16 inversion
— Myelomonocytic AML; good prognosis
7 11q23 (*MLL-1* gene) translocations
— Mixed-lineage leukemias (MLL), often (myelo)monocytic
8 5q-
— Myelodysplastic syndrome (MDS, refractory anemia, 'preleukemia')
9 5q-/7q-
— Iatrogenic AML* (second malignancy; poor prognosis)

* Seen following radiotherapy, and also in airline flight staff

MULTIPLE MYELOMA

Minimal diagnostic criteria for myeloma
1 Characteristic marrow aspirate
— % Plasmacytosis (e.g. > 30%)
— Morphology (plasmacytoma)
2 Monoclonal immunoglobulin spike, e.g.
— IgG > 3.5 g/dL/24 h urine EPG
— IgA > 2.0 g/dL/24 h urine EPG
— κ/λ light chains > 1.0 g/dL/24 h urine EPG

3 Demonstration of *multiple* lesions
— e.g. Repeated aspirations, skeletal survey

NB: Although the diagnosis will be supported by demonstration of a serum and/or urine paraprotein, such a finding is not sufficient for diagnosis, nor (given the occurrence of non-secretory myeloma) is it strictly necessary

Major prognostic variables in myeloma
1 Presence of renal impairment*
2 β_2-microglobulin levels‡
3 Plasma cell labelling index¶
4 Response to therapy

* NB: A minority of patients who present with renal failure recover function following rehydration; some others with irreversible failure may do quite well on dialysis
‡ Reflect disease bulk and/or renal function
¶ Measured using tritiated thymidine, thymidine kinase, or BuDR

Paraprotein-related clinical patterns in myeloma
1 Hyperviscosity
— IgG_3
2 Hypercalcemia; platelet dysfunction
— IgA
3 Plasma cell leukemia
— IgE
4 Renal failure
— IgD
— Bence-Jones only
5 Hepatosplenomegaly
— μ Heavy-chain disease

INVESTIGATING MYELOPROLIFERATIVE DISEASE

Thrombocytosis: factors favoring myeloproliferative disease
1 Physical examination
— Splenomegaly
2 Platelets
— Platelet count $> 1000 \times 10^9/L$
— Giant platelets on film
— Abnormal aggregation $\rightarrow \uparrow$ bleeding time
3 Blood film:
— Basophilia
— Neutrophilia
4 Other laboratory studies
— $\uparrow$ NAP score
— $\uparrow B_{12}$
— $\uparrow$ Uric acid
5 Clinical course
— Hemorrhage
— Thrombosis*

* Sudden increment in platelet count may indicate splenic vein thrombosis

Polycythemia? Laboratory features of polycythemia vera
1 Coexisting leukocytosis and/or thrombocytosis
2 HbO_2 saturation $> 92\%$*
3 $\uparrow$ NAP score
4 $\uparrow$ Plasma B_{12}
5 Low erythropoietin levels (limited assay availability)

* cf. chronic airways disease, smoking, altitude: HbO_2 saturation $< 90\%$ (plus high erythropoietin levels)

CHRONIC MYELOID (GRANULOCYTIC) LEUKEMIA

Diagnosis of chronic myeloid leukemia (CML)
1 Clinical
— Splenomegaly ± pain/rub (infarct)
— Hemorrhagic or thrombotic phenomena (e.g. priapism)
— *No* predisposition to infection (normal WBC function)
2 Blood film
— WCC often $> 100 \times 10^9/L$
— Predominant cells: neutrophils, myelocytes
— Left shift; basophilia ± eosinophilia
— Normochromic anemia ± thrombocytosis
3 Other laboratory studies
— $\downarrow$ NAP score (often zero)
— $\uparrow B_{12}$ ($\uparrow$ TC-I)
— $\uparrow$ Uric acid
4 Bone marrow
— $< 10\%$ myeloblasts (cf. blastic transformation)
— M:E ratio $> 10:1$ (usually)
— Rarely: Gaucher cells, sea-blue histiocytes
5 Philadelphia chromosome (Ph'; $\rightarrow > 90\%$)
— Main reason for performing marrow examination
— If negative, consider chronic myelomonocytic leukemia (CMML)

Signs of acute (blastic) transformation of CML
1 Symptoms
— Fever
— Bone pain
2 Signs
— Increasing splenomegaly
— Lymphadenopathy
3 Laboratory
— $\uparrow$ WCC/platelets
— Rising NAP score
— Appearance of circulating TdT+ or CALLA+ blasts*
4 Bone marrow
— $> 10\%$ blasts
— New cytogenetic aberrations
5 Clinical course
— Sensitive to imatinib (STI-571, Gleevec) *if* Bcr/Abl- or Kit-positive
— Refractoriness to busulfan

* Implies *lymphoblastic* transformation

Differential diagnosis of normal or high NAP score in CML
1 Partial remission
2 Intercurrent infection (or other stress)
3 Pregnancy
4 Development of myelofibrosis
5 Blastic transformation
6 Leukemoid reaction (i.e. misdiagnosis)

Characteristics of Ph'-negative CML
1 'Juvenile' CML
— Age of onset typically < 5 years
— May be inherited

— A subacute form of chronic myelomonocytic leukemia and subset of malignant histiocytosis
— May be responsive to isotretinoin
2 Adult Ph'-negative CML
— Tends to be later onset than Ph+ CML
— Smaller spleen
— Lower WCC
— Higher lysozyme and Hb F
— Poorer prognosis

NB: 'Ph-negative' CML may be clinically indistinguishable from Ph'-positive CML if chromosome 22 *Bcr* rearrangement is subtle

CHRONIC LYMPHOCYTIC LEUKEMIA (CLL)

Significance of anemia in CLL
1 Marrow suppression ('chronic disease') in 95%
2 Autoimmune hemolysis (in 5%)
3 Hypersplenism (rare)

Immunologic considerations in CLL
1 Impaired humoral immunity
— 50% have hypogammaglobulinemia (esp. ↓ IgM)
2 Impaired cell-mediated immunity
— CD4:CD8 (helper-suppressor) ratio often inverted
3 Effect of therapy on immunity
— Steroids increase the risk of infectious complications
— Hypogammaglobulinemia may improve with chemo
— IV gammaglobulin reduces the incidence of bacterial infections in hypogammaglobulinemic patients
4 Paraproteins and hemolysis
— 5% of patients have a paraprotein
— 5–10% have a positive direct antiglobulin (Coombs) test
— Significant hemolysis/thrombocytopenia affects < 5%
— Thrombocytopenia *usually* indicates marrow failure (rather than autoimmune destruction)

OTHER LEUKEMIAS

Clinicopathologic hallmarks of selected leukemic subtypes
1 Acute myelogenous leukemia
— Clinical: chloromas (greenish skin lesions due to myeloperoxidase)
2 Acute promyelocytic leukemia
— Clinical: DIC-like coagulopathy* (in 90%)
— Film: Auer rods (see below)
— t(15:17) chromosomal translocation‡
3 Acute (myelo)monocytic leukemia
— Clinical: gingival hyperplasia (± CNS/skin disease)
— Laboratory: lysozymuria (± hypokalemia)
4 B cell (Burkitt-type) leukemia
— t(14:18) translocation (i.e. same as Burkitt's lymphoma)

5 T cell leukemia/lymphoma
— Mediastinal mass (poor prognosis)
6 Prolymphocytic leukemia (PLL)
— Clinical: massive splenomegaly; *absent* lymphadenopathy
— Marked anemia and leukocytosis
7 Chronic lymphocytic leukemia
— 'Smudge' cells and/or 'basket' cells on film
— Distinguished from well-differentiated lymphocytic lymphoma by degree of peripheral lymphocytosis
— May transform to PLL or diffuse lymphoma
8 Hairy cell leukemia
— Clinical: massive splenomegaly (DD$_x$: CML, myelofibrosis, PLL)
— Thrombocytopenia (due to hypersplenism)
— Anemia/leukopenia (due to marrow fibrosis/failure)

* Hyperfibrinolytic bleeding disorder with normal AT III and protein C levels (cf. DIC) but high levels of the fibrinolytic (plasminogen and tPA) receptor annexin II. It is associated with hemorrhagic lethality in 10–20% of APL patients; *no* evidence for efficacy of heparin
‡ Affects retinoic acid receptor-α locus

Leukemias commoner in men than women
1 T cell leukemia/lymphoma
2 Chronic lymphocytic leukemia
3 Hairy cell leukemia
4 Prolymphocytic leukemia

Laboratory features of leukemias and lymphomas
1 Light microscopy
— Auer rods (in circulating blasts)
• AML (esp. APL)
— Reed-Sternberg cells
• Hodgkin's disease
— Pautrier microabscesses
• Mycosis fungoides
2 Electron microscopy
— Cerebriform nuclei
• Sézary syndrome
3 (Immuno)cytochemistry
— Anti-CALLA
• Good-prognosis ALL subtype
— Anti-CD4 (defines helper T cell phenotype)
• Sézary syndrome, mycosis fungoides
— Anti-CD8 (defines suppressor T cell phenotype)
• T cell CLL (some exceptions)
— Anti-light chains (κ, λ)
• Confirms monoclonality (malignant lineage) of immunocytes in effusions, CSF, marrow
— TdT
• ALL (except rare B-cell subtype)
• Lymphoblastic transformation of CML
— Acid phosphatase (tartrate-resistant: TRAP)
• T cell ALL
• Hairy cell leukemia
— PAS
• ALL
— Peroxidase/Sudan black
• AML

LEUKEMIAS: CLASSIFICATION, STAGING AND PROGNOSIS

Acute myeloid leukemias: the WHO (REAL) classification
1 Acute myeloid leukemias with recurrent cytogenetic translocations
   — AML with t(8:21)(q22:q22); *CBFα/ETO*
   — APL with t(15:17)(q22:q11–12); *PML/RARα*
   — AML with inv(16)(p13:q11); *CBFβ/MYH11*
   — AML with 11q23 (*MLL*) mutations
2 Acute myeloid leukemias with multilineage dysplasia
   — ± Preceding myelodysplastic syndrome
3 Acute myeloid leukemias, iatrogenic
   — Related to alklylating agent chemotherapy
   — Related to topoisomerase II inhibitors (e.g. etoposide)
4 Acute myeloid leukemias, miscellaneous
   — Includes acute (myelo)monocytic leukemias
   — Undifferentiated AML

Lymphocytic leukemias: the WHO (REAL) classification
1 Precursor B-lymphoblastic leukemia
   — Precursor B cell ALL
2 Mature (peripheral) B cell leukemias
   — B cell CLL
   — Plasma cell leukemia
   — Hairy cell leukemia
3 Precursor T lymphoblastic leukemia
   — Precursor T cell ALL
4 Mature (peripheral) T cell leukemias
   — T cell PLL
   — NK cell leukemia
   — HTLV+ adult T cell leukemia
5 Burkitt's cell leukemia

Poor prognostic signs in acute lymphoblastic leukemia
1 Adult onset
2 Male sex
   — Associated with T cell leukemia and mediastinal mass
   — Increased testicular relapse
3 CALLA negative (T cell, B cell, null cell)
4 Presentation with
   — Initial WCC > 100 × 10^9/L
   — Massive extramedullary disease
   — CNS leukemia
5 Philadelphia chromosome-positive*‡

* cf. CML: *better* prognosis
‡ cf. AML: poor prognosis indicated by 5q– or 7q– chromosomal deletion

CLL staging: modified Binet criteria
1 Stage A — < 3 enlarged lymphoid regions*
2 Stage B — ≥ 3 enlarged lymphoid regions
3 Stage C — Anemia and/or thrombocytopenia

NB: All have lymphocytosis (> 15 × 10^9/L; > 40% in marrow)
* Including liver and/or spleen

Life expectancy from diagnosis in CLL
1 Stage A disease   — 6 years
2 Stage B disease   — 3 years
3 Stage C disease   — 18 months

LYMPHOMAS

Pros and cons of staging laparotomy in Hodgkin's disease
1 Pros
   — Absent splenomegaly does not imply absent splenic disease, nor must splenomegaly imply splenic involvement; hence, of diagnostic value*
   — Morbidity of radiotherapy may be reduced by excluding splenic irradiation, thus preventing irradiation of left kidney, left lung base, and cardiac apex
   — Oophoropexy enables preservation of fertility in young women requiring pelvic irradiation
   — WBC/platelet counts may improve following splenectomy, thus improving treatment tolerance
2 Cons:
   — Invasive, potentially morbid and hazardous
   — Increased risk of infection post-splenectomy (p. 195)
   — Popularity of staging laparotomy in stage IA/IIA patients (esp. those with lymphocyte predominant disease) has declined, with close follow-up post-radiotherapy now being widely accepted

* Since 20% of patients with clinical stage II disease (normal abdominal CT) actually have abdominal disease (incl. liver, nodes), staging laparotomy remains the best way to confirm such disease and hence to determine need for chemotherapy in some cases

Staging of Hodgkin's disease: simplified Ann Arbor criteria
1 Stage 1 — Involvement of a single site (incl. extranodal)
2 Stage 2 — Involvement of > 1 lymph node region on the *same* side of the diaphragm
3 Stage 3 — Node involvement on *both* sides of diaphragm
4 Stage 4 — Extranodal disease (esp. marrow or liver)

Clinical staging of Hodgkin's disease: 'A' vs 'B' criteria
1 'A' — Asymptomatic
2 'B' — Fevers > 38°C
   — Sweats
   — > 10% weight loss in last 6 months

Non-Hodgkin's lymphomas: Kiel histologic subtypes*
1 Indolent
   — Follicular (nodular)
     • Centrocytic
     • Centroblastic
   — Diffuse small-cell
     • Lymphocytic (WDLL, CLL-like)
     • Centrocytic
     • Immunocytic (lymphoplasmacytoid)
2 Aggressive
   — Diffuse large cell
     • Lymphoblastic (T cell or Burkitt-type)
     • Centroblastic
     • Immunoblastic

* Superseded by REAL (WHO) classification, but easier to remember

Assessing prognosis in lymphoma

1 Hodgkin's disease*
   — Prognosis determined by disease *stage*, e.g.
     • Stage IA/IIA disease → 90% cure
     • Stage IIIB/IV disease → 30% cure
   — Other poor prognosticators
     • Advanced age
     • Elevated ESR (> 30 mm/h) following definitive R_x
2 Non-Hodgkin's lymphoma
   — Prognosis mainly determined by *histology*, e.g.
     • Indolent histology → median survival 5 years
     • Aggressive histology → median survival 1 year‡

* Note that *older* patients with Hodgkin's disease have a markedly worse prognosis than do young patients with the same disease stage
‡ Paradoxically, *chemocurability* is greatest in 'aggressive' histology

HYPERCOAGULABLE STATES

Indications for investigation of hypercoagulability

1 Family history of venous thrombosis
2 Recurrent venous thrombosis or pulmonary embolism
3 Single episode of venous thrombosis in a young patient
4 Unusual site of thrombosis
   — Retinal vein thrombosis
   — Renal vein thrombosis
   — Hepatic vein thrombosis
   — Arterial thrombosis

Molecular basis of genetic hypercoagulability

1 Factor V Leiden ($G^{1691}A$) mutation → activated protein C resistance*
   — Affects 5% Caucasian population
   — Affects 30% Caucasians with thromboembolism
2 Prothrombin $G^{20210}A$ mutation*
   — Affects 5% Caucasians with thromboembolism
3 Hereditary deficiencies of
   — AT III (heparin resistance) *or* protein C *or* protein S‡
   — Affects 5% Caucasians with thromboembolism
4 Hyperhomocystinemia (*also* prone to atherosclerosis)¶
   Hyperfibrinogenemia
5 ↑ Factor VIII plasma levels
   ↑ Factor XI plasma levels

* Predispose to thrombosis particularly in pregnant women and oral contraceptive users
‡ Both conditions prone to superficial thrombophlebitis and/or warfarin-induced skin necrosis
¶ cf. polymorphisms of the factor VII and/or factor XIII gene may protect against myocardial infarction *despite* atherosclerosis, presumably by reducing coronary thrombosis

Causes of acquired hypercoagulability

1 Antiphospholipid antibodies
2 Paroxysmal nocturnal hemoglobinuria
3 Thrombotic thrombocytopenic purpura
4 Myeloproliferative disorders
5 Carcinomatosis

When to screen for genetic hypercoagulability

1 Family history of thromboembolism
2 Thromboembolism at an early age (esp. neonatal)
3 Thrombosis associated with pregnancy or oral contraceptive use
4 Odd location of thrombosis, esp. arterial*
5 Recurrent thrombosis, esp. if despite anticoagulation
6 Thrombosis associated with thrombocytopenia
7 Recurrent miscarriages
8 Warfarin-induced skin necrosis

* May suggest antiphospholipid syndrome

Laboratory characterization of suspected hypercoagulability

1 Exclude hyperviscosity
   — Hb/PCV (polycythemia), platelets (thrombocytosis)
   — Paraproteinemia ± whole blood viscosity
2 Exclude defective fibrinolysis
   — FDPs, D-dimers*, hypofibrinogenemia (DIC)
   — Schistocytes (TTP, DIC)
   — Euglobulin clot lysis time (tPA deficiency/inhibitor)
   — Abnormal fibrinogen or plasminogen (activator)
3 Exclude primary deficiency of endogenous anticoagulation
   — Antithrombin III, protein C, protein S
4 Exclude inhibitors of endogenous anticoagulants
   — e.g. Factor V Leiden mutation
5 Exclude acquired inducers of hypercoagulability
   — Prothrombin gene mutation
   — Lupus anticoagulant
   — Acid hemolysis test (PNH)
   — Fibrin monomers/fibrinopeptide A (malignancy)
   — Prothrombin activation fragments 1 and 2

* Normal values make thrombosis unlikely

Antithrombin III deficiency: causes

1 Hereditary
2 Estrogens (pregnancy, OCs, Ca prostate)
3 Liver disease
4 Nephrotic syndrome
5 Disseminated thrombosis*
6 Heparin therapy

* Since heparin acts via AT III, massive thrombosis (which depletes AT III levels) may be associated with relative heparin resistance

Investigation of suspected deep venous thrombosis

1 First presentation
   — Ultrasonography *plus* plasma D-dimer
   — Repeat ultrasound after 1 week, if first study negative *and* clinical suspicion still moderate
2 Negative ultrasound *plus*
   — *either* symptoms and signs of distal thrombosis
   — *or* recurrent symptoms after earlier confirmed DVT
     • Venogram
3 High risk of pulmonary embolism
   — Spiral CT chest

HEMOSTATIC DISORDERS

Investigation of thrombocytopenia
1 Check automated count by direct vision (exclude clotting)
2 Film
   — Schistocytes (DIC, TTP)
   — Blasts (acute leukemia)
3 Coagulation screen
   — Helps further exclude DIC
4 Marrow aspirate
   — Hypoplastic etiology
   — Abundant megakaryocytes (ITP, hypersplenism)

Prolonged PT, APTT and thrombocytopenia?
1 Disseminated intravascular coagulation
2 Liver disease with hypersplenism
3 Intravenous heparin therapy* (pp. 158–9)

* NB: the APTT is *not* prolonged by subcutaneous low-dose heparin therapy

Platelet function tests: clinical correlations
1 Von Willebrand's disease (VWF mutations)
   — Normal aggregation in vitro
   — Defective ristocetin aggregation
   — Defective endothelial adhesion
     • Corrected by addition of normal plasma
2 Glanzmann's thrombasthenia (glycoprotein IIb/IIIa mutations)
   — Defective aggregation in vitro*
   — Normal ristocetin aggregation
   — Normal endothelial adhesion
3 Bernard–Soulier syndrome (glycoprotein 1B mutations)
   — Giant platelets → 'thrombocytopenia'
   — Normal aggregation in vitro
   — Defective ristocetin aggregation
   — Defective endothelial adhesion
     • *Not* corrected by addition of normal plasma
4 Aspirin ingestion
   — Defective aggregation in vitro
     • Impaired release reaction to ADP
5 Dysproteinemia
   Myeloproliferative disease
   Uremia, liver disease
   — Defective aggregation *and* adhesion

* i.e. to ADP, adrenaline, collagen

Differential diagnosis of giant platelets
1 Congenital platelet disorder
   — Bernard–Soulier syndrome
   — Alport's syndrome
   — May-Hegglin anomaly
2 Acquired platelet disorder
   — Myeloproliferative disease

Contraindications to platelet transfusions
1 Thrombotic thrombocytopenic purpura
2 Hemolytic uremic syndrome
3 Heparin-induced thrombocytopenia

Hemophilia A: levels of severity
1 > 50% F VIII_c
   — Normal hemostasis
2 20–40% F VIII_c
   — Excess bleeding after major trauma
3 5–20% F VIII_c
   — Excess bleeding after surgery or minor trauma
4 2–5% F VIII_c
   — Moderate hemophilia; severe post-traumatic and occasional spontaneous bleeding
5 < 2% F VIII_c
   — Severe hemophilia; frequent spontaneous bleeds into muscles and joints

Diagnosis of hemophilia
1 Low F VIII_c
2 Normal or increased F VIII_{Ag}
3 Normal F VIII_{VWF} (cf. VWD: ↓)
4 Normal bleeding time (cf. VWD: ↑)
5 Carrier status? VIII_c:VIII_{Ag} < 70%

Bleeding tendency with normal coagulation screen?
1 Vascular disorder
   — Hereditary hemorrhagic telangiectasia
   — Vasculitis, scurvy
2 Platelet dysfunction
   — Aspirin ingestion
   — Dysproteinemia (esp. IgA)
   — Inherited platelet dysfunction
   — Platelet factor 3 deficiency
3 Mild coagulopathy
   — von Willebrand's
   — Mild hemophilia
   — Factor XIII deficiency

Diagnosis of hereditary hemorrhagic telangiectasia
1 Clinical: at least two of
   — Autosomal dominant inheritance
   — Recurrent epistaxis
   — Non-nasal telangiectasia
   — Visceral involvement
2 Molecular diagnosis
   — Type I HHT: endoglin (chromosome 9q3) mutation
   — Type II HHT: type I TGF-β receptor (*ALK-1* gene) mutation

THE PORPHYRIAS

The acute porphyrias*: what do they have in common?
1 All three are autosomal dominant
2 All three are often precipitated by drugs
3 All three are potentially life-threatening

* Acute intermittent or variegate porphyria; hereditary coproporphyria

Approach to investigation of suspected acute porphyria
1 Urinary PBG absent
   — Excludes acute porphyrias
2 Urinary PBG absent
   Fecal screen negative
   — Excludes both acute and latent porphyrias

3 Urinary PBG present
   Fecal screen negative
   — Acute intermittent porphyria (acute or latent phase)
4 Urinary PBG present
   Fecal screen positive*
   — Variegate porphyria (acute phase)
5 Urinary PBG absent
   Fecal screen positive*
   — Variegate porphyria (latent phase)

NB: Urinary PBG and/or ALA are the hallmarks of porphyria-induced neurologic disease
* *Biliary* porphyrins may be positive in cases where fecal screen is negative

Investigation of suspected porphyria-induced photosensitivity

1 Urinary PBG absent
   Red cell screen negative   } Excludes porphyric
   Fecal screen negative   etiology
2 Urinary PBG present
   Fecal screen positive   } Variegate porphyria
   Biliary screen positive
3 Urinary PBG absent   Porphyria cutanea
   Red cell screen negative   }   tarda
   Fecal screen positive   Variegate porphyria
4 Urinary PBG absent
   Red cell screen positive   } Erythropoietic
   Fecal screen negative   coproporphyria
5 Urinary PBG absent   Erythropoietic
   Red cell screen positive   } uroporphyria/
   Fecal screen positive   protoporphyria

'Safe' drugs in patients with porphyria

1 Aspirin, paracetamol, codeine
2 Penicillin; low-dose chloroquine*
3 Chlorpromazine, metoclopramide; valproate
4 Propranolol, labetalol; digoxin
5 Insulin

* NB: *High-dose* chloroquine may precipitate porphyria cutanea tarda, whereas low-dose is therapeutic

Diagnostic significance of elevated RBC protoporphyrin

1 Porphyria
   — Erythropoietic protoporphyria
2 Ineffective erythropoiesis
   — Iron deficiency
   — Lead poisoning
   — Anemia of chronic disease

PRINCIPLES OF BLOOD SUPPORT

The leukopenic patient: principles of management

1 Assume fever represents infection until proven otherwise
2 Take urine and blood cultures if febrile
3 If prolonged leukopenia anticipated*, perform
   — Baseline HSV/CMV/toxoplasma titres
   — Regular swabs of throat/axillae/nose/perineum

   — Removal of IUD
4 Monitor chest and perineum for sepsis
5 Avoid pelvic examinations unless indispensable

* e.g. bone marrow transplant

Indications for recombinant hemopoietic growth factors

1 After febrile neutropenia in a previous chemotherapy cycle (if dose needs to be maintained for anticancer efficacy)
2 To reduce likelihood of febrile neutropenia in high-risk scenarios (e.g. high-dose regimens)
3 After high-dose chemotherapy and autologous stem-cell transplantation

Granulocyte transfusions

1 Sole potential indication
   — Fever > 48 h in a severely neutropenic patient (< 500 cells/μL) receiving optimal antibiotics, esp. if
      • Positive blood cultures (esp. *Pseudomonas aeruginosa*)
      • Imminent (< I week) marrow recovery unlikely
2 Problems
   — Questionable benefit*; expensive
   — Poor leukocyte function (esp. if obtained by filtration)
   — Transfusion reactions
   — Sensitization (alloimmunization)‡
   — Possible transmission of CMV
   — Pulmonary infiltrates (intravascular leukostasis)
   — Graft-versus-host disease if cells not irradiated

* Less important than prompt prescription of broad-spectrum antibiotics
‡ e.g. preventing increments to transfused platelets

Common drugs causing agranulocytosis

1 Phenylbutazone
2 Gold, penicillamine
3 Antithyroid drugs (e.g. carbimazole)
4 Clozapine
5 Sulfasalazine
6 Chloramphenicol*

* Though multilineage aplastic anemia is the greater risk

Morbidity of massive stored blood transfusions

1 Infection
   — Hepatitis (HCV, HBV, CMV)
   — HIV seroconversion
2 Coagulopathy
   — Low in factors V, VIII and platelets*
3 Citrate toxicity (usually subclinical)
   — Metabolic alkalosis with hypocalcemia
4 Tissue hypoxia (reversible after 24 h)
   — Due to low 2,3-DPG of stored blood
5 Metabolic acidosis and/or K+ (esp. if renal impairment)
   — Due to low pH of stored blood
6 Fever, fluid overload, hemolysis, DIC

* i.e. assuming packed cells (not whole blood) is used

Clinical utility of autologous blood transfusion
1 Advantages
— No infective risk
— No incompatibility risk
2 Indications
— Elective surgery, esp.
• Orthopedic surgery
• Cardiac surgery
— Pregnancy – 3rd trimester
3 Contraindications
— Insufficient time prior to planned transfusion
— Anemia, frailty, infection
— Severe cardiac disease
• Left main disease and/or unstable angina
• Tight aortic stenosis

Therapeutic indications for phlebotomy
1 Polycythemia rubra vera
2 Idiopathic hemochromatosis
   Sideroblastosis with iron overload
3 Porphyria cutanea tarda
4 Polycythemia (Hb > 20 g/dL) due to chronic lung disease or cyanotic congenital heart disease; keep hematocrit ~ 65%

Constituents of fresh frozen plasma
1 Coagulation factors
2 Endogenous anticoagulants
3 C_1-esterase inhibitor
4 α_1-antitrypsin
5 Fibronectin
6 Immunoglobulins
7 Albumin

Indications for fresh frozen plasma
1 (Anti)coagulation factor deficiency *if* concentrate unavailable
2 Thrombotic thrombocytopenic purpura
3 Bleeding associated with thrombolytic therapy, warfarin overdosage or DIC

CLINICAL USE OF HEMOPOIETIC GROWTH FACTORS

Human recombinant colony-stimulating factors (CSFs)*
1 G-CSF (granulocyte colony-stimulating factor: filgrastim)
— Increases granulocytes
2 GM-CSF (granulocyte-macrophage CSF: ecogramostim)
— Increases granulocytes, monocytes, eosinophils
3 M-CSF (monocyte/macrophage CSF)
— Increases monocytes
4 IL-3 ('multi-CSF')
— Increases monocytes, granulocytes, eosinophils, basophils, erythrocytes
5 Erythropoietin
— Increases erythrocytes
6 Thrombopoietin
— Increases platelets

* cf. lymphoid growth factors (lymphokines, interleukins)

Potential indications for hemopoietic growth factor therapy
1 G-CSF
— Kostmann's (inherited) neutropenia
— Cyclic neutropenia
2 G-CSF *or* GM-CSF
— Mobilization and recruitment of peripheral blood stem cells (PBSC) for autologous marrow transplantation
— Marrow support in patients receiving cancer chemotherapy, but at high risk of sepsis (expected probability > 40%)
3 Erythropoietin
— Symptomatic anemia due to chronic renal failure (esp. if on dialysis)
— Symptomatic anemia due to myeloma
— Anemia prophylaxis in premature births
— Preoperative 'priming' prior to autologous blood banking
— HIV anemia in patients receiving AZT treatment
4 Thrombopoietin
— Thrombocytopenia (if *not* related to chemotherapy)

Toxicity of hemopoietic growth factor therapy
1 G-CSF
— Bone pain, fever
2 GM-CSF
— Bone pain, fever, malaise, arthralgias
— Skin rash at injection site
— Capillary leak syndrome*: serous effusions/ascites
— Large-vessel venous thrombosis*
3 Erythropoietin
— Thrombotic tendency if hematocrit rises too quickly
— Hypertension, hyperkalemia

* Seen with high dose treatment; may reflect secondary release of TNF or IL-1

SPLENECTOMY

Splenectomy: common indications in hematologic disease
1 Hereditary spherocytosis
2 Chronic ITP
3 Hairy cell leukemia
4 Occasional indications
— Hodgkin's disease (staging laparotomy)
— Idiopathic 'warm' autoimmune hemolytic anemia
— Massive enlargement: pain, hypersplenism*

* e.g. in myelofibrosis or thalassemia

Specific indications for splenectomy in myelofibrosis
1 Painful spleen
2 Thrombocytopenia (requiring transfusion)
3 Frequent blood transfusions

Management of the splenectomy patient
1 Patient selection
— *Avoid* splenectomy if possible in children, esp. < 5 years (greatest risk of subsequent life-threatening sepsis)

2 Children requiring splenectomy
   — Prophylactic oral penicillin V until adulthood
3 All patients
   — Pneumococcal vaccination, *prior* to splenectomy
     if possible

HEMOLYTIC ANEMIAS

Management of warm autoimmune hemolytic anemia

1 Exclude drug-induced cause
2 Exclude B cell malignancy (bone marrow, EPG)
3 Treat underlying autoimmune disease if present
4 *Avoid* transfusion if possible
5 Trial of medical therapy
   — Steroids (prednisolone 60 mg/day)
   — Folate 5 mg/day
   — ± Azathioprine
6 Consider splenectomy if
   — Steroids ineffective or unacceptable
   — DAT → IgG only (no C_3)
   — ^{51}Cr-RBC studies confirm spleen as site of
     sequestration
7 Other therapies
   — Danazol
   — High-dose intravenous IgG
   — Ciclosporin

Management of cold autoimmune hemolytic anemia

1 Keep patient warm
2 Exclude *Mycoplasma pneumoniae*, infectious
   mononucleosis
3 Exclude B cell malignancy
4 Avoid steroids and splenectomy (they generally
   don't work)
5 If transfusion absolutely necessary
   — Use washed packed cells (less complement)
   — Infuse via blood warmer
6 Investigational therapy
   — High-dose IV methylprednisolone
   — Plasmapheresis/plasma exchange

Clinical significance of oxidant and antioxidant drugs

1 Oxidant drugs
   — Precipitate favism (hemolysis in G6PD
     deficiency)
   — Exacerbate methemoglobinemia
   — Include*
     • Nitrates (incl. nitroprusside)
     • Paracetamol
     • Sulfonamides, nitrofurantoin, primaquine
2 Antioxidant (reducing) drugs
   — Used for treatment of severe
     methemoglobinemia (e.g. levels > 20%; may
     cause cerebral ischemia)
   — Include
     • Ascorbic acid
     • Methylene blue (IV in emergencies)*

* NB: Notwithstanding its therapeutic role in
methemoglobinemia, methylene blue may also stimulate
hemolysis in G6PD deficiency

MANAGING HEMATOLOGIC MALIGNANCIES

Treatment options in acute lymphoblastic leukemia (ALL)

1 Induction/consolidation (95% → complete
   remission)
   — Vincristine/prednisone
   — Daunorubicin
   — ± L-asparaginase, cytosine arabinoside
2 Maintenance (50% → cure) therapy
   — Methotrexate/6-MP* (3 years)
3 Routine CNS prophylaxis‡
   — Cranial irradiation
   — Intrathecal methotrexate
4 Marrow transplant
   — In second remission
   — In first remission *if*
     • Poor prognosis ALL, *or*
     • Availability of HLA-identical donor

* Pharmacokinetics of 6-MP should be checked at beginning of
maintenance to confirm adequate bioavailability for individual
dosage schedule
‡ NB: Some centers also advocate prophylactic testicular
irradiation, while others monitor this potential sanctuary site for
relapse

Late complications of ALL treatment

1 Abnormal bone development
   — Short stature
   — Avascular necrosis
   — Osteoporosis
2 Intellectual impairment
   Encephalopathy
3 Cardiomyopathy
4 Second malignancy
   — Acute myeloid leukemia
   — Brain tumor
5 Metabolic
   — Hypothyroidism
   — Obesity

Treatment options in acute myeloblastic leukemia (AML)

1 Induction/consolidation (70% → complete
   remission)
   — Cytosine arabinoside + daunorubicin
     ± 6TG/VP-16
2 Marrow transplant*
   — In first remission (or *early* relapse if age > 30)
3 Promyelocytic leukemia
   — All-*trans*-retinoic acid (ATRA): induction and
     maintenance
   — Low-dose arsenic trioxide‡: post-relapse
     remission induction
   — Platelets, FFP, tranexamic acid (for
     coagulopathy)
4 CNS prophylaxis
   — Acute (myelo)monocytic leukemias only
5 Maintenance therapy, late intensification
   — Doubtful value in AML

* Relatively more valuable for AML than ALL
‡ Watch out for unexplained death during the first cycle of
treatment, however

Treatment of chronic lymphocytic leukemia (CLL)

1 Stage I/II disease
   — Observe if indolent (unless *massive* adenopathy)
2 Stage III/IV disease
   — Chlorambucil ± vincristine/prednisone (CVP)
   — 2nd-line
      • Fludarabine
      • Pentostatin (deoxycoformycin)
      • 2-chlorodeoxyadenosine
3 Immune hemolysis/thrombocytopenia
   — Steroids
   — Splenectomy in selected patients
4 Recurrent infections
   — Gammaglobulin (IV)

Indications for cytotoxic therapy in CLL

1 Symptomatic lymphadenopathy
2 Refractory constitutional symptoms
3 Non-immune cytopenia

Therapeutic approach to chronic myeloid leukemia (CML)

1 Chronic phase
   — Hydroxyurea (daily)*
   — Interferon-α‡
   — Imatinib (STI-571, Gleevec, a Bcr-Abl kinase inhibitor)
   — Bone marrow transplantation
2 Myeloblastic transformation (75%)
   — Imatinib (STI-571, Gleevec, a Bcr-Abl kinase inhibitor)
3 Lymphoblastic transformation (25%)
   — Vincristine/prednisone

* Busulfan now usually reserved for refractory disease
‡ 10% achieve cytogenetic remission while treatment continues

Management modalities in hairy cell leukemia

1 Splenectomy
   — For massive splenomegaly *or* hypersplenism
   — Improves cytopenia; may improve survival
2 Pentostatin (deoxycoformycin), *or* 2-chlorodeoxyadenosine
   — Impressive remission rates and durations
3 Interferon-α

Managing polycythemia vera

1 Mild disease, young patient (< 50), preoperative
   — Phlebotomy
      • May be technically difficult due to clotting
      • Aim to keep hematocrit in normal range (≤ 0.45)*
2 Older patients (50–65), or associated thrombocytosis
   — Hydroxyurea
      • Alternatives: busulfan, chlorambucil (may cause leukemia)
3 Elderly or non-compliant patients
   — ^{32}P
      • Takes 6–12 weeks to work
      • Risk of leukemia
4 Non-specific measures
   — Allopurinol
   — H_2-blockers

NB: *Pruritus* may or may not respond to normalization of hematocrit; if not, antihistamines may help
* cf. secondary polycythemia: do *not* venesect unless PCV > 0.54

Managing the dysproteinemias

1 Myeloma
   — Melphalan (or cyclophosphamide) ± prednisone
   — Thalidomide
   — Doxorubicin/BCNU
   — Interferon-α
   — Apheresis for hyperviscosity
   — Erythropoietin for symptomatic anemia
   — IV immunoglobulin for infection prophylaxis*
   — Bisphosphonates for bone fracture prophylaxis
2 Macroglobulinemia
   — Chlorambucil, CVP
   — Plasmapheresis

* esp. for patients with poor IgG responses to pneumococcal vaccination

Management options in cutaneous lymphoma*

1 Topical nitrogen mustard
2 Whole skin electron beam therapy
3 PUVA (or home UVB)
4 Oral steroids
5 Combination cytotoxic therapy
6 Ciclosporin; interferon-α; retinoids

* None is regularly effective

Management modalities in non-Hodgkin's lymphomas

1 Low-grade (indolent, usually nodular) lymphomas
   — CVP and/or local irradiation
   — Fludarabine
   — Treated with palliative intent
2 High-grade (aggressive, usually diffuse) lymphomas
   — CVP + doxorubicin (CHOP)
   — Treated with curative intent
3 Lymphoblastic lymphoma
   — Treated as for T cell ALL (incl. CNS prophylaxis)
4 Remission after first relapse
   — High-dose chemotherapy with marrow transplant
5 Refractory end-stage disease
   — Total body irradiation (palliative only)

Approach to the management of Hodgkin's disease

1 Pathologic stage IA
   — Local irradiation
2 Pathologic stage IIA (above diaphragm)
   — 'Mantle' irradiation*
3 Pathologic stage IIA (below diaphragm)
   — 'Inverted Y' irradiation‡
4 Pathologic stage III or IV
   Bulky disease (irrespective of stage)
   'B' symptoms, irrespective of stage
   'E' (extranodal) disease
   — Combination chemotherapy (e.g. ABVD, MOPP)

* Supradiaphragmatic + upper para-aortic nodes
‡ All para-aortic, iliac and pelvic nodes

Toxicity of therapy for Hodgkin's disease

1 Induced by radiotherapy (e.g. mantle)
   — Hypothyroidism
   — Lhermitte's phenomenon (radiation myelitis)

— Radiation pneumonitis/pericarditis
— Reduced hemopoietic reserve
2 Induced by chemotherapy (e.g. MOPP)
— Sterility (esp. in males)
— Second malignancies (esp. if prior radiation)

Chemoresistance in Hodgkin's disease
1 Occurs in 25%
2 More common with
— 'B' symptoms
— Nodular sclerosing histology ($\rightarrow$ frequent relapses)

Tumor lysis syndrome: features and clinical significance
1 Occurs after initial chemotherapy for sensitive tumors*, esp.
— Burkitt's lymphoma; other lymphomas
— ALL
— Germ-cell tumors (esp. with mediastinal mass or retroperitoneal disease)
2 Metabolic effects
— Hyperuricemia + urate nephropathy
— Hyperphosphatemia + reciprocal hypocalcemia
— Hyperkalemia (esp. if azotemic or acidotic)
3 Complications
— Renal failure (typically irreversible: may be fatal)
— Arrhythmias, cardiac arrest (due to hyperkalemia)
— Tetany, weakness, paralytic ileus (hypocalcemia)
— Severe metabolic acidosis

* NB: Can also occur following treatment of 'aleukemic' leukemias

BONE MARROW TRANSPLANTATION

Curative potential of allogeneic bone marrow transplantation
1 Acquired chronic bone marrow disorders
— Aplastic anemia (preferably untransfused)
— CML in chronic phase
— Myelodysplasia
— Paroxysmal nocturnal hemoglobinuria (severe)
2 Hemoglobinopathies
— β-thalassemia major
— Sickle-cell disease
3 Primary immunodeficiencies
— Severe combined immunodeficiency
— Wiskott–Aldrich syndrome
— Chronic granulomatous disease
4 Inborn errors of metabolism
— Hurler's syndrome
— Osteopetrosis

Indications for autologous stem cell transplantation
1 Hodgkin's or non-Hodgkin's lymphoma in complete remission
2 Acute leukemia (lymphoblastic or myeloid)
3 Myeloma
4 Refractory teratoma or neuroblastoma

Prerequisites for allogeneic marrow transplantation*
1 HLA- and MLC-compatible sibling
2 Recipient's age < 40 years (preferably < 20)

* Cord blood from unrelated donors may also be effective, and is associated with lower frequencies of both acute and chronic GVHD

Autologous transplantation: peripheral stem cells vs marrow reinfusion
1 Stem cell harvest less traumatic than bone marrow harvest
2 Stem cells $\rightarrow$ accelerated recovery of transplant hemopoiesis
3 Stem cells $\rightarrow$ lower risk of disease relapse in neoplastic disorders

Complications of bone marrow transplantation
1 High-dose cyclophosphamide
— Cystitis
— Cardiomyopathy
2 Total body irradiation
— Pancreatitis
— Pneumonitis
— Parotitis
— Hepatic veno-occlusive disease
— Cataracts
3 Combined toxicity
— Sterility
— Second malignancy
4 Other
— Infection
— Cardiac tamponade (?due to infection)
— Graft-versus-host disease
— Disease relapse; graft failure

Differential diagnosis of CXR infiltrates in marrow transplants
1 Pneumonia, esp.
— CMV
— Parainfluenza virus
— Respiratory syncytial virus (RSV)
2 Radiation pneumonitis
3 Graft-versus-host disease

GRAFT-VERSUS-HOST DISEASE (GVHD)

Prerequisites for developing GVHD
1 Graft must contain immunologically competent cells
2 Host must express antigens foreign to the graft
3 Host must be immunologically incapable of destroying the grafted immunocytes

Patients at high risk of GVHD
1 Older transplant recipients
2 Recipients of HLA-mismatched transplants
3 Recipients of grafts from allosensitized donors
4 Recipients of small-intestinal transplants
5 Recipients of unirradiated blood transfusions

Features and management of GVHD
1 Acute GVHD (occurs < 100 days post-transplant)
— Mediated by cytotoxic T-cells; affects ~ 50%
  • Dermatitis (bullous, morbilliform)
  • Hepatitis; abnormal LFTs $\rightarrow$ liver failure
  • Enterocolitis, diarrhea, nausea

2 Chronic GVHD (occurs > 100 days post-transplant)
  — Affects 30% long-term survivors, esp. if older
    • Dermatitis (scleroderma/lichen planus-like)
    • Conjunctivitis, stomatitis, esophagitis
    • Wasting, recurrent infections (bacterial, zoster)
3 Patients who have survived an episode of GVHD have a significantly lower risk of leukemic relapse
4 Prophylaxis
  — Ciclosporin (agent of choice in aplastic anemia)
  — ± Methotrexate
  — ± Autologous marrow purging with anti-T_H antibodies
5 Established disease
  — Symptomatic treatment
  — Steroids, azathioprine
  — Thalidomide

Diagnostic criteria for hepatic veno-occlusive disease*
1 Jaundice before day 30 post-transplant
2 Tender hepatomegaly
3 Ascites and weight gain

* Due to chemoradiotherapy-induced hepatic endothelial damage

THROMBOCYTOPENIA

Points to remember in managing the thrombocytopenic patient
1 Precautions on the ward
  — No aspirin
  — No intramuscular injections
  — No routine blood pressure measurements
2 Precautions at the bedside
  — Inspect skin and oral mucosa daily
  — Examine fundi daily
  — Remove IUD if prolonged cytopenia anticipated
3 Precautions in the laboratory
  — Check coagulation screen (esp. to exclude DIC)

What minimum platelet count mandates platelet transfusion?
1 For asymptomatic patients without bleeding or fever
  — $5–10 \times 10^9$/L
2 For patients with bleeding manifestations or fever
  — 10×10^9/L
3 For patients with coagulopathy, high-risk anatomical lesions, or on heparin
  — 20×10^9/L

Predictors of response to splenectomy for ITP
1 Age < 60 years
2 Short history of ITP (i.e. not chronic)
3 Initial promising response to steroids*
4 Good or excellent response to IV gammaglobulin
5 Post-operative platelet count > 500×10^9/L

* Note that the diagnosis should be confirmed by marrow examination first

Failed splenectomy for ITP?
1 Look at the blood film
  — Absent Howell–Jolly bodies suggest accessory spleen

2 Short-term control measures
  — IV gammaglobulin (esp. if recent onset ITP)
  — Vincristine or vinblastine
  — Plasmapheresis
3 Longer-term control measures
  — Azathioprine (best)
  — High-dose pulse corticosteroids, oral or IV (for 2 months)
4 Still refractory?
  — Cyclophosphamide 2 mg/kg (for 1–2 months)
  — Danazol (esp. in post-menopausal women)

Post-transfusion (thrombocytopenic) purpura
1 Occurs in susceptible 2–3% of population lacking Pl^{A1} antigen
2 Prior sensitization required (e.g. transfusion, pregnancy)
3 Usually occurs in older women 2–10 days post-transfusion
4 Widespread purpura and mucosal bleeding (10% mortality)
5 Diagnosis may be confirmed by direct detection of anti-Pl^{A1}
6 Management:
  — Pl^{A1}-negative transfusions
  — High-dose IV IgG
  — Steroids, plasmapheresis if necessary

Features of heparin-induced thrombocytopenia (HIT)
1 General
  — Reports of overall incidence average ~ 1–4%
  — Incidence is not dose-dependent
  — Commoner with bovine than porcine heparin
  — Occurs less often with low-molecular-weight heparin (LMWH)
2 Type I: early-onset (mild, common) HIT
  — Occurs within 1 week of starting
  — Typically asymptomatic; bleeding *rare*
  — Platelet count usually > 100×10^9/L
  — Due to platelet-aggregating effect of heparin
  — Treatment: continue heparin therapy
3 Type II: delayed-onset (severe, unusual) HIT
  — Typically occurs 1–3 weeks after heparin commenced
  — Can occur earlier if previous heparin exposures
  — May cause
    • Severe thrombocytopenia, bleeding
    • Limb-threatening paradoxical arterial thromboembolism in 0.5% (due to platelet aggregation), possibly resulting in limb gangrene, stroke, or death
  — Caused by immune mechanism: heparin-IgG complexes bind platelets, causing
    • Reduced survival and thrombocytopenia
    • Aggregation and thrombosis (may precede thrombocytopenia)
  — Diagnosis: clinical picture (most important) *plus*
    • In vitro platelet aggregometry studies
    • Two-point platelet ^{14}C-serotonin release assay
    • Antibody to platelet factor 4/heparin complex
  — Treatment
    • Cease intravenous heparin immediately
    • Commence warfarin ± dextran, *or*

- Substitute LMWH, or hirudin, or danaparoid sodium, *or*
- Add IV immunoglobulin

MANAGING COAGULOPATHIES

Long-term complications of hemophilia A
1 AIDS
2 Chronic hepatitis (esp. non-A non-B)
3 Arthropathy
4 Narcotic addiction
5 F VIII antibodies (inhibitors: seen in 10%)

Replacement factor levels required in hemophilia
1 Minor hemarthrosis
   — 10–20%
2 Dental extraction
   Major joint/muscle bleed
   — 20–50% (may need multiple transfusions)
3 Surgery, major trauma (esp. cranial)
   — 50–100%

Management of bleeding in patients with factor VIII$_c$ inhibitors*
1 For *serious* hemorrhage, or preoperatively
   — Plasmapheresis
   — Extracorporeal protein A adsorption of patient plasma
2 If inhibitor levels *low*
   — Porcine factor VIII$_c$
   — Alternate-day human factor VIII 'desensitization'
3 If inhibitor levels *high*
   — Activated prothrombin complex concentrates (APCCs)
   — Contain factor IX, II, X (but not VII) + proteins C and S
   — These factor IX concentrates may be riskier for virus transmission
4 Other measures
   — *Megadose* factor VIII plus APCCs
   — Recombinant activated factor VII (factor VIIa)
   — IV gammaglobulin + cyclophosphamide

* 25% of all hemophilia A patients (50% of severe cases) develop inhibitors

Indications for antifibrinolytic treatment* of bleeding
1 Menorrhagia
2 Acute promyelocytic leukemia
3 Dental extraction in coagulopathy patients
4 Upper gastrointestinal hemorrhage

* Tranexamic acid, EACA

Possible indications for desmopressin treatment of bleeding
1 Mild bleeding in hemophilia or VWD
2 Congenital or acquired platelet function defects*
3 Uremia‡ or cirrhosis

* Including drug-induced
‡ Delayed effects may also be achievable using conjugated estrogens or erythropoietin

ANTICOAGULATION

Duration of therapeutic anticoagulation: the rough guide
1 Prosthetic heart valve, *or*
   Arterial emboli + mitral valve disease/atrial fibrillation, *or*
   Recurrent thromboses or emboli, *or*
   Paroxysmal nocturnal hemoglobinuria (severe)
   — Treat lifelong
   — Aim for INR > 3
2 Single episode of life-threatening pulmonary embolism, *or*
   Single episode of extensive proximal (ileofemoral) DVT
   — Treat for 12 months
   — Aim for INR 2.5–3
3 Uncomplicated pulmonary embolus, *or*
   Localized proximal DVT, *or*
   Carotid TIA in a female
   — Treat for 6 months
   — Aim for INR 2.5–3
4 Uncomplicated calf DVT
   — Treat for 6 months
   — Aim for INR 2.0–2.5
   — Consider prophylactic use of orthopedic stockings

Mechanisms of antithrombotic drugs
1 Heparin
   — Binds to and activates AT III; this complex
     • Inhibits thrombin-induced activation of factors V and VIII
     • Inactivates factor Xa
     • (Thus) prevents fibrin formation from fibrinogen
   — Does *not* efficiently inactivate fibrin-bound thrombin (cf. hirudin)
   — Is neutralized by other (non-AT III) heparin substrates (e.g. vitronectin, platelet factor 4); elevated plasma levels of these may cause heparin resistance
2 Warfarin
   — Prevents activation of vitamin K, thereby inhibiting γ-carboxylation of factors II, VII, IX and X*
3 Streptokinase/urokinase
   Tissue plasminogen activator (tPA)
   — Activate plasminogen
4 Hirudin
   — AT III-independent anticoagulant, formerly from leeches (*Hirudo medicinalis*); now recombinant
   — Inactivates fibrin-bound thrombin; hence, more effective than heparin in preventing extension of preformed thrombi

* And also of the anticoagulant proteins C and S; hence, if deficiency of these proteins is suspected as a possible cause of thrombosis, assay should be undertaken *prior* to commencing warfarin

Side-effects of heparin therapy
1 Bleeding ± thrombocytopenia (see above)
2 Osteoporosis (*if* full-dose treatment > 6 months)

3 Burning sensation of hands and feet
4 Alopecia

Indications for heparin therapy
1 Prophylaxis of thromboembolism
2 Treatment of established deep venous thrombosis
3 Unstable angina
4 Acute myocardial infarction
   — Prevention of mural thrombus and/or reinfarction
5 Following thrombolytic therapy
   — Maintenance of vessel patency

Advantages of low-molecular-weight heparin (LMWH)*
1 Outpatient self-administration possible
2 Once-daily administration
3 More consistent therapeutic levels
4 Fewer hemorrhagic complications
5 Less osteoporosis with long-term use
6 Lower incidence of heparin-induced thrombocytopenia

* i.e. over intravenous (unfractionated) heparin

Mechanisms of warfarin potentiation
1 ↑ Catabolism of coagulation factors
   — Fever, thyrotoxicosis, post-operative
   ↓ Hepatic drug metabolism
   — Liver disease, cardiac failure, acute alcoholic binge
   ↓ Renal excretion
   — Renal failure, old age
2 ↑ Bleeding tendency (independent of coagulation)
   — Aspirin, indometacin, phenylbutazone
3 Potentiation of hypoprothrombinemia
   — Aspirin; quin(id)ine
   — Tetracycline, chloramphenicol:
      → ↓ Bacterial vitamin K synthesis
4 Drugs inhibiting hepatic metabolism
   — Antibiotics (isoniazid, chloramphenicol, metronidazole, sulfonamides)
   — Amiodarone; cimetidine; allopurinol; valproate
   — Phenylbutazone (inhibits S-enantiomer metabolism)
5 Plasma protein displacement
   — Clofibrate

Drugs inducing hepatic metabolism of warfarin
1 Phenytoin, phenobarbital, carbamazepine
2 Chronic alcohol ingestion; cigarette smoking
3 Rifampicin; griseofulvin

Relatively 'safe' drugs in warfarinized patients
1 Analgesics
   — Paracetamol (unless prolonged)
2 Sedatives, anticonvulsants
   — Benzodiazepines
3 Antibiotics
   — Penicillins, cephalosporins, aminoglycosides

NB: Caution must *always* be exercised when *changing* therapy of patients stabilized on warfarin

---

ANTIPLATELET THERAPY

Mechanisms of antiplatelet drugs
1 Platelet thromboxane A_2 synthesis antagonists
   — Aspirin (irreversibly acetylates cyclo-oxygenase)
   — Sulfinpyrazone (reversibly acetylates cyclo-oxygenase)
2 Platelet cAMP agonists
   — Epoprostenol (prostacyclin, PGI_2): activates adenyl cyclase
   — Dipyridamole (inhibits phosphodiesterase)
3 Platelet ADP receptor antagonists (thienopyridines)
   — Clopidrogel
4 Platelet glycoprotein IIb/IIIa receptor antagonists
   — Abciximab (antibody)
   — Eptifibatide, tirofiban

Proven benefits of antiplatelet therapy
1 Fatal vascular event
   — Risk reduced by 15% in high-risk groups
2 Non-fatal myocardial infarction
   — Risk reduced by 30% in all groups
3 Stroke or vascular event
   — Risk reduced by 30% in high-risk groups
   — Net benefit *not* proven in low-risk groups
4 Graft (e.g. CABG) occlusion
   — Risk reduced by 40% in high-risk groups
5 Thromboembolism
   — Risk reduced by 50% in high-risk groups

UNDERSTANDING HEMATOLOGIC DISEASE

Hereditary syndromes predisposing to leukemias/lymphomas
1 DNA repair/chromosomal stability defects
   — Ataxia telangiectasia
   — Bloom's syndrome
   — Fanconi's syndrome
2 Down's syndrome
3 Klinefelter's syndrome
4 Osteogenesis imperfecta
5 Wiskott–Aldrich syndrome

Clinical varieties of B cell neoplasms
1 Dysproteinemias*
   — Benign monoclonal gammopathy
   — Multiple myeloma, solitary plasmacytoma
   — Waldenström's macroglobulinemia
   — Heavy chain disease (α and γ)
   — 'Primary' amyloidosis
2 Leukemias
   — ALL (most cases)
   — CLL (98% cases)
   — Hairy cell leukemia
3 Lymphomas
   — Most subtypes, incl. Burkitt's

* Characterized by M proteins

Clinical varieties of T cell neoplasms
1 Mycosis fungoides
2 Sézary syndrome

3 T cell leukemia/lymphoma
4 Lymphoblastic lymphoma

The myelodysplastic syndromes ('preleukemias')
1 Classification
   — Refractory anemia with (30%) or without (40%) ringed sideroblasts
   — Refractory anemia with excess blasts (RAEB: 25%)
   — 5q– syndrome (5%)
2 Acute leukemia (often myelomonocytic) supervenes in 10%
3 Risk of leukemia is not reliably predicted by marrow features
4 Overall prognosis is inversely proportional to
   — Transfusion requirement (i.e. ± leukemic transition)
   — % Marrow blasts ($\rightarrow$ $\uparrow$ AML transition, $\uparrow$ infection)
5 Low-dose cytosine arabinoside may help 'differentiate' dysplastic marrow precursors

MULTIPLE MYELOMA

Relative incidence of myeloma subtypes
1 IgG   — 50%
2 IgA   — 30%
3 Light-chain (BJP) only   — 10%
4 IgM   — 5%
5 IgD   — 2%
6 Biclonal   — 2%
7 Non-secretory   — 1%

Mechanisms of renal failure in myeloma
1 Intratubular precipitation of Bence-Jones protein
2 Prerenal (e.g. dehydration with IVP)
3 Sepsis (e.g. pyelonephritis) ± nephrotoxic antibiotics
4 Amyloid; plasma cell infiltration
5 Hypercalcemia, urate nephropathy
6 Hyperviscosity

Mechanisms of anemia in myeloma
1 Marrow failure (leukoerythroblastic)
2 Marrow failure (iatrogenic)
3 'Chronic disease' (± azotemia)
4 Dilutional
5 Bleeding (reduced platelet number and function)
6 Iatrogenic sideroblastosis (? preleukemic)

Spectrum of bony involvement in myeloma
1 Lytic lesions esp. ($\rightarrow$ 60%)
   — Vertebral bodies (cf. carcinoma $\rightarrow$ pedicles)
   — Skull (usually painless; cf. carcinoma)
   — Mandible (classical)
2 Diffuse osteoporosis ($\rightarrow$ 20%)
3 Skeletal survey more sensitive than isotope bone scan Osteosclerotic lesions are very rare; when present they may be associated with neuropathy (POEMS syndrome)*
4 Serum alkaline phosphatase typically *normal*

* *Polyneuropathy, organomegaly, endocrinopathy, M spike, skin changes*

Neurologic manifestations of myeloma
1 Spinal cord compression
   — Usually due to vertebral collapse
2 Confusion
   — Hyperviscosity
   — Hypercalcemia
   — Steroid-induced
3 Peripheral neuropathy
   — Amyloid
4 Cranial nerve palsies
   — Base of skull lesions

HEMOLYTIC ANEMIAS

Paroxysmal nocturnal hemoglobinuria: features
1 Pathogenesis
   — A clonal stem-cell defect
   — Red cell subpopulation develops with abnormal affinity and/or sensitivity to complement
   — May terminate in leukemia, aplasia, myelofibrosis
2 Clinical features
   — Episodic 'smoky' urine
   — Abdominal/back pain
   — Thrombotic events (esp. $\rightarrow$ portal and hepatic veins)
3 Laboratory diagnosis
   — Anemia
     • Usually normochromic, but may be hypochromic
     • Macrocytes may be present
   — Hemoglobinuria, hemosiderinuria
   — Positive Ham's (acid hemolysis) test*
   — $\downarrow$ NAP; $\downarrow$ red cell acetylcholinesterase
   — Bone marrow hypoplastic in 25%
4 Management principles
   — Transfusion of washed packed red cells
   — Avoidance of whole blood or iron supplements
   — ± Androgens, folate, warfarin

* Sucrose lysis/sugar-water tests now outmoded

Causes of intravascular hemolysis
1 Paroxysmal nocturnal hemoglobinuria
   Paroxysmal cold hemoglobinuria (IgG-mediated)
   Cold hemagglutinin disease (IgM-mediated)
2 Intracardiac prostheses
   — Aortic valve replacements
   — Patch repair of ostium primum ASD
3 Incompatible blood transfusion
   Burns, snake venom, 'march' hemoglobinuria

Causes of microangiopathic hemolytic anemia
1 Thrombotic thrombocytopenic purpura (TTP)*
   Hemolytic uremic syndrome (HUS)*
2 Malignant hypertension
   Pregnancy-associated hypertension
3 Mucinous adenocarcinoma
4 Vasculitis
5 Transplant rejection

* Designates clinical syndrome which tends to be diagnosed TTP by hematologists and HUS by nephrologists

Bacterial precipitants of hemolytic uremic syndrome (HUS)

1 *E. coli* O157: H7 diarrhea
   — Produces shigella-like toxins
   — Causes hemorrhagic colitis in children under 5
2 *E. coli* O103: H2 urinary tract infection
   — Produces shiga toxins (causes diarrhea in rabbits)
   — May be non-bacteremic; no diarrhea associated
3 *Shigella dysenteriae* serotype I
   — Renal failure more likely if treated with ampicillin

Precipitants of adult HUS/TTP syndromes

1 Drugs
   — Hypersensitivity: ticlopidine, clopidogrel, quinine
   — Cumulative, dose-related risk: mitomycin
2 Pregnancy
3 Autoimmune disease
   — SLE, scleroderma, antiphospholipid syndrome
4 Transplantation
   — Allogeneic (esp. with ciclosporin treatment)

Features of thrombotic thrombocytopenic purpura (TTP)

1 Pathogenesis (distinguishes TTP from HUS)
   — Familial: primary deficiency of VWF-cleaving protease
   — Sporadic: inhibitory antibodies to VWF-cleaving protease
2 Diagnostic pentad
   — Thrombocytopenic purpura
   — Microangiopathic hemolytic anemia
   — Bizarre neurologic signs
   — Fever
   — Renal failure
3 Investigations
   — Blood film: schistocytes, no spherocytes
   — Coombs-negative
   — PI, PTTK, FDPs, D-dimers, fibrinogen usually normal
   — ANA negative in 80%
4 Management
   — Large-volume plasma exchange ± FFP/steroids
   — Antiplatelet therapy *if* platelet count $> 50 \times 10^9$/L
   — Splenectomy

Features favoring TTP over hemolytic uremic syndrome

1 Usually affects adult *women* (may be autoimmune)
2 Usually *relapsing* clinical course
3 *Neurologic* involvement is more characteristic
4 Benefit from steroids or antiplatelet therapy*

* But note that thieneopyridine derivatives such as clopidogrel may (like ticlopidine) predispose to TTP

Differential diagnosis of HUS/TTP

1 Exotic infectious disease
   — Malaria (± DIC)
   — Viral hemorrhagic fever (e.g. Dengue)
   — Leptospirosis
2 Septicemia with DIC
   — Gram-negative sepsis
   — Pneumococcus, meningococcus
   — *Staphylococcus aureus*
   — *Mycoplasma pneumoniae*

Disseminated intravascular coagulation

1 Major causes
   — Sepsis (Gram-negative septicemia, *Plasmodium falciparum*)
   — Malignancy (e.g. disseminated prostate cancer, pancreatic cancer)
   — Obstetric disaster
2 Diagnosis
   — Film: RBC fragments, thrombocytopenia
   — ↑ PI, PTTK, TT
   — ↑ FDPs ($\rightarrow$ ↓ thrombin, ↓ platelet function), ↑ D-dimers
   — ↓ Fibrinogen, factors V and VIII, AT III
   — + Ethanol gelation/soluble fibrin monomer complexes

HEMOGLOBINOPATHIES

Thalassemias: basic concepts

1 Thalassemias are a heterogeneous group of disorders due to abnormal production of globin chains
2 Anemia in (say) β-thalassemia results from
   — Ineffective erythropoiesis (insufficient β-chains)
   — Hemolysis (precipitation of relative α-chain excess)
3 Predominant genetic basis
   — α-thalassemias
      • Usually due to gene deletions (chromosome 16)
      • Become symptomatic when α-globin production drops below ~ 25% normal
   — β-thalassemias
      • Usually due to complex (non-deletional) lesions on chromosome 11* (e.g. causing abnormal β-globin mRNA splicing/translation)
4 Incidence
   — About 100 000 homozygotes world-wide
   — Most of these are β-thalassemics

* In addition to β-globin, most of the other non-α globin genes (γ — Hb F — δ, ε) are in this chromosome 11 cluster

Clinical categorization of thalassemias

1 Thalassemia trait
   — Asymptomatic condition; may be detected on screening
2 Thalassemia minor
   — Mild anemia with minimal symptoms
3 Thalassemia intermedia
   — Moderate anemia and splenomegaly
   — e.g. Hb C, Hb Lepore; HbE plus β-thal trait
4 Thalassemia major
   — Severe transfusion-dependent anemia

Features of α-thalassemia

1 αα/α-
   — Asymptomatic carrier (α-thalassemia-2 trait)
   — Occurs in 15–20% blacks
   — Low normal MCV/MCHC, but rarely anemic
   — Hb A_2, Hb F levels normal (cf. β-thal trait)
   — 1–2% Hb Bart's (γ_4 tetramers) in cord blood

2 α-/α-
— Homozygous α-thalassemia-2 trait
— Mild anemia and microcytosis, but usually asymptomatic
— 5–10% Hb Bart's; normal Hb A$_2$; ± ↓ MCV
3 αα/--
— Heterozygous α-thalassemia (α-thalassemia-1 trait)
— Low MCV, mild anemia; normal Hb A$_2$
— Blood film
  • Target cells
  • Some Hb H (β4 tetramers) inclusion bodies (Hb H < 1%)
4 α-/--
— Hb H disease; offspring of α-thal-2 and α-thal-1 traits
— Moderate/severe hemolytic anemia (similar to β-thal intermedia)
— Typical Hb H cells visible on cresyl violet stain (20–40% Hb Bart's)
— Presentations in adult life: gallstones, splenomegaly
— 10–30% Hb H ± ↓ Hb A$_2$
— May improve with splenectomy
5 --/--(α°)
— Hydrops fetalis (→ stillbirth, perinatal death)
— 80% Hb Bart's, 20% Hb Portland (i.e. absent Hb A$_2$)

Features of β-thalassemia
1 β-thalassemia minor
— ↓ MCV (< 75 fL) but hematocrit > 30%*
— Basophilic stippling; targets, few teardrops
— ↓ Osmotic fragility (cf. spherocytosis)
— ↑ Hb A$_2$ ± ↑ Hb F
— Definitive diagnosis by Hb EPG
2 Suspected thalassemia minor with normal Hb A$_2$
— α-thalassemia
— δβ-thalassemia (heterozygous; suspect if ↑ Hb F)
3 β-thalassemia major
— ↑ Hb F (> 70%) ± ↑ Hb A$_2$ (cf. β-thal minor)
— β°-thalassemia: no detectable Hb A
— β$^+$-thalassemia: up to 30% Hb A
— Blood film: teardrops, targets, nucleated red cells

* i.e. microcytosis excessive for degree of anemia, e.g compared with iron deficiency anemia

Approach to the patient with thalassemia
1 Thalassemia trait
— Test partner (spouse-to-be) for trait; refer for genetic counselling if positive
— Educate patient against accepting oral iron on basis of ↓ MCV interpreted by doctors unaware of diagnosis
— Prescribe prophylactic folate and/or iron supplements during marrow stress (e.g. menorrhagia, pregnancy)
2 Thalassemia intermedia
— Similar phenotype to thal major, but no need for chronic hypertransfusion

— Transfusion requirement may increase in infection, puberty; may benefit from splenectomy
3 Thalassemia major
— Hypertransfuse to maintain Hb > 10 g/dL
— Folate supplements; hepatitis B vaccination
— Splenectomy for hypersplenism or discomfort; presplenectomy pneumococcal vaccination
— Iron chelation regimen at earliest possible age*
— Genetic counselling, amniocentesis
— Hydroxyurea to increase Hb F (investigational)
— Monitor for siderosis-induced endocrine deficiency
— Bone marrow transplantation work-up

* Subcutaneous desferrioxamine; organ damage (e.g. hepatic fibrosis) otherwise begins after first 50–100 units (10–20 g Fe) transfused

SICKLE-CELL ANEMIA

Clinical spectrum of sickle-cell disease
1 Hb AS (sickle trait)
— 60% Hb A, 35% Hb S
— Normal life expectancy
— Hyposthenuria, nocturia, papillary necrosis
— Painless (micro)hematuria
— Bacteriuria in pregnancy; zinc wasting
— Hypoxia (e.g. unpressurized aircraft at high altitude) may precipitate splenic/retinal infarction
2 Hb SS (sickle-cell disease)*
— No Hb A; 85% Hb S, 10% Hb F
— Dactylitis, leg ulcers, cerebrovascular disease, gout, priapism (→ impotence), retinopathy
— Autosplenectomy usually supervenes before age 3
3 Hb SC (sickle-C disease)
— Sickle and target cells on film
— Thrombotic tendency
  • Proliferative retinopathy
  • Aseptic necrosis of femoral head or shoulder
  • Hematuria
  • Complications during pregnancy
4 Hb S + α-thal
— *Less* severe than Hb SS

* Manifestations due to fibrous polymerization of Hb S ($\alpha_2\beta_2^{6Val \to Glu}$) on deoxygenation

Hepatic manifestations of sickle-cell anemia
1 Complications related to transfusion
— Hemochromatosis
— (Chronic) hepatitis B/C
2 Complications related to chronic hemolysis
— Gallstones
3 Complications related to repeated vascular occlusion
— Hepatic fibrosis or infarction
— Liver failure

REVIEWING THE LITERATURE: HEMATOLOGIC DISEASE

5.1 Kearon C et al (1999) A comparison of three months of anticoagulation with extended anticoagulation for a first episode of idiopathic venous thromboembolism. N Engl J Med 340: 901–907

Schulman S et al (1997) The duration of oral anticoagulant therapy after a second episode of venous thromboembolism. N Engl J Med 336: 393–398

Two randomized studies showing greater efficacy of longer anticoagulation in the prevention of subsequent thrombotic events. As expected, however, both studies confirmed a higher incidence of bleeding complications in those assigned to longer-term anticoagulation.

5.2 Brandjes D et al (1997) Randomised trial of effect of compression stockings in patients with symptomatic proximal-vein thrombosis. Lancet 349: 759–762

Agnelli G et al (1998) Enoxaparin plus compression stocking compared with compression stockings alone in the prevention of venous thromboembolism after elective neurosurgery. N Engl J Med 339: 80–85

The former of these two studies showed a 50% reduction in the incidence of post-phlebitic syndrome conferred by the use of correct-size compression stockings. The latter study showed that the efficacy of compression stockings in preventing subsequent thrombosis was enhanced by concomitant use of low-molecular-weight heparin (enoxaparin).

5.3 Pulmonary Embolism Prevention (PEP) Trial Collaborative Group (2000) Prevention of pulmonary embolism and deep vein thrombosis with low dose aspirin. Lancet 355: 1295–1302

Randomized study of over 17 000 perioperative patients, showing that 160 mg aspirin/day reduced the incidence of venous thromboembolism by 36% in all groups, including those also receiving heparin prophylaxis. A 58% reduction in fatal pulmonary emboli was also seen, but there was an excess risk of 6 bleeding events per 1000 patients treated.

5.4 Cromheecke ME et al (2000) Oral anticoagulation self-management and management by a specialist anticoagulation clinic: a randomized cross-over comparison Lancet 356: 97–102

Small randomized study of 50 patients, showing that most patients can be trained to manage their anticoagulation themselves: better control and greater satisfaction were apparent in the self-managed cohort.

5.5 Reling MV et al (2000) Adverse effect of anticonvulsants on efficacy of chemotherapy for acute lymphoblastic leukaemia. Lancet 356: 285–290

Evans WE et al (1998) Conventional compared with individualized chemotherapy for childhood acute lymphoblastic leukemia. N Engl J Med 338: 499–505

Two studies looking at chemotherapy optimization in ALL. In the former cohort study of 716 children treated for acute lymphoblastic leukemia, 5.6% of whom received anticonvulsants, increased hepatic clearance of antileukemic drugs was apparent in those being treated for B cell (but not T cell) leukemias, and was associated with reduced survival in this group. The latter randomized study of 182 children with ALL showed that patients in whom methotrexate levels (but not teniposide or cytarabine) were optimized incurred fewer relapses.

5.6 Kadir RA et al (1998) Frequency of inherited bleeding disorders in women with menorrhagia. Lancet 351: 485–489

Coagulopathy screening of 150 women referred for investigation of menorrhagia revealed clotting defects in 17%. These defects included von Willebrand's disease, factor XI deficiency, hemophilia A heterozygosity, and platelet dysfunction.

5.7 Preston FE et al (1996) Increased fetal loss in women with heritable thrombophilia. Lancet 348: 913–916

Kupferminc MJ et al (1999) Increased frequency of genetic thrombophilia in women with complications of pregnancy. N Engl J Med 340: 9–13

Martinelli I et al (2000) Mutations in coagulation factors in women with unexplained late fetal loss. N Engl J Med 343: 1015–1018

Gerhardt A et al (2000) Prothrombin and factor V mutations in women with a history of thrombosis during pregnancy and the puerperium. N Engl J Med 342: 374–380

Four studies of pregnancy-associated thrombotic complications, attesting to the recent rapid improved understanding of thrombotic predisposition. The first study followed a cohort of 1384 women with known defects of factor V, proteins C or S, or antithrombin III, and found a 3.6-fold increased risk of stillbirth. The second analyzed a cohort of 110 women with obstetric complications, and confirmed a 3-fold relative increased frequency of mutations in the factor V or prothrombin genes; the same conclusions were reached in the last two studies.

5.8 Sarasin FP, Bounameaux H (1998) Decision analysis model of prolonged oral anticoagulant treatment in factor V Leiden carriers with first episode of deep vein thrombosis. Br Med J 316: 95–99

Theoretical study showing lack of evidence for factor V mutation screening among patients treated for DVT: anticoagulation exceeding a year in duration appears of no net benefit in this cohort, given the increase in bleeding complications.

5.9 Wells PS et al (1998) SimpliRED D-dimer can reduce the diagnostic tests in suspected deep vein thrombosis. Lancet 351: 1405–1406

Bernardi E et al (1998) D-dimer testing as an adjunct to ultrasonography in patients with clinically suspected deep vein thrombosis. Br Med J 317: 1037–1040

Perrier A et al (1999) Non-invasive diagnosis of venous thromboembolism in outpatients. Lancet 353: 190–195

Three studies suggesting a sea-change in the traditional reliance on venographic diagnosis of venous thrombosis: the combination of D-dimer and ultrasonography seems sufficiently reliable to guide management in most clinical contexts.

5.10 Taskinen M et al (2000) Impaired glucose tolerance and dyslipidaemia as late effects after bone marrow transplantation in childhood. Lancet 356: 993–997

Case-control study showing that 12 of 23 long-term marrow transplant survivors had developed insulin resistance, while 9 of 23 had developed full-blown syndrome X (hyperglycemia + hypertriglyceridemia).

5.11 Kraaijenhagen RA et al (2000) Travel and risk of venous thrombosis. Lancet 356: 1492–1493

Scurr JH et al (2001) Frequency and prevention of symptomless deep-vein thrombosis in long-haul flights. Lancet 357: 1485–1489

Two studies of DVT in the air, with different, but not mutually exclusive, conclusions. The former showed no increase in symptomatic DVT, whereas the latter showed up to 10% occurrence of symptomless DVT.

CHAPTER 6

HIV-related disease

Physical examination protocol 6.1   You are asked to examine a patient with HIV infection

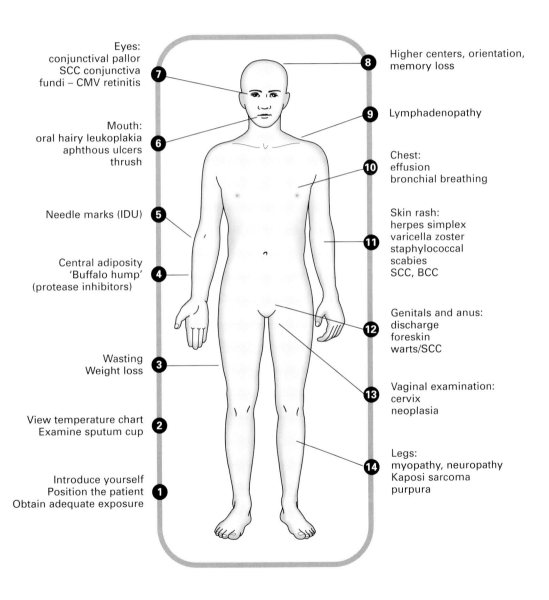

Eyes:
conjunctival pallor
SCC conjunctiva
fundi – CMV retinitis
7

Mouth:
oral hairy leukoplakia
aphthous ulcers
thrush
6

Needle marks (IDU) **5**

Central adiposity
'Buffalo hump'
(protease inhibitors) **4**

Wasting
Weight loss **3**

View temperature chart
Examine sputum cup **2**

Introduce yourself
Position the patient
Obtain adequate exposure **1**

8 Higher centers, orientation,
memory loss

9 Lymphadenopathy

10 Chest:
effusion
bronchial breathing

11 Skin rash:
herpes simplex
varicella zoster
staphylococcal
scabies
SCC, BCC

12 Genitals and anus:
discharge
foreskin
warts/SCC

13 Vaginal examination:
cervix
neoplasia

14 Legs:
myopathy, neuropathy
Kaposi sarcoma
purpura

COMMON AND CLASSIC HIV-RELATED PROBLEMS

Common HIV-related problems in clinical practice
1 Treatment side-effects
2 Opportunistic infections (e.g. thrush, herpes, scabies)
3 Weight loss

Classic HIV-related problems in clinical exams
1 Kaposi's sarcoma
2 Oral hairy leukoplakia
3 Non-Hodgkin's lymphoma

EMERGENCIES IN HIV-RELATED DISEASE

HIV-related emergencies
1 Fulminant infection, esp. *Pneumocystis carinii* pneumonia
2 Acute psychosis or encephalopathy (exclude abnormal brain scan or CSF)
3 Cytomegalovirus retinitis*
4 Possible HIV exposure of uninfected individual

* Treat with intravenous ganciclovir or foscarnet via central line

Post-exposure prophylaxis (PEP): principles and practice
1 Few hard data are available for formulating evidence-based policies
2 Common exposures: sexual, blood, needlestick
3 HIV status of the exposure may not be known
4 Regimens include: zidovudine + lamivudine + indinavir for up to 4 weeks, but cost and toxicity often prevent completion
5 Baseline and subsequent serology should be monitored

CLINICAL ASSESSMENT OF HIV-RELATED DISEASE

High-risk transmission modes for HIV infection
1 Blood-borne transmission
   — Blood transfusions
   — Transplacental/peripartum (3rd trimester) neonatal infection*
   — Needle sharing (e.g. heroin addicts)
2 Venereal transmission, in absence of condom usage
   — By semen (receptive anal > vaginal > oral intercourse)
   — By blood (esp. sex during menstruation or post-partum)
   — By vaginal secretions (esp. if uncircumcised or genital ulcers)
3 Breast-feeding
   — Duration-dependent increased risk beyond 3 months

* Risk can be reduced from 20% to 5% by use of antiretroviral therapy

Highly transmissible HIV-positive body fluids
1 Blood
2 Semen

3 Vaginal secretions
4 Amniotic fluid
5 Cerebrospinal fluid
6 Peritoneal, pleural, or bronchoalveolar fluids

Average risk quantification per HIV exposure episode
1 Blood transfusion: 95%
2 Peripartum: 25% (no prophylaxis)
                          5% (+ zidovudine prophylaxis)
3 Needle-sharing/-stick: 0.5%
4 Sex (receptive anal): 0.5%
5 Sex (vaginal):   0.1%

Clinical spectrum of HIV infection
1 Mononucleosis-like ('seroconversion') syndrome
   — Fever, rash, ± neuropathy, encephalitis
2 Asymptomatic phase (~ 7–10 years)*
   — CD4 count drops below 200/mm^3
   — Active HIV replication continues, but largely confined to fixed lymphoid tissue (nodes, Kupffer cells)
3 AIDS-related complex (ARC)‡
   — e.g. adenopathy¶, diarrhea, fever, weight loss, thrush
4 AIDS ('full-blown')
   — e.g. *P. carinii* pneumonia, cerebral toxoplasmosis, *Cryptosporidium* diarrhea§

* Unless HIV acquired by *transfusion* → average latency ~ 4 years
‡ Persistent generalized lymphadenopathy + sweats, fever, weight loss; = 'AIDS prodrome'
¶ i.e. 2 extrainguinal nodes > 1 cm diameter
§ Typically resistant to treatment; symptomatic measures such as octreotide may be tried

AIDS-defining malignancies
1 Kaposi's sarcoma
   — Risk increased 1000-fold by HIV positivity
   — Incidence has declined dramatically since advent of HAART (p. 168)
2 Non-Hodgkin's lymphoma
   — Risk increased 300-fold by HIV positivity
   — Incidence has declined slightly since advent of HAART
3 Cervix cancer
   — Risk increased 3-fold by HIV positivity
   — Incidence has not declined measurably* since advent of HAART

* i.e. in HIV-infected cohorts

HIV-associated malignancies unassociated with immunodeficiency
1 Lung cancer
2 Skin cancers (squamous and basal cell)
3 Squamous cell carcinoma of the conjunctiva
4 Squamous cell carcinoma of the anus
5 Germ-cell tumors
6 Hodgkin's disease
7 Pediatric leiomyosarcoma

Occurrence of Kaposi's sarcoma in HIV-infected cohorts
1 Seen commonly in homosexuals with AIDS*
2 Seen occasionally in intravenous drug abusers with AIDS

3 Seen rarely in hemophiliacs with AIDS

* Fecal–oral contact may predispose

Diseases caused by HHV-8 (KSHV)
1 Kaposi's sarcoma (in AIDS, esp. homosexually acquired)
2 Multicentric Castleman's disease (HIV > non-HIV)
3 Primary effusion lymphoma (PEL)*

* A rare B-cell lymphoma also known as body cavity lymphoma (BCL)

Neurologic complications of HIV infection
1 Subacute diffuse encephalitis
2 Meningitis (incl. cryptococcal)
3 Progressive multifocal leukoencephalopathy
4 Space-occupying lesion(s)
   — Cerebral toxoplasmosis*
   — Non-Hodgkin's lymphoma
5 Myelitis (CMV, HSV type 2)
6 Neuropathies

* Negative serology makes diagnosis unlikely

Clinical features of progressive multifocal leukoencephalopathy (PML)
1 Commonest predisposition
   — HIV infection (1–5% incidence), esp. male IV drug addicts
   — Occasionally seen in leukemias (esp. CLL), lymphomas
2 Pathology and pathogenesis
   — Deep corticocerebellar demyelination due to JC virus (JCV)
   — JCV is a polyomavirus which targets myelin-synthesizing oligodendrocytes
   — 80% of normal individuals have latent JCV in lymph and kidney
3 Presentation
   — Progressive cortical (visual, speech, higher centers) and cerebellar deficits
   — Tends to be unassociated with other opportunistic infections
4 Diagnosis
   — CSF: microscopy, culture and pressure typically normal
   — CSF: positive PCR for JCV supports the diagnosis
   — MRI: lesions in frontal lobe, cerebellum ± basal ganglia, brainstem
   — Autopsy: brain biopsy for JCV and other viral studies
5 Course
   — Survival averages 4 months from diagnosis

Indirect sequelae of HIV infection*
1 Progressive multifocal leukoencephalopathy (JC virus)
2 Cerebral lymphoma (EBV)
3 Kaposi's sarcoma (see ref. 6.8)
4 Hairy leukoplakia
5 Cardiomyopathy‡
6 Aphthous ulcers¶

* i.e. may be precipitated by immunodeficiency (e.g. via a second viral infection) rather than directly by HIV

‡ Infective basis unproven; also may occur with interferon-α therapy
¶ Respond to thalidomide treatment

Infective complications of early HIV infection
1 Oral candidiasis
2 Herpesviruses (esp. zoster, recurrent herpes simplex)
3 Staphylococcal infections
4 Oral hairy leukoplakia* (EBV)
5 Antibiotic hypersensitivity reactions

* Virtually pathognomonic of HIV infection

Infective complications of advanced HIV infection
1 *P. carinii* pneumonia*
2 CMV infection, esp. pneumonitis/retinitis/colitis‡
3 Invasive mucosal candidiasis, esp. esophageal
4 Cryptococcosis, aspergillosis, histoplasmosis
5 Intestinal cryptosporidiosis, isosporiasis (esp. in Haitians)
6 Disseminated (extraintestinal) strongyloidiasis
7 Toxoplasmosis, esp. CNS
8 Mycobacterial infections, esp. *avium–intracellulare* ¶
9 Recurrent *Salmonella* bacteremias
10 Chronic ulcerative herpes simplex, or disseminated zoster

* Presentation of AIDS in 50%; affects 80% of patients at least once; 10% die with first infection; 50% relapse within 12 months
‡ Treat with ganciclovir (oral prophylaxis is effective); cf. CMV adrenalitis, treat with steroid replacement
¶ May cause marrow depression; infection confirmed in 50% of AIDS autopsies

INVESTIGATING HIV-RELATED DISEASE

DIAGNOSIS AND PROGNOSIS OF HIV INFECTION

HIV antibody tests: who should you screen?
1 Donors of blood, semen, ova or transplant tissues
2 Regular clients of VD and drug detoxification clinics*
3 Prostitutes; rapists
4 Patients in whom HIV status is clinically relevant*
5 Patients whose blood has inadvertently contaminated a health professional (needlestick‡, mucosal exposure)
6 Anybody requesting a test (may be confidential or anonymous)

* Refusal of such patients to give informed consent for testing may be interpreted as signifying HIV-positivity until proven otherwise
‡ Note that HBV is a far more frequent complication of needlestick; seroconversion occurs in only ~ 1% of needlestick injuries involving HIV-positive patients (cf. HIV blood *transfusion*: almost 100% seroconversion after one unit)

HIV seropositivity: screening and confirmation
1 HIV ELISA* is the best screen (cf. definitive test: Western blot)

2 ELISA may remain negative for 3–6 months post-infection (i.e. negative test does *not* exclude HIV infection)
3 ELISA is 99% sensitive if performed > 6 months post-infection
4 ELISA has a significant false-positive rate; hence, all positives need to be confirmed using Western blot
5 ELISA+ neonates of infected mothers may not have HIV
6 Some patients with AIDS do not have positive ELISA

* Note that there are different ELISA varieties available: indirect, competitive, double antigen

Predictors of poor prognosis in HIV infection
1 Advanced disease, late presentation, frail condition
2 Marked anemia
3 CD4$^+$ lymphocyte count* < 100/mm^3
4 Viral load > 100 000 copies/mL
5 Loss of p24 antibody; p24 antigenemia
6 Female sex (prognosis may be worse than for males)

* NB: Rate of decline may predict likely long-term onset of AIDS

Sequence of serological events post-infection
1 First 2–4 weeks: Rise in viral RNA copies*
2 First 3–6 weeks: Rise in HIV-specific cytotoxic T cells
3 First 4–8 weeks: Rise in antibodies to HIV *env* protein
                    Rise in antibodies to HIV p24 antigen
4 First 10–15 years: Progressive decline in CD4 T cell count

* May exceed 10^7 copies/mL at this stage, reflecting lack of antibody response; hence, this is a highly infectious period. RNA copy number subsequently declines, up to the onset of full-blown AIDS

Helper T cell (T$_H$) thresholds predicting infectious complications
1 CD4 cell count < 200 cells/mL (T$_H$:total lymphocyte ratio < 1:5)
   — *Pneumocystis carinii* pneumonia
   — Refractory (chronic) cryptosporidiosis diarrhea
2 CD4 cell count < 100 cells/mL
   — Cerebral *Toxoplasma gondii*
   — *Cryptococcus neoformans* (e.g. pulmonary, cerebral)
3 CD4 cell count < 50 cells/mL
   — *Mycobacterium avium* complex*
   — CMV (e.g. retinal, pulmonary)
   — Microsporidium

* cf. tuberculosis: can occur at any CD4 cell level

MANAGING HIV-RELATED DISEASE

ANTIRETROVIRAL THERAPY

Classification of antiretroviral drugs
1 Reverse transcriptase inhibitors
   Nucleoside analog inhibitors
   — Zidovudine (azidothymidine; AZT)
   — Lamivudine
   — Didanosine (DDI)
   — Zalcitabine, stavudine, abacavir
   Non-nucleoside inhibitors
   — Nevirapine
   — Efavirenz
2 Protease inhibitors
   — Indinavir
   — Ritonavir
   — Saquinavir (best tolerated but least active)
   — Nelfinavir, amprenavir

Mechanism of zidovudine (AZT) action
1 Structural analog of thymidine
2 Phosphorylated to zidovudine phosphates on entering cells
3 Zidovudine monophosphate inhibits production of important HIV metabolites, thymidine di- and triphosphate
4 Zidovudine triphosphate inhibits HIV reverse transcriptase

Major toxicities of antiretroviral drugs
1 Zidovudine
   — Gastrointestinal intolerance (nausea), esp. initially
   — Mitochondrial myopathy*
   — Macrocytic anemia, neutropenia
   — Lactic acidosis
2 Lamivudine, zalcitabine, stavudine
   — Peripheral neuropathy
3 Didanosine
   — Diarrhea, pancreatitis, impaired indinavir absorption
4 Nevirapine (and other non-nucleoside inhibitors)
   — Rash (serious in 10%), abnormal LFTs, drug interactions
   — Rapid development of resistance as a single agent
5 Protease inhibitors
   — Diarrhea
   — Hyperlipidemia + insulin resistance + lipodystrophy: 'buffalo hump'
   — Renal stones (in 4%) or renal failure – indinavir

* DD$_x$: polymyositis, primary HIV myopathy. Hence, proceed to biopsy if no improvement after 2 weeks' zidovudine cessation; inflammatory infiltrates may indicate steroids plus zidovudine reintroduction

HIGHLY ACTIVE ANTIRETROVIRAL THERAPY (HAART)

Indications for considering HAART
1 Onset of HIV-related symptoms
2 CD4 count < 500 cells/mL
3 Viral load (plasma HIV RNA) > 30 000 copies/mL

Indications for altering the HAART regimen
1 Development of new symptoms
2 Sustained new decline in CD4 count
3 Viral load rises to 70% pretreatment value

Subjective benefits of HAART

1 Improved functional capacity and quality of life
2 Reduced frequency of opportunistic infections
3 More rapid recovery from major infective complications*
4 Slowed disease progression‡
5 Improved survival from HIV encephalopathy

* May also hasten neuropathy resolution during initial seroconversion phase
‡ Also in ARC, but not in asymptomatic phase

Quantitative indices of therapeutic benefit

1 ↑ Weight
2 ↑ CD4+ lymphocyte number
3 ↓ HIV p24 antigenemia
4 ↑ Platelets (if thrombocytopenic)

Typical composition of HAART protocol

1 Zidovudine, *plus*
2 Second nucleoside analog lacking overlapping toxicity*
   — e.g. lamivudine *or* didanosine, *plus*
3 Protease inhibitor (e.g. indinavir) *or*
   Non-nucleoside reverse transcriptase inhibitor (e.g. nevirapine)

* Combination with a second inhibitor greatly reduces acquisition of resistance (e.g. to zidovudine or lamivudine alone) and thus prolongs reduction in viral load

Varying HAART protocol based on viral load

1 < 50 000 HIV RNA copies/mL
   — 2 nucleoside analogs, *plus*
   — *Either* non-nucleoside *or* protease inhibitor
2 > 50 000 HIV RNA copies/mL
   — 2 nucleoside analogs, *plus*
   — *One or two* (e.g. saquinavir + ritonavir) protease inhibitors

Switching HAART from current therapy? Some examples

1 Current zidovudine monotherapy
   — Add lamivudine *or* didanosine, *or*
   — Change to zalcitabine *plus* saquinavir
2 Current zidovudine + didanosine duotherapy
   — Add nevirapine, *or* ritonavir if CD4 count < 100 cells/mL

MANAGEMENT OF INFECTIONS IN HIV-RELATED DISEASE

Approach to infective complications in the AIDS patient

1 Infections for which effective therapy exists
   — *P. carinii* pneumonia (commonest infection)
     • Prophylaxis: oral co-trimoxazole, *or* nebulized pentamidine (less effective, better tolerated)
     • Treatment: IV or oral co-trimoxazole depending on infection severity
     • Adjunctive steroids may be of value in respiratory failure (PaO_2 < 9 kPa)
   — Toxoplasmosis (e.g. cerebral mass lesions)
     • R_x: sulfadiazine + pyrimethamine
   — Cryptococcosis (e.g. meningitis or disseminated)
     • R_x: (oral) fluconazole *or* (IV) amphotericin B

   — Candidiasis
     • R_x: fluconazole
2 Infections for which promising therapy exists
   — CMV
     • Ganciclovir, foscarnet, cidofovir
   — *M. avium–intracellulare*
     • Rifabutin, azithromycin/clarithromycin, ethambutol
3 Infections for which no effective therapy exists
   — Cryptosporidiosis

Clinical indications for co-trimoxazole prophylaxis

1 Oral thrush
2 Unexplained fever
3 Kaposi's sarcoma
4 Prior *P. carinii* pneumonia or cerebral toxoplasmosis

UNDERSTANDING HIV-RELATED DISEASE

HIV AND ACQUIRED IMMUNODEFICIENCY

Immunological abnormalities in the AIDS patient

1 T cells
   — ↓ Helper (CD4+) T cell number*
   — ↓ T cell function (↓ IL-2/IFN-response to Ag)
   — ↓ Cytotoxic (CD8+) T cell response to HIV-infected cells
   — Cutaneous anergy
2 B cells
   — ↓ Function (↓ humoral response to vaccination)
   — Activation → polyclonal hypergammaglobulinemia
3 NK cells
   — ↓ Number and function
4 Monocytes/macrophages
   — ↓ Function (↓ IL-1, chemotaxis, antigen presentation)

* Normally > 0.7×10^9/L; falls to < 0.2×10^9/L

Molecular biology of HIV

1 Structurally related to animal lentiviruses, and contains
   — Core protein (p24)
   — Reverse transcriptase
   — Envelope (*env*) glycoproteins (gp120, gp41)
   — HIV protease
2 HIV-1 (group M*) is currently responsible for 99% of human infections
   HIV-2 (West Africa) expresses different *env* region; hence, 'false-negative' serology
3 The *env* protein gp120 binds to the T_H marker CD4
   The homodimeric HIV protease is encoded by the 5' end of the *pol* gene (i.e. part of the Gag-Pol polyprotein); proteolytic cleavage of the latter to p24 permits virion maturation
4 Macrophage-tropic (R5) HIV-1 enters T_H cells via CD4 *plus* the chemokine coreceptor CCR5; this is the usual mode of primary infection
   T cell-tropic (X4) HIV-1 enters T_H cells via CD4 *plus* the chemokine coreceptor CXCR4

5 Most AIDS manifestations reflect consequent T_H dysfunction

* 'M' for 'main'; cf. group O ('outlier')

Resistance and sensitivity to HIV infection or progression

1 Individuals who lack wild-type CCR5* exhibit resistance to primary HIV infection
2 HIV-positive individuals who are *homozygous* for HLA-B35/-Cw04 progress rapidly
   HIV-positive individuals who are fully *heterozygous* for HLA-B35/-Cw04 survive longer
3 HIV-positive individuals who are positive for GBV-C ('hepatitis G') survive longer

* The common polymorphism is a 32-bp deletion

REVIEWING THE LITERATURE: HIV-RELATED DISEASE

6.1 Pauk J et al (2000) Mucosal shedding of human herpesviruses 8 in men. N Engl J Med 343: 1369–1377

Showed that oral sex efficiently transmitted HHV8 infection among homosexuals. Thirty percent of salivary samples contained HHV8, as opposed to 1% of anogenital samples. Use of amyl nitrite, and contact with a partner with Kaposi's sarcoma, were also risk factors for infection.

6.2 Sun X et al (1997) Human papillomavirus infection in women infected with the human immunodeficiency virus. N Engl J Med 337: 1343–1349

Eighty-three percent of HIV-seropositive women screened positive for HPV DNA in a New York gynecological clinic. Twenty percent were persistently positive for HPV-16, though sexual activity was not implicated in the interval acquisition of HPV.

6.3 Cardo DM et al (1997) A case-control study of HIV seroconversion in health care workers after percutaneous exposure. N Engl J Med 337: 1485–1490

Study of 33 cases and 665 controls showing that risk of needlestick HIV acquisition varies directly with the volume of inoculum and the HIV titre of infected blood. Post-exposure prophylaxis (PEP) using zidovudine appeared to confer protection.

6.4 Quinn TC et al (2000) Viral load and heterosexual transmission of human immunodeficiency virus type 1. N Engl J Med 342: 921–929

Study of 415 Ugandan couples with one HIV-positive partner. Rates of male-to-female and female-to-male transmission were similar (seroconversion about once per 10 person-years), but were higher in younger individuals. Circumcised men seroconverted significantly less often than uncircumcised men. Serum HIV-1 RNA levels ('viral load') was the chief predictor of infectivity.

6.5 Cameron DW et al (1998) Randomized placebo-controlled trial of ritonavir in advanced HIV-1 disease. Lancet 351: 543–549

Palella FJ et al (1998) Declining morbidity and mortality among patients with advanced human immunodeficiency virus infection. N Engl J Med 338: 853–860

Two studies documenting the benefit of protease inhibitors in HIV infection. In the former study, 1090 patients were randomly assigned to receive nucleoside-based treatment alone or with the addition of the protease inhibitor ritonavir; the ritonavir arm had fewer complications and lived longer. The second study of 1255 HIV-positive patients confirmed the survival benefit of more intensive (protease inhibitor-containing) antiretroviral therapy.

6.6 Leroy V et al (1998) International multicentre pooled analysis of late postnatal mother-to-child transmission of HIV-1 infection. Lancet 352: 597–600

International prospective cohort study of 4000 children born to HIV-positive mothers, showing that prolonged breastfeeding (exceeding 4–6 months' duration) is a major mechanism of post-natal HIV transmission (about 5% seroconverted).

6.7 Benn PD et al (2001) Prophylaxis with a nevirapine-containing triple regimen after exposure to HIV-1. Lancet 357: 687–688

High rate of adverse reactions, particularly drug-induced hepatitis, with this regimen, suggesting that routine PEP (post-exposure prophylaxis) may not justify inclusion of nevirapine.

6.8 International Collaboration on HIV and Cancer (2000) Highly active antiretroviral therapy and incidence of cancer in human immunodeficiency virus-infected adults. J Natl Cancer Inst 92: 1823–1830

Survey of 47 936 HIV-infected patients who developed 2702 incident cancers, showing that HAART reduced the frequency of Kaposi's sarcoma, cerebral lymphoma and immunoblastic lymphoma, but not of Burkitt's lymphoma, Hodgkin's disease, or cervical cancer.

6.9 Benhamou Y et al (2001) Safety and efficacy of adefovir dipivoxil in patients co-infected with HIV-1 and lamivudine-resistant hepatitis B virus: an open-label pilot study. Lancet 358: 718–723

35 co-infected patients received 48 weeks of adefovir, with good effect and relatively little toxicity other than transient transaminitis.

6.10 Scheer S et al (2001) Effect of highly active retroviral therapy on diagnoses of sexually transmitted diseases in people with AIDS. Lancet 357: 432–435

Study showing that patients on HAART were twice as likely to develop another sexually transmitted disease, suggesting that these patients were failing to use safe sex once they were on HAART.

6.11 Kral AH et al (2001) Sexual transmission of HIV-1 among injection drug users in San Francisco, USA. Lancet 357: 1397–1401

Case-control study of 1200 drug users, showing that the risk of HIV seroconversion in this at-risk subset was more strongly linked to sexual behavior than to injection practices.

6.12 Gray RH at el (2001) Probability of HIV-1 transmission per coital act in monogamous, heterosexual, HIV1-discordant couples in Rakai, Uganda. Lancet 357: 1149–1153

HIV transmissibility was increased in proportion to viral load, and occurred four times more often in those with 'genital ulcer disease' (usually HSV2). Overall probability of transmission per coital act was 0.001. Information about condom usage was not supplied.

CHAPTER 7

Immunology, autoimmune disease and transplantation

Physical examination protocol 7.1 You are asked to examine a patient suspected of having a collagen-vascular disease

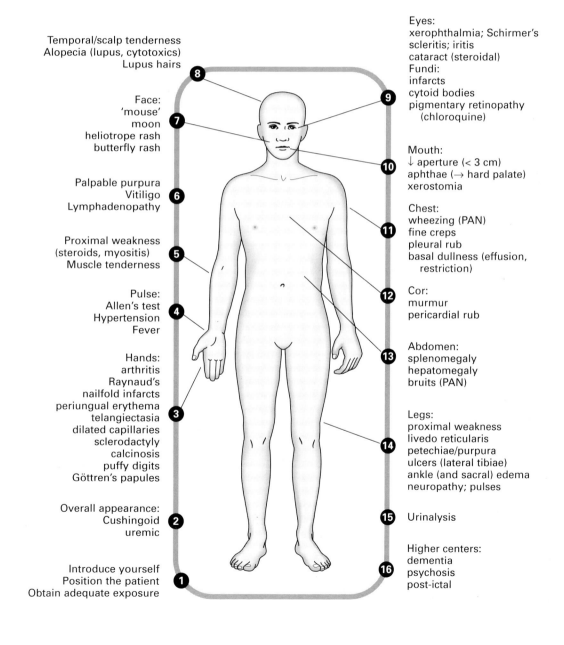

Temporal/scalp tenderness
Alopecia (lupus, cytotoxics)
Lupus hairs
⑧

Face:
'mouse'
moon
heliotrope rash
butterfly rash
⑦

Palpable purpura
Vitiligo
Lymphadenopathy
⑥

Proximal weakness
(steroids, myositis)
Muscle tenderness
⑤

Pulse:
Allen's test
Hypertension
Fever
④

Hands:
arthritis
Raynaud's
nailfold infarcts
periungual erythema
telangiectasia
dilated capillaries
sclerodactyly
calcinosis
puffy digits
Göttren's papules
③

Overall appearance:
Cushingoid
uremic
②

Introduce yourself
Position the patient
Obtain adequate exposure
①

Eyes:
xerophthalmia; Schirmer's
scleritis; iritis
cataract (steroidal)
Fundi:
infarcts
cytoid bodies
pigmentary retinopathy
(chloroquine)
⑨

Mouth:
↓ aperture (< 3 cm)
aphthae (→ hard palate)
xerostomia
⑩

Chest:
wheezing (PAN)
fine creps
pleural rub
basal dullness (effusion,
restriction)
⑪

Cor:
murmur
pericardial rub
⑫

Abdomen:
splenomegaly
hepatomegaly
bruits (PAN)
⑬

Legs:
proximal weakness
livedo reticularis
petechiae/purpura
ulcers (lateral tibiae)
ankle (and sacral) edema
neuropathy; pulses
⑭

Urinalysis
⑮

Higher centers:
dementia
psychosis
post-ictal
⑯

Physical examination protocol 7.2 You are asked to examine a patient suspected of having Sjögren's syndrome

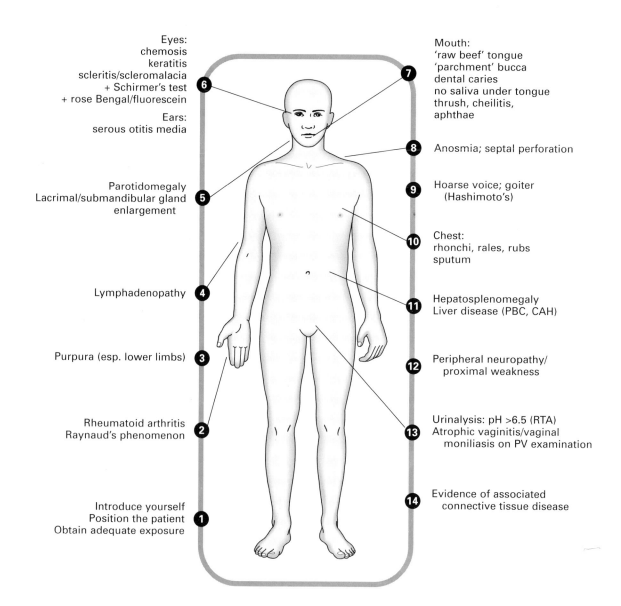

Eyes:
chemosis
keratitis
scleritis/scleromalacia
+ Schirmer's test
+ rose Bengal/fluorescein

Ears:
serous otitis media

Parotidomegaly
Lacrimal/submandibular gland
enlargement

Lymphadenopathy

Purpura (esp. lower limbs)

Rheumatoid arthritis
Raynaud's phenomenon

Introduce yourself
Position the patient
Obtain adequate exposure

Mouth:
'raw beef' tongue
'parchment' bucca
dental caries
no saliva under tongue
thrush, cheilitis,
aphthae

Anosmia; septal perforation

Hoarse voice; goiter
(Hashimoto's)

Chest:
rhonchi, rales, rubs
sputum

Hepatosplenomegaly
Liver disease (PBC, CAH)

Peripheral neuropathy/
proximal weakness

Urinalysis: pH >6.5 (RTA)
Atrophic vaginitis/vaginal
moniliasis on PV examination

Evidence of associated
connective tissue disease

Physical examination protocol 7.3 You are asked to examine a patient with Raynaud's phenomenon and esophageal reflux

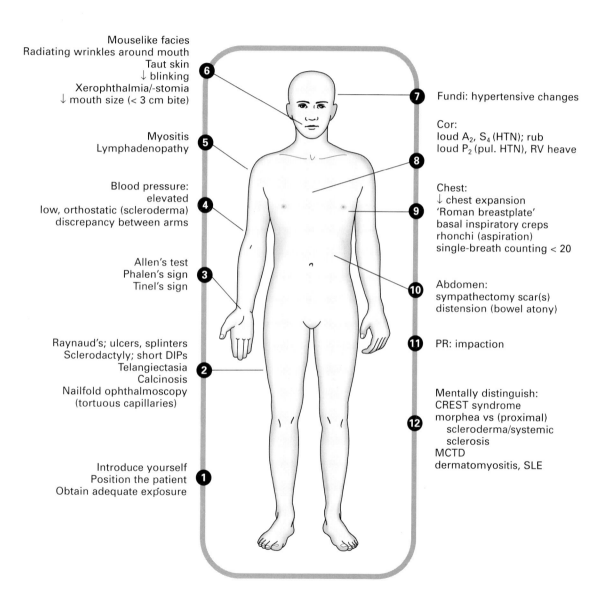

Mouselike facies
Radiating wrinkles around mouth
Taut skin
↓ blinking
Xerophthalmia/-stomia
↓ mouth size (< 3 cm bite)

6

7 Fundi: hypertensive changes

Myositis
Lymphadenopathy

5

Cor:
loud A_2, S_4 (HTN); rub
loud P_2 (pul. HTN), RV heave

8

Blood pressure:
elevated
low, orthostatic (scleroderma)
discrepancy between arms

4

Chest:
↓ chest expansion
'Roman breastplate'
basal inspiratory creps
rhonchi (aspiration)
single-breath counting < 20

9

Allen's test
Phalen's sign
Tinel's sign

3

Abdomen:
sympathectomy scar(s)
distension (bowel atony)

10

Raynaud's; ulcers, splinters
Sclerodactyly; short DIPs
Telangiectasia
Calcinosis
Nailfold ophthalmoscopy
(tortuous capillaries)

2

11 PR: impaction

Mentally distinguish:
CREST syndrome
morphea vs (proximal)
   scleroderma/systemic
   sclerosis
MCTD
dermatomyositis, SLE

12

Introduce yourself
Position the patient
Obtain adequate exposure

1

Physical examination protocol 7.4 You are asked to examine a patient for stigmata of amyloidosis

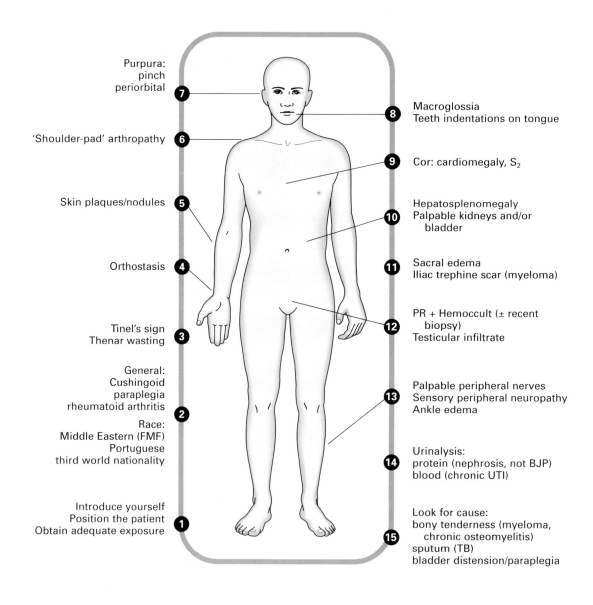

Purpura:
pinch
periorbital **7**

8 Macroglossia
Teeth indentations on tongue

'Shoulder-pad' arthropathy **6**

9 Cor: cardiomegaly, S_2

Skin plaques/nodules **5**

10 Hepatosplenomegaly
Palpable kidneys and/or
bladder

Orthostasis **4**

11 Sacral edema
Iliac trephine scar (myeloma)

Tinel's sign
Thenar wasting **3**

12 PR + Hemoccult (± recent
biopsy)
Testicular infiltrate

General:
Cushingoid
paraplegia
rheumatoid arthritis
2
Race:
Middle Eastern (FMF)
Portuguese
third world nationality

13 Palpable peripheral nerves
Sensory peripheral neuropathy
Ankle edema

14 Urinalysis:
protein (nephrosis, not BJP)
blood (chronic UTI)

Introduce yourself
Position the patient **1**
Obtain adequate exposure

15 Look for cause:
bony tenderness (myeloma,
chronic osteomyelitis)
sputum (TB)
bladder distension/paraplegia

COMMON AND CLASSIC

Common immunologic problems in clinical practice
1 Atopy
2 Renal transplant
3 Systemic lupus erythematosus

Classic immunologic problems in clinical exams
1 Raynaud's (± SLE, MCTD, CREST, etc.)
2 Fibrosing alveolitis
3 Palpable purpura

IMMUNOLOGIC EMERGENCIES

Acute management of anaphylaxis
1 For acute life-threatening profound shock
   — Slow intravenous adrenaline (epinephrine)
      1:100 000 solution, *plus*
   — Cardiac monitoring if possible
2 For acute but non-life-threatening anaphylaxis
   — Intramuscular adrenaline (epinephrine) 1:10 000
3 No improvement within 5 min
   — Repeat adrenaline (epinephrine) dose
4 IV fluids (crystalloid > colloid)

CLINICAL ASSESSMENT OF IMMUNOLOGIC DISEASE

VASCULITIS

Clinical stigmata of vasculitis
1 Leukocytoclastic vasculitis
   — Palpable purpura
2 Non-inflammatory obliterative endarteritis
   — Nailfold infarcts
   — Splinter hemorrhages
3 Necrotizing vasculitis
   — Purpura with skin ulceration
   — Mononeuritis multiplex
   — Motor neuropathy
   — Aneurysmal dilatations overlying arterial
     bifurcations
4 Cutaneous signs *sometimes* indicating vasculitis
   — Livedo reticularis
   — Atrophie blanche
   — Hemorrhagic bullae/vesicles/ulcers
   — Panniculitis; pustulonecrotic nodules
   — Scarring alopecia
   — Urticarial lesions > 24 h duration
5 Non-cutaneous signs *sometimes* indicating
   vasculitis
   — Hypertension
   — Microscopic hematuria
   — Retinal vasculopathy, cytoid bodies

Vasculitides with characteristic anatomic distributions
1 Cranial arteritis
   — Temporal, external carotid, other extracranial
     arteries

2 Takayasu's arteritis
   — Aortic arch
3 Behçet's syndrome
   — Ocular vessels, skin and mucosa, CNS
4 Degos disease
   — Gastrointestinal tract
5 Sneddon's syndrome
   — Skin, CNS

Differential diagnosis of purpura in collagen-vascular diseases
1 Vasculitis (see above)
2 Corticosteroid therapy
3 Thrombocytopenia
   — Immune (SLE) ± hypersplenism (Felty's)
   — Iatrogenic (penicillamine, gold)
   Platelet dysfunction
   — Iatrogenic (aspirin, other NSAIDs)
4 Amyloidosis
5 Cryoglobulinemia
6 Factor VIII antibodies (SLE, RA)

Conditions mimicking vasculitis
1 Infective endocarditis
2 Left atrial myxoma
3 Cholesterol embolism
4 Amyloidosis

SCLERODERMA

Raynaud's phenomenon: features suggesting secondary cause*
1 Symptoms
   — Abrupt onset
   — Digital edema, ulceration, gangrene
   — Thumb involvement
   — Dry eyes/mouth, dysphagia, breathlessness
   — Joint pain or swelling
2 Signs
   — Abnormal Allen's test
   — Telangiectasia
   — Puffy finger thickening
   — Tight skin around mouth
3 Nailfold capillaroscopy
   — *Avascular areas* with tortuous capillaries‡
4 Serology
   — Strongly positive autoantibody profile
     (esp. ANA)
   — Autoantibodies: topo I, dsDNA, centromere,
     nucleolar
   — Cryoglobulins; EPG and immunoglobulins
   — Hypocomplementemia (incl. C_7 deficiency)
   — Grossly elevated ESR ± elevated whole blood
     viscosity
5 Radiology
   — Digital artery occlusion on Doppler
     study/arteriogram
   — Subcutaneous calcinosis on plain X-ray
   — Abnormal barium swallow

* Systemic diseases are responsible for ~ 20% of Raynaud's
phenomenon; most cases are primary
‡ Highly specific for scleroderma or dermatomyositis

Criteria for scleroderma diagnosis

1 Major criterion
   — Bilateral skin thickening proximal to MCP joints associated with Raynaud's phenomenon
2 Supporting clinical findings
   — Sclerodactyly, pitted fingertip scars, finger pulp loss
   — Bibasilar pulmonary fibrosis
3 Supporting investigations
   — Nailfold capillaroscopy: enlarged and distorted capillary loops, reduced in number, plus hemorrhages
   — Positive ANA, esp. if nucleolar or centromeric pattern
   — Abnormal esophageal motility on barium swallow

Differential diagnosis of scleroderma

1 'Overlap' syndrome
   — Mixed connective tissue disease
   — CREST syndrome (strictly, a subtype of scleroderma)
   — Dermatomyositis, SLE
2 Eosinophilic fasciitis
   — Spares hands and feet (no Raynaud's)
   — No visceral complications
3 Morphea
   — Localized sclerodermatous plaques
   — No systemic features
4 Other sclerosing diseases
   — Carcinoid syndrome
   — Graft-versus-host disease
   — Amyloidosis
5 Sclerosant exposure, e.g.
   — Bleomycin
   — Silica; vinyl chloride monomer

Spectrum of pulmonary disease in scleroderma

1 Interstitial fibrosis ± (secondary) pulmonary hypertension
2 Primary pulmonary hypertension, esp. in CREST variant
3 Pleurisy
4 Aspiration pneumonitis
5 Restriction of chest wall expansion
6 Bronchioloalveolar cell carcinoma

Mechanisms of cardiac failure in scleroderma

1 Left ventricular failure
   — Severe hypertension
   — Myocardial fibrosis (scleroderma cardiomyopathy)
   — Reperfusion necrosis (?due to myocardial Raynaud's)
2 Right ventricular failure
   — Pulmonary hypertension (primary or secondary)
3 Pericarditis
   — Tamponade (acute)
   — Constriction (chronic)
4 Arrhythmias

Differential diagnosis of anemia in scleroderma

1 Normocytic
   — 'Chronic disease' ± uremia
2 Microcytic
   — Esophagitis, telangiectasia
3 Macrocytic
   — Bacterial overgrowth
4 Microangiopathic
   — Renal involvement with severe hypertension

Gastrointestinal presentations of scleroderma

1 Reflux esophagitis
   — Regurgitation
   — Epigastric pain; dysphagia
2 Post-prandial 'bloating'
   — Gastric dilatation, delayed emptying
   — Malabsorption
3 Steatorrhea
   — Bacterial overgrowth (due to gut hypomotility)
   — Lymphatic fibrosis
4 Anemia
   — Severe esophagitis ± peptic ulceration telangiectasia
   — Bacterial overgrowth
5 Constipation
   — Chronic intestinal pseudo-obstruction
   — Fecal impaction; barium impaction

Esophageal abnormalities in the scleroderma patient

1 Distal hypoperistalsis (in 70%)
2 Reflux (in 60%)
3 Esophageal dilatation (in 50%)
4 Absent lower esophageal sphincter tone (in 40%)
5 Positive Bernstein (acid perfusion) test (in 30%)
6 Hiatus hernia (in 20%)
7 Stricture (in 10%)

Radiology of the lower gastrointestinal tract in scleroderma

1 Plain abdominal film
   — Fluid levels, dilated loops of bowel
   — Pneumoperitoneum*
2 Small bowel series
   — Flocculated barium ('moulage' sign)
   — Close-packed valvulae coniventes‡
   — Dilatation of second and third parts of duodenum
3 Barium enema
   — Megacolon; pneumatosis intestinalis
   — Wide-mouthed diverticulae on antimesenteric border
   — Reduced motility, slow transit time

* = Pneumatosis intestinalis with cyst rupture
‡ 'Hidebound' or 'accordion' appearance

SYSTEMIC LUPUS ERYTHEMATOSUS

Clinical associations of SLE

1 IgA deficiency
2 C_2 deficiency (and other complement components)
3 α_1AT deficiency
4 Thymoma
5 Porphyria cutanea tarda
6 Klinefelter's syndrome

Adverse prognostic indicators in SLE

1 Associations of more aggressive disease
   — Male sex; youth (esp. children)
   — High-titre dsDNA Ab; ↓↓ complement (esp. C_3)*
   — Sm Ab (predicts development of renal disease)
   — IgG 'lupus band' on (uninvolved) skin biopsy‡
   — Cryoglobulinemia; phospholipid antibody
2 Clinical evidence of established disease
   — Renal involvement
     • Heavy proteinuria
     • Proliferative/membranous nephritis on biopsy
3 Development of infectious complications
   — Gram-positive cocci, *Neisseria, Salmonella*, due to
     • Autoimmune leukopenia/leukocyte dysfunction
     • Hypocomplementemia, hyposplenism
   — Opportunistic infections, due to
     • Steroid/immunosuppressive therapy

* Note that primary deficiencies of C_4 or other complement components (e.g. C_2) may cause a degree of hypocomplementemia unrelated to prognosis
‡ cf. IgM/A

Indicators of active disease in SLE

1 Clinical indicators
   — Acute arthritis or vasculitis
   — Worsening rash, mucosal ulceration, hair loss
   — Pleurisy or pericarditis
   — Hematuria, active urinary sediment (esp. red cell casts)
   — Systolic hypertension
   — Fits, psychosis, 'lupus headache'
2 Laboratory indicators
   — Recent rise in dsDNA antibody titre
   — ↓C_3, ↓ THC (if recent)
   — Leukopenia, lymphopenia, anemia, reticulocytosis, thrombocytopenia

Indications for renal biopsy in SLE

1 Exclusion of reversible renal failure in atypical disease
2 Confirmation of irreversible disease

Incidence, therapy and prognosis of lupus nephritis

1 40% of SLE patients develop clinical nephritis within 1 year
2 65% of SLE patients develop clinical nephritis within 5 years
3 90% of SLE patients have abnormal renal histology on biopsy
4 WHO type II or V (p. 320): 10–15% → renal failure in 5 years
5 WHO type III, IV: 20–30% → renal failure in 5 years

Pathophysiology of CNS lupus

1 Frank CNS vasculitis is *rare*; commonest pathology is a non-inflammatory vasculopathy with microinfarcts (i.e. bland thrombosis, often due to phospholipid antibodies; p. 185)
2 Vasculitis (± immune-complexes) may cause
   — *Extracerebral* disease (e.g. cranial nerve palsies) *or*
   — *Focal cerebral* disease (e.g. chorea, stroke)*

3 CSF *antineuronal antibodies* are present in up to 80% of patients with 'diffuse' CNS lupus (fits, psychosis)
4 Antibodies to *ribosomal P antigen* in neuronal cytoplasm may be detectable in 90% of psychotic lupus patients
5 Such autoantibodies may prove to be useful in distinguishing primary CNS lupus from iatrogenic *steroid psychosis*

* NB: Phospholipid antibodies may also cause focal cerebral sequelae

Features of drug-induced SLE

1 Occurrence
   — Older patients than primary SLE
   — More frequently male (40% vs 10% in primary SLE)
   — Increases with dosage and duration of drug therapy
   — Most cases are due to procainamide
   — Primary SLE is not exacerbated by such drugs
2 Clinical patterns
   — Lung, joint and serosal (esp. pleural) disease common
   — Arthralgias, maculopapular rash, fever, cytopenias
   — Renal disease *uncommon*; CNS disease *rare*
3 Serology
   — ANA against histones (homogeneous pattern) in 95%
   — Double-stranded DNA antibodies typically *absent*
   — Complement levels *normal*
4 Slow acetylation status usual
   — Incidence approaches 100% in hydralazine lupus
   — Less marked association in primary SLE
5 HLA association
   — DR4
   — cf. primary SLE: DR2, DR3
6 Course
   — Symptoms persist for 1–3 months after drug ceased
   — ANA can remain positive for 6–12 months

Features of neonatal SLE

1 Cutaneous type
   — Commoner in female neonates (75%)
   — Transient photosensitive skin eruptions, often discoid
   — Associated thrombocytopenia, liver dysfunction
2 Cardiac type
   — Commoner in male neonates
   — Causes perinatal complete heart block in 95%
   — Anti-Ro (SS-A) present in virtually 100%*
   — La (SS-B), nRNP antibodies also often present
   — 20% of affected neonates will need pacemaker insertion
   — 15% will die of associated myocarditis
   — Pathology: endomyocardial fibrosis → AV block
3 *Mothers* of affected neonates
   — 70% asymptomatic at time of neonatal diagnosis
   — 90% develop collagen disease (e.g. SLE) in 10 years

— Anti-Ro in a pregnant woman is an indication for fetal monitoring using echocardiography
— Fetal myocarditis is treated with dexamethasone (not inactivated by placenta) or plasmapheresis

* Of all anti-Ro-positive pregnant women (i.e. whether symptomatic or not), fewer than 3% have children with congenital heart block. Active maternal SLE causes far greater morbidity from intrauterine fetal death (± pre-eclampsia, phospholipid antibodies) or neonatal lupus

When to suspect primary complement deficiency in SLE
1 Early-onset disease
2 Absent total hemolytic complement (THC, CH_{50})*
3 Normal C_3, C_4 despite persistently active disease
4 Parental consanguinity

* DD_x: Blood sample left on bench in immunology laboratory over weekend

SJÖGREN'S SYNDROME

Clinical concomitants of Sjögren's syndrome
1 Dry mouth and eyes; also nose, throat, trachea, skin
2 Secondary otitis, bronchitis, pneumonitis
3 Dental caries
4 Vulvovaginitis → dyspareunia, pruritus vulvae
5 Atrophic gastritis
6 Recurrent parotidomegaly
7 Lymphadenopathy, splenomegaly; 'pseudolymphoma'
8 Lymphoma, thymoma
9 Cryoglobulinemia; Waldenström's macroglobulinemia
   Benign hyperglobulinemic purpura of Waldenström
10 Pulmonary atelectasis (esp. post-operative)
   Renal tubular acidosis (esp. post-partum)
11 Drug hypersensitivity
12 Autoimmune disease, esp. PBC, Raynaud's, Hashimoto's

Distinction of primary from secondary Sjögren's syndrome
1 No other evident connective tissue disease, esp.
   — Rheumatoid arthritis
   — SLE
   — Scleroderma
2 Autoantibody profile
   — ANA more commonly positive (90% vs 50%)
   — La (SS-B) antibodies* more positive (50% vs 10%)
   — Ro (SS-A) antibodies‡ more positive (80% vs 50%)
   — Antisalivary duct antibodies *less* positive (15% vs 60%)
3 Associated with HLA-DR3
   — cf. secondary type: HLA DR4

NB: Rheumatoid factor is positive in almost 100% of *both* primary and secondary Sjögren's syndrome
* Most specific
‡ Less specific; also commonly positive in SLE

Diagnosis of Sjögren's syndrome
1 Clinical sicca syndrome (± connective tissue disease, e.g. RA)
   — Gritty eyes, dry mouth*
2 Ophthalmological examination
   — Positive Schirmer's test
     • < 15 mm in 5 min
   — Abnormal rose Bengal stain
     • Punctate uptake in conjunctival/corneal erosions
   — Slit-lamp examination
     • Reduced tear film; erosions
3 Serology
   — High-titre IgM rheumatoid factor
   — High-titre ANA (± Ro, La)
4 Salivary/labial gland biopsy‡
   — Lymphocytic infiltrate
   — Acinar atrophy
   — Myoepithelial islands

* Note that similar symptoms can occur due to other causes such as sarcoidosis, anticholinergic side-effects. Additional symptoms such as night sweats, adenopathy, weight loss may suggest lymphoma development
‡ Salivary gland scintigraphy may obviate the need for biopsy in centers where this expertise is available

OTHER CONNECTIVE TISSUE DISEASES

Diagnosis of polymyositis
1 Clinical
   — Proximal weakness > wasting
   — Muscle tenderness
   — Heliotrope rash, Göttren's papules
2 Laboratory
   — CPK
   — EMG
   — Muscle biopsy

Diagnosis of polyarteritis nodosa
1 Clinical
   — Hypertension
   — Mononeuritis multiplex
   — Asthma (?Churg–Strauss variant)
2 Laboratory
   — Neutrophilia, eosinophilia (?Churg–Strauss variant)
   — ↑ ESR
   — Biopsy of clinically involved tissue
   — Angiography (e.g. celiac axis) → aneurysms

Diagnosis of 'mixed connective tissue disease'
1 Clinical
   — Raynaud's; puffy fingers/hands (scleroderma-like)
   — Arthralgias/itis; lymphadenopathy (SLE-like)
   — Myositis, serositis, pneumonitis (polymyositis-like)
   — Renal involvement rare
2 Laboratory
   — High-titre (> 1:1024) speckled ANA
   — High-titre (cf. SLE) anti-RNP Ab
   — Negative dsDNA Ab; negative Sm Ab
   — Normal complement levels

— Polyclonal hypergammaglobulinemia
— Abnormal upper (polymyositis-like) and/or lower (scleroderma-like) esophageal motility
— ↓ DL_{CO}
3 Therapy
— Steroid-responsive features
• Myositis
• Pleurisy
• Depression
• Interstitial lung fibrosis, pulmonary hypertension
• Esophageal dysmotility
4 Clinical course
— 5–10% 10-year mortality
— Indiscriminate steroid use may cause osteoporosis

Clinical significance of mixed connective tissue disease (MCTD)

1 The diagnosis of MCTD is important because it implies the presence of *myositis*
2 Myositis is an indication for *steroids* even in cases with only *mild* symptoms
3 Even if only mild myositis symptoms, initial steroid therapy should be *aggressive* (e.g. prednisone 1 mg/kg)
4 Despite being traditionally regarded as 'mild' disease, complications such as fibrosing alveolitis may be *fatal* if undertreated

AMYLOIDOSIS

Clinical significance of amyloid components

1 AL
— Amyloid L-(light-chain) component
— Causes amyloid of monoclonal immunocytic origin
— Derived from light-chain (BJP) fragments, λ > κ*
— Occurs in
• 10% Myeloma cases (overall)
• 25% BJP-only myeloma
• 5% Benign monoclonal gammopathy
2 AA
— Amyloid A-component
— Causes amyloidosis of reactive systemic origin
— Derived from the acute phase plasma protein SAA
— Occurs in
• Familial Mediterranean fever‡
• *Long-standing* (> 10 years) rheumatoid arthritis (10%), juvenile chronic arthritis (5%), Hodgkin's (5%), TB, leprosy, osteomyelitis
3 AP
— Amyloid P-component
— Pathogenetic significance unknown
— Resembles the acute phase reactant C-reactive protein
— Occurs with all amyloid subtypes *except* cerebral
— ^{123}I-AP scanning may be useful in diagnosis

* cf. most paraproteins and normal immunoglobulins: κ > λ
‡ May *present* with amyloid

Classification of clinical amyloidosis variants

1 Monoclonal immunocytic dyscrasia (AL-amyloidosis)
— Incl. myeloma-associated and 'primary' amyloidosis*
2 Reactive systemic (AA-) amyloidosis due to amyloid A
— 'Secondary' amyloidosis (similar to FMF type)
3 Endocrine amyloid (affects APUD cells), e.g. from
— Calcitonin-related fibrils in medullary thyroid Ca
— Amylin (amyloid islet polypeptide) in type II DM
4 Senile amyloid (affects heart, joints, seminal vesicles)
— Amyloid from plasma prealbumin ASc
5 Hemodialysis-associated (AH) amyloid (→ bones, kidneys)
— Amyloid derived from plasma β_2-microglobulin‡
6 Cerebral amyloid (Alzheimer's, Down's, senile dementia)
— Amyloid from β/A4-protein (APP derivative)
— Also → Dutch hereditary cerebral angiopathy
7 Hereditary (Icelandic) cerebral amyloid (→ CVA)
— Amyloid from cystatin C (γ-trace protein)
8 Hereditary neuropathic (ATTR) amyloid (e.g. familial Portuguese amyloid)
— Amyloid from plasma transthyretin ('prealbumin') mutants
9 Familial amyloid polyneuropathy and nephropathy (Iowa, USA)
— Amyloid from apolipoprotein A1
10 Hereditary nephropathic amyloid¶ (FMF; similar to AA)
— Autosomal recessive; colchicine prophylaxis effective
11 Finnish hereditary (Agel) amyloid
— Amyloid from abnormal gelsolin (binds actin)
— Lattice corneal dystrophy and corneal neuropathy

* Both respond to melphalan and prednisone (better than to colchicine!)
‡ Not removed by dialysis; causes arthropathy, bone cysts, fracture, carpal tunnel syndrome
¶ Caused by mutations affecting the proinflammatory *pyrin* gene product. However, nephropathy is also caused by familial amyloidoses affecting lysozyme or fibrinogen A α

AL- ('primary') vs AA- ('secondary') amyloidosis

1 AL-amyloidosis → *mesenchymal* tissue deposition
— Macroglossia*
— Acquired factor X deficiency*
— Neuropathy
• Peripheral (incl. carpal tunnel syndrome)
• Autonomic
— Arthropathy
• Large joints (e.g. 'shoulder-pads')
• Carpal tunnel syndrome
— Purpura
• 'Pinch' (non-thrombocytopenic) purpura
• Post-proctoscopic periorbital purpura
— Cardiomyopathy (restrictive or HOCM)
• Often associated with low-voltage ECG
— Hyposplenism
2 AA-amyloidosis → *parenchymal* tissue deposition:
— Nephrotic syndrome‡
— Hepatosplenomegaly‡
— Goiter

* *Highly* specific for AL-amyloidosis
‡ Also occur in 'primary' amyloid

Diagnosis of amyloidosis
1 Paraproteinemia, *plus*
2 Biopsy (Congo red stain) of
   — Routinely biopsied site (e.g. marrow in myeloma)
   — Affected site* (e.g. sural nerve in neuropathy)
   — Deep rectal biopsy
   — Aspirated abdominal fat
3 Biopsy (polarized light microscopy)
   — 'Apple-green' birefringence
4 Electron microscopy
   — β-pleated sheets
5 Direct immunofluorescence of bone marrow plasma cells
   — Light chain antibodies → monoclonal immunocytes
   — Polyclonality (e.g. in reactive systemic amyloidosis)

* NB: Due to increased risk of bleeding in amyloidosis, suspected renal amyloid is usually considered an indication for *rectal* biopsy

INVESTIGATING IMMUNOLOGICAL DISEASE

B lymphocytes: laboratory characteristics
1 Phenotype
   — Surface immunoglobulin (IgM, IgD) present
   — $\kappa:\lambda$ chains = 2:1
2 Function
   — IgG, A, M levels
   — Isohemagglutinins (IgM)
   — Antibodies to
     • Pneumococcus (IgM)
     • Tetanus/polio/diphtheria (IgG)
3 In vitro blastogenesis (T cell dependent)
   — Inducible with pokeweed mitogen
4 Lymph node localization
   — Follicles, medullary cords

Phenotypic characterization of T cell subtypes
1 T cells (general)
   — Express CD3 (pan T cell*) cell-surface marker
2 Helper/inducer (T_H)
   — Normally comprise 70–80% T cells
   — Express CD4 (T cell receptor for HIV)
   — Lineage causing T cell leukemia (HTLV-1+)
3 Suppressor/cytotoxic (T_S)
   — Normally comprise about 30% T cells
   — Express CD8

* cf. Ia antigen; expression excludes T cell origin

Characterization of T cell function in vitro and in vivo
1 Phenotype
   — Spontaneous E-rosette formation with sheep RBCs
2 Function
   — Primary response: DNCB sensitization
   — Lymphokine (MIF, LIF) production
   — 'Memory': DTH skin testing to tuberculin, *Candida*, mumps, trichophyton, tetanus, streptokinase

3 In vitro blastogenesis
   — Inducible with Con A, PHA
   — Specific antigen (e.g. herpes simplex type II)
4 Lymph node localization
   — Paracortical

T_H:T_S ratios in health and disease
1 *Normal* T_H:T_S
   — CD4:CD8 = 1.5–2.0
2 *Inverted* ratio ($T_H < T_S$)
   — With lymphopenia
     • AIDS*
   — With normal lymphocyte count
     • Common variable hypogammaglobulinemia
     • X-linked lymphoproliferative (Duncan's) disease
   — With lymphocytosis
     • CLL
3 *Exaggerated* ratio ($T_H \gg T_S$)
   — SLE
   — Sjögren's syndrome
   — Juvenile chronic arthritis
4 *Relative variations* of T_H:T_S ratio
   — Leprosy
     • Tuberculoid: ↑ T_H:T_S
     • Lepromatous: ↓ T_H:T_S
   — Renal transplant
     • Acute rejection: ↑ T_H:T_S
     • Homograft infection (e.g. CMV): ↓ T_H:T_S
   — Graft-versus-host disease‡
     • Acute: ↑ T_H:T_S
     • Chronic: ↓ T_H:T_S
   — Active sarcoid¶
     • Bronchoalveolar lavage: ↑ T_H:T_S
     • Peripheral blood: ↓ T_H:T_S

* T_H:T_S ratio normal in SCID, WAS, Nezelof's (i.e. despite lymphopenia)
‡ Acute GVHD is associated with hypergammaglobulinemia, chronic GVHD with hypogammaglobulinemia
¶ Bronchoalveolar lavage fluid in active sarcoid is associated with lymphocytosis; cf. peripheral blood → lymphopenia

INVESTIGATION OF HYPERSENSITIVITY STATES

Drugs for which prick testing is reliable
1 β-lactams
2 Local anesthetics

Radioallergosorbent testing ('RAST'): indications*
1 Known high risk of anaphylaxis
   — e.g. Hypersensitivity to penicillin or insect sting
2 Pre-existing skin hypersensitivity
   — Dermatitis, dermatographia, other skin disease
3 Recent (< 72 h) exposure to drugs inhibiting prick test
   — Esp. antihistamines, sympathomimetics‡
4 Highly suggestive history with negative prick test
   — e.g. Inhalant allergy (i.e. suspected false-negative)
5 Small children (< 5 years)

* = Relative contraindications to prick testing
‡ Note that oral steroids do *not* significantly interfere with prick tests

Elevated IgE: differential diagnosis

1 Metazoan parasitic infestation
   — Trichinosis
   — Toxocariasis
   — Filariasis
   — Schistosomiasis
2 Pulmonary disease
   — Atopic asthma
   — Bronchopulmonary aspergillosis
   — Churg–Strauss syndrome
   — Löffler's syndrome
3 Skin disease
   — Pemphigus
   — Pemphigoid
4 Rare causes
   — Wiskott–Aldrich syndrome
   — Job's syndrome
   — Hodgkin's disease
   — Sézary syndrome
   — Selective IgA deficiency

NB: IgE is *not* elevated in the hypereosinophilic syndrome or in extrinsic allergic alveolitis (hypersensitivity pneumonitis)

IgA excess states

1 Elevated serum levels
   — Wiskott–Aldrich syndrome
   — Berger's (IgA nephropathy) disease
   — Henoch–Schönlein purpura
   — Alcoholic cirrhosis
   — Wegener's granulomatosis
2 Positive direct immunofluorescence
   — Extrarenal
      • Celiac disease
      • Dermatitis herpetiformis
      • Pyoderma gangrenosum
   — Renal
      • Berger's disease
      • SLE (IgA$_1$)
      • Henoch-Schönlein (IgA$_2$)
      • Alcoholic cirrhosis (IgA$_2$)

ABNORMALITIES OF PLASMA PROTEINS

Differential diagnosis of polyclonal hypergammaglobulinemia

1 Liver disease
2 Autoimmune disease, connective tissue disease
3 Sarcoidosis
4 Chronic infection
5 Hodgkin's disease, angioimmunoblastic lymphadenopathy
6 AIDS

Dominant polyclonal gammopathy in liver disease

1 Primary biliary cirrhosis — IgM
2 Chronic active hepatitis   — IgG
3 Alcoholic cirrhosis   — IgA (not invariably)

Secondary causes of hypogammaglobulinemia

1 Hematologic malignancy
   — Myeloma

— Chronic lymphocytic leukemia
   — Non-Hodgkin's lymphoma
2 Some infections (e.g. EBV, rubella)
3 Nephrotic syndrome
4 Protein-losing enteropathy (e.g. intestinal lymphangiectasia)
5 Thymoma
6 Myotonic dystrophy

Paraproteinemia: differential diagnosis

1 Benign monoclonal gammopathy (diagnosis of exclusion)
2 Myeloma (IgG > A > BJP only > D > non-secretory > M > E)
3 Plasmacytoma
4 Macroglobulinemia
5 Heavy chain disease*‡
6 Non-Hodgkin's lymphoma
7 Chronic lymphocytic leukemia
8 Essential cryoglobulinemia
9 Cold hemagglutinin disease (IgM)
10 Primary amyloidosis

* λ-heavy chain disease → lymphoma-like syndrome in elderly men
‡ α-heavy chain disease → malabsorption in young Mediterranean patients

Benign monoclonal gammopathy: diagnostic criteria

1 No increase with time
2 No immune paresis (i.e. other Ig levels normal)
3 Normal skeletal survey
4 Paraprotein level
   — < 20 g/L (IgG)
   — < 10 g/L (other)
   — Absent Bence-Jones protein
5 Marrow plasmacytosis < 10%

Components of normal serum protein electrophoresis

1 α_1 band
   — α_1AT; α_1 acid glycoprotein (orosomucoid)
   — αFP
2 α_2 band
   — Haptoglobin
   — Ceruloplasmin
   — AT III
3 β_1 band
   — Transferrin
   β_2 band
   — C_3

Abnormal electrophoretic patterns: clinical significance

1 α_1 pallor
   — α_1AT deficiency
2 β pallor
   — Frozen/stored specimen → in vitro C_3 activation
3 γ pallor
   — Hypogammaglobulinemia (primary or secondary)
4 β–γ fusion
   — IgA paraproteinemia
   — FDPs (DIC)
   — Alcoholic liver disease
   — Hemoglobinemia (intravascular hemolysis)

5 ↓ Albumin
↑ Gammaglobulin
— Chronic liver disease (any etiology)
6 ↓ Albumin
↑ α_2 globulins
↓ Gammaglobulin
— Nephrosis
7 Discrete band cathodal to γ region in serum and urine
— Lysozyme (e.g. in AMOL, CGL)

Electrophoretic abnormalities of urine and CSF
1 In urine
— ↑ IgG: transferrin clearance
• Glomerular disease
— ↑ β_2 microglobulin: transferrin clearance
• Tubular disease
— Bizarre EPG
• Bladder cancer
• Factitious contamination
2 In CSF
— Strong prealbumin bands
— ↑ IgG:albumin ratio
— Oligoclonal IgG bands
• Multiple sclerosis, neurosyphilis, SSPE

THE COMPLEMENT CASCADE

Complement abnormalities in disease
1 Acute phase reaction
— ↑ C_3 ↑ C_4 ↑ total hemolytic complement (THC)
2 Classical pathway activation
— ↓ C_3 ↓ C_4 ↓ THC
3 Alternate pathway activation
— ↓ C_3
— Normal C_4
— Normal or reduced THC
4 Fluid phase activation
— Normal C_3
— ↓↓ C_4 ↓ THC
— ↓ C_1-INH (in hereditary angioedema)
5 Deficiency of classical pathway component
— ↓↓ THC
6 Poorly collected specimen
— ↓ THC ± ↓ $C_{3,4}$
Idiopathic angioneurotic edema
— *Normal* complement profile (cf. hereditary)

The alternate pathway: its pathogenetic significance
1 Function
— Antibody-independent resistance (e.g. via opsonization)
2 Activation
— Endotoxin (bacterial lipopolysaccharide)
3 Defectiveness
— Hyposplenism (p. 195)
4 Pathogenicity
— Post-infective glomerulonephritis
— Mesangiocapillary glomerulonephritis type II ('dense deposit disease') ± partial lipodystrophy
— Paroxysmal nocturnal hemoglobinuria

Phenotypes associated with primary complement deficiencies
1 C_1-esterase inhibitor (C_1-INH) deficiency
— Hereditary angioneurotic edema (see below)
2 C_2 deficiency (commonest deficiency; → 1 in 10 000)
— One-third → asymptomatic
— One third → mild or atypical SLE
— One-third → recurrent pyogenic infections*
3 $C_{1q,r,s}$, C_2 or C_4 deficiency
— Mild SLE, glomerulonephritis, Henoch–Schönlein
4 C_3 deficiency (most serious deficiency)
— Life-threatening infections (encapsulated bacteria)
— May reflect deficiency of factor H/I or C_3b inactivator
5 Factor H deficiency
— Associated with hemolytic uremic syndrome
6 C_5 dysfunction (Leiner's syndrome; presents in infancy)
— Eczema, Gram-negative infections, diarrhea
7 C_7 deficiency
— Raynaud's phenomenon
8 C_{5-9} deficiency
— *Neisseria* (meningococcal/gonococcal) infections

NB: Total hemolytic complement may be undetectable in C_{1q} or C_2 deficiency (confusing in clinically mild SLE). All homozygous complement deficiencies are *rare* except for C_1-INH and C_2 deficiencies
* e.g. pneumococcal/*Haemophilus influenzae* sepsis, esp. meningitis

Features of hereditary angioneurotic edema (C_1-INH deficiency)
1 Presentations
— Non-pruritic skin swellings lasting at least 48–72 h
— Recurrent abdominal colic
— Upper respiratory tract obstruction
— Intestinal pseudo-obstruction
— Family history of asphyxiation (glottal edema)
2 Diagnostic clues
— *No* inflammation, itching or urticaria with attacks
— Normal histamine levels during attacks
— Interictal low C_4
3 Acute management
— Purified C_1-esterase inhibitor (if available)
— Fresh plasma*
— Tracheostomy
4 Prophylaxis
— Danazol, stanozolol
— EACA, tranexamic acid
5 *Acquired* C_1-INH deficiency may be associated with B cell malignancy or glomerulonephritis

* NB: Contains C_2/C_4 which may precipitate or worsen glottal edema

PATHOPHYSIOLOGY OF AUTOIMMUNE DISORDERS

Vasculitis: clinicopathological correlations
1 Large arteries
— Giant cell arteritis, Takayasu's arteritis

2 Medium arteries
  — Polyarteritis nodosa, Kawasaki's disease
3 Medium arteries and veins
  — Buerger's disease
  — Behçet's disease
4 Small arteries and veins
  — Churg–Strauss, Wegener's (granulomatous)
  — Microscopic polyangiitis (non-granulomatous)
5 Arterioles, capillaries, post-capillary venules
  (leukocytoclastic)
  — Cutaneous vasculitis → intradermal capillaries
  — Henoch–Schönlein purpura
  — Essential mixed cryoglobulinemic vasculitis
  — Rheumatoid vasculitis

Ultrastructural features of the vasculitides
1 Giant-cell arteritis
  — Absent fibrinoid necrosis
  — Moderate giant cell infiltrate
  — Mononuclear infiltration
2 Wegener's granulomatosis
  — Marked fibrinoid necrosis
  — Marked giant cell infiltrate
  — Polymorph/mononuclear infiltration
3 Churg–Strauss syndrome
  — Moderate fibrinoid necrosis
  — Moderate giant cell infiltrate
  — Eosinophil infiltration
4 Polyarteritis nodosa
  — Marked fibrinoid necrosis
  — Absent giant cells
  — Polymorph/eosinophil infiltration
5 Hypersensitivity vasculitis
  — Slight fibrinoid necrosis
  — Absent giant cells
  — Polymorph/lymphocyte infiltration
6 Miscellaneous
  — Intercellular cement Ab (pemphigus)
  — Anticollagen type II (relapsing
    polychondritis)
  — Glutamic acid decarboxylase Ab ('stiff-man'
    syndrome)

ANTINEUTROPHIL CYTOPLASMIC ANTIBODIES (ANCA)

Disease associations of ANCA
1 Cytoplasmic (cANCA) staining against α-
  proteinase 3
  — Wegener's granulomatosis (80% sensitivity)
2 Perinuclear (pANCA) staining against
  myeloperoxidase or elastase
  — Microscopic polyangiitis (*not* PAN) – 50%
  — Churg–Strauss syndrome, SLE
  — Idiopathic crescentic (rapidly progressive)
    glomerulonephritis*
  — Kawasaki syndrome

* Anti-GBM antibodies also may be present

ANCA variation with disease activity
1 ANCA levels often (but not always) parallel
  activity

2 Can be used to monitor treatment efficacy
3 Clinical relapses may be prevented by treating
  presumptively when ANCA rises
4 Pathogenetic role of ANCA remains unproven

Diagnostic interpretation of negative ANCA
1 ANCA-negative vasculitis
  — Leukocytoclastic vasculitis
  — Henoch–Schönlein purpura
  — Cryoglobulinemic vasculitis
2 Vasculitis is local, *not* systemic
3 Patient already commenced on therapy
4 Patient does *not* have vasculitis after all
5 Suboptimal assay system

Differential diagnosis of false-positive ANCA
1 Infection, esp.
  — HIV
  — Infective endocarditis
  — Amebic abscess
2 Inflammatory bowel disease
  — Esp. with sclerosing cholangitis
3 Malignancy, e.g.
  — Atrial myxoma
  — Lung cancer
4 Sweet's syndrome (p. 399)

Clinical implications of positive ANCA
1 Diagnosis
  — Wegener's, Churg–Strauss, microscopic
    polyarteritis
2 Complications
  — Prone to renal failure
3 Management
  — Tend to respond to cyclophosphamide

KAWASAKI SYNDROME

Diagnosis of Kawasaki syndrome*
1 High fever > 5 days in a child aged < 5 years,
  plus
2 At least 4 of the following signs
  — Bilateral non-purulent conjunctival injection
  — Unilateral, painful, non-purulent, single cervical
    node > 15 mm
  — Oral mucosal erythema, strawberry tongue,
    cracked lips
  — Painful hand/foot erythema or edema‡
  — Polymorphic skin rash¶
3 Exclusion of
  — Scarlet fever (gp A strep§), rheumatic fever
  — Staphylococcal infection with toxin release$
  — Leptospirosis, Rocky Mountain spotted fever
  — EBV infection, measles
  — Juvenile rheumatoid arthritis
  — Drug rash, Stevens–Johnson syndrome

* An epidemic systemic vasculitis of children
‡ Desquamates in convalescence
¶ Incl. 'reactivation' of previous BCG vaccination site
§ But note that positive culture does not exclude Kawasaki's
$ e.g. staphylococcal scalded skin syndrome, toxic shock
syndrome

Management of Kawasaki syndrome

1 Monitor for potentially lethal vasculitic complications
   — Echocardiographic detection of coronary aneurysms (usually detectable 2–4 weeks after symptom onset)
   — Myocarditis, pancarditis; acute myocardial infarction
2 Therapy
   — IV gammaglobulin (up to 2 g/kg over 10 h, single infusion)
   — High-dose aspirin (30 mg/kg/day in divided doses) for 14 days helps fever
   — Low-dose aspirin (3–5 mg/kg/day as single antiplatelet dose) for 8 weeks*

* Unless coronary lesions detected, in which case continue long term

AUTOANTIBODIES

Autoantibodies causing neuromuscular disorders

1 AChRAb (acetylcholine receptor antibody)
   — Myasthenia gravis
2 Antibody to voltage-gated calcium channels
   — Eaton–Lambert (myasthenic) syndrome
3 Antibody to membrane potassium channels
   — Acquired neuromyotonia (Isaacs' syndrome)
4 Antibody to glutamic acid decarboxylase (GAD)
   — Stiff-man syndrome*

* GAD occurs in both GABA-ergic nerve terminals and in pancreatic islet cells. Hence, GAD antibodies (to a distinct antigenic epitope) may occur in type I diabetes, and many stiff-man patients also have diabetes

Autoantibodies causing paraneoplastic disorders

1 Anti-Yo (Purkinje cell antibody)
   — Cerebellar degeneration (rarely, temporal lobe epilepsy)
2 Anti-Jo-1 (muscle cell antibody)
   — Polymyositis
3 Anti-Ri (neuronal nuclear antibody)
   — Opsoclonus–myoclonus

Autoantibodies causing connective tissue disorders

1 Antibody to type II collagen
   — Bilateral progressive sensorineural hearing loss
2 Anti-GBM (glomerular basement membrane antibody)
   — Goodpasture's syndrome
3 Anti-Ro (SS-A)
   — Congenital heart block (maternal SLE)
4 Antiphospholipid
   — Thrombotic tendency in SLE

Endocrine disorders caused by autoantibodies

1 Endocrinopathies mediated by *agonistic* antibodies, e.g.
   — TSH receptor Ab
     • Graves' disease (→ goiter)
   — β islet cell Ab
     • Spontaneous hypoglycemia

2 Endocrinopathies mediated by *blocking* antibodies, e.g.
   — TSH receptor* Ab
     • 1° myxedema, Hashimoto's
   — ACTH receptor Ab, 21-hydroxylase Ab
     • Addison's
   — Gastrin receptor Ab
     • Pernicious anemia
   — FSH receptor Ab
     • Premature menopause
   — Insulin receptor Ab
     • Type B insulin receptor abnormality (diabetes)
     • Associated with acanthosis nigricans

* *Mutations* affecting this receptor may also cause congenital hypothyroidism

Intestinal disorders caused by autoantibodies

1 Celiac disease
   — α-gliadin Ab
   — Transglutaminase Ab
2 Autoimmune polyendocrinopathy type 1 with intestinal symptoms
   — Tryptophan hydroxylase*

* Involved in serotonin biosynthesis

Diagnostic patterns of antinuclear antibodies

1 Rim (peripheral)
   — Associated with native (double-stranded) DNA antibodies to DNA sugar-phosphate backbone, base pairs, or specific double-helical conformations
   — Titre parallels disease activity
2 Homogeneous (diffuse)
   — Associated with histone* (or ssDNA) antibodies
   — Rarely associated with dsDNA antibodies
3 Nucleolar
   — Associated with antibodies to nucleolar RNA
4 Speckled
   — Associated with antibodies to non-histone antigens
   — Ribonucleoproteins
     • U1 RNP (nRNP)
     • rRNP
     • Sm
     • Ro (SS-A)
     • La‡ (SS-B)
   — Jo-1 (aminoacyl tRNA synthetase)
   — Topoisomerase I (Scl-70)
   — Centromere
   — Ku¶

* Histones are DNA-binding chromatin proteins
‡ A nucleic acid-binding ATPase which terminates RNA transcription
¶ DNA-binding protein; associated with sclerodactyly

Features of ANA-negative SLE

1 Subacute presentation
2 Major skin involvement (e.g. photosensitive dermatitis)
3 Thrombocytopenia common
4 Renal and CNS disease unusual
5 Lupus band negative
6 Antibodies to Ro (SS-A) positive in ~ 50%*

NB: Only 5% of SLE cases are ANA-negative; hence, difficult to be sure of diagnosis in this situation. *Discoid* LE is usually ANA-negative
* Standard ANA immunofluorescence does *not* reliably detect anti-Ro (or antiphospholipid)

Serologic subsets of SLE
1 Specific SLE markers predictive of renal disease, hypocomplementemia
— dsDNA antibodies (in 60% SLE patients)
— Sm antibodies* (in 20%; → membranous GN)
— PCNA antibodies (in 5%)
2 Drug-induced SLE (e.g. due to procainamide)
— Homogeneous ANA (in 95%)
3 Sjögren's/scleroderma, overlap
— Nucleolar ANA
4 Mixed connective tissue disease (pp. 178–9)
— Anti-U1 (anti-RNP)
5 Polymyositis/pulmonary fibrosis overlap
— Jo-1‡

* Particularly common in Asians with SLE
‡ 25% of dermatomyositis patients will have anti-Jo-1; of these, 80% will have both myositis and lung fibrosis

Serologic subsets of scleroderma
1 Diffuse scleroderma
— Antitopoisomerase I (Scl-70); Ku
2 Limited scleroderma, CREST syndrome
— Anticentromere antibody*
3 Sicca syndrome/Sjögren's
— La, Ro

* Indicates a good prognosis in scleroderma but *not* in Raynaud's (i.e. suggests progression to scleroderma)

Clinical associations of anti-Ro antibodies
1 Neonatal SLE
— Esp. congenital heart block
2 Subacute cutaneous SLE (SCLE)
— 'Polycyclic' lesions in photosensitive distribution
3 ANA-negative SLE
4 SLE due to homozygous C_2 deficiency
5 Sicca syndrome* ± arthritis
6 Pneumonitis, hyperglobulinemia

* 'Primary' Sjögren's syndrome

PHOSPHOLIPID ANTIBODIES

Detection of phospholipid antibodies
1 'Lupus anticoagulant' test*
— Detects autoantibody-dependent interference with prothrombin activation in vitro
— This in vitro *anticoagulant* effect has a paradoxical *procoagulant* effect in vivo
2 Anticardiolipin antibody tests
— Detect and identify target-specific autoantibodies to this phospholipid
3 Reaginic tests for syphilis
— Biological false-positives

* Detects the presence, but not identity, of all phospholipid antibodies. A positive lupus anticoagulant *test* thus implies the presence of any one of several so-called 'lupus anticoagulant' antiphospholipid *autoantibodies* (see below)

What are phospholipid antibodies?
1 Anticardiolipin antibody
— One of the family of antibodies that bind phospholipids in plasma
— Binds cardiolipin when complexed with a cofactor, the plasma protein β_2-glycoprotein I (β_2GPI, apolipoprotein H), thereby activating factor XII, platelets, and endothelial membrane binding
2 Lupus anticoagulant(s)
— Denotes the presence in plasma of any uncharacterized autoantibody* responsible for prolongation of in vitro coagulation‡
— Detectable in ~ 30% lupus (SLE) patients, incl. drug-induced
— Paradoxical *thrombosis* in vivo¶, including arterial; usually *no* bleeding
3 False-positive syphilis reagins
— Distinct from lupus anticoagulants and anticardiolipin
— Distinguishable serologically from *true* syphilis reagins
— Do *not* cause thrombosis

* i.e. including anticardiolipin
‡ → Prolonged PTTK *uncorrected* by in vitro addition of normal plasma (i.e. a true 'anticoagulant')
¶ Esp. with IgG phospholipid antibody; risk correlates with plasma level

Phospholipid-binding protein cofactors for autoantibodies
1 β_2-glycoprotein I (β_2GPI, apolipoprotein H)
2 Prothrombin
3 Protein C, protein S
4 Annexin V
5 Lamins

Major features of antiphospholipid syndrome
1 Thrombosis (arterial as well as venous)
2 Thrombocytopenia
3 Recurrent miscarriages
4 Brain involvement (rich in phospholipids)

Vascular complications of phospholipid antibodies*
1 Placental arterial insufficiency
— Recurrent abortions (1st and 2nd trimester)
— Intrauterine fetal death (2nd and 3rd trimester)
2 CNS arterial insufficiency
— TIAs, stroke, multi-infarct dementia
— Vascular myelopathy (?ant. spinal artery thrombosis)
— Migraine, amaurosis fugax, CRA occlusion
3 Cardiac insufficiency
— Acute myocardial infarction
— Coronary graft thrombosis
4 Pulmonary arterial insufficiency
— Recurrent pulmonary emboli
5 Peripheral arterial insufficiency
— Aortic arch syndrome
— Axillary arterial thrombosis
— Mesenteric arterial thrombosis
— Peripheral vascular disease (incl. gangrene)

6 Venous thrombosis
— Superficial thrombophlebitis
— Deep venous thrombosis
— Renal vein thrombosis (± bilateral)
— Retinal vein thrombosis
— Budd–Chiari syndrome
— Portal vein thrombosis

* NB: Only 50% cases have SLE; the others represent 'primary antiphospholipid syndrome'. Note also that arterial insufficiency in this context is *not* mediated by vasculitis, but by bland intimal thickening

Forms of hypertension associated with phospholipid antibodies
1 'Primary' pulmonary hypertension
2 Labile systemic hypertension
3 Portal venous hypertension

Additional manifestations of phospholipid antibodies
1 Thrombocytopenia, Coombs-positive hemolytic anemia
2 Chorea, epilepsy, psychiatric disturbance
3 Guillain–Barré syndrome
4 Libman–Sachs cardiac valve degeneration*
5 Splenomegaly
6 Livedo reticularis, splinter hemorrhages
7 Adrenal infarction, Addison's disease
8 Avascular necrosis of bone

* Vegetations → regurgitation

Bleeding in patients with lupus anticoagulant? Exclude
1 Thrombocytopenia
2 Hypoprothrombinemia
3 Factor VIII antibodies

Management of antiphospholipid syndrome
1 Low-dose aspirin (e.g. 75 mg/day)
2 History of thrombosis?
— Long-term warfarin (keep INR > 3)
3 Recurrent miscarriages?
— Add low-molecular-weight heparin to low-dose aspirin
4 Steroids/immunosuppressives
— Not useful *except* in management of cytopenias

'COLD' AUTOANTIBODIES

The cryopathies: clinicopathological background
1 Cryoglobulinemia
— May be monoclonal or polyclonal (usually IgM)
— Clinical manifestations arise due to precipitation of immunoglobulins at low temperatures (i.e. < 37°C)
— Sequelae include
• Raynaud's (may progress to gangrene)
• Purpura (esp. legs)
• Hepatosplenomegaly; abnormal LFTs
• Arthralgias, fever
• Confusion, weakness (hyperviscosity)
• Renal failure, uremia (glomerulonephritis)
— Etiological associations
• Connective tissue disease (e.g. SLE)

• Myelo-/lymphoproliferative disease (e.g. CLL)
• Infections (e.g. HBV, post-infectious nephritis)
2 Cold agglutinins
— Clinical manifestations due to IgM binding red cells at low temperatures → complement activation on rewarming to 37°C → hemolysis
— Less often, red cell *autoagglutination* may supervene → vascular obstruction (Raynaud's, acrocyanosis)
— Etiological associations
• *Mycoplasma pneumoniae* (anti-I; Rh specificity)
• Infectious mononucleosis (anti-i)
• Diffuse large-cell lymphoma
• Waldenström's macroglobulinemia
3 Paroxysmal cold hemoglobinuria
— Clinical manifestations due to low-temperature IgG (Donath–Landsteiner antibody) binding P antigen of red cell membrane → complement fixation → intravascular hemolysis on rewarming to 37°C
— Hemoglobinemia/transient leukopenia may also occur
— Etiological associations
• Measles, mumps, varicella
• Congenital syphilis
4 Cryofibrinogenemia
— Manifestations may include cold urticaria (pp. 398–9)
— Etiological associations
• Diabetes mellitusi
• Prostate cancer

TISSUE TYPING

Gene loci in the major histocompatibility complex (MHC)
1 HLA determinants (see below)
2 Complement components
— e.g. C_2, C_4; C_3 convertase
3 Tumor necrosis factor
— Proinflammatory cytokine implicated in rheumatoid arthritis and other autoimmune disorders
4 Heat-shock proteins (HSPs)
— Molecular chaperones controlling protein folding
5 Genes affecting antigen processing and presentation
— Located between DP and DQ loci
6 Unrelated ('class III') genes responsible for some 'HLA-linked' disorders, e.g.
— Narcolepsy*
— 21–hydroxylase
— Hemochromatosis*

* Though responsible gene not yet identified

HLA antigens: patterns of expression and function
1 HLA A, B, and C antigens (*class I* antigens) are found on most nucleated cells (not RBCs) except trophoblast
— Function: present foreign antigen (usually viral) to *cytotoxic T cells*
— Mediate graft rejection

2 D-related (DR, or *class II*) antigens are found on
  • B cells (basis of pretransplant MLC)
  • Activated T cells
  • Monocytes and macrophages
  • Sperm, epididymal cells
  — Function: present foreign antigen to *helper T cells*
  — Mediate immune-responsiveness

Prevalence of HLA-antigens in Caucasian populations
1 HLA-A3   — 25%
2 HLA-B8   — 10%
3 HLA-B27 — 5–10%
4 HLA-DR4 — 20–40%

HLA allele linkage disequilibrium: common haplotypes
1 A1, B8, DR3
  — Often occur together in Caucasians
  — May include deletion for C_4 complement component
2 A2, B35, DR4
  — Often occur together in American Indians
3 A30, B13, DR7
  — Often occur together in Chinese

HLA antigens: strongest disease associations
1 HLA-DQw6
  — Present in 20% controls
  — Present in > 95% *narcolepsy* cases (50-fold ↑ risk)
  — Also present in 80% Goodpasture's (anti-GBM disease)
2 HLA-B27
  — Present in 5–10% controls
  — Present in 90% *ankylosing spondylitis* (80-fold ↑ risk)
  — Also present in 80% *Reiter's syndrome* (40-fold ↑ risk)
3 HLA-A29
  — Predisposes to birdshot retinochoroidopathy (100-fold ↑ risk)

Other disease associations with HLA antigens
1 A3
  — Idiopathic hemochromatosis (in 75%)
  — B7, B14 also linked to IHC
2 B5
  — Behçet's disease with ocular or colonic involvement
  — Takayasu's arteritis
3 B12
  — Minimal lesion nephrosis
4 B27
  — Psoriatic arthritis ± sacroiliitis
  — Juvenile chronic arthritis with sacroiliitis
  — Reactive arthritis
  — Acute anterior uveitis
  — Chronic balanitis; chronic prostatitis
  — 'Frozen shoulder'
  — Asbestosis
5 B35
  — Subacute (de Quervain's, viral) thyroiditis
  Bw47
  — 21–hydroxylase deficiency

B51
  — Behçet's syndrome (4× ↑ risk; also B12, B5)
  Bw53
  — Malarial resistance
6 Cw6
  — Psoriasis vulgaris (15× ↑ risk)
  Cw7
  — Guillain–Barré syndrome (chronic relapsing subtype)
7 DP
  — Beryllium hypersensitivity
8 DQ
  — Pemphigus vulgaris
  DQw3
  — Ca cervix
9 DR2
  — Goodpasture's syndrome (15× ↑ risk)
  — Multiple sclerosis (4× ↑ risk; also B7, DQw1)
  — SLE (esp. with C_2 deficiency)
10 DR3 (and B8)
  — Primary Sjögren's (sicca) syndrome (10× ↑ risk)
  — Celiac disease/dermatitis herpetiformis (12× ↑ risk; also B8, DQw2)
  — SLE (esp. neonatal or subacute cutaneous SLE; 6× ↑ risk)
  — Addison's disease (6× ↑ risk); Graves' disease (4× ↑ risk)
  — Insulin-dependent diabetes (also DR4, B8, B15; 3× ↑ risk)
  — Post-partum thyroiditis (5× ↑ risk)
  — HBsAg-negative chronic active hepatitis
  — Myasthenia gravis (3× ↑ risk)
  — Buerger's disease
  — Idiopathic membranous nephropathy (12× ↑ risk)
11 DR4
  — Seropositive RA (4× ↑ risk); secondary Sjögren's syndrome
  — Polyarticular (RA-like) juvenile chronic arthritis
  — Chronic (antibiotic-resistant) Lyme arthritis
  — SLE (iatrogenic)
  — Pre-eclampsia (familial)
  — Pemphigus (15× ↑ risk among Ashkenazis)
12 DR5
  — Pernicious anemia
  — Hashimoto's thyroiditis (also DR11)
  — Early-onset systemic (Still's) juvenile chronic arthritis
  — HIV-associated sicca syndrome

MANAGING IMMUNOLOGICAL DISEASE

INDICATIONS FOR IMMUNOMODULATORY THERAPY

Indications for cytokine therapy
1 Interferon-α
  — Chronic hepatitis B and C
  — Kaposi's sarcoma, melanoma, myeloma, chronic granuloyctic leukemia, renal cell carcinoma

2 Interferon-β
— Multiple sclerosis
3 Interferon-γ
— Chronic granulomatous disease
4 Interleukin-2
— Renal cell carcinoma
5 Interleukin-11
— Chemotherapy-induced thrombocytopenic purpura

Indications for plasmapheresis/plasma exchange

1 Autoantibody removal
— Idiopathic thrombocytopenic purpura
— Non-oliguric anti-GBM disease (Goodpasture's)
— Myasthenia gravis: crisis or prethymectomy
— Fulminant Guillain–Barré syndrome
2 Antibody removal
— ABO-incompatible transplantation
3 Immunoglobulin or cryoglobulin removal
— Hyperviscosity syndrome (acute or maintenance)
— Cryoglobulinemia with vasculitis
4 Factors replaced
— Thrombotic thrombocytopenic purpura
— Acquired factor X deficiency

Potential indications for intravenous immunoglobulin

1 Immune thrombocytopenia
— Recent-onset ITP*
— Post-transfusion purpura
2 Symptomatic hypogammaglobulinemia
— Primary (incl. IgG subclass deficiencies)
— Secondary (e.g. in CLL; but see below)
3 Infection
— Neonatal sepsis‡
— Prophylaxis for marrow transplants, ICU patients
— CMV pneumonia (with ganciclovir)
— Pediatric AIDS
4 Autoimmune/vasculitis
— Kawasaki syndrome (with aspirin; pp. 183–4)
— Acute Guillain–Barré syndrome
— Refractory myasthenia gravis
— Pure red cell aplasia
— Reduction of F VIII antibodies in hemophilia
— Severe allergic asthma in childhood

NB: High-dose IV IgG can cause transient hyperviscosity, aseptic meningitis and/or renal impairment; but rarely transmits hepatitis or HIV. It does not appear *cost-effective* for chronic disorders such as CLL
* Or autoimmune neutropenia/hemolysis; esp. presplenectomy
‡ Or prophylaxis for this in premature neonates

Therapeutic monoclonal antibodies

1 Rituximab
— anti-CD20 (for B-cell lymphoma)
2 Abciximab
— anti-GP IIa/IIIb (for coronary disease)
3 Trastuzumab
— anti-ErbB2 (for metastatic breast cancer)
4 Daclizumab, basiliximab
— anti-CD25 (for organ transplantation)
5 Muronomab
— anti-CD3 (for graft rejection)

Indications for hyposensitization

1 Bee/wasp sting anaphylaxis, *or* Severe reaction with strongly positive prick test
2 Severe allergic rhinitis if due to pollen/grass/housedust-mite hypersensitivity*
3 (Major) penicillin allergy *if essential* for management‡

* *Not* in food allergy
‡ e.g. life-threatening enterococcal endocarditis

Therapeutic modalities in allergic rhinitis

1 Prophylaxis
— Sodium cromoglicate (mast cell stabilizer), esp. in children
— Ketotifen*, astemizole (antihistamine)
2 Sneezing or itch
— Intranasal steroids
— Oral antihistamines
3 Nasal obstruction
— Intranasal steroids
— Topical decongestants
4 Watery rhinorrhea
— Ipratropium bromide (antimuscarinic anticholinergic)
— Intranasal steroids, oral antihistamines
5 Refractory symptoms (e.g. obstruction prevents inhalation)
— Oral prednisone (prednisolone) 20 mg/day for 5 days
— Hyposensitization (e.g. to grass pollen)‡

* Mast cell stabilizer and antihistamine with other actions including PAF (platelet-activating factor) and leukotriene $C_4/D_4/E_4$ inhibition
‡ Note that allergen injection immunotherapy is contraindicated if coexisting asthma

Antihistamines: indications and toxicities

1 Main indications
— Allergic rhinoconjunctivitis
— Chronic urticaria, angioedema
2 Toxicities
— Somnolence (esp. first-generation antihistamines)*
— Q-T_c prolongation (esp. second-generation antihistamines‡)
3 Interactions to be avoided with terfenadine or astemizole
— Liver or cardiac disease
— Imidazole antifungals (e.g. ketoconazole)
— Macrolide antibiotics (e.g. erythromycin)
— Grapefruit juice

* Hence, avoid diphenhydramine and chlorphenamine in schoolchildren
‡ Use cetirizine, loratidine, or fexofenadine in preference to terfenadine or astemizole *if* any of the contraindications listed are present

Potential toxicity of inhaled/intranasal steroids in childhood

1 Growth retardation (may need to monitor height)
2 Decreased bone mineral density
3 Adrenal suppression (prolonged or high-dose treatment)
4 Cataract, glaucoma

DRUG-INDUCED IMMUNOLOGIC DISORDERS

Pathogenesis of drug fever
1 Hypersensitivity reactions
  — Penicillins, sulfonamides
  — Methyldopa; hydralazine (SLE)
  — D-penicillamine
2 Antituberculosis drugs
  — INH, PAS, rifampicin, streptomycin
3 Cytotoxics
  — Bleomycin, L-asparaginase
4 Dose-related pyrogens
  — Amphotericin B
5 Thermoregulatory dysfunction
  — Anticholinergics (impaired sweating)
  — Phenothiazines (hypothalamic effect)
6 Overdosage
  — Aspirin
  — Iodine (may → transient hyperthyroidism)
7 Drug abuse
  — Amphetamines, LSD, barbiturates, IV cocaine
  — Laxatives
8 Drug withdrawal
  — Corticosteroids
9 Malignant hyperthermia
  — Anesthetic agents, esp. inhalational
10 Rare (unlikely) causes
  — Digoxin
  — Chloramphenicol, tetracycline
  — Monocomponent insulin

Anaphylaxis: frequent iatrogenic causes
1 Penicillins* (and other protein-binding haptens)
2 Insulin
3 Heterologous antisera (e.g. tetanus antitoxin)
4 Intravenous vitamin K
5 Iron dextran infusion
6 Streptokinase, protamine

* Frequency of penicillin-induced anaphylaxis is ~ 0.2%, with
~ one-quarter of these proving fatal

Precipitants of anaphylactoid reactions*
1 Aspirin and other NSAIDs
2 Opiates: codeine, morphine
3 Gammaglobulin administration, blood transfusions
4 Anesthetics and muscle relaxants (e.g. thiopentone, curare)
5 Iodinated contrast agents (esp. in venography)
6 Hydrocortisone (rare but occasional)

* i.e. not IgE-dependent and not requiring prior antigen exposure; cf. anaphylaxis

Radiocontrast reactions: occurrence and outcome
1 For iodinated media, incidence is about 5%*
2 Anaphylaxis occurs in 1%, death in 0.01%
3 Atopy predisposes
4 Previous reaction indicates a 25% risk on re-exposure
5 Premedication with oral steroids and antihistamines reduces the risk

* Less with newer low-osmolarity agents

Clinical spectrum of aspirin reactions
1 Anaphylactoid reactions
2 Uriticaria, asthma, rhinitis
3 Angioedema
4 Lyell's syndrome; purpura; photodermatitis

Cross-reactive drug sensitivity
1 p-Aminobenzoates
  — Sulfonamides
  — Sulfonylureas
  — Thiazides
  — Phenothiazines
  — Procainamide
  — Acetazolamide
2 Penicillins
  — Penicillin G
  — Semisynthetic penicillins
  — Penicillamine
  — Cephalosporins
3 Allopurinol-induced maculopapular rash is commoner if past history of ampicillin rash, esp. if renal dysfunction (ampicillin rash also commoner in allopurinol patients)

Clinical aspects of penicillin hypersensitivity
1 *Allergic* reactions most commonly occur with semisynthetic penicillins; such reactions represent *major determinant* (i.e. penicilloyl group of the cleaved β-lactam ring) hypersensitivity mediated by IgG/IgM antibodies
2 True IgE-dependent *anaphylactic* reactions are rare (incidence 0.05%, mortality 0.0002%); such reactions commoner with parenteral administration, esp. of benzylpenicillin, and represent *minor determinant* (penilloate, penicillin or penicilloic acid), or hapten, hypersensitivity
3 *Fatal* anaphylactic reactions usually occur in patients with *no* past history of penicillin allergy or atopy. To confirm a past history of anaphylaxis, prick testing is indicated
4 85% of patients with history of minor reactions can be re-exposed without toxicity, perhaps indicating transient sensitization; only major contraindication is anaphylaxis
5 Cephalosporin cross-sensitization occurs, but is uncommon
6 If penicillin is required for a serious bacterial infection in a patient with a history of penicillin-induced anaphylaxis, temporary desensitization may be undertaken and completed within 4 h*

* NB: Desensitization works by raising the cell threshold to IgE; it cannot be performed using steroid or antihistamine cover

IMMUNOMODULATORY THERAPY

Potency of steroid dose relative to prednisolone
1 Betamethasone: 0.5
2 Methylprednisolone: 2.5
3 Dexamethasone: 3

Alternate-day steroids: guidelines for use

1 Benefits
   — Less growth retardation in children
   — Less HPA axis suppression
   — Fewer infective complications
   — Less aseptic necrosis, cataracts
2 Problems
   — Less likely to be effective in remission induction
3 Useful in
   — Polymyositis
   — Myasthenia gravis
4 Ineffective in
   — Giant cell arteritis
   — Severe rheumatoid arthritis
   — Chronic active hepatitis
   — Asthma

Therapeutic immunomodulation: which drug?

1 Azathioprine
   — Renal transplantation
   — HBsAg-negative chronic active hepatitis
   — SLE
   — Behçet's syndrome (esp. with uveitis)
2 Cyclophosphamide
   — Wegener's*, lymphomatoid granulomatosis
   — PAN, systemic vasculitis, SLE with renal involvement
3 Methotrexate
   — Severe psoriasis (e.g. pustular)
   — Reiter's syndrome
   — Dermatomyositis, pemphigus (steroid-sparing)
4 Immunophilin-binding drugs
   — Ciclosporin (binds ciclophilin)
     • Marrow transplantation (prevents graft rejection in aplasia, GVHD in leukemia)
     • Immunosuppression in renal transplantation
     • Refractory psoriasis, rheumatoid arthritis, uveitis/Behçet's
   — Tacrolimus (FK506; binds FKBP, or tacrolimus-binding protein)
     • Organ transplantation
   — Sirolimus (rapamycin; antifungal which binds TOR‡)
     • Organ transplantation
5 Mycophenolate mofetil (antifungal; inhibits IMP dehydrogenase)
   — Renal and cardiac transplantation
   — Systemic vasculitis, rheumatoid arthritis
   — Idiopathic retroperitoneal fibrosis
   — IgA nephropathy
   — Refractory psoriasis, bullous pemphigoid
6 Biological lymphocyte inhibitors
   — Antilymphocyte (-thymocyte) globulin
     • Organ transplantation
     • Aplastic anemia
   — Anti-CD25 monoclonal antibodies (daclizumab, basiliximab)
     • Organ transplantation
   — Anti-CD3 monoclonal antibodies (muromonab)
     • Threatened graft rejection

* Addition of co-trimoxazole further reduces relapse rate
‡ TOR = target of rapamycin, a kinase which together with the PP2A phosphatase, controls mRNA translation and hence the cell cycle

Mechanisms implicated in therapeutic immunomodulation

1 Corticosteroids
   — Polymorphs
     • ↓ Extravascular egress (impaired chemotaxis)
     • Post-phagocytic defect (↓ intracellular killing)
   — Mononuclears
     • Extravascular trapping (↓ T cell number/function)
     • Impaired antibody–antigen uptake
     • ↓ Immunoglobulin synthesis
   — Eosinopenia
   — ↓ Interleukin II levels
2 Azathioprine
   — Prodrug for 6MP (metabolized in liver)
   — Reduced lymphocyte proliferation
   — Impaired lymphokine release
   — Reduced antibody synthesis
3 Ciclosporin
   — Fungal cyclic polypeptide
   — Binds peptidyl prolyl isomerases*
   — No lympholytic action; no myelosuppression
   — ↓ IL-2 release (→ ↓ T cell activation)
   — ↓ IL-1 levels, ↓ helper T cell number
4 Tacrolimus, sirolimus
   — Binds peptidyl prolyl isomerases (like ciclosporin)
   — 100 times more potent than ciclosporin
5 Antilymphocyte globulin
   — Reduction of circulating lymphocyte pool
   — Suppression of cell-mediated immunity

* Enzymes that mediate both protein folding and lymphocyte activation

General indications for cytotoxic immunosuppression

1 Uncontrolled disease despite non-cytotoxic therapy, esp. if major organ involvement (e.g. in vasculitis, sarcoid)
2 Unacceptable steroid side-effects
3 Organ transplantation
4 Wegener's granulomatosis, PAN

Comparative morbidity of immunomodulatory therapy

1 Azathioprine
   — Neutropenia; impaired cell-mediated immunity
   — Cholestasis, pancreatitis
   — Lymphomas; SCC (skin/cervix)
   — 4-fold ↑ bioavailability (hence, toxicity) if given with allopurinol (also true for oral 6MP)
2 Cyclophosphamide
   — Myelosuppression, sterility, alopecia
   — Cystitis, bladder fibrosis/cancer (avoided with MESNA)
   — AML (less frequent than with chlorambucil)
3 Methotrexate
   — Hepatotoxicity (liver fibrosis) with long-term therapy
   — No demonstrated second malignancy rate
4 Ciclosporin*
   — Nephrotoxicity (esp. older patients on high doses)
     • Manifests as prolonged post-transplant oliguria

— Lymphoma
  • May regress on dose reduction (?EBV-induced)
— Hypertension
  • Despite normal renal function/renin levels
— CNS syndrome
  • Cortical blindness, confusion, pyramidal lesions
— Other: hepatotoxicity, hirsutism, gum hypertrophy‡, tremor, breast lumps, hyperuricemia, gout
5 Antilymphocyte globulin
  — Transfusion reactions
  — CMV viremia

* Toxicity potentiated by ketoconazole
‡ NB: Some cases reported of gingival carcinoma arising on ciclosporin

Patient evaluation prior to glucocorticoid therapy
1 Urinalysis (glycosuria), urine culture
2 Blood pressure
3 Chest X-ray
4 Measurement of intraocular pressure in patients with diabetes, severe myopia or family history of glaucoma

INTERFERONS

Varieties of interferon
1 Interferon-α ('leukocyte')
  — Derived originally from human monocytes
  — Now mainly produced using recombinant techniques
2 Interferon-β (fibroblast)
  — Derived from human fibroblasts
  — 30% amino acid homology with interferon-α
3 Interferon-λ ('immune')*
  — Derived from human T cells
  — No homology with interferon-α or β

* May offer effective prophylaxis against infection in chronic granulomatous disease

Physiological actions of interferons
1 Inhibit viral replication (e.g. in chronic HBV infection)
2 Activate NK cells and macrophages
3 Increase HLA antigen expression
4 Increase plasma membrane rigidity

Indications for interferon-α immunotherapy
1 Established indications
  — Hairy cell leukemia (90% response rate)
  — CML (chronic phase)
  — Lymphoma (cutaneous T cell, aggressive NHL)
  — Kaposi's sarcoma (HIV+)
  — Metastatic renal cell carcinoma (with IL-2)
  — Chronic active hepatitis B or C
  — Juvenile laryngeal papillomatosis (HPV-induced)
2 Investigational indications
  — Essential mixed cryoglobulinemia*
  — Islet cell tumors, esp. VIPoma
  — Genital warts

* Esp. if associated with anti-HCV

Toxicity of interferon
1 'Flu-like syndrome; lethargy, somnolence
2 Nausea, vomiting, anorexia, diarrhea
3 Thrombocytopenia and/or neutropenia
4 Dysgeusia, xerostomia
5 Abnormal liver function tests
6 Reversible cardiac dysfunction

TRANSPLANTATION

Renal transplantation: predictors of successful engraftment
1 Essential
  — ABO compatibility
  — Negative cytotoxic crossmatch (MLC)
2 Desirable
  — HLA-B/DR matching (esp. DR)
  — Prior transfusions

Marrow transplantation: predictors of successful engraftment
1 Negative cytotoxic crossmatch
2 HLA-B/DR matching
3 Satisfactory number of transplanted marrow cells
4 No prior transfusions

Key distinctions between organ and bone marrow transplant (BMT)
1 BMT requires immunoablation of host tissue
2 HLA matching is more important for BMT
3 Immunosuppression is more important for organ transplant
4 GVHD more often complicates BMT
5 Rejection more often complicates organ transplant

Disease-specific hazards of bone marrow transplantation
1 For immunodeficiency (e.g. Wiskott–Aldrich)
  — Graft-versus-host disease (GVHD) especially
2 For aplastic anemia
  — Graft rejection especially
3 For acute leukemia
  — GVHD, rejection and disease relapse constitute approximately equivalent risks to survival

Classification of transplant rejection
1 Hyperacute
  — Complement-fixing antibodies in recipient serum prior to transplant → irreversible Ag-Ab reaction usually presenting as graft thrombosis
2 Acute
  — Potentially reversible reaction due to cell-mediated immunity; occurs unpredictably and at any time
3 Chronic
  — Irreversible process due to subendothelial antibody deposition and arteriolar narrowing

Post-transplant malignancies
1 Squamous cell carcinoma of skin
2 Squamous cell carcinoma of cervix (usually in situ)

3 Non-Hodgkin's lymphoma
— In azathioprine-treated patients → CNS
— In ciclosporin-treated patients → GIT/Lung
4 Acute myeloblastic leukemia*

* NB: Only occurs after therapy with alkylators and/or irradiation

VASCULITIS THERAPY

Drug therapy in SLE: a rough guide
1 Minimally symptomatic disease
— Withhold medication
2 Tenosynovitis, arthralgias, pleurisy
— NSAIDs (except aspirin: potentially hepatotoxic)
3 Skin disease and/or joint symptoms resistant to NSAIDs
— Topical steroids (for rash)
— Hydroxychloroquine 200–400 mg/day
4 Refractory arthritis (sepsis excluded)
Immune leukopenia/thrombocytopenia
Fevers
— Prednisone 0.5 mg/kg/day
5 Immune hemolysis
Pneumonitis, peritonitis
Myositis
— Prednisone 0.75 mg/kg/day
6 Myopericarditis
Focal glomerulonephritis
Vasculitis, neuropathy
— Prednisone 1 mg/kg/day*
7 Diffuse proliferative glomerulonephritis
Membranous glomerulonephritis
— Acute phase (first 12 weeks)
• Pulse IV methylprednisolone 1 mg/kg/day, *plus*
• Cyclophosphamide* (2–3 mg/kg/day orally)
— Maintenance phase
• Azathioprine 1 mg/kg/day
8 Cerebral lupus
— Exclude infection, use anticonvulsants, and tailor immunosuppression as above

NB: If prolonged therapy > 10 mg/day prednisone is required, azathioprine may be added as a steroid-sparing agent
* May prolong survival

General measures in Raynaud's phenomenon
1 Cold avoidance (effective in 50% of all patients)
— Thermal underwear
— Gloves, warm socks (may be electrically heated)
— Maintenance of *steady* ambient temperature
2 Other general measures
— Arm exercises, biofeedback
— Stop smoking (esp. in Buerger's disease)
— Cessation of β-blockers, ergotamine

Specific therapies for Raynaud's disease
1 Oral nifedipine 20–60 mg/day
— Drug of choice: reduces attack frequency and severity
— Inhibits both vasospasm and platelet aggregation

— Effective in 50% of patients requiring medication
Alternative calcium blockers:
— Diltiazem 60 mg t.d.s.
— Nicardipine, felodipine, isradipine
2 Glyceryl trinitrate 2% ointment
— Useful for Raynaud's affecting odd sites (e.g. nipples)
— Works only transiently; causes headaches
3 Iloprost (prostacyclin analog)
— Particularly useful in aborting prolonged severe attacks (e.g. to prevent digital ulceration/necrosis)
— Requires IV administration in hospital
4 Second-line approaches in mild disease
— ACE inhibitors
— Alpha-blockers (moxisylyte/thymoxamine, prazosin)
— Ketanserin, naftidrofuryl (serotonin antagonists)
— Sympathectomy (for Raynaud's of the feet)
5 Plasma exchange
— Cryoglobulinemia patients esp.
6 Unproven therapies popular with patients
— Evening primrose oil (linolenic/gamolenic acid)
— Fish oil

UNDERSTANDING IMMUNOLOGICAL DISEASE

Classification of hypersensitivity reactions
1 Type I (immediate)
— IgE-mediated → *eosinophil chemotaxis*, e.g.
• Atopic asthma
• Hay fever
2 Type II (membrane-bound antigen)
— IgM/IgG-mediated → cell lysis (*cytotoxicity*) due to granulocyte/complement activation, e.g.
• Transfusion reactions
• AIHA, ITP, methyldopa hemolysis
• Anti-GBM disease (Goodpasture's syndrome)
— IgM/IgG-mediated → *receptor blocking*, e.g.
• Pernicious anemia
• Myasthenia gravis
• Hashimoto's disease
— IgM/IgG-mediated → *receptor activation*, e.g.
• Graves' disease
3 Type III (circulating immune-complexes)
— IgA/IgG-mediated → *Arthus reaction* (antibody excess)
• Hypersensitivity pneumonitis
• Allergic bronchopulmonary aspergillosis
— IgA/IgG-mediated → *serum sickness* (antigen excess)
• Rheumatic fever
• Post-infectious glomerulonephritis
• Secondary syphilis
• Lepromatous leprosy
• Henoch–Schönlein purpura
4 Type IV (delayed)
— T cell-mediated → *mononuclear chemotaxis*
• Graft rejection, graft-versus-host disease
• Contact dermatitis
• Tuberculin reaction; TB gumma/caseation
• Tuberculoid leprosy

Isotypes, idiotypes, and anti-idiotypic antibodies
1 The class of an antibody (IgG, IgM, etc.) is its *isotype*
2 Highly variable heavy and light chain regions (where antigen and antibody combine; i.e. in the Fab fragment) constitute a unique antibody specificity termed *idiotype*
3 Particular structural antigenic determinants comprising a given idiotype are termed *idiotopes*
4 An immunoglobulin contains many idiotopes which can generate a large number of *anti-idiotypic antibodies* raised against these antigens (cf. rheumatoid factors: antibodies raised against the constant Fc portion of the antibody)
5 Circulating idiotype/anti-idiotype immune complexes have been demonstrated (e.g. in cryoglobulinemia, SLE)

Regulatory functions of interleukins
1 Interleukin 1 (IL-1)
    — Following antigen recognition, IL-1 is released by activated macrophages, leading to stimulation of helper (CD4+) T cells with release of IL-2
    — Also induces proliferation of activated B cells
2 Interleukin-2 (IL-2), 'T cell growth factor'
    — Mitogenic for T cells and natural killer (NK) cells
    — Released by CD4+ (helper) T cells*
    — Stimulates IFN-production
3 Interleukin-3 (IL-3, multi-CSF)
    — Released by T cells and other cells
    — Stimulates growth of most hemopoietic stem cells

* cf. IL-1; released by monocytes/macrophages

Lymphocytes: functional aspects
1 B cells
    — Defence against extracellular bacteria, protozoa
    — Prevention of viral reinfection in immune host
2 T cells
    — Defence against intracellular bacteria
    — Defence against viruses (esp. herpes), fungi, protozoa
3 K ('killer') cells
    — Mediate antibody-dependent cell-mediated cytotoxicity (ADCC; e.g. against measles)
4 NK ('natural killer') cells
    — Non-antigen specific action
    — Postulated but unproven role in 'tumor surveillance'

Symptom mechanisms in mast cell-mediated diseases
1 Capillary leakage
    — Angioedema
    — Urticaria
    — Hypotension
2 Mucosal edema
    — Rhinitis, conjunctivitis
    — Laryngeal edema (stridor, asphyxia)
3 Smooth muscle spasm
    — Acute asthma

Common allergens underlying asthma
1 Housedust mite
2 Cockroach allergen
3 Cat allergen

Food allergy: common dietary culprits
1 Milk
2 Eggs
3 Peanuts (peas, beans)
4 Shrimp, prawns (crab, lobster)
5 Wheat (rye, corn)
6 Cod (mackerel, herring, plaice)

IMMUNE DEFECTS

Molecular defects underlying SCID
1 X-linked SCID
    — Mutation affecting cytokine receptor γ-chain
2 Autosomal recessive SCID
    — *JAK3* mutation
3 T- and B-cell-deficient SCID*
    — Mutation affecting adenosine deaminase
    — *RAG-1* or *-2* mutation

* The X-linked and autosomal recessive SCIDs are associated with T cell deficiency but normal B cell function

Clinical patterns of lymphocyte dysfunction
1 Ataxia–telangiectasia (Louis-Bar syndrome)
    — ↓ IgA
    — ↓ Cell-mediated immunity
    — Causes recurrent sinopulmonary infections
    — May terminate as lymphoma
2 Wiskott–Aldrich syndrome (WAS)
    — ↓ IgM; ↑ IgA/E
    — ↓ Cell-mediated immunity
    — ↓ Platelets
    — Causes eczema, abscesses, bleeding
    — May terminate as lymphoma

Infective complications of compromised immunity
1 Defective cell-mediated immunity (incl. Hodgkin's, sarcoid)
    — Intracellular bacteria (TB, *Listeria* spp.)
    — Candidiasis, cryptococcosis
    — CMV, HZ; toxoplasmosis
    — *Pneumocystis*, atypical mycobacteria
2 Hypogammaglobulinemia (incl. CLL, myeloma)
    — Extracellular bacteria (e.g. pneumococcus, *Staphylococcus aureus*)
    — *Mycoplasma* (septic arthritis, pneumonia)
    — CNS enteroviruses (e.g. ECHO in Bruton's)
    — Warts (↓ IgM); giardiasis, *Campylobacter* enteritis
3 Hyposplenism/post-splenectomy
    — Encapsulated bacteria (pneumococci, *H. influenzae, Salmonella* spp., *Neisseria meningitidis, Capnocytophaga canimorsus –* DF2); babesiosis*, malaria
4 Hypocomplementemia
    — ↓ $C_{2,3}$ → recurrent pyogenic infections, esp.
      • *S. aureus*
      • Streptococci
      • *H. influenzae*
    — ↓ $C_{6,7,8}$ → *Neisseria* spp. esp.
5 Combined B and T cell defects (CLL, SCID, WAS, Louis-Bar)
    — Recurrent sinopulmonary infections (CMV, Gram-negatives, anerobes, *S. aureus*)

6 Steroid therapy
— Aspergillosis
— *Pneumocystis carinii*

* In endemic areas, e.g. Massachussetts

PROBLEMS WITH POLYMORPHS

Clinical patterns of leukocyte dysfunction
1 Chédiak-Higashi syndrome
— Autosomal recessive; mutation of *LYST* gene (chr. 1q43)
— ↓ Neutrophil function (↓ intracellular killing) and myeloperoxidase deficiency
— Also defective T cell signalling; may lead to lymphoproliferative disease
— Associated with partial oculocutaneous albinism
— Treatable with vitamin C
2 Chronic granulomatous disease of childhood (CGDC)
— ↓ Intracellular killing (post-phagocytic defect)
— ↓ H_2O_2 generation
— + NBT test (diagnostic)
— *S. aureus*/Gram-negatives/*Nocardia* spp./*Serratia*
3 Job's/hyper-IgE syndrome
— ↓ Intracellular killing
— ↓ T cell number
— ↑ IgE
— Recurrent staphylococcal abscesses; herpes
4 'Lazy leukocyte' syndrome
— ↓ Chemotaxis
5 Leukocyte adhesion deficiency (LAD)
— Defective β-chain of LFA-1 integrin
— Associated with neutrophilia, but absent pus formation
— Severe bacterial childhood infections (e.g. pneumonia)

Infective complications of neutrophil dysfunction
1 Neutropenia
— Pneumonia (enterococci, Gram-negatives, *S. aureus*)
— Perirectal suppuration
— Pharyngostomatitis (esp. candidal)
— Recurrent bacteremias
2 Defective neutrophil chemotaxis (steroids, diabetes, alcohol)
— Abscesses, cellulitis (*S. aureus*, strep, *Pseudomonas aeruginosa*)
3 Defective intracellular killing (CGDC, Job's, Chédiak-Higashi)
— Abscesses (*Escherichia coli, S. aureus*)
— Septic arthritis/osteomyelitis (*Salmonella, Serratia*)

PRIMARY IMMUNE-DEFICIENT STATES

Varieties of primary immunoglobulin deficiency
1 X-linked (Bruton's) agammaglobulinemia*
2 IgG subclass deficiencies
3 Selective IgA deficiency
4 Common variable immunodeficiency

* Prone to enteroviral (esp. echovirus) infections; antibody-deficient patients are otherwise not usually troubled by viral infections

Selective IgA deficiency*: clinical features
1 Sinopulmonary infections (± otitis media)
2 Giardiasis (severe and prolonged)
3 Autoimmune diathesis (e.g. thrombocytopenia), atopy
4 Anaphylactic reactions triggered by small amounts of IgA in transfusions (blood or plasma) or gammaglobulin

* Surface IgA present *but* B cells fail to differentiate to plasma cells; may be associated with ↓ IgG_2. Often asymptomatic; affects 1 in 700

Common variable hypogammaglobulinemia*: complications
1 Allergies; autoimmune diathesis
2 Gastrointestinal complications
— Giardiasis
— Gluten-sensitive enteropathy/dermatitis herpetiformis
— Nodular lymphoid hyperplasia
— Achlorhydria/atrophic gastritis; 50× ↑ gastric cancer
3 Splenomegaly; lung/liver granulomata
4 Polyarthritis
5 Thymoma esp. in late-onset disease (i.e. onset after 40 years)

* *Normal* B cell number – cf. Bruton's – but fail to differentiate into plasma cells and secrete immunoglobulins; hence, low serum IgG and IgA

AUTOIMMUNE DISEASE

Clinical associations of thymoma
1 Myasthenia gravis (40%)
2 Pure red cell aplasia (*not* corrected by thymectomy)
3 Common variable hypogammaglobulinemia
4 Chronic mucocutaneous candidiasis
5 Autoimmune disease
— Sjögren s syndrome
— SLE
— Dermatomyositis
— Hashimoto's/Graves' disease
— Pemphigus

Female population prevalence of autoimmune disorders
1 Myasthenia gravis — 0.02%
2 Primary biliary cirrhosis — 0.1%
3 Multiple sclerosis — 0.2%
4 SLE — 0.2%
5 Rheumatoid/Sjogren's — ~ 2%
6 Graves'/Hashimoto's — ~ 3%

SECONDARY IMMUNE DEFECTS

Etiology of acquired hyposplenism
1 Splenectomy
   — Trauma (incl. operative)
   — Hypersplenism, esp.
     • ITP
     • Hereditary spherocytosis
     • Thalassemia
   — Hodgkin's staging (now uncommon)
2 Autosplenectomy
   — Repeated infarction in sickle cell disease
3 Celiac disease
4 Rare
   — SLE
   — Ulcerative colitis
   — Amyloidosis
   — Sarcoidosis
   — Thyrotoxicosis
   — Lymphoma, CML

Recommended prophylaxis for the hyposplenic patient
1 Pneumococcal vaccine
   — preferably 2 weeks before splenectomy, and every 5 years thereafter
2 Hib (*H. influenzae* type b) vaccine
3 Meningococcal groups A and C vaccine
4 Penicillin 250 mg b.d. for life

Features of overwhelming post-splenectomy infection (OPSI)
1 Incidence of OPSI is 1% in children, 0.1% in adults
2 Incidence is greatest in first 3 years post-splenectomy;
   10-year OPSI incidence is ~ 7%
3 Pneumococcal OPSI is a particular risk if age < 20
4 Incidence of OPSI varies with indication for splenectomy
5 10–20% of OPSI cases are polymicrobial

Effective antibiotic prophylaxis regimens post-splenectomy
1 Phenoxymethylpenicillin
   • 125 mg b.d. (age < 6)
   • 250 mg b.d. (age 6–12)
   • 500 mg b.d. (age > 12)
2 Amoxycillin
   — Covers *H. influenzae* as well as pneumococcus
     • 250 mg b.d. (age < 10)
     • 500 mg b.d. (age > 10)
3 Erythromycin
   — If penicillin-allergic
     • 125 mg b.d. (age < 3)
     • 250 mg b.d. (age > 3)

Predispositions to recurrent localized infections
1 Recurrent candidiasis
   — Steroids (incl. estrogens, pregnancy)
   — Broad-spectrum antibiotic therapy
   — T cell defects
2 Recurrent boils (furunculosis)*
   — Hypogammaglobulinemia

   — Hypocomplementemia
   — Job's/hyper-IgE syndrome
3 Recurrent candidiasis *or* boils
   — Diabetes mellitus
   — Iron deficiency‡
   — HIV infection

* Usually idiopathic
‡ Often subclinical; no anemia

Skin infections in immunosuppressed patients
1 'Transplant elbow'
   — *S. aureus*
2 Cellulitis
   — Streptococci
3 Opportunistic bacteria
   — *Nocardia*, atypical mycobacteria
4 Fungi
   — *Aspergillus, Cryptococcus*
5 Viruses
   — Herpes simplex, varicella-zoster; HPV

REVIEWING THE LITERATURE: IMMUNOLOGY, AUTOIMMUNE DISEASE AND TRANSPLANTATION

7.1 International Study of Asthma and Allergies in Childhood (ISAAC) Steering Committee (1998) Worldwide variation in prevalence of symptoms of asthma, allergic rhinoconjunctivitis, and atopic eczema: ISAAC. Lancet 351: 1225–1232

Study of 463 801 children in 155 countries, showing striking prevalence differences in atopic disorders: the highest were in UK, Australia, New Zealand and Ireland, whereas the lowest were in Eastern Europe and East Asia.

7.2 Gereda JE et al (2000) Relation between house-dust endotoxin exposure, type 1 T-cell development, and allergen sensitisation in infants at high risk of asthma. Lancet 355: 1680–1683

Prick testing of 61 infants aged 9–24 months was undertaken in parallel with measurement of house-dust endotoxin. The homes of allergen-sensitized infants contained significantly *less* housedust endotoxin than did those of non-sensitized infants, suggesting a possible role for early exposure to endotoxin in protecting against later sensitization.

7.3 Taylor MA et al (1991) Randomized controlled trial of homeopathy versus placebo in perennial allergic rhinitis with overview of four trial series. Br Med J 321: 471–476

Randomized double-blind placebo-controlled trial of 50 hay fever patients. No significant difference was apparent between the groups based on visual analog symptom scores.

7.4 Legendre C et al (1997) Transfer of symptomatic peanut allergy to the recipient of a combined liver-and-kidney transplant. N Engl J Med 337: 822–824

Case report documenting transmission of IgE-dependent peanut allergy via liver transplant. The transplant caused microchimerism within recipient skin, suggesting the escape of stem cells and/or dendritic cells from the graft.

7.5 Tamaoki et al (2000) Effect of suplatast tosilate, a Th2 cytokine inhibitor, on steroid-dependent asthma: a double-blind randomised study. Lancet 356: 273–278

Interesting early study of 77 asthmatic patients, showing symptomatic improvement in those receiving this novel IL-4/5 synthesis inhibitor; IL-5 promotes eosinophilia, whereas gain-of-function mutations in the IL-4 receptor have been linked to atopy.

7.6 Adkinson NF et al (1997) A controlled trial of immunotherapy for asthma in allergic children. N Engl J Med 336: 324–331

Double-blind placebo-controlled study of 121 allergic children receiving appropriate medical treatment, showing no additional benefit of putative aeroallergen extract injections on symptom control over 2 years.

7.7 Rai R et al (1997) Randomised controlled trial of aspirin and aspirin plus heparin in pregnant women with recurrent miscarriage associated with phospholipid antibodies. Br Med J 314: 253–257

Small study of 90 women with recurrent miscarriages and phospholipid antibodies, suggesting a possible increase in live births for those receiving heparin in addition to aspirin.

7.8 Kahan BD et al (2000) Efficacy of sirolimus compared with azathioprine for reduction of acute renal allograft rejection: a randomized multicentre study. Lancet 338: 1471–1475

In this study of 719 renal transplant recipients, use of the potent calcineurin inhibitor sirolimus (rapamycin) reduced the frequency and severity of acute rejection events.

7.9 Weiner JM et al (1998) Intranasal corticosteroids versus oral H1 receptor antagonists in allergic rhinitis: systematic review of randomized controlled trials. Br Med J 317:1624–1629

Meta-analysis of 2267 hay fever sufferers in 16 studies, showing that intranasal steroids were better than oral antihistamines.

7.10 Chan TM et al (2000) Efficacy of mycophenolate mofetil in patients with diffuse proliferative lupus nephritis. N Engl J Med 343: 1156–1162

Stewart SF et al (2001) Mycophenolate mofetil monotherapy in liver transplantation. Lancet 357: 609–611

Two studies reporting the immunosuppressive efficacy of this lymphocyte-inhibitory drug.

7.11 Hatakka K et al (2001) Effect of longterm consumption of probiotic milk on infections in children attending day care centres. Br Med J 322: 1327–1329

Kalliomaki M et al (2001) Probiotics in primary prevention of atopic disease: a randomised placebo-controlled trial. Lancet 357: 1076–1079

Two studies of probiotic therapy, the former showing modest apparent efficacy in preventing respiratory infections, and the second showing a halving of incidence of atopic eczema.

CHAPTER 8

Infectious disease

Physical examination protocol 8.1   You are asked to examine a patient with fever of unknown origin

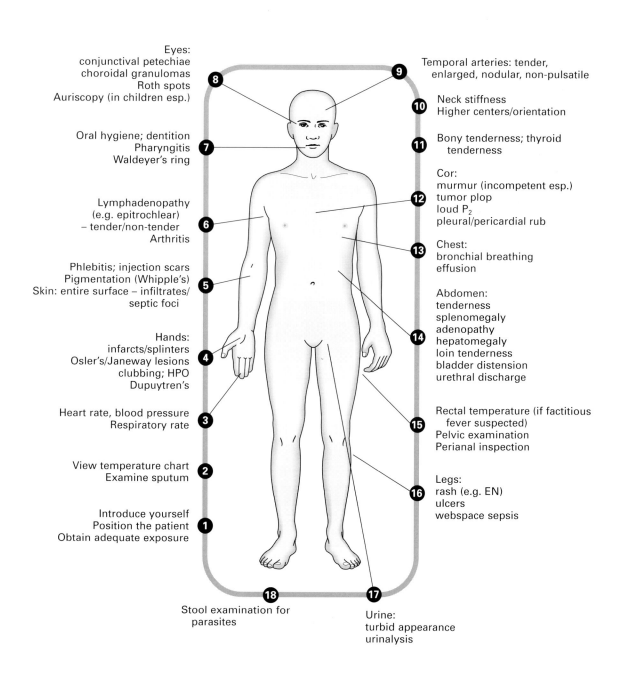

Eyes:
conjunctival petechiae
choroidal granulomas
Roth spots
Auriscopy (in children esp.)

Temporal arteries: tender,
enlarged, nodular, non-pulsatile

Neck stiffness
Higher centers/orientation

Oral hygiene; dentition
Pharyngitis
Waldeyer's ring

Bony tenderness; thyroid
tenderness

Cor:
murmur (incompetent esp.)
tumor plop
loud P_2
pleural/pericardial rub

Lymphadenopathy
(e.g. epitrochlear)
– tender/non-tender
Arthritis

Chest:
bronchial breathing
effusion

Phlebitis; injection scars
Pigmentation (Whipple's)
Skin: entire surface – infiltrates/
septic foci

Abdomen:
tenderness
splenomegaly
adenopathy
hepatomegaly
loin tenderness
bladder distension
urethral discharge

Hands:
infarcts/splinters
Osler's/Janeway lesions
clubbing; HPO
Dupuytren's

Rectal temperature (if factitious
fever suspected)
Pelvic examination
Perianal inspection

Heart rate, blood pressure
Respiratory rate

View temperature chart
Examine sputum

Legs:
rash (e.g. EN)
ulcers
webspace sepsis

Introduce yourself
Position the patient
Obtain adequate exposure

Stool examination for
parasites

Urine:
turbid appearance
urinalysis

Diagnostic pathway 8.1 The patient has an enlarged spleen. Which etiologies would you suspect?

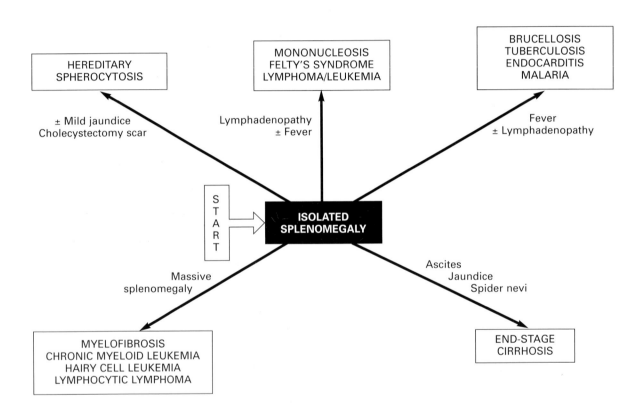

COMMON AND CLASSIC INFECTIOUS DISEASE CASES

Common infectious problems in clinical practice

1 Fever of uncertain origin
2 Management of antibiotic-resistant organisms
3 Tuberculosis

Classic infectious problems in clinical exams

1 Pneumonia and/or empyema
2 Zoonoses
3 Opportunistic infections

INFECTION-RELATED EMERGENCIES

Emergency treatment of *Plasmodium falciparum* malaria

1 For fulminant or cerebral malaria: admit to intensive care unit
2 Infusion of quinine dihydrochloride 20 mg/kg (= 15 mg/kg quinine base), diluted in crystalloid, over 4 h; then 10 mg/kg q 8 h; 5% dextrose to obviate risk of hypoglycemia; *or*
3 IMI artesunate or artemether if quinine causes difficult arrhythmias or hypotension
4 Measure blood parasite levels every 6 h

Adjunctive therapeutic measures in severe *P. falciparum* malaria

1 Exchange transfusion (5–10 units) if parasitemia > 10%
2 Dichloracetate (for lactic acidosis)
3 Desferrioxamine
4 Anticonvulsants
5 Dextrose infusion

CLINICAL ASSESSMENT OF INFECTIOUS DISEASE

Fever of unknown origin*: direct questions

1 Past medical history
   — Rheumatic fever
   — Tuberculosis
   — Splenectomy
2 Recent drug use
   — Antibiotics
   — Alcohol
   — Intravenous narcotics
3 Recent foreign travel
4 Recent sexual contacts and practices
5 Animal exposure (occupational or domestic)
6 Recent insect or tick bites
7 Recent ingestion of unusual or exotic food (or water)
8 Family history and racial background

* Defined here as fever with negative signs, CXR, MSU, and blood cultures

Common fevers in patients returning from tropical countries

1 Malaria
2 Dengue (and Lassa, Ebola, etc.; p. 207)
3 Typhoid
4 Tick typhus
5 Amebic liver abscess
6 Schistosomiasis; visceral leishmaniasis
7 Tuberculosis
8 Brucellosis

Factitious fever: clinical clues

1 Patient's apparent well-being
2 Normal physical examination, cool skin, no sweating
3 No correlation between fever spikes and heart rate
4 Consistently normal rectal temperature
5 Dramatic fluctuations of temperature, often > 41°C
6 Absence of normal diurnal variation
7 Normal WCC, ESR
8 Recovery of multiple and/or unusual organisms
9 Typical patient profile: young, female, (para)medical

Classical fever patterns

1 Fevers recurring every 48 h
   — 'Tertian' malaria
     • *P. vivax* (± *ovale*): 'benign tertian'
     • *P. falciparum*: 'malignant tertian'
2 Fevers recurring every 72 h
   — 'Quartan' malaria
     • *P. malariae*
3 Fevers lasting 1–2 weeks, alternating with afebrile periods of similar duration
   — Hodgkin's disease (Pel–Ebstein fever; rare)
4 Fevers recurring every 3 weeks
   — Cyclic neutropenia

Differential diagnosis of night sweats

1 Pulmonary tuberculosis
2 Lymphoma
3 Brucellosis; abscess; endocarditis
4 Alcoholic withdrawal
5 Nocturnal hypoglycemia
   Nocturnal dyspnea
   Nightmares

Diagnostic significance of localized lymphadenopathy

1 Inguinal adenopathy
   — Venereal diseases* (p. 201)
   — Perianal sepsis or malignancy
   — Lymphoma
2 Occipital adenopathy
   — Scalp infection (e.g. fungal) or neoplasm
   — Viral infection (e.g. rubella)
3 Cervical adenopathy
   — Mononucleosis; other viral infection
   — Streptococcal infection
   — TB (scrofula)
   — Lymphoma
   — Kikuchi's histiocytic necrotizing lymphadenitis
4 Axillary adenopathy
   — Catscratch disease; dogbite
   — Lymphoma; lung or breast cancer

5 Epitrochlear adenopathy
— Miliary TB
— Local pyogenic infection
— Lymphoma

* 'Groove sign' (adenopathy above and below inguinal
ligament) is said to be classical of LGV

TUBERCULOSIS: CLINICAL

Skin manifestations of TB
1 Primary skin inoculation
— Ulcer with regional adenopathy
2 Lupus vulgaris
— Nodules, scarring, face and neck
3 Scrofuloderma
— Cervical adenopathy, skin fixation
4 Erythema nodosum
— Signifies onset of Mantoux reactivity
5 Erythema induratum (Bazin's disease)
— Cyanotic nodules with central necrosis on calves

Manifestations commoner in primary TB infections
1 Chest
— Pleurisy and/or large pleural effusion*
— Lower zone infiltrate + ipsilateral hilar
adenopathy
2 Cervical adenopathy
3 Erythema nodosum
4 Phlyctenular conjunctivitis
5 Acute miliary dissemination

* May follow rupture of peripheral caseous foci

Time-course of sequelae following untreated primary TB
1 First 3–4 weeks post-inoculation
— Positive tuberculin test
— Erythema nodosum, fevers
— Phlyctenular conjunctivitis
• Esp. in children
2 After 4–8 weeks
— Appearance of primary focus on CXR
3 After 2–6 months
— Pleural effusion
4 After 3–12 months
— Bronchial rupture (erosion by caseating nodes)
— Tuberculous meningitis
— Miliary TB
5 After 1–3 years
— Bone and joint involvement
6 After 5 years
— Skin involvement
— Renal involvement

Misleading clinical presentations of TB
1 Night sweats, hilar adenopathy
Misdiagnosis: lymphoma
2 PUO, granulomas, splenomegaly, erythema
nodosum
Misdiagnosis: sarcoidosis*
3 Right iliac fossa mass and/or ileitis on barium
studies
Misdiagnosis: Crohn's disease, yersiniosis,
actinomycosis

4 Ureteric stricture(s)
Misdiagnosis: idiopathic retroperitoneal fibrosis*
5 Headache, meningism, CSF lymphocytosis, neg.
Gram-stain
Misdiagnosis: viral meningitis
6 Constrictive pericarditis
Misdiagnosis: restrictive cardiomyopathy‡
7 Bloodstained ascites
Misdiagnosis: abdominal malignancy
8 Scrotal (epididymal) mass
Misdiagnoses: tumor, syphilitic (testicular) gumma

* NB: Treated with steroids
‡ Attributable to (for example) endomyocardial fibrosis in
African migrant

Clinical features of tuberculous meningitis
1 Significance
— Potentially life-threatening
2 Onset
— Subacute (days → weeks)
3 Symptoms and signs
— Fever
— Headache, meningism
— Impaired consciousness
4 Complications
— Hydrocephalus, cerebral edema, convulsions
— Cranial nerve palsies
— Arachnoiditis; hemiparesis
— SIADH

NON-TUBERCULOUS MYCOBACTERIA

Clinical significance of non-tuberculous mycobacteria
1 Rarely transmitted between humans
2 Clinical pattern of involvement similar to that of TB
3 Positive culture does not necessarily indicate
pathogenicity in non-immunosuppressed patients
4 Clinical infection may indicate need for HIV
serologic testing

Clinical spectrum of non-tuberculous mycobacterial disease
1 Pulmonary
— *M. avium–intracellulare*
• Commonest and most serious pathogen
• Predilection for diseased lungs or AIDS
• Resistant to therapy (> 20% die)
— *M. fortuitum/chelonei*
• Predilection for diseased lungs
• Responds poorly to therapy
— *M. kansasii*
• Responds well to therapy
— *M. xenopi*, *M. szulgai*, *M. simiae* (rare)
2 Skin/soft tissue
— *M. marinum*
• Swimming-pool granuloma
• Responds poorly to drug therapy
• Usually resolves spontaneously
— *M. ulcerans*
• Responds poorly to drug therapy
• Treat by excision

— *M. fortuitum/chelonei*
  - Occurs following trauma or surgery
  - Best treated by initial debridement
3 Lymphadenitis (esp. cervical)
— *M. scrofulaceum*
  - Occurs in healthy children
  - Best treated by excision
  - Responds poorly to drug therapy
— *M. avium–intracellulare*
  - Treat by excision (see also p. 213)

SEXUALLY TRANSMITTED DISEASES

Post-exposure time-course of syphilitic presentations

1 Primary chancre
— 3–6 weeks
2 Secondary (skin) lesions
— 6 weeks–4 months
3 Meningitis
— 2–12 months
4 Meningovascular syphilis
— 4–8 years
5 General paresis of the insane (GPI)
— 5–25 years
6 Tabes dorsalis
— 10–50 years

Skin signs of secondary syphilis

1 Symmetric papulosquamous psoriasiform rash involving palms and soles; ± paronychia
2 Condylomata lata
3 Mucous patches (buccal)
   Mucosal erosions ('snail track' ulcers)
   Split papules
4 Leukoderma ('necklace of Venus')
5 Erythema nodosum
6 'Moth-eaten' alopecia

Clinical features of disseminated gonococcal infection

1 Typically occurs in young women or male homosexuals
   Symptoms of (primary) gonococcal infection may be absent
   Complicates approximately 2% of gonorrhea cases
2 Symptoms and signs include
— Fever
— Arthralgias/arthritis ± tenosynovitis
  - Asymmetrical; polyarticular, predilection for small joints of hands/wrists (cf. Reiter's)
— Pustular hemorrhagic skin lesions, esp. on limbs
— Myocarditis (may simulate rheumatic fever)
— Hepatitis (may simulate hepatitis B, cholecystitis)
— Perihepatitis (Fitz-Hugh Curtis syndrome*); if laparotomy is carried out in error, 'violin-string' adhesions are classically seen between the liver and abdominal wall (spread from fallopian tubes)
3 Laboratory investigations
— Cultures of urethra, endocervix, rectum, pharynx
— Blood and synovial fluid cultures: positivity of one tends to exclude the other; only 25% of clinically involved joints will yield gonococci

— Culture of skin lesions (positive only occasionally)
4 Pathogen characteristics
— Auxotype requires hypoxanthine/uracil for culture
— Serum-resistant (i.e. resists serum antibody/C_3)
— Penicillin-sensitive (exquisitely and regularly so)

* Also seen in chlamydial infection; rarely, occurs in bacteremic males

Vaginal discharges: typical presentations

1 *Candida albicans*
— Predispositions
  - Oral contraceptives
  - Antibiotics (esp. tetracyclines)
  - Diabetes mellitus
— Presentation
  - Marked pruritus vulvae
  - Perineal erythema
— Discharge
  - Scanty, cheesy, little odor
— Diagnosis
  - Gram-stain
2 *Trichomonas vaginalis*
— Venereally transmitted
— Presentation
  - Foul-smelling discharge
  - Pruritus often absent
  - Variable skin irritation
— Discharge
  - Yellow, foamy, offensive; often profuse
— Diagnosis
  - Direct microscopy: dark-field illumination
3 *Gardnerella vaginalis*
— Venereally transmitted
— Presentation
  - Malodorous discharge
  - No skin irritation
— Discharge
  - Greyish, foul-smelling ('fishy' odor)
— Diagnosis
  - Positive amine test
  - 'Clue cells' on microscopy
4 Gp B streptococci
— Uterine discharge post-partum
— Discharge
  - Foul-smelling lochia

ANAEROBIC INFECTION

Common anaerobic infections

1 Dental infections
2 Gynecological sepsis (e.g. septic abortion)
3 Abscesses: cerebral, lung, liver
4 Aspiration pneumonia
5 Biliary tract sepsis
6 Bite wounds

Factors predisposing to anaerobic infection

1 Mucosal injury
2 Microvascular disease
3 Tissue necrosis
4 Foreign bodies

ZOONOSES

Zoonoses: diseases transmitted to humans by animals
1 Leptospirosis/Weil's disease
  (*L. icterohemorrhagica*)
  'Plague' (*Yersinia pestis*)
  — From rats
2 Brucellosis (esp. *B. melitensis*)
  Q fever (*Coxiella burnetii*)
  Leptospirosis (*L. hardjo*)
  — From cattle
3 Salmonellosis (esp. *S. enteritidis*)
  — From cattle, poultry (esp. hens' eggs)*
4 Toxocariasis (*Toxocara canis*)
  Canicola fever (*Leptospira canicola*)
  Blastomycosis, leptospirosis
  Hydatids (*Echinococcus granulosus*)
  Bite wounds (*Pasteurella multocida*)
  Capnocytophagia canimorsus (DF-2)
  — From dogs
5 Toxoplasmosis (*T. gondii*)‡
  Tularemia; catscratch disease
  Bite wounds (*Pasteurella multocida*)
  — From cats
6 Campylobacter enteritis (*C. jejuni, C. coli*)
  — *C. jejuni* is the common human pathogen
  Yersiniosis (*Y. enterocolitica*)
  — From birds, poultry, pigs, dogs, cats
7 Rabies (rabiesvirus; a rhabdovirus)
  — From foxes, bats, small carnivores (in the wild)
  — From infected domestic dogs (or cats) in urban centers
8 Anthrax (*Bacillus anthracis*)
  — From goats, sheep
9 Equine morbillivirus (paramyxovirus) encephalitis
  — From horses

* cf. *Shigella* spp.: man is the natural host
‡ Commonest overall source is undercooked meat

Clinical features of specific zoonoses
1 Toxocara canis ('visceral larva migrans')
  — Transmitted to children by dogs
  — Systemic presentation ($\rightarrow$ age 1–4): rash, fever, cough, failure to thrive, eosinophilia
  — Retinal presentation ($\rightarrow$ older children): strabismus, unilateral loss of visual acuity, no eosinophilia
  — Diagnosis: ELISA or biopsy
  — R_x: tiabendazole* (if symptomatic), plus steroids for allergic manifestations
2 *Toxoplasma gondii*
  — Presentation: usually subclinical; may present with isolated non-tender adenopathy (DD_x: lymphoma)
  — Systemic presentation: malaise, fever, headache, mononucleosis-like syndrome
  — Ocular presentation: posterior uveitis (usually due to reactivation of in utero infection)
  — Severe congenital presentation (maternal infection in 1st/2nd trimester) may cause thrombocytopenia, hepatosplenomegaly, hydrocephalus

— Other presentations: CNS toxoplasmosis (e.g. in AIDS)
  — Diagnosis
    • Sabin–Feldman dye test (if available)
    • IgM antibody (for acute infections only)
  — R_x: sulfadiazine/pyrimethamine and folinic acid
3 *Echinococcus granulosus* (hydatid disease)
  — Transmitted to humans by dogs (definitive host) from sheep and cattle (intermediate hosts)
  — Presentation: enlarging cyst(s), esp. in liver and lung
  — Diagnosis: serology, biopsy (Casoni test non-specific)
  — Indications for surgery
    • Lung cyst   } *unless* calcified
    • Liver cyst > 5 cm }
  — Needle aspiration contraindicated
4 Brucellosis
  — Presentation: back pain, arthralgias, epididymo-orchitis, scrotal pain, cough, splenomegaly, endocarditis, weight loss, chronic fatigue, depression
  — Diagnosis: blood cultures, marrow culture, serology
  — R_x: doxycycline *plus* streptomycin (or rifampicin)
5 Leptospirosis
  — Septicemic phase: fever, aches and pains, conjunctival injection; renal involvement (pyuria, hematuria); diagnose by finding leptospires in blood or CSF
  — 'Immune phase': meningism, uveitis, rash; diagnose by demonstrating leptospiruria
  — Weil's disease (i.e. severe leptospirosis): jaundice, renal failure, cardiovascular collapse; with any serotype
  — Diagnosis (general): serology
  — R_x: parenteral penicillin or doxycycline‡
6 Yersiniosis
  — Organisms multiply in Peyer's patches
  — Ileitis/enterocolitis (esp. in children)
  — Mesenteric adenitis (may mimic appendicitis)
  — Reactive polyarthritis, erythema nodosum
  — Diagnosis: stool culture, paired sera
  — R_x: symptomatic ± co-trimoxazole
7 *C. canimorsus* (DF-2)
  — Immotile Gram-negative bacillus; normal in dogs, transmitted by dogbite
  — Predispositions to active infection: alcoholism (25%), splenectomy (25%), chronic airways disease or immunosuppression (25%)
  — Sepsis $\rightarrow$ meningitis/pneumonia/endocarditis
  — R_x: penicillin G (resistant to aminoglycosides)

* cf. 'cutaneous larva migrans' – caused by *Ancylostoma caninum/braziliense* – is treated with *topical* tiabendazole
‡ NB: Efficacy uncertain; may precipitate Herxheimer reaction

Organisms transmitted by human bite injuries
1 Streptococci, staphylococci
2 *Bacteroides* spp.
3 *Eikenella corrodens*
4 *Fusobacterium* spp.
5 *Peptostreptococcus* spp.

Organisms transmitted by dog bites*
1 Streptococci
2 *Staphylococcus aureus*
3 Anaerobes
4 *Pasteurella multocida*
5 *Capnocytophaga canimorsus*

* Best antibiotic cover is a macrolide

FOOD POISONING

Clinical spectrum of food poisoning
1 *Salmonella* (esp. *enteritidis, typhimurium*)
— Incubation period 12–48 h (toxin and infection)
— Source: raw meat/chicken/eggs/milk powder
— Fever, pain, diarrhea; may last several days (cf. typhoid)
— Incubation period 1–3 weeks
— Source: human fecal–oral transmission, polluted water
— Causes headache, initial constipation, fever (cf. cholera), cough, orchitis
2 *Staphylococcus aureus*
— Short incubation period 1–6 h (preformed toxin)
— Source: cold food (dairy products, sliced meats, salads)
— Vomiting prominent, no fever
3 Shigellosis
— Source: houseflies
4 *Listeria monocytogenes* ('Vacherin cheese disease')
— Incubation period 1 week
— Source: hot dogs/chicken, soft cheese, coleslaw
— Pregnancy infection → intrauterine fetal death
— Meningitis (30% die)
— Septicemia (esp. in T cell defects)
5 *Bacillus cereus*
— Incubation period 1–6 h (preformed toxin)
— Source: fried rice (→ vomiting; incubation 1–5 h)
— Diarrheal form → incubation 10–12 h
6 *Clostridium botulinum*
— Incubation period 12–36 h (preformed toxin)
— Source: canned food
— Vomiting, paralysis, apnea; constipation; nerve palsies
7 *Clostridium perfringens* (formerly *welchii*) – type A strain
— Incubation period 12–24 h (pre-formed toxin)
— Source: undercooked meat, poultry, vegetables
— Abdominal pain, diarrhea
8 Cryptosporidiosis
— Source: water, milk, raw sausages/offal
— Predispositions: travel, livestock exposure
— Causes watery diarrhea
— Common in AIDS (± isosporiasis)
9 Yersiniosis (see above)
— Source: pigs, raw pork

Seafood poisoning: specific pathogens and syndromes
1 *Vibrio parahemolyticus*
— Incubation period 24 h (toxin and infection)
— Source: seafood/shellfish (esp. shrimp)
— Vomiting, diarrhea; may last up to 5 days
2 *Vibrio vulnificus*
— Source: oysters, other raw shellfish
— Septicemic illness, shock, hepatitis, osteomyelitis, DIC
— Sensitive to ciprofloxacin
3 Domoic acid poisoning
— Source: mussels
— Excitotoxic encephalopathy
4 Eustrongylidiasis; gastric anisakiasis
— Source: eating sushi
5 *Diphyllobothrium latum*
— Finnish infestation
— Secondary B$_{12}$ deficiency
6 Ciguatera fish poisoning
— Toxin from flagellate *G. toxicus*
— Causes nausea, abdominal cramps, oropharyngeal paresthesiae, shooting pains in legs, pain in teeth
7 Scombroid fish poisoning (with mackerel, tuna; anchovies)
— Scombrotoxin = histamine (from fish histidine)
— Nausea, flushing, diarrhea, dizziness
— Treatable with cimetidine
8 Norwalk virus (p. 204), hepatitis A
— Source: raw shellfish, cold foods prepared by handlers

INFECTIVE DIARRHEAS

Common pathogens implicated in travellers' diarrhea*
1 Gram-negative bacilli
— Enterotoxigenic *E. coli*
— *Salmonella* spp.
— *Shigella* spp.
2 Curved motile Gram-negative bacilli
— *Vibrio* spp.
— *Campylobacter* spp.
— *Plesiomonas shigelloides*‡
— *Aeromonas hydrophila*
3 Protozoa
— *Giardia lamblia*
— Amebiasis
— Cryptosporidiosis
4 Viruses
— Norwalk (parvovirus)

* Therapy/prophylaxis: (1) ciprofloxacin (2) doxycycline
‡ From eating oysters

Clinical spectrum of *E. coli* diarrhea
1 Enterotoxigenic *E. coli* (ETEC)
— Clinically resembles cholera
— Commonest cause of travellers' diarrhea
— Organisms adhere to small bowel mucosa and release toxins
2 Enterohemorrhagic *E. coli* (EHEC)
— *E. coli* O157:H7 releases verotoxins*, causing
  • Hemorrhagic colitis (mimics ulcerative colitis)
  • Hemolytic uremic syndrome, TTP
3 Enteroinvasive *E. coli* (EIEC)
— Clinically resembles shigellosis (dysentery)
— Colonic invasion → mucosal ulceration

4 Enteropathogenic *E. coli* (EPEC)
— Adhere to gut mucosa, destroy microvilli
— Common cause of infantile diarrhea

* a.k.a. shigatoxins

Features of *Campylobacter** enteritis
1 Source: chickens (esp. fast-food)
— Illness resembles salmonellosis, shigellosis
— Affects older children and young adults
2 Rapid onset; duration less than 1 week
— Relapses in 25%
3 Severe abdominal pain, fever, myalgia, backache
— May simulate acute abdomen
— Bloody diarrhea in 60% ± toxic megacolon
4 Reactive arthritis (esp. if HLA B27+)
— May simulate inflammatory bowel disease
May also be complicated by Guillain–Barré syndrome
— Slow recovery and residual disability common
5 Culture requires special conditions ($\uparrow CO_2$, $\downarrow O_2$)
6 Antibiotics usually *not* indicated
— Erythromycin in severe disease
— Asymptomatic carriers *rare*

* *C. jejuni, C. coli*

Features of viral gastroenteritis
1 Rotavirus, esp. group A (DD_x = *Pestivirus*)
— Affects infants, young children (6 months–2 years)
— Incubation period 1–3 days; illness duration 1 week
— Mucosal IgA production confers lifelong immunity
— Vomiting prominent, dehydration common
2 Parvoviruses (esp. Norwalk virus)
— Affects all ages (esp. older children and adults)
— Produces winter epidemics ('winter vomiting disease')
— Fever, vomiting, abdominal pain common
— Illness duration ~ 48 h; incubation period 1–2 days
— No predictable development of immunity
— Asymptomatic carriage may occur (cf. *Campylobacter*)
— Frequently transmitted via shellfish ingestion
3 Astroviruses
— Usually affect children; may coinfect with rotavirus
— Cause mild, rotavirus-like diarrheal illness
4 Enteric adenoviruses
— Affect children (~ 3% of infantile gastroenteritis)

PRESENTATIONS OF INFECTIOUS DISEASE

'Spot' diagnosis of infectious diseases
1 Horder's spots
— Facial macules in psittacosis
2 Forschheimer's spots
— Soft palate lesions in rubella
3 Koplik's spots
— Bluish-grey buccal nodules in measles

4 Roth spots
— Pale-centered retinal infarcts in SBE*
5 Rose spots
— Truncal rash in 20% typhoid patients
6 Target lesions (erythema multiforme)
— *M. pneumoniae*, herpes simplex (esp.)

* Due to either septic microemboli or vasculitis

Features of staphylococcal toxic shock syndrome
1 Toxic (fever > 39°C)
2 Shock (systolic BP < 90 mmHg)
3 Rash
— Initially a diffuse 'sunburn-like' macular erythroderma
— About 10 days post-onset generalized desquamation supervenes, particularly affecting palms and soles
4 At least three of
— Vomiting or diarrhea
— Mucosal (conjunctival/pharyngeal/vaginal) hyperemia
— Myalgias ± rhabdomyolysis ($\uparrow$ CPK)
— Sterile pyuria and/or azotemia
— Abnormal liver function tests
— Thrombocytopenia
— Confusion (in absence of shock or high fever)
5 Vaginal/endocervix cultures for *S. aureus* (phage gp 1) are positive in about 98% of untreated patients*
Cultures of blood, throat and CSF are generally negative (very occasionally blood cultures may grow *S. aureus*). Staphylococcal exotoxin may be identified
6 Treatment consists of supportive measures (since symptoms are primarily toxin-mediated) ± flucloxacillin

* Not all cases occur in tampon users; e.g. nasal surgery may also predispose

Presentations of invasive group A streptococcal infections
1 Necrotizing fasciitis ('flesh-eating' disease)
2 Streptococcal toxic shock syndrome

UNUSUAL MICROORGANISMS

The rickettsioses: clinical syndromes
1 *R. rickettsi*
— Rocky Mountain spotted fever
2 *R. tsutsugamushi*
— Scrub typhus
3 *R. prowazekii*
— Epidemic typhus (louseborne; human reservoir)
— Brill–Zinser disease (recrudesence of latent disease)
4 *R. typhi*
— Endemic typhus (fleaborne; rodent reservoir)

Lyme disease (*Borrelia burgdorferi*): features
1 Skin lesions
— Erythema migrans (EM)
— Acrodermatitis chronica atrophicans
— Lymphocytoma

2 Neurological
— Meningism, cranial nerve (esp. VII) palsies, neuropathy
3 Cardiac
— AV block, myopericarditis
4 Arthritis
— Recurrent, asymmetric, often affects knee

Clinical spectrum of *Mycoplasma pneumoniae* infection
1 Community-acquired pneumonia, esp. in young patients
2 Cold agglutinin production ± hemolytic anemia
3 Erythema multiforme, Stevens–Johnson syndrome
4 Musculoskeletal and/or gastrointestinal upset
5 Neurologic effects: Guillain–Barré, aseptic meningitis
6 D_x: rising CFT, *M. pneumoniae* IgM/IgA, sputum ELISA

Microbial spectrum of venereal *Mycoplasma* spp. infections
1 *Mycoplasma hominis*
— Bacterial vaginosis
— Premature labor, miscarriage
2 *Mycoplasma genitalium*
— Non-gonococcal urethritis
— Pelvic inflammatory disease
3 *Ureaplasma urealyticum*
— Reactive arthritis (esp. in hypogammaglobulinemia)
— Non-gonococcal urethritis, epididymitis, PID
— Premature labor, miscarriage

Clinical spectrum of *Bartonella* spp. infections
1 *Bartonella henselae*
— Catscratch disease
2 *Bartonella quintana*
— Trench fever
3 *B. henselae* or *B. quintana* in HIV patients
— Bacillary angiomatosis-peliosis

Catscratch disease
1 Presentation
— Red papule with regional adenopathy
— Adenopathy suppurative in 30%
2 Differential diagnosis
— Mycobacterial lymphadenitis
3 Diagnosis
— Biopsy with Warthin–Starry stain
4 Treatment
— Symptomatic

MALARIA AND OTHER PARASITES

Malarial subtypes: the clinical distinction
1 *P. falciparum*
— Causes 75% malaria in Africa (+ almost all deaths)
— Presents within 3 months of exposure (cf. *vivax*)
— High mortality; dense parasitemia; often drug-resistant

— Presentations
• 'Cerebral malaria' (RBCs aggregate) ± hypoglycemia
• 'Blackwater fever'*
• Acute renal failure, DIC; pulmonary edema
— Does *not* relapse following effective treatment
2 *P. vivax*
— Responsible for 90% malaria in Asia
— Difficult to eradicate (due to exoerythrocytic phase)
— 10% of cases present over a year after exposure
— Manifests with persistent splenomegaly and/or anemia
— Prone to splenic rupture (may be spontaneous)
— Blood film: Schüffner's dots within parasitized red cell
— Symptoms may recur every few months for 10 years
3 *P. ovale*
— Contracted only in Africa
— Also exhibits exoerythrocytic phase and Schüffner's dots (hence primaquine treatment required; p. 214)
4 *P. malariae*
— Long incubation; prodromal symptoms common
— Red cell parasitization may persist for decades
— Late recrudescences may occur for up to 50 years; splenomegaly persists; symptoms usually mild
— Hematuria, nephrotic syndrome may occur

NB: *Quinine* R_x has been linked to both hypoglycemia and hemoglobinuria
* Intravascular hemolysis → hemoglobinuria

Endogenous protective factors in malarial regions
1 Acquired immunity (partial)
2 HLA Bw53*
3 Hemoglobinopathy
— HbS heterozygosity‡
— Ovalocytosis
— G6PD deficiency
— Increased HbF levels¶
4 ?Malnutrition
— ?Due to accompanying iron deficiency

* Allelic frequency in Africa is 40-fold greater than in Europe
‡ Confers 80% protection
¶ e.g. thalassemia minor

Predispositions to severe malaria
1 Extremes of age
2 Pregnancy
3 Hyposplenism*

* Incl. autosplenectomy in sickle-cell disease; cf. HbS heterozygotes

Laboratory markers of severe malaria
1 Hypoglycemia
2 Renal failure
3 Neutrophilia*
4 Markedly deranged LFTs
5 Elevated CSF protein (+ lactate)

* WCC more commonly low or normal in mild disease; anemia, thrombocytopenia may also be associated

Classical presentations of parasitic disease
1 'Duodenal ulcer' type pain
  — *Strongyloides stercoralis*
2 Iron-deficiency anemia ± hypoalbuminemia
  — Hookworm (*Ancylostoma/Necator*)
3 Intestinal/biliary obstruction
  — *Ascaris lumbricoides*
4 Rectal prolapse (+ bloody diarrhea, anemia)
  — *Trichostrongylus*; *Trichura* (whipworm)
5 Malabsorption
  — *Giardiasis* (a protozoon), capillariasis
6 Pruritus ani
  — *Enterobius* (pinworm, threadworm)
7 Hemoptysis (lung abscesses)
  — Paragonomiasis (may simulate TB)
  'Anchovy sauce' expectoration
  — Amebiasis (a protozoon) (hepatic)
8 'Grape skin' expectoration
  — Echinococcosis (hydatid disease)
9 Terminal hematuria
  — *Schistosoma hematobium*
10 Portal hypertension
  — *Schistosoma japonicum*
11 Pulmonary hypertension
  — *Schistosoma mansoni*
12 'Swimmer's itch'
  — Non-human schistosome cerceriae*
13 Cholangitis, pancreatitis, cholangiocarcinoma
  — *Clonorchis sinensis*
14 Lymphedema, elephantiasis
  — Filariasis
15 Vitamin B_{12} deficiency
  — *Diphyllobothrium latum*
16 Megaesophagus/-colon, cardiomyopathy
  — Chagas' disease (*Trypanosoma cruzi*)

* cf. 'swimming pool granuloma': from *Mycobacterium marinum*

VIRAL DISEASES

Lymphotropic viruses
1 EBV
2 CMV
3 HHV-6 (human herpesvirus-6)*
4 Adenoviruses

* Also known as human B cell lymphotropic virus (HBLV); resembles CMV

Distinguishing features of mononucleosis-like syndromes
1 EBV
  — Affects mainly adolescents (12–25 years)
  — Pharyngitis/tonsillitis prominent, may be exudative
  — Palatine petechiae characteristic, fever common
  — Tender cervical lymphadenopathy usual
  — Splenomegaly frequent
  — Lymphocytosis in 90% of cases
    • Relative lymphocytosis > 50%
    • Atypical lymphocytosis > 10%
  — Liver function tests abnormal in 90% (jaundice 5–10%)
  — Ampicillin rash in 90% of exposed cases

2 CMV
  — Affects mainly young adults (25–35 years)
  — Pharyngitis absent; fever prominent
  — Lymphadenopathy/splenomegaly unusual
  — Hepatomegaly usual (granulomatous hepatitis on biopsy); liver function tests often abnormal (esp. alkaline phosphatase); jaundice rare
  — Implicated in Rasmussen's encephalitis (refractory partial epilepsy + focal neurologic defects)
  — Atypical lymphocytosis less common than with EBV
  — Virus isolable from urine long after infection
  — Virus also isolable from secretions (e.g. saliva) or from buffy coat (i.e. leukocyte) blood fraction (best test)
  — Ampicillin rashes occur with same frequency as EBV
3 Toxoplasmosis (a protozoon)
  — Affects all age groups
  — Systemic symptoms unusual (usually subclinical)
  — Pharyngitis absent
  — Non-tender 'rubbery' lymphadenopathy common, may persist for up to 12 months
  — Splenomegaly unusual
  — Liver dysfunction, atypical lymphocytosis absent
  — Ampicillin rash not associated
  — May respond to antibiotics (spiramycin; co-trimoxazole, pyrimethamine/sulfadimidine)
4 HHV-6 (human herpesvirus-6)
  — Mononucleosis-like syndrome affects adults
  — Children → exanthem subitum (roseola infantum)
  — Fever unusual; non-specific viral syndrome
  — Non-tender cervical adenopathy
  — Virus persists in salivary glands
  — Atypical lymphocytosis usual
  — May cause pneumonia in immunosuppressed
5 Early HIV infection
  — Affects mainly homosexuals (> IV drug abusers)
  — Occurs within 2–6 weeks of primary HIV infection
  — Sudden onset (cf. EBV: insidious)
  — Short duration (about 2 weeks)
  — Prominent *rash* (± fever/pharyngitis/ adenopathy)
  — Often associated with oral/genital/anal *ulcers* ?reflecting portal of virus entry
  — Cough and/or watery diarrhea also common
  — No atypical lymphocytosis
  — No hepatosplenomegaly or abnormal liver function
  — Neurologic abnormalities unusual (cf. later HIV)
  — Patients usually well for 2–3 years subsequently

Parvovirus B19: the clinical spectrum
1 Erythema infectiosum
  — Fifth disease ('slapped-cheek' syndrome)
  — Often misdiagnosed as rubella; peak age 4–11
2 Anemia
  — Aplastic crises (e.g. in sickle-cell, spherocytosis)
  — In AIDS, ALL, Nezelof's syndrome*

3 Symmetric polyarthropathy (esp. in adult women)
— Rubella-like; rheumatoid factor negative
4 Fetal abnormalities
— Hydrops fetalis
— Intrauterine fetal death

* Treatable with IV gammaglobulin

Human papillomavirus (HPV): clinical associations
1 Type 1
— Plantar warts
2 Type 3
— Flat warts
3 Type 5/8
— Skin SCCs in transplant patients
4 Type 7
— Common warts in food handlers
5 Types 6 and 11
— Condylomata acuminata (genital warts)
— Juvenile laryngeal papillomatosis
6 Type 13
— Oral leukoplakia
7 Types 16 and18* > types 31, 33, 35, 51, 52, 58 > 45, 56, 59, 67
— SCC cervix
— SCC penis
— SCC anus
— SCC vulva
8 Type 30
— SCC larynx

* HPV-18 is associated with younger onset of cervix cancer, more aggressive histology and stage, higher frequency of adenocarcinoma and more frequent implication in South-East Asian cohorts, compared with the more prevalent HPV-16

Complications of viral infections
1 Influenza A
— Staphylococcal/pneumococcal pneumonia
— Meningococcal disease
2 Measles
— Reactivation of pulmonary TB
— Bacterial pneumonia
— Encephalomyelitis, SSPE
3 Mumps
— Meningitis, deafness, thyroiditis, pancreatitis
— Paroxysmal cold hemoglobinuria
— Orchitis (common), sterility (rare)
4 Varicella-zoster
— Miliary calcification on CXR
— DIC
5 CMV
— Guillain–Barré syndrome
— Myopericarditis
— Necrotizing pneumonitis in transplant patients
6 Coxsackie A
— Aseptic meningitis, paralysis
— Herpangina
— 'Hand, foot and mouth' disease (esp. A16)
— Acute hemorrhagic conjunctivitis (esp. A24)*
7 Coxsackie B
— Pleurodynia; myopericarditis
— Pancreatitis, orchitis
— ?Diabetes mellitus
8 JC virus (a papovavirus)
— Progressive multifocal leukoencephalopathy

9 Parvovirus
— Fifth disease ('slapped cheek' syndrome)
— Aplastic crisis in sickle-cell disease

* Also caused by enterovirus 70

VIRAL HEMORRHAGIC FEVERS

Classification of the viral hemorrhagic fevers
1 Togaviruses
— Alphaviruses (mosquito-borne)
• Chikungunya fever (Asia)
• O'nyong nyong (Africa)
— Flaviviruses (mosquito- and tick-borne)
• Dengue fever (Asia, Africa, Pacific, Caribbean)
• Yellow fever (Africa, S. America)
• Kyasanur Forest disease (Asia)
• Omsk hemorrhagic fever (Central Asia)
2 Bunyaviruses (mosquito- and tick-borne)
— Congo–Crimean fever (Africa, Asia)
— Rift Valley fever (Africa)
— Korean hemorrhagic fever (Hantaan virus: Asia)
3 Arenaviruses (rodent-borne)
— Lassa fever (Africa)
— Argentinian hemorrhagic fever (Junin virus)
— Bolivian hemorrhagic fever (Machupo virus)
— Venezuelan hemorrhagic fever (Guanarito virus)
— Brazilian hemorrhagic fever (Sabla virus)
4 Filoviruses (nosocomial transmission)
— Marburg virus disease (Europe, Asia, Africa)
— Ebola virus disease (Africa)

The viral hemorrhagic fevers: differential diagnostic features
1 Marburg/Ebola viruses
— Filoviruses; African endemicity
— Nosocomial spread (transmissible by blood products)
— Different incubations, similar manifestations
— Presentation (abrupt onset)
• Headache, conjunctivitis, back pain, arthralgias
• Diarrhea ± melena
• Pleurisy, psychosis, proteinuria
• DIC; characteristic hemorrhagic rash
2 Lassa fever
— An arenavirus*; African endemicity
— Rodent-borne; transmission similar to filoviruses
— Presentation (insidious onset; may be subclinical)
• Pharyngitis, lymphadenopathy, nephrosis
• Hypoxic death, esp. in pregnancy
— Management: barrier nursing, ribavirin‡
3 Dengue fever
— A flavivirus (four serotypes); South Pacific endemicity
— Presentation
• Rash, DIC
• Shock (esp. in infants with previous infection)
4 Korean hemorrhagic fever with renal syndrome
— Due to Hantaan virus; rodent-borne¶
— Presentation
• Nephrosis, acute renal failure
• *Mild* hemorrhagic signs in Korean variant

Hantavirus pulmonary syndrome (a distinct hantavirus)
- Fulminant non-cardiogenic pulmonary edema

5 Congo–Crimean fever
— Tick-borne
— Similar to Kyasanur Forest disease (India)
— Presentation
- Severe hemorrhagic sequelae
- Chest pains, oropharyngitis

6 Yellow fever
— Mosquito-borne
— Similar to Rift Valley fever (also in Africa)
— Presentation
- Arthritis
- Retinal damage
- Jaundice (hence 'yellow') in convalescent phase
- Black vomitus (+ other hemorrhagic signs)

* Similar syndromes seen with other arenaviruses, notably Junin (Argentinian) and Machupo (Bolivian) fevers
‡ NB: For Junin-type disease, give 500 mL high-titre immune plasma
¶ Same virus probably responsible for *nephropathica epidemica* in Scandinavia (a related bunyavirus may cause Balkan nephropathy)

INVESTIGATING INFECTIOUS DISEASE

Diagnoses suggested by direct microscopy

1 Acid-fast bacteria to Ziehl–Neelsen staining
— *Mycobacteria* spp.
Catalase-positive, niacin-negative, INH-resistant
— Atypical (non-tuberculous) mycobacteriosis

2 Weakly acid-fast organisms
— *Nocardia* (aerobic) spp.
— *Actinomyces* (anaerobic) spp.

3 Dark-field examination
— *Treponema pallidum*

4 Silver methenamine stain
— *P. carinii*

5 Indian ink stain (CSF)
— *Cryptococcus neoformans*

6 Romanowsky stained thick and thin films*
— *Plasmodia* spp.

7 Gram-negative diplococci in WBCs (cervical/urethral swab)
— *Neisseria gonorrheae*

8 Inclusion bodies within urethral epithelial cells
— *Chlamydia trachomatis*

9 Pyogenic meningitis in adults: Gram-positives in CSF
— Pneumococcal meningitis (presumptive)
Pyogenic meningitis in adults: Gram-negatives in CSF
— Meningococcal meningitis (presumptive)

* Antigen capture assays are now a popular alternative

Diagnostic value of throat swabs

1 Gp A β-hemolytic strep (see below)
2 Gonococcal pharyngitis
3 *Mycoplasma pneumoniae*
4 Diphtheria, pertussis
5 Some viral infections: polio, rubella

Diagnosis of streptococcal pharyngitis

1 Throat swab (culture)
— Heavy growth confirms diagnosis
— Diagnosis excluded by negative swab
— 'Light growth' unhelpful

2 Throat swab (rapid antigen test)
— ELISA directly confirms strep antigen presence
— 90% specificity and sensitivity

3 Supportive tests
— C-reactive protein (p. 367)
- Levels higher in bacterial than viral infections
— ASO titre
- Rising titre useful if retrospective D_x needed
— Heterophile antibody ('Mono spot')
- Useful in excluding EBV

Diagnostic utility of bone marrow culture

1 Miliary tuberculosis
2 Brucellosis
3 Typhoid
4 Kala-azar

TUBERCULOSIS: INVESTIGATIONS

Diagnostic criteria in pulmonary tuberculosis

1 Suggestive
— Clinical context
— Radiographic appearance*
— Positive tuberculin test, esp. if converts
— Positive antibody to 38 kDa TB antigen

2 Presumptive
— Acid-fast bacilli in sputum/gastric washings
— Caseating granulomata on biopsy

3 Definitive
— *Mycobacterium tuberculosis* isolated on culture

* NB: *Activity* of TB *cannot* be assessed from CXR

Diagnosis of tuberculous meningitis

1 Routine CSF examination
— ↑ Mononuclears
— ↑ Protein
— ↓ Glucose

2 Special CSF examination
— ↓ Chloride
— ↓ Serum/CSF bromide partition ratio
— Positive tryptophan assay

3 Diagnostic CSF examination
— Acid-fast bacilli on Ziehl–Neelsen staining, confirmed as tuberculous on culture (NB: usually negative)

4 CXR, tuberculin test
— Useless (negative in up to 50%)

The false-negative tuberculin test: differential diagnosis

1 Extremes of age
2 Very recent infection (< 10 weeks since inoculation)
3 Viremia (e.g. measles, influenza)
Following live vaccination (e.g. rubella)
4 Severe systemic disease
— Septicemia (incl. miliary tuberculosis)
— Carcinomatosis and/or cytotoxic therapy
— Uremia, malnutrition
— Tuberculous meningitis

5 Defective T cell function
— Hodgkin's disease and/or thymic irradiation
— Sarcoidosis
— Wiskott–Aldrich, di George, SCID
— AIDS (NB: test hazardous to perform)
6 Drugs
— Steroids, other immunosuppressives
7 Technical problems
— Inadvertent subcutaneous injection
— Adsorption of antigen to syringe
— Substandard potency of preparation

SYPHILIS SEROLOGY

What tests are available for diagnosing syphilis?
1 Dark-field examination
— For direct spirochetal identification
2 Reaginic (flocculation) tests
— VDRL (best test; quantitative)
— WR (little used now)
— RPR (used in outlying areas)
3 Specific treponemal serologic tests*
— FTA-ABS
— TPI
— TPHA

* Positive for life after initial infection; hence, not appropriate for monitoring therapeutic adequacy

Positive dark-field examination: differential diagnosis
1 Primary syphilitic chancre
2 Secondary syphilis (mucosal lesions)
3 Congenital syphilis (mucosal lesions)
4 Non-pathogenic oral or rectal treponemes

Sensitivity of reaginic tests (e.g. VDRL) in established syphilis
1 Primary syphilis
— Positive in 80% (reliably negative within 2 years of R_x)
2 Secondary syphilis
— Positive in 99%
3 Late/latent syphilis
— Positive in 70% (may remain positive long after R_x)
4 Neurosyphilis
— CSF positive in 50% (i.e. 50% false-negative rate*)

* cf. CSF VDRL: false-positives *rare* unless 'bloody tap' contaminates sample

Causes of chronic reaginic false-positives
1 Non-treponemal bacterial infections
— Leprosy*, leptospirosis*, malaria*
— Venereal: LGV, chancroid
— Tuberculosis, psittacosis, rickettsial disease
2 Viral infections
— Infectious mononucleosis*
— Viral hepatitis
— HIV
3 Autoimmune disease
— SLE*
4 Narcotic abuse

5 Chronic liver disease
6 Pregnancy
7 Neoplasia
— Carcinomatosis
— Myeloma, lymphoma
8 Multiple blood transfusions

* May also cause false-positive treponemal serology (e.g. FTA-ABS)

Choosing the most appropriate test in suspected syphilis
1 Primary (recent) exposure
— Dark-field examination of primary chancre
— FTA-ABS is the first test to become positive
2 Secondary syphilis
— Dark-field examination if skin/mucosal lesions present
— VDRL
3 Screening (pregnant women, prostitutes, contacts of cases)
— VDRL
— If positive, do FTA-ABS
4 Follow-up (of primary/secondary/late syphilis) after therapy
— VDRL at 3, 6, 12 months*
— If titre unchanged after 12 months, re-treat
5 Exclusion of neurosyphilis
— CSF FTA-ABS (negativity reliably excludes diagnosis)

* Titer should decline 4-fold by 3 months and 8-fold by 6 months

Diagnostic significance of syphilis serology
1 Positive VDRL
Positive FTA-ABS
— Syphilis (yaws, pinta, bejel)
2 Positive VDRL
Negative FTA-ABS
— Biological false-positive
3 Negative VDRL
Positive FTA-ABS
— Early, latent, late or treated syphilis
4 Positive FTA-ABS (IgM)
— Congenital syphilis*

* cf. IgG only: implies passive transfer of maternal antibody

Neurosyphilis: CSF monitors during treatment
1 Total protein
2 Mononuclear cell count
3 Quantitative VDRL titre *if* positive prior to treatment*

* CSF VDRL is 100% specific but only 50% sensitive

FEVER OF UNKNOWN ORIGIN

Considerations in the investigation of unexplained fever
1 Exclude
— Drug allergy
— Surreptitious drug abuse
— Factitious fever

2 Bone marrow examination
— Aspiration/trephine (lymphoma)
— Bone marrow culture
3 Unusual organism suspected
— Acid-fast stains, etc.
— Thick and thin blood films
— Plasma immunoassays
• *Candida* enolase antigenemia
• *Aspergillus* antigenemia
4 Abscess suspected
— CT/ultrasound
— Scintigraphy
• ^{67}Gallium-scanning
• ^{111}Indium-leukocyte (or IgG) scanning
5 Invasive fungal infection suspected (e.g. post-transplant)
— Plasma (1→3) β-D-glucan
— Candida enolase antigenemia
6 HIV serology or PCR

Possible indications for gallium scanning
1 Fever of unknown origin (?abscess, e.g. subphrenic; ?lymphoma)
2 Monitor activity of sarcoidosis
3 Detect AIDS complications
4 Evaluation of chronic osteomyelitis

Infections causing profound peripheral eosinophilia
1 Trichinosis (diagnosis by serology or muscle biopsy)
2 Visceral larva migrans (*Toxocara canis*) esp. in children
3 Tropical pulmonary eosinophilia (filariasis)

Discrepancies in antibiotic predictivity testing
1 Infection 'sensitive' to prescribed antibiotic, but does not respond
— Bugs isolated are not the cause of the infection
— Antibiotics do not reach site of infection
— Inadequate antibiotic dose
— Infection is too advanced
2 Infection 'resistant' to prescribed antibiotic, but resolves
— Bugs isolated are not the cause of the infection
— Infection resolves anyhow

DIAGNOSTIC STUDIES IN OTHER INFECTIONS

Infectious mononucleosis: making sense of the serology
1 VCA (viral capsid antibody; IgG)
— Positivity indicates past or present infection
2 EA (antibody to EBV 'early antigen')
— Appears within 2–3 weeks of symptom onset
— 'D' (diffuse) component disappears within months; useful marker of current infection if positive
— 'R' (restricted) component may persist for years, esp. in relapsing disease
3 EBV specific IgM (i.e. to viral capsid antigen)
— Tends to parallel heterophile antibody rise (see below)
— Usually becomes negative within 3 months of onset

— Extremely useful in heterophile-negative cases; the best test for confirming acute disease
4 EBNA (EB virus-associated nuclear antigen)
— Viral antigen detected by immunofluorescence
— Indicates infected cells harboring viral genome
5 EBNA antibody (IgG)
— Appears late
— Indicates previous infection; persists lifelong
6 Heterophile antibody (IgM)
— i.e. heterophile agglutinins for sheep erythrocytes
— Basis of Paul–Bunnell test (diagnostic); present in 90%
— Similar (Forssman-type) agglutinins seen in hepatitis, lymphomas, etc; adsorbed out by guinea pig kidney*
— May be misleadingly negative for up to a month after symptom onset; tedious and expensive to perform

* cf. positive Paul–Bunnell: antibodies adsorbed out by ox (beef) erythrocytes

Weil–Felix reactions: diagnostic significance
1 Epidemic (*R. prowazekii*) typhus
— OX-19 positive
Brill–Zinsser disease (recurrent epidemic typhus)
— All negative
2 Scrub (*R. tsutsugamushi*) typhus
— OX-K positive
3 Rocky Mountain (*R. rickettsii*) spotted fever
— OX-19 and OX-2 positive
4 Q (*Coxiella burnetii*) fever
— All negative (see below)
5 *Proteus* spp. infections, brucellosis, typhoid, leptospirosis
— False-positives

Diagnosis of Q fever
1 Complement fixation test (CFT)
2 Acute disease → 4× ↑ phase II antibody titre
3 Chronic disease → persistent ↑ phase I and II Ab titre
4 Endocarditis → > 1:200 phase I Ab titre

Diagnosis of genital ulcers ± inguinal adenopathy
1 Positive dark-field examination
— Primary syphilis
2 *H. ducreyi* on microscopy/culture
— Chancroid
3 Donovan bodies on microscopy
— Granuloma inguinale*
4 *Chlamydia* on culture/serology
— Lymphogranuloma venereum
5 *H. simplex* on viral culture
— Genital herpes
6 Negative microbiology
— Consider Behçet's/Reiter's syndrome

* Bipolar staining bacilli visible within monocytes, reflecting presence of *Calymmatobacterium inguinale*

Laboratory diagnosis of specific infections
1 Gonorrhea
— Immediate plating and Gram-stain
— Urethral culture in chocolate (blood) agar
— Endocervical/anorectal/pharyngeal culture in Thayer-Martin (antibiotic-enriched) medium

2 Typhoid
   — Blood cultures; stool and urine cultures
   — Widal test: > 4× ↑ antibody titre to 'O' (cell wall) antigen
3 Cryptococcal meningitis
   — Cryptococcal antigen in CSF (most sensitive test)
   — CSF culture (most specific test)
   — Indian ink stain (quickest test)

MANAGING INFECTIOUS DISEASE

PRINCIPLES OF ANTIBIOTIC CHEMOTHERAPY

Mechanisms underlying antibiotic activity
1 Interference with bacterial cell wall synthesis
   — β-lactams (penicillins, cephalosporins)
     • Prevent proteoglycan crosslinking by inhibiting transpeptidases
   — Vancomycin
     • Inhibits proteoglycan formation by sequestering substrate (D-Ala-D-Ala terminus of peptidoglycan)
2 Interference with fungal cell wall synthesis
   — Imidazoles (ketoconazole, miconazole, clotrimazole)
     • Inhibit ergosterol synthesis (making cells 'leaky')
3 Interference with bacterial protein synthesis
   — Aminoglycosides
     • Distorts bacterial 30S ribosomal subunit → ↓ mRNA attachment and translation
   — Tetracycline
     • Blocks aminoacyl-tRNA binding to 30S ribosome
   — Chloramphenicol; oxazolidinones (e.g. linezolid)
     • Block 50S ribosome transpeptidation
   — Macrolides
     • Block bacterial 50S ribosomal translocation
   — Fusidic acid
     • Inhibits ribosomal GTPase (= elongation factor)
4 Interference with folate metabolism
   — Sulfonamides (PABA analogs → ↓ dihydropteroate)
   — Trimethoprim (inhibits bacterial DHFR)
   — 5-Flucytosine (fungal antimetabolite)
5 Interference with DNA gyrase (bacterial topoisomerase II)
   — Nalidixic acid
   — Fluoroquinolones*
6 Other mechanisms
   — Metronidazole: inhibits anaerobic electron transfer
   — Nitrofurantoin: interferes with bacterial acetyl CoA
   — Rifampicin: inactivates bacterial RNA polymerase
   — Aciclovir: inhibits viral DNA polymerase‡

* Both contraindicated in children
‡ Drug is selectively activated by viral thymidine kinase

Bioavailability of antibiotics at specific sites of infection
1 CSF
   — Cefotaxime, cefuroxime, ceftriaxone*
   — Penicillins (during meningitis only)
   — Chloramphenicol; erythromycin; metronidazole
   — Isoniazid/rifampicin/pyrazinamide
   — 5-FC (flucytosine), fluconazole
2 Bile
   — Penicillins (e.g. mezlocillin)
   — Cephalosporins
   — Erythromycin
3 Urine
   — Penicillins, cephalosporins
   — Sulfonamides, trimethoprim
   — Aminoglycosides
   — Nitrofurantoin, nalidixic acid
   — Ethambutol
   — Fluoroquinolones
   — Fluconazole, flucytosine

* i.e. *unlike* other cephalosporins

Non-absorbable antibiotics
1 Nystatin
2 Neomycin
3 Colistin
4 Framycetin
5 Vancomycin

Bactericidal antibiotics
1 β-lactams*
   — Penicillins
   — Cephalosporins
   — Imipenem (a carbapenem)
   — Aztreonam (a monobactam)
2 Aminoglycosides
3 Rifampicin
4 Metronidazole
5 Fluoroquinolones

* cf. β-lactamase *inhibitors*: negligible antibacterial activity

Relative indications for bactericidal antibiotic therapy
1 Infective endocarditis
2 Bacterial meningitis
3 Febrile neutropenia

TREATMENT OF ANAEROBIC INFECTIONS

Antibiotics with anaerobic specificity

1	Metronidazole Imipenem Chloramphenicol Co-amoxiclav*	Good activity against *Bacteroides fragilis*
2	Clindamycin Cefoxitin Piperacillin	Moderate activity against *Bacteroides fragilis*
3	Penicillin G Tetracycline Erythromycin	Poor activity against *Bacteroides fragilis*

* Amoxicillin + clavulanic acid

Metronidazole: indications for parenteral administration

1 Prior to urgent surgery if anaerobic sepsis suspected
2 Proven anaerobic infections resistant to oral or rectal therapy
3 Patients with vomiting, diarrhea and known anaerobic sepsis
4 Life-threatening sepsis in patients with anaerobic source

PROPHYLACTIC ANTIBIOTICS

Antibiotic prophylaxis regimens

1 Rheumatic fever (maintenance prophylaxis)
   — 1.2×10^6 U penicillin G IM monthly, or
   — 250 mg penicillin V orally b.d. until adulthood; lifelong prophylaxis if significant valve disease
2 Infective endocarditis (intermittent prophylaxis)
   — Dental work
     • Amoxicillin 3 g p.o. 1 h pre-, 6 h post, or
     • Clindamycin 300 mg IV pre, 150 mg p.o. 6 h post
   — Genitourinary/colonic instrumentation
     • Ampicillin 1 g IV + gentamicin 2 mg/kg IV 30 min pre-, then amoxicillin 1 g orally q 6 h
   — Penicillin allergy
     • Clindamycin 600 mg p.o. 1 h before, or
     • Vancomycin 1 g slow IV + gentamicin, or
     • Teicoplanin 400 mg IV + gentamicin
3 Tuberculosis
   — Isoniazid 300 mg daily p.o. for 6–12 months, plus
   — Pyridoxine 25 mg daily p.o. for 6–12 months
4 Pneumocystis carinii (in marrow transplant recipients)
   — Trimethoprim/sulfamethoxazole (best)
   — Aerosolized pentamidine (expensive, less effect)
5 Infant contacts of epiglottitis (H. influenzae type B)
   — Rifampicin 20 mg/kg daily for 4 days

Malarial prophylaxis: general measures

1 Minimize or avoid travel to endemic regions
2 Avoid mosquito bites
   — Cover exposed skin with clothing, esp. at night
   — Use repellents and (within bedrooms/tents) insecticide
   — Use bednets if mosquitos cannot be excluded

Prophylactic antimalarial chemotherapy regimens*

   — Non-resistant area, or during pregnancy‡:
     • Chloroquine
   — Endemic non-falciparum chloroquine resistance
     • Chloroquine + pyrimethamine/dapsone
   — Falciparum area
     • Mefloquine (in highly resistant areas) or
     • Chloroquine + proguanil
     • Primaquine
     • Doxycycline (investigational)

* NB: Recommendations change often
‡ Ideally, pregnant women should avoid elective travel to malarious areas

MANAGING MYCOBACTERIAL DISEASE

Relative indications for BCG vaccination

1 Medical or laboratory workers exposed to tubercle bacilli
2 Neonates exposed to active TB
3 Tuberculin-negative children/adolescents in endemic areas

Therapeutic indications for tuberculin skin testing

1 To assess need for isoniazid prophylaxis in non-BCG-treated contacts (esp. children) of active tuberculosis cases
2 To assess need for BCG immunization in children
3 To assess TB prevalence in different communities
4 To investigate individuals suspected of having active TB

Indications for prophylactic isoniazid therapy

1 A tuberculin-positive individual younger than 50 (esp. a child):
   — Is a member of a household in which a recent diagnosis of TB has been made
   — Has a chest X-ray suggesting TB
2 A tuberculin-positive individual
   — Is about to commence immunosuppressive treatment
   — Has a predisposition to TB
     • Hodgkin's disease, leukemia (e.g. CLL, hairy cell)
     • Silicosis, sarcoidosis, alcoholism
     • Poorly controlled insulin-dependent diabetes
     • Post-gastrectomy
3 An anergic HIV-positive individual
   — Is exposed to active tuberculosis
4 Any individual
   — Undergoes recent tuberculin conversion in absence of BCG vaccination

Chemotherapy of established tuberculosis

1 Standard (presensitivity) regimen for pulmonary TB
   — 6 months* INH + rifampicin (strongly bactericidal) plus
   — 2 months pyrazinamide (weakly bactericidal) plus
   — 2 months ethambutol (bacteriostatic) or
   — 2 months streptomycin (weakly bactericidal)
2 Sputum cultures still positive after 4 months of above?
   — Reculture and check for acquired resistance
   — If no resistance, recommence R_x for 9 months
   — If resistance demonstrated, use second-line drug(s)
3 Pulmonary TB in pregnancy or during lactation
   — Isoniazid (plus pyridoxine supplements) for 9 months
   — Add ethambutol for 2 months if resistance suspected
   — Rifampicin probably safe in 2nd and 3rd trimesters
   — Avoid streptomycin at all stages
4 Pulmonary TB in child < 16 years old
   — Isoniazid and rifampicin for 9 months
   — Third drug not mandatory unless resistance suspected

5 Immunosuppressed patients
 — Isoniazid and rifampicin for 12 months
 — Ethambutol and pyrazinamide for 2 months
6 Renal TB
 — Avoid streptomycin and ethambutol if azotemic

* NB: If *cavities* on initial CXR, continue isoniazid and rifampicin for 9 months

Indications for corticosteroids in tuberculosis*
1 Absolute indication
 — Acute hypoadrenalism due to tuberculous ablation of adrenal glands
2 Life-threatening tuberculous meningitis
3 Controversial indications
 — Spinal or ureteric stenosis
 — Pericarditis
 — Acute miliary dissemination with septic shock
 — Refractory large pleural effusion(s)

* NB: Steroids absolutely contraindicated *unless* the patient is receiving antituberculous chemotherapy

Therapies useful for multiple-drug-resistant TB (MDRTB)*
1 Ciprofloxacin, ofloxacin
2 Amikacin, capreomycin
3 Cycloserine
 Protionamide, ethionamide
 PAS
4 Clofazimine
5 Clarithromycin/azithromycin ± rifabutin‡
6 Surgical excision of tuberculous foci

* Resistant to INH, rifampicin, pyrazinamide, ethambutol and streptomycin. Try to use at least 3 non-resistant drugs together, don't just add one at a time to a failing regimen
‡ As prophylaxis or active therapy against *M. avium–intracellulare* in HIV disease

Toxicity of antituberculous chemotherapy
1 Isoniazid
 — Hepatitis (see below)
 — SLE
 — Pyridoxine deficiency (rare)
  • Pellagra-like rash
  • Neuropathy; optic neuritis ($\downarrow$ green vision)
  • Sideroblastosis*
 — *Potentiation* of phenytoin, warfarin
2 Rifampicin
 — Daily administration
  • *Antagonism* of oral contraceptives, warfarin, steroids, digoxin and sulfonylureas
  • Asymptomatic elevation of transaminases
 — Intermittent administration
  • Flu-like illness: affects Caucasians receiving R_x < 3 times/week for 3–6 months (20% mortality)
  • Hepatitis‡
  • Venous thrombosis
  • Hemolysis, thrombocytopenia; azotemia
3 Streptomycin
 — Hypersensitivity reactions
  • Rash, malaise, PUO; eosinophilia
 — Vestibular damage (esp. if renal impairment)
 — Teratogenicity
4 Ethambutol
 — Optic neuritis, esp. in renal impairment

5 Pyrazinamide
 — Hepatotoxicity in ~ 10%
6 Less commonly used antituberculous drugs
 — Cycloserine
  • Fits, psychoses, pyridoxine deficiency
 — Ethionamide
  • Hepatotoxicity
 — Protionamide
  • Neuropathy; nausea; psychoses

* Commoner in (1) high dosage schedule (> 15 mg/kg/day), (2) slow acetylation status, (3) alcoholism and (4) pregnancy
‡ NB: Also colors urine orange

Features of isoniazid-associated hepatotoxicity
1 Occurs in about 1%; usually within 3 months (may be fatal)
2 *Not* dose-related
 Not consistently related to acetylator phenotype*
3 Risk factors
 — Male sex
 — Age > 35 years (8-fold increase if > 65 years)
 — Alcoholism
 — Other hepatotoxic R_x (e.g. rifampicin, pyrazinamide)
4 Clinically indistinguishable from viral hepatitis
5 Liver function tests should only be *routinely* performed in the latter 'at-risk' group, or in symptomatic patients
6 Cease R_x if ALT/AST exceed 3 times upper limit of normal

* Though an association with rapid acetylation has been reported

Problems in managing the alcoholic with TB
1 Poor compliance necessitating supervised (intermittent) treatment schedule; predisposes to rifampicin toxicity
2 Increased risk of hepatotoxicity
3 Increased risk of toxic amblyopia
4 Increased risk of pyridoxine deficiency
5 Neuropathy/optic neuritis, rash, and sideroblastosis may arise due to other (non-iatrogenic) alcohol-related causes

Therapy of non-tuberculous mycobacteria
1 *Mycobacterium avium–intracellulare*
 — Indolent disease
  • Standard anti-TB regimens (for up to 2 years)
  • Azithromycin, clarithromycin
 — Aggressive local disease
  • Surgery (lobectomy)
 — Aggressive widespread disease
  • Multidrug combinations (e.g. clofazimine, ciprofloxacin and ethambutol)
2 *Mycobacterium marinum*
 — Expectant (conservative) management
 — Excision of involved skin
 — Rifampicin, ethambutol, doxycycline
3 *Mycobacterium scrofulaceum*
 — Lymphadenectomy
4 *Mycobacterium fortuitum-chelonei*
 — Excision of soft-tissue abscesses
 — Doxycycline; amikacin, sulfonamides, erythromycin

5 *Mycobacterium kansasii*
  — Isoniazid ⎫
  — Rifampicin ⎬ for 2 years
  — Ethambutol ⎭
6 *Mycobacterium xenopi*
  — Standard anti-TB therapy

Leprosy: therapeutic options
1 Dapsone + rifampicin + clofazimine
2 Sparfloxacin + clarithromycin
3 Fusidic acid (or rifampicin) + ciprofloxacin
4 Thalidomide (for reactions following antibiotics in males)

Diseases that may respond to dapsone
1 Leprosy
2 Dermatitis herpetiformis
3 Pyoderma gangrenosum
4 Relapsing polychondritis

ANTIBIOTIC PRESCRIBING STRATEGIES

When to consider prescribing penicillin V for sore throat*
1 Pharyngeal/tonsillar exudate, *or*
2 Palpable tender anterior neck nodes, *or*
3 Fever > 38°C, *and*
4 *No* cough, *and*
5 Infectious mononucleosis *not* suspected

* i.e. factors suggesting streptococcal rather than viral etiology

Antibiotic therapy of venereal disease
1 Genital gonorrhea
  — Ceftriaxone 250 mg IMI *or* (oral) cefixime 800 mg stat
  — Tetracycline 500 mg q.i.d. for 5 days, *or*
  — Single-dose oral amoxicillin 3 g (*if* sensitive)
  — Single-dose ciprofloxacin 100 mg (*if* penicillin-resistant)
  — Spectinomycin (*if* ciprofloxacin-resistant)
2 Gonococcal pharyngitis*
  — Trimethoprim/sulfamethoxazole for 5 days
3 Gonococcal proctitis‡
  — Single-dose ciprofloxacin 100 mg, *or*
  — Spectinomycin 4 g IM
  Gonococcal proctitis with positive VDRL
  — Procaine penicillin (see below)
4 Syphilis¶
  — Procaine penicillin 600 000 U IM daily
  — Primary/secondary: for 10 days
  — Latent/gummatous: for 15 days
  — Neurological/aortitic: for 20 days
5 Chlamydial urethritis
  — Azithromycin 1 g stat, *or*
  — Doxycycline 100 mg b.d. for 7 days, *or*
  — Tetracycline 500 mg q.i.d. for 14 days

* Usually unresponsive to amoxicillin or spectinomycin
‡ Unresponsive to tetracycline in males and, usually, to amoxicillin
¶ *Resistant* to spectinomycin; cf. gonorrhea

Antibiotic therapy of vaginitis
1 Candidal vulvovaginitis
  — Vaginal clotrimazole/miconazole/nystatin, *or*
  — Oral fluconazole (150 mg single dose)
2 Trichomonal vaginitis
  — Metronidazole or tinidazole (2 g single oral dose)
3 Bacterial vaginosis (*Gardnerella* spp., *Mycoplasma hominis*)
  — Oral metronidazole (2 g single dose *or* 800 mg/day for 1 week), *or*
  — Topical metronidazole gel *or* topical clindamycin

Treatment strategies in uncomplicated malaria
1 Non-severe *P. falciparum*: consider oral treatment using
  — Mefloquine 25 mg/kg single dose, *or*
  — Atovaquone–proguanil (1 g/400 mg) daily for 3 days, *or*
  — Pyrimethamine–sulfadoxine (75/1500 mg) single dose
2 Drug-sensitive malaria (most *vivax, ovale, malariae*)
  — Chloroquine (base) 600 mg stat orally, then 300 mg 6 h later, then 300 mg daily for 2 days, *or*
  — Pyrimethamine–sulfadoxine as above
3 *P. vivax/ovale*
  — Due to exoerythrocytic (cryptobiotic) phase, add primaquine (base) 7.5 mg orally b.d. for 2 weeks to the chloroquine-based regimen; inadequate treatment may otherwise lead to late relapse
4 *P. malariae*
  — Relapse *not* prevented by primaquine; relapses may occur decades later and must be fully retreated

Antibiotic chemotherapy of infection in the AIDS patient
1 *P. carinii*
  — Co-trimoxazole; pentamidine
2 *C. albicans* (mucosal)
  — Topical clotrimazole
  — Oral ketoconazole
  C. albicans (esophageal, invasive or disseminated)
  — IV amphotericin B ± 5-FC
3 *T. gondii*
  — Pyrimethamine/sulfadiazine
4 *C. neoformans*
  — Amphotericin B* *plus* 5-FC
  — Maintenance fluconazole
5 *Salmonella/Shigella* spp.
  — IV ampicillin
6 Herpes simplex, varicella-zoster
  — Aciclovir (nucleoside analog of guanosine, a herpesvirus thymidine kinase substrate)
  — Valaciclovir (an aciclovir prodrug), famciclovir (penciclovir prodrug)
7 CMV
  — Ganciclovir (dihydroxypropoxymethylguanine)
  — Foscarnet (phosphonoformic acid)

* Oral fluconazole may also be effective in acute management of non-life-threatening cryptococcal meningitis

OPTIMIZING ANTIBIOTIC THERAPY

Indications for fluoroquinolone therapy

1 Serious Gram-negative infections
   — Acute Gram-negative osteomyelitis (IV ciprofloxacin)
   — Severe necrotizing otitis externa (oral ciprofloxacin)
   — Infective exacerbations of cystic fibrosis
2 Bacterial gastroenteritis
   — Travellers' diarrhea
   — Invasive salmonellosis
3 Complicated urinary tract infections, e.g.
   — Pyelonephritis
   — Trimethoprim-resistant cystitis
   — Indwelling catheter in situ
   — Chronic or relapsing prostatitis
   — Penicillinase-producing *N. gonorrhea* urethritis
4 Prophylaxis
   — Eradication of *Salmonella* carrier state
   — Asymptomatic contacts of meningococcal infection

Which macrolide?

1 Clarithromycin*
   — Undiagnosed community-acquired pneumonia, e.g.
     • Legionnaires' disease
     • *Mycoplasma* pneumonia
     • Psittacosis
2 Azithromycin
   — *Chlamydia trachomatis* keratitis
   — Toxoplasmal encephalitis
   — *M. avium–intracellulare* infections (500 mg/day)
   — Single-dose (1 g) therapy of chlamydial NSU‡
3 Erythromycin
   — Penicillin-allergy + Gram-positive cocci, e.g.
     • Strep throat
     • Pneumococcal pneumonia
   — Prophylactic or cautionary use
     • *C. diphtheriae* carrier state
     • *B. pertussis* (preparoxysmal)
     • Severe *Campylobacter* enterocolitis¶

* Improved activity against *H. influenzae*, and high serum levels; hence, preferred for undiagnosed respiratory illnesses (if *severe*; if not, an aminopenicillin may be preferable)
‡ NB: Far more expensive than doxycycline or erythromycin
¶ *If* treatment indicated; ciprofloxacin is also effective

Drug of choice: tetracycline

1 Chlamydial disease (doxycycline)
   — ('Non-specific/non-gonococcal') urethritis
   — Non-gonococcal pelvic inflammatory disease
   — Epididymo-orchitis
   — Trachoma
   — Lymphogranuloma venereum
   — TWAR pneumonia
2 Zoonoses
   — Brucellosis (doxycycline*)
   — Lyme disease (doxycycline)
   — Rickettsioses
3 Small intestinal infections‡
   — Whipple's disease (due to *Tropheryma whippelii*)

   — Severe *Yersinia* enteritis¶
   — Bacterial overgrowth
4 Mild-to-moderate acne vulgaris/rosacea
5 Broad-spectrum cover in renal failure (doxycycline)

* As part of combination therapy
‡ Efficacy due to poor gastrointestinal absorption; hence, high fecal levels
¶ Extraintestinal manifestations may be better treated with co-trimoxazole

Drug of choice: chloramphenicol

1 Pyogenic meningitis/encephalitis (in children < 5)
2 Cerebral abscess
3 Severe (para)typhoid fever*
4 Acute epiglottitis
5 High oral bioavailability required‡

* Resistant strains now recognized; ciprofloxacin may be better
‡ e.g. refractory chest infections due to cystic fibrosis

Drug of choice: co-trimoxazole*

1 Major indications
   — *Pneumocystis carinii* (treatment or prophylaxis)
   — Nocardiosis (treatment or prophylaxis)
2 Other susceptible pathogens
   — Toxoplasmosis
   — *Klebsiella* spp.
   — *Serratia/Enterobacter* spp.
   — Yersiniosis, cyclosporiasis, melioidosis
   — Chancroid, granuloma inguinale

* Trimethoprim/sulfamethoxazole

Drug of choice: co-amoxiclav*

1 Bite wounds (human or animal)
   — *P. multocida*
   — *Eikenella corrodens*
   — Streptococci, anaerobes
2 Resistant respiratory tract infections
   — Staphylococcal
   — *Moraxella catarrhalis*
   — *H. influenzae*
3 Complicated urinary tract or pelvic infections
   — *Proteus* spp.
   — *Klebsiella* spp.
   — Anaerobes, *E. coli*

* Amoxicillin plus clavulanic acid

Drug of choice: vancomycin

1 Methicillin-resistant staphylococci (MRSA)
2 Bacterial endocarditis
   — (Major) penicillin allergy
   — Prosthetic valve involvement
3 Shunt infections in dialysis patients*

* Vancomycin *not* dialysable

Drug of choice: metronidazole (or tinidazole)

1 Giardiasis
2 Trichomoniasis, *Gardnerella* vaginitis
3 Amebic dysentery
4 Anaerobic infections
5 Pseudomembranous colitis
6 Abscesses (incl. hepatic, cerebral)*

* NB: Many liver abscesses are due to *microaerophilic* strep – *St. milleri* – and may therefore be resistant

Drugs of choice: miscellaneous diseases
1 Trachoma
   — Azithromycin
2 Bacterial meningitis*
   — Ceftriaxone *or* cefotaxime
3 Shigella dysentery; anthrax chemoprophylaxis; neutropenia prophylaxis
   — Ciprofloxacin

* Pending the results of culture

Chemoprophylaxis for meningococcal disease
1 Rifampicin
2 Ciprofloxacin
3 Ceftriaxone

CEPHALOSPORINS

A rough guide to the cephalosporins
1 First generation: strong Gram-positive activity
   — Cephalothin, cefazolin (IV); cefalexin (oral)
      • Active against β-lactamases, incl. *S. aureus*
      • Weak Gram-negative activity
2 Second generation: intermediate activity spectrum
   — Cefoxitin
      • Moderate Gram-positive and Gram-negative activity (but not to *S. aureus, Ps. aeruginosa*)
   — Cefuroxime
      • Penetrates CSF; active against *H. influenzae*
3 Third generation: strong Gram-negative activity
   — Cefotaxime
      • Weak Gram-positive activity*
      • Does not cover anaerobes or *Ps. aeruginosa*
      • Good CSF penetration‡
   — Ceftazidime
      • Gram-negative cover includes *Ps. aeruginosa*

* Fails to cover *St. fecalis* or *S. aureus*
‡ Currently the drug of choice for undiagnosed childhood bacterial meningitis

Common problems with cephalosporin therapy
1 Poor penetration of sputum and CSF
2 Development of Gram-negative resistance
3 Significant incidence of cross-sensitivity in penicillin allergy
4 Expense

PENICILLINS

Microorganisms highly sensitive to penicillin G
1 Non-enterococcal (gp A and B) streptococci
2 *Clostridia* spp. (except *C. difficile*)
3 *Actinomyces* spp., *Corynebacteria* spp., *L. monocytogenes*
4 *Neisseria meningitidis*
5 *Leptospira*
6 *Borrelia burgdorferi**
7 *Treponema pallidum*
8 *C. canimorsus* ('DF-2'), *Pasteurella multocida*

* In *complicated* Lyme borreliosis; rash alone can be treated with tetracycline

Ampicillin/amoxicillin as first-line therapy?
1 Non-life-threatening community-acquired pneumonia
2 Acute bacterial exacerbations of chronic bronchitis
3 Meningitis due to *Listeria monocytogenes*
4 Urinary tract infections in pregnancy
5 Dental/surgical prophylaxis of bacterial endocarditis

Penicillin allergy or resistance: which antibiotic?
1 Pyogenic meningitis
   Aspiration pneumonia
   — Cefotaxime
   — Chloramphenicol
2 Typhoid
   — Ciprofloxacin
   — Chloramphenicol
3 Lobar pneumonia
   — Clarithromycin
   Rheumatic fever prophylaxis
   — Erythromycin
4 Acute bronchitis
   Sinusitis, otitis
   — Co-trimoxazole
   — Ciprofloxacin
5 Osteomyelitis
   — Ciprofloxacin
   — Clindamycin
6 Gonorrhea
   — Ciprofloxacin
   — Spectinomycin
7 Syphilis
   — Erythromycin
8 Empirical use in life-threatening staph infections
   — Vancomycin ± aztreonam

Antibiotics for endocarditis in penicillin allergy
1 Prophylaxis
   — Vancomycin
2 Staphylococcal or non-enterococcal streptococcal endocarditis
   — Vancomycin
   — Oral ciprofloxacin* + rifampicin
3 Enterococcal endocarditis
   — Penicillin desensitization → ampi- + aminoglycoside *or*
   — Vancomycin (pending MIC, MBC) + aminoglycoside
4 Right-sided *S. aureus* endocarditis
   — Flucloxacillin + tobramycin
   — Oral ciprofloxacin + rifampicin (on discharge)

* NB: Pneumococci also usually resistant

Pneumococcal infections: approximate duration of therapy
1 Otitis media   — 5 days
2 Pneumonia   — 10 days
3 Meningitis   — 2 weeks
4 Septic arthritis — 4 weeks
5 Empyema   — 6 weeks

Clinical features of Jarisch–Herxheimer reactions
1 Occurs due to rapid release of microbial endotoxin
2 Typically occurs within 1–6 h of bactericidal antibiotic therapy, esp. penicillins

3 Manifests with abrupt onset of fever, chills, myalgias, hyperventilation, tachycardia (± hypotension)
4 Classically occurs following initial treatment of *secondary syphilis*, but also occurs in other infections (esp. penicillin-treated spirochetal diseases, e.g. leptospirosis)

ANTIBIOTIC SENSITIVITY AND RESISTANCE

Important patterns of antibiotic resistance
1 Enterobacteriaceae (*E. coli, Proteus, Klebsiella, Shigella, Salmonella* spp.)
   — Aminoglycosides, β-lactams, tetracyclines
   — Vancomycin, chloramphenicol
2 *S. aureus*
   — β-lactams, ciprofloxacin, rifampicin, tetracycline
3 *H. influenzae*
   — Penicillin G, cephalosporins; ampicillin
   — Erythromycin
   — Chloramphenicol, tetracycline, co-trimoxazole
4 *Pseudomonas* spp.
   — Aminoglycosides, β-lactams, chloramphenicol, sulfonamides
5 Streptococci, anaerobes
   — Aminoglycosides*, tetracycline
6 Listeriosis
   — Cephalosporins

* NB: Enterococcal strep are only 'sensitive' to aminoglycosides when used with a penicillin

Patterns of bacterial susceptibility to antibiotics
1 *Pseudomonas aeruginosa*
   — Combination therapy (for serious infections)
     • Aminoglycoside + antipseudomonal penicillin
   — Extended-spectrum penicillins
     • Piperacillin (most potent)
   — Other β-lactams
     • Imipenem/cilastatin
     • Ceftazidime
     • Aztreonam
2 *Staphylococcus aureus*
   — Drug of choice
     • Flucloxacillin
     • Nafcillin (for staphylococcal meningitis)
   — Second-line regimens
     • Clindamycin, erythromycin
     • Amoxicillin/clavulanic acid (co-amoxiclav)
   — Multiresistant ('methicillin-resistant': MRSA)
     • Vancomycin
     • Fusidic acid, rifampicin
3 *Haemophilus influenzae**
   — Cefotaxime (drug of choice for invasive disease)
   — Co-amoxiclav
   — Chloramphenicol; clarithromycin; ciprofloxacin

* Note that *corticosteroids* may confer additional therapeutic benefit in comatose children with *H. influenzae* meningitis

Established synergy of antibiotic combinations
1 *Pseudomonas* infections
   — Aminoglycoside + antipseudomonal penicillin
2 *Strep. fecalis* endocarditis
   — Ampicillin + gentamicin
3 Cryptococcal meningitis
   — Amphotericin B + 5-FC

Microorganisms commonly expressing β-lactamases
1 Staphylococci (95%)
2 Gonococci
3 Enterococci*
4 Enterobacteriaceae‡
5 *H. influenzae*

* Intestinal commensals which are pathogenic in immunocompromised hosts
‡ Normal enteric bacteria (e.g. *E. coli, Proteus, Klebsiella*) which are conditional pathogens in normal hosts, causing urinary tract infections, wound infections, septicemia. Related pathogens include enterotoxigenic *E. coli, Shigella, Salmonella* spp.

β-lactamase inhibitors
1 Clavulanic acid
2 Sulbactam
3 Tazobactam

Antibiotics rapidly engendering resistance if used alone
1 *M. tuberculosis*
   — Rifampicin, streptomycin, pyrazinamide
2 *S. aureus*
   — Fusidic acid, rifampicin, erythromycin
   — 2nd- and 3rd-generation cephalosporins*
3 *Ps. aeruginosa*
   — Piperacillin, imipenem‡, aztreonam
4 Gram-negatives
   — Nalidixic acid, ciprofloxacin (esp. IV)
5 Fungi (e.g. *C. neoformans*)
   — Flucytosine (5-FC), fluconazole
6 Viruses
   — Ganciclovir

* e.g. Cefoxitin (induces β-lactamase)
‡ Usually combined with cilastatin, a renal dipeptidase inhibitor (→ ↑ urinary imipenem levels, ↓ nephrotoxicity); has the broadest activity spectrum of any antibiotic

Mechanisms of antibiotic resistance to *S. aureus*
1 'Plasmid resistance'
   — Express β-lactamases (e.g. TEM-1) → cleave antibiotic (β-lactam) ring
   — These plasmid-encoded β-lactamases confer antibiotic insensitivity rather than frank resistance
   — Certain bacteria (e.g. *Klebsiella, Ps. aeruginosa, Serratia, Enterobacter*) induce β-lactamases only in response to antibiotic exposure; these inducible enzymes are *resistant* to clavulanic acid
2 Reduced bacterial cell wall permeability
   — e.g. Decreased expression of porin-F (normally permits entry of cephalosporins)*
   — Similar mechanism underlies vancomycin resistance
   — β-lactamase-resistant drugs (or inhibitors) do *not* help

3 'Methicillin resistance' (MRSA)‡
   — Chromosomally–dependent ('intrinsic') resistance due to expression of penicillin-binding proteins (PBP 2a)
4 'Tolerance'
   — Development of MBC:MIC ratio > 32 (reflecting failure of autolytic bacterial enzyme activation by β-lactam)
5 Staphylococcal DNA gyrase mutations
   — Confer ciprofloxacin resistance

* cf. imipenem: enters via different porin, hence still works
‡ Resist not only methicillin but also all other penicillins, cephalosporins, aminoglycosides, quinolones, erythromycin and clindamycin

Major indications for specific aminoglycosides
1 Gentamicin
   — Suspected Gram-negative sepsis
   — Adjunctive to β-lactams as broad-spectrum cover
2 Amikacin
   — Gentamicin resistance
3 Tobramycin
   — Suspected *Pseudomonas aeruginosa*
4 Streptomycin
   — TB, brucellosis
5 Netilmicin
   — Concern over nephrotoxicity

Drug therapy of miscellaneous infections and infestations
1 Giardiasis
   — Metronidazole 2 g once daily for 3 days, *or*
   — Tinidazole 2 g stat (single dose)
2 Hepatic amebiasis
   — Metronidazole 400 mg t.d.s. for 5 days (or chloroquine)
   Cecal amebiasis
   — Metronidazole 800 mg t.d.s. for 5 days* (or emetine)
3 Toxoplasmosis
   — Pyrimethamine/sulfadiazine; spiramycin
4 Scabies, lice
   — Topical permethrin (or benzylbenzoate, malathion)
5 Hookworm, whipworm; echinococcus (may need surgery)
   — Mebendazole
6 *Strongyloides, Toxocara*
   — Tiabendazole
7 *Ascaris, Trichuris*
   — Pyrantel pamoate and/or albendazole
8 *Schistosoma japonicum* (plus all 3 other schistosomes): paragonomiasis, clonorchiasis, neurocysticercosis
   — Praziquantel
9 Onchocerciasis ('river blindness'), bancroftian filariasis
   — Ivermectin + albendazole
   Other filariases
   — Diethylcarbamazine (single-dose)
10 *Trypanosoma brucei gambiense*
   — Eflornithine (IV)
   Trypanosoma brucei rhodesiense
   — Suramin

* Colonic amebiasis requires higher doses than hepatic, because metronidazole is very efficiently absorbed in the small intestine

ANTIBIOTIC TOXICITY

Potential morbidity of antibiotic use
1 Nitrofurantoin
   — Neuropathy (esp. with renal impairment)
   — Pulmonary fibrosis
   — Hemolytic anemia; megaloblastosis
   — Cholestasis → chronic active hepatitis
2 Chloramphenicol
   — Idiosyncratic aplastic anemia (→ 1:25 000)
   — Dose-related myelosuppression
   — Neuropathy, optic atrophy
   — Depression of antibody synthesis
3 Erythromycin
   — Abdominal pain*
   — Phlebitis (with IV use)
4 Ticarcillin
   — Fluid (sodium) overload; hypokalemia
   — Impaired platelet function, seizures
   — Inactivation of gentamicin/tobramycin if admixed
5 Metronidazole
   — Dysgeusia
   — Disulfiram-type reactions
   — Painful neuropathy
6 Amphotericin B
   — Fever, rigors; vomiting; phlebitis
   — Azotemia (75%); hypokalemia, renal tubular acidosis
   — Anemia
7 Ciprofloxacin
   — May precipitate theophylline toxicity
   — Arthralgias in children
   — Photosensitivity, psychosis, transaminitis, crystalluria
8 Vancomycin
   — Rapid infusion → 'red-man' syndrome (histamine release); hydroxyzine prophylaxis may help
   — Phlebitis, ototoxicity, nephrotoxicity

* Activates gastrointestinal tract motilin receptors

Antibiotics that may precipitate seizures
1 High-dose β-lactams
   — e.g. Ticarcillin, piperacillin
2 Imipenem
3 Fluconazole
4 Fluoroquinolones

Tetracyclines: toxic manifestations
1 Common
   — Diarrhea
   — Esophagitis
   — Moniliasis
2 Benign intracranial hypertension
3 Photosensitization (demeclocycline)
   Vertigo (minocycline)
4 Worsening of renal failure

5 Hepatotoxicity, esp.
— Intravenous use
— In pregnant women
— With pre-existing renal impairment
6 Teeth staining when administered to children aged < 8 years*

* Or to pregnant women; ingestion during the 3rd trimester may result in staining of the child's secondary (permanent) dentition

Aminoglycoside toxicity: variations between drugs
1 Deafness (cochlear VIII toxicity)
— Amikacin (most)
— Neomycin, gentamicin, tobramycin (moderate)
2 Ataxia (vestibular VIII toxicity)
— Streptomycin, gentamicin, tobramycin (most)
— Amikacin (moderate)
— Netilmicin (least)
3 Nephrotoxicity*
— Gentamicin, tobramycin (most)
— Amikacin (moderate)
— Netilmicin, streptomycin (least)

* Worsened by concurrent furosemide (frusemide) or cephalothin

Disadvantages of aminoglycosides
1 Narrow therapeutic range (must monitor levels)
2 Ineffective against anaerobes and Strep/Staph*
3 Failure to penetrate CSF, bile, abscesses
4 Must be given IV

* But synergistic with concomitant β-lactams

IATROGENIC INFECTIONS

Infections occurring in prosthetic appliances
1 Prosthetic valves, arterial grafts
— S. albus
— S. aureus
— St. viridans
— Gram-negative bacilli
2 Prosthetic joints
— S. albus
— S. aureus
— Gram-negative bacilli
3 CSF shunts
— S. albus (75%)
— S. aureus
— Gram-negative bacilli
4 Intraocular lens implant
— S. albus
— S. aureus

Microorganisms transmissible by blood transfusion
1 Hepatitis viruses
— HCV, HBV, δ agent
2 HIV
3 CMV
4 Syphilis
5 Malaria, babesiosis
6 Trypanosoma cruzi (Chagas' disease)
7 Rare
— Brucellosis, yersiniosis
— EBV, HAV

Approach to the febrile neutropenic patient
1 Culture blood, urine and other relevant sites
2 Commence presumptive treatment with either
— Antipseudomonal β-lactam (e.g. piperacillin) *plus* an aminoglycoside (e.g. gentamicin); *or*
— Oral ciprofloxacin *if* neutropenic duration expected to be short (investigational)
3 If penicillin-allergic or uremic, substitute
— Ceftazidime, *or*
— Imipenem/cilastatin
4 Add amphotericin B if
— Fever and neutropenia persist > 1 week, *or*
— Fever persists > 3 days and condition deteriorating, *or*
— Fever persists despite resolution of neutropenia, *or*
— Sinus tenderness, nasal ulcers, CXR focal lesion, *or*
— Central line cultures are positive for *Candida*
5 Add vancomycin if
— S. albus identified on blood culture, *or*
— Endemic MRSA and persistent fever
6 Add metronidazole (or clindamycin) if
— Perianal tenderness, *or*
— Necrotizing gingivitis
7 Add aciclovir if
— Ulcerative or vesicular mouth lesions

ANTIFUNGAL DRUGS

Principles of antifungal chemotherapy
1 For *any* disseminated or life-threatening fungal infection (e.g. invasive aspergillosis, rhinocerebral mucormycosis)
— Intravenous amphotericin B ± 5-FC
— AIDS patients: maintenance oral fluconazole
For visceral leishmaniasis
— Liposomal amphotericin B
— Pentavalent antimony; aminosidine
2 Candiduria with indwelling catheter in situ
— Oral 5-FC ± amphotericin B bladder washouts
3 Chronic mucocutaneous candidiasis Paracoccidioidomycosis
— (Oral) ketoconazole
4 Less serious infections
— Oropharyngeal candidiasis
• Amphotericin lozenges ± nystatin/clotrimazole
— Oropharyngeal candidiasis in AIDS; esophageal candidiasis
• Fluconazole
— Vaginal candidosis
• Itraconazole
— Superficial dermatophytes
• Terbinafine
— Petriellidosis; *Pseudallescheria boydii*
• Miconazole (IV)
— Tinea capitis
• Oral griseofulvin (or ketoconazole)
— Tinea corporis
• Topical clotrimazole/tolnaftate
— Pityriasis ('tinea') versicolor
• Selenium sulfide (topical) shampoo

5 Cryptococcal meningitis
— IV (or intraventricular) amphotericin B *plus*
— Oral (or intravenous) 5-FC (at least 6 weeks)
— *Maintenance* fluconazole in HIV patients

Indications for itraconazole
1 Invasive mycoses
— Histoplasmosis, blastomycosis
— Sporotrichosis, chromomycosis
— Non-life-threatening invasive aspergillosis
2 Dermatophyte infections
— Onychomycosis (toenail tinea)
3 Vaginal candidosis

Indications for fluconazole
1 Mucosal candidiasis *or* systemic candidemia
— In non-neutropenic patients*
2 Coccidioidomycosis
3 CNS cryptococcosis
— Definitive therapy for non-life-threatening infections
— Maintenance therapy for HIV-infected patients

* Including AIDS patients

Disadvantages of ketoconazole therapy
1 Toxicity
— Nausea, hepatotoxicity
— Inhibition of steroid hormone synthesis*
  • Impotence (antiandrogenic; useful in Ca prostate)
  • Dysfunctional uterine bleeding
  • Hypoadrenalism (useful in Cushing's)
2 Drug interactions (also common with itraconazole)
— Antagonism of ketoconazole by coadministered drug
  • Absorption inhibited by antacids, H_2-blockers
  • Mutual antagonism by rifampicin ($\uparrow$ liver metabolism), isoniazid, phenytoin
— Potentiation of coadministered drug
  • Cyclosporin A toxicity (esp. in renal transplants)
  • Phenytoin toxicity (?warfarin, tolbutamide)
— Disulfiram-like effect with alcohol

* cf. triazoles (fluconazole, itraconazole): specific for fungal cytochrome P450, *no* effect on steroid metabolism

ANTIVIRAL CHEMOTHERAPY

Antibiotic regimens for viral infections
1 Herpes simplex
— Keratitis: 3% aciclovir ointment five times daily
— Genital: oral aciclovir (valaciclovir, famciclovir)
— Lip: oral aciclovir *or* topical penciclovir
— Encephalitis: IV aciclovir (10 mg/kg q 8 h)
— Aciclovir resistant disease in AIDS? Foscarnet
2 Varicella-zoster
— Disseminated: IV aciclovir (10 mg/kg q 8 h)*
— Ophthalmic: 3% ointment *plus* oral aciclovir 4 g/day

3 Influenza A
— Amantadine/rimantidine (prophylaxis)
— Neuraminidase inhibitors (therapy)
4 Influenza B, RSV
— Ribavirin aerosol, *or*
— Neuraminidase inhibitors
5 Lassa fever
— Ribavirin orally
6 HPV (in juvenile laryngeal papillomatosis)
— Interferon-α
7 Rhinovirus (for the common cold)
— Interferon (intranasally)‡
8 CMV in the immunosuppressed patient
— Ganciclovir (prevents retinitis, pneumonitis, colitis)
9 Hepatitis B
— Interferon-α *or* lamivudine
10 Hepatitis C
— Interferon-α *plus* ribavirin

* NB: Aciclovir therapy has *not* yet been proven to affect subsequent incidence or severity of post-herpetic neuralgia, or to reduce analgesic intake
‡ Doesn't work for colds due to RSV, adenovirus, or (para)influenza

VACCINES

Active immunization: mechanisms of vaccine action
1 Toxoids
— Tetanus, diphtheria, botulinum
2 Recombinant vaccines
— Hepatitis B (HBsAg)
3 Pooled surface proteins
— Pneumococcus
— *H. influenzae* type B ('Hib')
— Typhoid (parenteral Vi vaccine)
4 Attenuated (live) organisms*
— Viruses: polio, measles, rubella, mumps
— BCG
— Hepatitis A
— Cholera (CVD 103-HgR)‡
— Typhoid (oral Ty21a vaccine)‡
5 Killed organisms¶
— Influenza A
— Rabies

* *Hazardous* (hence, contraindicated) in immunosuppressed patients
‡ NB: Efficacy of cholera and typhoid vaccines for travellers remains modest
¶ *Ineffective* (hence, contraindicated) in immunosuppressed patients

Indications for pneumococcal vaccine
1 Patients aged 2–70
— Hyposplenism (all causes)
— HIV infection (any stage)
— Immunosuppression (e.g. transplant)
2 Patients aged 55–70
— Diabetes mellitus
— Chronic renal, liver, cardiac and/or pulmonary disease
— CSF leaks

Indications for passive immunization
1 Pooled gammaglobulin
  — Hepatitis A
    • Family contacts
    • Institutional outbreaks
    • Travellers in tropical/developing countries*
  — Measles
    • Immunosuppressed contacts of acute cases‡
2 Hyperimmune globulin
  — Hepatitis B
    • Percutaneous/mucosal exposure to positive sera
    • Sexual contacts of acute cases (optional)
    • Newborns of HBsAg+ mothers (at 0, 3, 6 months)
  — Rh isoimmunization (→ Rh(D)-negative mother)
    • After delivery of Rh+ infant
    • On abortion of pregnancy with Rh+ father
    • Following inadvertent transfusion of Rh+ blood
  — Varicella-zoster
    • Immunesuppressed contacts of acute case
    • Newborn contacts of acute case
  — Rabies
    • Subjects exposed to rabid animals
  — Tetanus
    • Prophylaxis (exposure of non-immune subject)
    • Therapeutic (on diagnosis of disease: urgent)

* Repeat passive immunization every 4 months
‡ *If* exposed less than a week previously

Efficacy of active immunization
1 Pneumococcal vaccination
  — Prevents 60% infections
2 Influenza vaccination
  — Prevents 70% infections
3 Hepatitis B vaccination
  — Prevents 90% infections
4 MMR (measles, mumps, rubella) vaccination
  — Prevents 95% infections
5 DPT (diphtheria, pertussis, tetanus) vaccination
  — Prevents 99% infections

UNDERSTANDING INFECTIOUS DISEASE

A simplified classification of microorganisms
1 Viruses
  — RNA
    • Myxoviruses (e.g. influenza)
    • Paramyxoviruses (e.g. measles, mumps, RSV)
    • Picornaviruses (e.g. enteroviruses*, hepatitis A)
    • Reoviruses (e.g. rotavirus)
    • Rhabdoviruses (e.g. rabies)
    • Arenaviruses (e.g. Lassa fever)
    • Togaviruses (e.g. rubella, dengue)
    • Retroviruses (e.g. HIV, HTLV)
  — DNA
    • Herpesviruses
    • Adenoviruses
    • Parvoviruses
    • Papovaviruses (e.g. HPV, JC virus)
    • Hepadnaviruses (e.g. hepatitis B)
2 Bacteria
  — Cell-wall-deficient
    • *Mycoplasma* spp.

  — Obligate intracellular
    • *Chlamydiae, Rickettsiae*
  — Helically coiled
    • Spirochetes (*Treponema, Leptospira, Borrelia*)
    • *Helicobacter pylori*
    • *Campylobacter* spp.
    • *Aeromonas* spp., *Plesiomonas* spp.
  — 'Higher' bacteria
    • *Mycobacteria* spp.
    • *Corynebacteria* spp.
    • *Actinomyces, Nocardia*
  — Eubacteria (the rest)
3 Fungi
  — Yeasts (grow as hyphae, increase by budding), e.g.
    • *Candida albicans*
    • *Cryptococcus neoformans*
  — Molds (grow as mycelia, increase by branching), e.g.
    • *Aspergillus fumigatus*
    • *Dermatophytes* (e.g. tinea)
  — Dimorphic, e.g.
    • *Histoplasma capsulatum*
4 Parasites
  — Protozoa
    • *Plasmodium* spp.
    • *Toxoplasma gondii*
    • *Entameba histolytica*
    • *Giardia lamblia*
    • *Pneumocystis carinii*‡
    • *Trichomonas vaginalis*
  — Multicellular (worms)
    • *Schistosoma* spp.
    • *Strongyloides stercoralis*
    • *Echinococcus granulosus*
    • *Toxocara canis*
    • *Filariasis*

* Includes ECHO, polio, Coxsackie viruses
‡ *Pneumocystis* may be genetically closer to *fungi* than protozoa

Gram-staining: clinically relevant organisms
1 Gram-positive cocci
  — *Staphylococcus* spp.
  — *Streptococcus* spp.
2 Gram-negative cocci
  — *Neisseria* spp. (gonococcus, meningococcus)
3 Gram-positive bacilli
  — *Clostridium* spp.
  — *Bacillus* spp.
  — *Corynebacterium diphtheriae*
  — *Actinomyces israeli*
  — *Gardnerella vaginalis*
  — *Listeria monocytogenes*
4 Gram-negative bacilli
  — Enterobacteriaceae*
  — *Pseudomonas aeruginosa*
  — *Haemophilus influenzae*
  — *Campylobacter jejuni/coli*
  — *Brucella* spp.
5 Acid-fast bacilli
  — *Mycobacteria* spp.
  — *Nocardia* spp., *Actinomyces* spp. (weakly acid-fast)

* Includes *E. coli, Proteus, Klebsiella, Salmonella/Shigella* spp.

Human herpesviruses (HHVs): classification
1 α-Herpesviruses
  — HHV1 (HSV1)
  — HHV2 (HSV2)
  — HHV3 (VZ)
2 β-Herpesviruses
  — HHV5 (CMV)
  — HHV6*
  — HHV7‡
3 γ-Herpesviruses
  — HHV4 (EBV)
  — HHV8 (KSHV)

* Implicated in exanthem subitum, febrile seizures (and, tentatively, in multiple sclerosis), interstitial pneumonitis, and infectious mono-like syndromes; and may coactivate EBV, CMV, HPV
‡ Tentatively implicated in pityriasis rosea

EPIDEMIOLOGY OF INFECTIOUS DISEASE

Seasonality of infectious disease
1 Summer/autumn
  — Legionnaires' disease
  — Leptospirosis
  — Polio; enteroviruses
  — Arboviruses (e.g. Ross River virus)
2 Autumn/winter
  — Hepatitis A
  — Coxsackie B
  — Coronaviruses; RSV
3 Winter/spring
  — Mumps
  — Infectious mononucleosis
  — Lymphocytic choriomeningitis
  — Rotavirus; Norwalk (parvovirus)
4 Spring or autumn
  — Rhinoviruses

Insect vectors of infectious disease
1 Malaria
  — *Anopheles* mosquito (female)*
2 Yellow fever, dengue
  — *Aëdes aegyptii* mosquito
3 Leishmaniasis
  — *Phlebotomus* sandfly
4 *Trypanosoma cruzi*
  — *Reduviid* arthropod
5 *Trypanosoma gambiense*
  — *Tsetse* fly
6 *Shigella* spp.
  — Housefly (*Musca domestica*)
7 Babesiosis
  — *Ixodes* tick

* Bite only between dusk and dawn

Incubation periods of various infective agents
1 Rapid-onset (incubation period often < 1 week)
  — Viruses
    • Herpes simplex (esp. type I)
    • Yellow fever
  — Bacterial
    • Cholera (*V. cholerae*)
    • Bacillary dysentery (*Shigella*)

• Scarlet fever (*St. pyogenes*)
  • Diphtheria (*C. diphtheriae*)
  • *Neisseria* spp. (gonococcus, meningococcus)
  • *H. influenzae*
  • Anthrax (*B. anthracis*)
2 Delayed-onset (incubation period often > 3 weeks)
  — Viruses
    • Hepatitis A/B
    • Epstein–Barr virus
    • Rabies
  — Bacteria
    • Syphilis (*T. pallidum*)
    • Leprosy (*M. leprae*)
  — Protozoa
    • Amebiasis (*E. histolytica*)
    • Chagas' disease (*T. cruzi*)
  — Worms
    • Filariasis
    • Schistosomiasis

Infectious disease: periods of infectivity
1 Hepatitis A
  — Prior to icteric phase
2 Measles
  — From prodrome until 4 days after onset of rash
3 Mumps
  — 3 days preparotitis until 1 week after
4 Rubella, chicken pox
  — 1 week prior to onset of rash until 1 week after
5 Scarlet fever, diphtheria
  — Onset until 3 weeks after (↓ by antibiotic therapy)

The childhood exanthemata
1 Measles (rubeola)
2 German measles (rubella)
3 Scarlet fever
  — Due to toxin-producing streptococci
4 Filatov–Dukes disease
  — Variant of scarlet fever, *or*
  — Due to toxin-producing staph infections
5 Erythema infectiosum ('Fifth disease')
  — Due to parvovirus B19 infection
6 Exanthem subitum (roseola, 'Sixth disease')
  — Due to HHV-6 infection

Pathogen or contaminant? A guide to normal flora
1 Mouth
  — Anaerobes
  — *St. viridans*
  — Pneumococcus
  — *H. influenzae*
2 Skin
  — *Propionibacterium acnes*
  — *Staphylococcus* spp.
3 Colon
  — Anaerobes
  — *Enterobacteriaceae*, esp. *E. coli*
4 Vagina
  — Lactobacilli
  — Anaerobes
  — Gp B streptococci

Infections that commonly persist in the host
1 Herpesviruses
2 Hepatitis B and C viruses

3 Toxoplasmosis
4 Malaria (esp. *P. malariae*)
5 *Strongyloides stercoralis*
6 TB

Etiologic significance of specific soft-tissue infections
1 *Staphylococcus aureus*
   — Injectable illicit drug use
2 Gp A β-hemolytic streptococci (*St. pyogenes*)
   — Can affect healthy adults; *no* predisposition needed
3 *Clostridia* spp.
   — Exposure to dirt or feces
   — Colorectal cancer
4 *Pasteurella multocida*
   — Cat bite
5 *Capnocytophaga canimorsus*
   — Dog bite
6 *Vibrio vulnificus*
   — Shellfish exposure
   — Cirrhosis

Etiologic significance of specific osteomyelitis subtypes*
1 *Bartonella henselae*
   — AIDS
2 *Salmonella* spp., pneumococcus
   — Sickle cell disease
3 *S. albus*, propionibacteria
   — Foreign body
4 *Ps. aeruginosa*, enterobacteriaceae
   — Nosocomial transmission
5 *M. avium–intracellulare*, *Candida* spp., *Aspergillus* spp.
   — Immunosuppression

* *S. aureus* is the 'usual suspect'

Dental caries: the most prevalent infectious disease of humans
1 *St. mutans* is the most cariogenic bacterium in plaque (an accretion on tooth enamel in which acid accumulates)
2 Dietary sucrose reduces plaque pH thus inducing demineralization of hydroxyapatite enamel
3 Immunization against *St. mutans* reduces plaque load and caries by stimulating production of secretory IgA (± IgG)
4 Fluoride also reduces caries
5 Necrotizing ulcerative gingivitis or chronic periodontal disease may occur due to treponemal spirochetes, esp. *Treponema denticola* and *T. socranskii*

OCCUPATIONAL EXPOSURE TO INFECTIOUS DISEASE

Nosocomial sources of infection
1 Air conditioners
   — Aspergilli, staphylococci
2 Humidifiers
   — *Acinetobacter* spp.
   — *Pseudomonas* spp.
3 Water cooling towers
   — *Legionella pneumophila*, *Pseudomonas* spp.
4 Foods (e.g. salads)
   — Gram-negatives, staphylococci, streptococci
5 Tongue depressors
   — *Rhizopus microsporus* (mucormycosis), *Penicillium* spp., *Aspergillus* spp.
6 Endogenous flora
   — *Enterobacteriaceae*, staphylococci (incl. MRSA)
7 Parenteral nutrition
   — Candidiasis, staphylococci
8 Blood transfusions
   — Hepatitis B and C, CMV, HIV, HTLV
   — Malaria, Chagas' disease (developing countries)
9 Hydrotherapy pools
   — *Ps. aeruginosa* folliculitis
10 Other patients and staff
   — Herpesviruses (esp. zoster)
   — *Listeria* spp.
   — *Cl. difficile*

Seroconversion risk after needlestick from viral index case
1 HIV
   — 0.5%
2 HCV
   — 5%
3 HBV
   — 25%*

* Risk varies widely depending on virion titer and HBeAg status

MECHANISMS OF INFECTIOUS DISEASE

Microorganisms that form spores
1 Fungi
2 *Clostridium* spp. (e.g. → botulism)
3 *Bacillus* spp. (e.g. → anthrax)

Diseases mediated by exotoxins
1 Clostridial disease
   — Tetanus (*Cl. tetani*)
   — Botulism (*Cl. botulinum*)
   — Gas gangrene (*Cl. perfringens*)
   — Antibiotic-associated colitis (*Cl. difficile*)
2 Diphtheria
3 Cholera
   Enterotoxigenic *E. coli* diarrhea
4 Staphylococcal food poisoning
   Toxic shock syndrome

Diseases in which prion proteins are implicated
1 Scrapie
2 Kuru
3 Creutzfeldt–Jakob disease
4 Gerstmann–Sträussler–Schenker syndrome
5 Familial fatal insomnia

Microbiological determinants of the 'gay bowel' syndrome
1 Pruritus ani
   — *Enterobius vermicularis* (pinworm)
   — *Pthirus pubis* (pubic lice)
   — *Sarcoptes scabiei* (scabies)

2 Perianal lesions
  — Condylomata acuminata (HPV 6, 11)
  — Condylomata lata (secondary syphilis)
  — Primary syphilitic chancre (simulates fissure)
  — Granuloma inguinale (*H. ducreyi*: donovanosis)
  — Herpetic vesicles
3 Proctitis
  — *C. trachomatis* (non-LGV serotypes)
  — *N. gonorrhea*
  — *T. pallidum*
  — Herpes simplex
4 Proctocolitis
  — *C. trachomatis* (LGV serotypes)
  — *Shigella flexneri*
  — *Campylobacter* spp.
  — *Entameba histolytica**
5 Enteritis
  — *Giardia lamblia*
6 AIDS-associated gastrointestinal infections
  — Cryptosporidiosis (small intestine)
  — Candidiasis (esophageal)
  — *M. avium–intracellulare* (may mimic Whipple's)
  — *Salmonella typhimurium*
  — *Isospora belli, Cyclospora* spp.
  — CMV

* NB: May be non-pathogenic commensal

Predispositions to mucormycosis (invasive zygomycosis)*
1 Diabetes (→ rhinocerebral)
2 Malnutrition (→ gastrointestinal)
3 Burns (→ cutaneous)
4 Leukemia (→ pulmonary)
5 Immunosuppression (→ disseminated)

* Caused by *Rhizopus microsporus*

Predispositions to osteomyelitis
1 'Standard-risk' individuals
  — *S. aureus* in 60%
2 Sickle cell disease
  — *Salmonella* spp.
3 Drug addiction
  — *Ps. aeruginosa* (→ pelvis, vertebrae)

Infectious agents sought by bioterrorists
1 Smallpox
2 Anthrax (*Bacillus anthracis*)
3 Bubonic plague (*Yersinia pestis*)
4 Botulism (*Clostridium botulinum*)
5 Ebola virus

DISEASE SUBTYPES

Diseases caused by HTLVs
1 HTLV-1
  — Tropical spastic paraparesis (HTLV1-associated myelopathy)
  — T-cell leukemia/lymphoma
2 HTLV-2
  — Hairy cell leukemia

Clinical manifestations of *Haemophilus influenzae* (HI) infection
1 Capsulated HI → children
  — Acute epiglottitis*
  — Meningitis
  — Septic arthritis
2 Non-capsulated HI → children
  — Otitis media
  — Conjunctivitis
3 Non-capsulated HI → adults
  — Exacerbation of chronic bronchitis

* Caused by type B *H. influenzae* which is often resistant to ampicillin

Varieties and features of chlamydial infection
1 Non-specific urethritis (NSU)
  — Caused by *C. trachomatis* serotypes D–K
  — Commonest sexually transmitted disease
  — Presentations
    • Seropurulent urethral discharge
    • Persistent symptoms after gonorrhea therapy
    • Failure of presumptive β-lactam therapy
    • Reiter's syndrome; Fitz-Hugh Curtis syndrome
    • Pelvic inflammatory disease, infertility
  — Diagnosis: chlamydial isolation
2 Lymphogranuloma venereum (LGV)
  — Caused by *C. trachomatis* serotypes L1–L3
  — Systemic venereal disease endemic in tropics
  — Commonest in males (5:1), esp. homosexuals
  — Presentations
    • Painful inguinal adenopathy (may suppurate)
    • 'Groove sign' (nodes indented by inguinal lig.)
    • Ulcerative proctitis; rectal stricture
    • Rectovaginal or rectovesical fistula
    • Genital elephantiasis (esp. in women)
  — Diagnosis: serology
3 Trachoma inclusion conjunctivitis (TRIC)
  — Caused by *C. trachomatis* serotypes A–C (hyperendemic)
  — Estimated to affect 500 million people
  — Commonest avoidable cause of blindness (→ keratitis)
  — Diagnosis: chlamydial isolation
4 Psittacosis
  — Caused by *C. psittaci*
  — Occupational hazard of bird-fanciers
  — Presentations
    • Atypical pneumonia
    • Myocarditis, endocarditis (rarely)
  — Diagnosis: serology
5 Epidemic pneumonia (TWAR)
  — Caused by *C. pneumoniae* *
  — Causes 10–30% of pneumonia in Finland
  — Presentations
    • Prolonged, often relapsing illness
    • Prominent pharyngitis, laryngitis
    • Atypical pneumonia (mimics psittacosis)
  — Resistant to erythromycin‡, responds to tetracycline
  — Diagnosis: serology (distinguishable from *C. psittaci*)

* Named TWAR after first two isolates, TW-183 and AR-39; morphologically resembles *C. psittaci*
‡ cf. other atypical pneumonias (p. 352)

STREPTOCOCCI

Pathogenicity of streptococci

1 *St. pyogenes* (= Gp A β-hemolytic strep; see below)
   — Acute invasive suppurative effects
     • Impetigo
     • Cellulitis, pyoderma
     • Pharyngitis
   — Other acute sequelae
     • Scarlet fever
     • Erysipelas
     • Puerperal sepsis
     • Wound infection
   — Late non-suppurative sequelae
     • Rheumatic fever
     • Post-infective nephritis
2 *St. pneumoniae* (pneumococci)
     • Pneumonia, esp. community-acquired lobar
     • Meningitis
     • Otitis media
3 *St. 'viridans'*: a broad term including
   — *St. sanguis*
     • Infective endocarditis (commonest strep cause)
   — *St. fecalis* (enterococci)
     • Urinary tract infection
     • Infective endocarditis (penicillin-resistant)
   — *St. bovis* (enterococci)
     • Infective endocarditis (penicillin-sensitive)
   — *St. milleri*
     • Liver and/or brain abscess
   — *St. mutans*
     • Dental plaque/caries

Characterization of streptococci

1 Diagnostically relevant Lancefield antigen groups
   — Gp A
     • *St. pyogenes*
   — Gp B
     • *St. agalactiae* (e.g. post-partum)
   — Gp D
     • Enterococci
2 Diagnostically relevant in vitro hemolysis
   — α-Hemolytic*
     • *St. viridans*
     • Pneumococci
   — β-Hemolytic‡
     • *St. pyogenes*

* α-Hemolytic organisms convert unlysed red cell hemoglobin in 5% blood agar to greenish (hence, 'viridans') compounds
‡ β-Hemolytic organisms lyse red cells in 5% blood agar

Pyogenic streptococci

1 *St. pyogenes*
   — i.e. Gp A β-hemolytic strep
   — Nephritogenic, skin and invasive (esp. M1) strains
2 Pneumococci
   — Gram-positive diplococci on microscopy
3 *St. milleri*
   — Anaerobic strep

NB: *St. pyogenes* and pneumococci *rarely* cause streptococcal endocarditis

Streptococcal infections: clinical correlations

1 Untreated Gp A streptococcal pharyngitis predisposes to rheumatic fever (cf. primary skin infections)
2 *Both* pharyngeal and cutaneous Gp A streptococcal infections predispose to post-strep glomerulonephritis
3 Prompt antibiotic therapy does *not* prevent post-strep glomerulonephritis (cf. rheumatic fever)
4 Latent periods between initial infection and complications
     • 4 weeks for rheumatic fever
     • 2 weeks for nephritis following impetigo
     • 1 week for synpharyngitic nephritis
5 ASO titres are strongly positive in strep pharyngitis, but only weak in impetigo (streptolysin O inactivated by skin lipids). Guttate psoriasis may also follow gp A strep infections
6 Elevated or changing ASO titres may also be associated with erythema nodosum or Henoch–Schönlein purpura

REVIEWING THE LITERATURE: INFECTIOUS DISEASE

8.1 Wald A et al (2000) Reactivation of genital herpes simplex virus type 2 infection in asymptomatic seropositive persons. N Engl J Med 342: 844–850

Prospective comparison of 53 individuals who had no history or symptoms of genital herpes, but who were seropositive for HSV2, with a control group of 90 genital herpes patients. The rate of genital viral shedding was in fact similar in both groups, indicating the presence of a large asymptomatic infectious reservoir in the community.

8.2 The MIST (Management of Influenza in the Southern Hemisphere Trialists) Study Group (1998) Randomized trial of efficacy and safety of inhaled zanamivir in treatment of influenza A and B virus infections. Lancet 352: 1877–1881

Hayden FG et al (1999) Use of the selective oral neuraminidase inhibitor oseltamivir to prevent influenza. N Engl J Med 341: 1336–1343

Two studies documenting the promising anti-influenza efficacy of neuraminidase inhibitors; unlike amantadine and rimantidine, which offer prophylaxis against only influenza A, the two new agents appeared efficacious against both influenza A and B. Since they actively inhibit viral replication, they appear also effective in shortening acute influenza.

8.3 Wong CS et al (2000) The risk of the hemolytic-uremic syndrome after antibiotic treatment of E. coli O157:H7 infections. N Engl J Med 342: 1930–1936

Prospective cohort study of 71 children with E. coli O157:H7 diarrhea, showing a 14-fold increase in the development of hemolytic uremic syndrome in those children treated with antibiotics.

8.4 Chavasse DC et al (1999) Impact of fly control on childhood diarrhoea in Pakistan. Lancet 353: 22–25

Application of insecticide significantly reduced the frequency of diarrhea in three 'sprayed' villages vs three 'unsprayed' villages, confirming the importance of fly control in limiting infectious disease.

8.5 Greif R et al (2000) Supplemental perioperative oxygen to reduce the incidence of surgical-wound infection. N Engl J Med 342: 161–167

Randomized study of 500 colorectal surgery patients, showing that those receiving 80% oxygen post-operatively had only half the number of wound infections when compared with those receiving 30% oxygen.

8.6 Steinhoff MC et al (1997) Effectiveness of clinical guidelines for the presumptive treatment of streptococcal pharyngitis in Egyptian children. Lancet 350: 918–921

Zwart S et al (2000) Penicillin for acute sore throat: randomised double blind trial of seven days versus three days treatment or placebo in adults. Br Med J 320: 150–154

Two studies of sore throat treatment. The first study suggested that antibiotic treatment is indicated in the presence of either tonsillar exudate or cervical node enlargement. The second study showed that seven days of penicillin therapy was superior to three days' therapy in such 'strep throat' patients.

8.7 van Rie A et al (1999) Exogenous reinfection as a cause of recurrent tuberculosis after curative treatment. N Engl J Med 341: 1174–1179

McKinney JD et al (2000) Persistence of Mycobacterium tuberculosis in macrophages and mice requires the glyoxylate shunt enzyme isocitrate lyase. Nature 406: 735–738

Two studies shedding light on the natural history of tuberculosis. The former study questions the role of TB 'reactivation' by showing that 12 of 16 patients with recurrent TB actually had different TB strains responsible for the original and subsequent infections. The latter study showed that the normal (human) macrophage enzyme, isocitrate lyase – which metabolizes fatty acids – is essential for TB persistence, indicating a critical interplay with the host immune defense system that is exploited by the bug.

8.8 Abraham E et al (1998) Double-blind randomized controlled trial of monoclonal antibody to human tumour necrosis factor in treatment of septic shock. Lancet 351: 929–933

Study of 1879 septic patients from 105 hospitals, showing that coagulopathy was improved in the treatment group but survival was not. The treatment was never licensed, representing a major failure for rational drug design.

8.9 Levin M et al (2000) Recombinant bactericidal/permeability-increasing protein as adjunctive treatment for children with severe meningococcal sepsis. Lancet 356: 961–967

Randomized study of 1287 patients, showing a trend towards improved survival and fewer limb amputations in the treatment group.

8.10 Gonzales RD et al (2001) Infections due to vancomycin-resistant *Enterococcus faecium* resistant to linezolid. Lancet 357: 1179

Tsiodras S et al (2001) Linezolid resistance in a clinical isolate of *Staphylococcus aureus*. Lancet 358: 207–208

Two studies reporting early cases of resistance to this potent oxazolidinone antibiotic which is reserved for vancomycin-resistant infections.

CHAPTER 9

Metabolic and nutritional disorders

Physical examination protocol 9.1   You are asked to assess the nutritional status of a patient with diarrhea

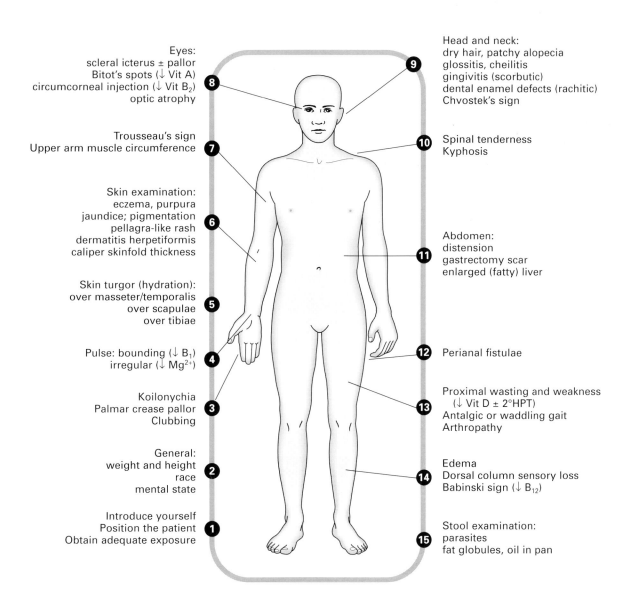

Eyes:
scleral icterus ± pallor
Bitot's spots (↓ Vit A)
circumcorneal injection (↓ Vit B_2)
optic atrophy

8

Head and neck:
dry hair, patchy alopecia
glossitis, cheilitis
gingivitis (scorbutic)
dental enamel defects (rachitic)
Chvostek's sign

9

Trousseau's sign
Upper arm muscle circumference

7

Spinal tenderness
Kyphosis

10

Skin examination:
eczema, purpura
jaundice; pigmentation
pellagra-like rash
dermatitis herpetiformis
caliper skinfold thickness

6

Skin turgor (hydration):
over masseter/temporalis
over scapulae
over tibiae

5

Abdomen:
distension
gastrectomy scar
enlarged (fatty) liver

11

Pulse: bounding (↓ B_1)
irregular (↓ Mg^{2+})

4

Perianal fistulae

12

Koilonychia
Palmar crease pallor
Clubbing

3

Proximal wasting and weakness
(↓ Vit D ± 2°HPT)
Antalgic or waddling gait
Arthropathy

13

General:
weight and height
race
mental state

2

Edema
Dorsal column sensory loss
Babinski sign (↓ B_{12})

14

Introduce yourself
Position the patient
Obtain adequate exposure

1

Stool examination:
parasites
fat globules, oil in pan

15

COMMON AND CLASSIC METABOLIC DISORDERS

Common metabolic and nutritional disorders in clinical practice
1 Obesity
2 Osteoporosis
3 Alcoholism

Classic metabolic and nutritional disorders in clinical exams
1 Paget's disease
2 Marfan's syndrome
3 Wernicke-Korsakoff syndrome

METABOLIC AND NUTRITIONAL EMERGENCIES

Metabolic diagnoses to exclude before certifying death
1 Hypothermia
2 Myxedema coma
3 Hyperosmolar coma
4 Hypoglycemia
5 Drug overdose causing coma, esp.
   — Tricyclic antidepressants
   — Barbiturates or benzodiazepines
6 Alcohol intoxication

CLINICAL ASSESSMENT OF METABOLIC DISEASE

WILSON'S DISEASE

Potential misdiagnoses in Wilson's disease
1 Coombs-negative hemolytic anemia due to hypersplenism
2 Idiopathic ('lupoid', HBsAg-negative) chronic active hepatitis
3 'Juvenile cirrhosis'
4 Schizophrenia, manic-depressive psychosis
5 Demyelination; primary cerebellar degeneration; Hallervorden–Spatz disease; idiopathic epilepsy

Other complications of Wilson's disease
1 Renal tubular acidosis (proximal type)
2 Amenorrhea, recurrent abortions
3 Chondrocalcinosis; pathological fractures
4 'Sunflower' cataracts
5 Pigmentation, blue lunules
6 Penicillamine toxicity

Diagnosis of Wilson's disease
1 Clinical signs
   — Hepato/splenomegaly
   — Kayser–Fleischer rings*
   — Slurred speech, 'batswing' tremor, rigidity, chorea
2 Copper metabolism
   — ↑ *Free* serum copper
   — ↓ *Total* serum copper

   — ↓↓ Serum ceruloplasmin (false-negatives in hepatitis)
   — ↑ 24-h urinary copper (usually > 100 g; *not* pathognomonic), esp. post-penicillamine
   — Delayed rate of radiocopper incorporation into ceruloplasmin (definitive but rarely performed)
3 Liver biopsy (prone to sampling error)
   — ↑ Liver copper (> 60 g/g dry weight)‡
   — Histology: fatty infiltration, hepatitis, cirrhosis
4 CT brainscan
   — Cortical atrophy, basal ganglia hypodensities

* Exclusion may require slit-lamp examination; absence excludes Wilson's as cause of neurological signs, but presence is *not* pathognomonic
‡ Most diagnostic test, though positives also may be seen in PBC

Drugs preventing clinical manifestations of Wilson's disease
1 Oral zinc (blocks gastrointestinal copper uptake)
2 Trientine (triethylene dihydrochloride)*
3 D-penicillamine

* An alternative to D-penicillamine in Wilson's, but *not* in cystinuria or rheumatoid arthritis

SKELETAL DISORDERS

Diagnostic criteria for Marfan's syndrome
1 Major criteria
   — Mitral valve prolapse with regurgitation
   — Dilated aortic root with regurgitation
   — Dissecting ascending aortic aneurysm
   — Lens dislocation with iridodonesis (shaky iris)
2 Minor criteria
   — Isolated mitral valve prolapse
   — Severe myopia (> 4 dioptres)
   — High arched palate
   — Scoliosis, 'funnel' chest, asthenic build
   — Spontaneous pneumothorax
   — Arachnodactyly; flat feet
   — Joint hypermobility (esp. ankle)
   — Positive family history

The patient with Paget's: clinical examination
1 Deformity of long bone(s), e.g. tibia
2 Bruit over deformity
3 Skull enlargement; associated bruit
4 Cervical spondylosis
5 Deafness (usually nerve)
6 Hyperdynamic circulation ± congestive cardiac failure

Presentations of primary hyperparathyroidism
1 Asymptomatic (in 30%)
   — Hypercalcemia detected on 'routine' biochemical test
2 Renal calculi (in 50%)
3 'Acute' presentations
   — Polydipsia/polyuria/dehydration
   — Nausea, vomiting, anorexia, constipation
   — Lethargy, dementia, psychosis

4 'Chronic' presentations
  — Nephrocalcinosis
  — Band keratopathy
5 Rare presentations
  — **P**eptic ulcer
  — **P**ancreatitis
  — **P**roximal myopathy
  — **P**athological fracture (of 'brown tumor')
  — **P**seudogout
  — **P**ituitary tumors ⎫
  — **P**ancreatic tumors ⎬ MEN1
  — **P**heochromocytoma ⎭

NUTRITIONAL DISORDERS

Clinical presentations of vitamin deficiency
1 Vitamin A deficiency
  — Xerophthalmia, night blindness, Bitot's spots
  — Hyperkeratosis
2 Thiamine deficiency
  — Beri-beri (esp. in Asians)
    • Muscle weakness
    • Tachycardia, heart failure
  — Wernicke–Korsakoff syndrome*, esp. in
    • Alcoholics ($\downarrow$ erythrocyte transketolase activity)
    • Also → hemodialysis/renal transplant patients
    • May be precipitated by IV glucose
    • May be mimicked by niacin deficiency
3 Pellagra (niacin deficiency)
  — Dermatitis (and glossitis)
  — Diarrhea
  — Dementia
4 Strachan's syndrome (? vitamin B-complex deficiency)
  — Orogenital dermatitis
  — Amblyopia
  — Painful peripheral neuropathy
5 Scurvy (vitamin C deficiency)
  — Weakness, fatigue, arthralgias
  — Ulcers, poor wound healing
  — Gingivitis, purpura
  — Subperiosteal hemorrhages (may be palpable)
6 Osteomalacia/rickets (vitamin D deficiency)
  — Tetany (in children)
  — Bone disease
  — Proximal myopathy
7 Vitamin E deficiency (e.g. cystic fibrosis, ileal resection)
  — Peripheral neuropathy, areflexia
  — Spinocerebellar degeneration, ataxia
  — Hemolysis

* NB: IV thiamine treatment usually reverses coma and ocular palsies, but nystagmus or ataxia often persist

Clinical presentations of trace element deficiency
1 Zinc deficiency (genetic, short bowel, alcoholism, TPN, or malnutrition)
  — Acrodermatitis enteropathica; alopecia
  — Poor wound healing
  — Impaired taste (hypogeusia); photophobia
2 Selenium deficiency (may occur in TPN)
  — Muscle pain, hemolytic anemia

  — Keshan disease → childhood cardiomyopathy in China
  — Kashin-Beck disease* → iodine and selenium deficiency in Tibet
3 Copper deficiency
  — Hypochromic microcytic anemia
4 Chromium deficiency
  — Glucose intolerance
  — Peripheral neuropathy; encephalopathy
5 Manganese deficiency
  — Nausea, dermatitis

* Degenerative osteoarthropathy arising between ages 5 and 15

Differential diagnosis of a pellagra-like rash
1 Pellagra (dietary niacin deficiency)
  — Esp. with high-maize (leucine-rich, tryptophan-poor) diet; leucine inhibits tryptophan → niacin
2 Hartnup disease (inherited aminoaciduria)
  — Tryptophan malabsorption → nicotinamide deficiency
3 Carcinoid syndrome
  — $\uparrow\uparrow$ 5-hydroxytryptamine → $\downarrow\downarrow$ tryptophan (precursor)
4 Isoniazid toxicity
  — Prevents pyridoxine activation → $\downarrow\downarrow$ niacin precursors

Sorting out vitamin B_6 metabolism
1 'Niacin' = vit. B_3 = nicotinic acid = pyridine 2-carboxylic acid
2 Nicotinic acid is a precursor of *nicotinamide* which is in turn a precursor of NAD (nicotinamide adenine dinucleotide) and NADP (NAD phosphate), both of which participate in cellular oxidation/reduction reactions
3 'Pyridoxine' (vitamin B_6) = one of three pyridine (niacin precursor) moieties in the diet; it is converted to the active coenzyme, pyridoxal phosphate
4 Pyridoxal phosphate is involved in intermediary amino acid metabolism, and binds to muscle glycogen phosphorylase

Common predispositions to acquired folate deficiency
1 Alcoholism
2 Blind loop syndrome
3 Celiac disease

Differential diagnosis of B_{12} deficiency and a laparotomy scar
1 Postgastrectomy
2 Ileal resection for Crohn's

HYPOTHERMIA

Predispositions to hypothermia
1 Environmental
  — Any severe or immobilizing illness
  — Poverty, poor housing, advanced age
  — Exposure
2 Reduced heat production
  — Hypothyroidism, adrenal failure

— Malnutrition
— Exhaustion (decreased shivering)
3 Increased heat loss
— Erythroderma
— Extensive burns
— Vasodilatation, esp. if alcohol-induced
4 Impaired heat regulation/poikilothermia
— Stroke
— Autonomic neuropathy
5 Drug overdose, esp.
— Phenothiazines
— Barbiturates

Systemic complications of profound hypothermia
1 Metabolic
— Acidosis, hyperkalemia
— Hypoglycemia
2 Cardiovascular
— Reduced cardiac output, BP, heart rate
— ECG: 'J' waves, ventricular dysrhythmias, asystole
— Myocardial infarction*
3 Renal
— Initial diuresis → hypovolemia → oliguria
4 Respiratory
— Reduced oxygen consumption *and/or* tissue hypoxia
— Pulmonary edema, pneumonia; apnea
5 Gastrointestinal
— Erosive gastritis, pancreatitis
— Drug toxicity ($\uparrow$ hepatic metabolism on rewarming)
6 CNS
— Amnesia, mydriasis
— Hallucinations, paradoxical undressing
— Reduced cerebral blood flow, coma

* e.g. if externally rewarmed without IV fluid replacement

HYPERTHERMIA

Differential diagnosis of hyperthermia
1 Fever (due to infection)
2 Heat stroke (exacerbated by anticholinergic therapy)
3 Iatrogenic (general)
— Bleomycin, L-asparaginase, interferon
— MAOI or sympathomimetic overdose ± tricyclics
4 Malignant hyperthermia
5 Neuroleptic malignant syndrome

Malignant hyperthermia or neuroleptic malignant syndrome?
1 Malignant hyperthermia (MH)
— Autosomal dominant etiology
— Caused by *many* inhalational anesthetics (e.g. halothane, suxamethonium*)
— *Peripheral* origin (post-synaptic muscle contraction)
— High fever develops within minutes; may be fatal
— Often complicated by metabolic acidosis/hyperkalemia

— Muscle necrosis → myoglobinuria, renal failure, $\uparrow$ Ca^{2+}
— Associations: central core disease, myotonic dystrophy
— Prophylaxis or therapy: dantrolene sodium
2 Neuroleptic malignant syndrome (NMS)
— Idiosyncratic etiology (impossible to predict)
— Precipitated by phenothiazines/butyrophenones‡
— *Central* origin (CNS dopaminergic inhibition)
— Develops insidiously over 1–3 days: fluctuating consciousness, dystonias, autonomic instability
— 20% mortality due to aspiration pneumonitis, acute myoglobinuric renal failure, arrhythmias
— Neuromuscular blockers (e.g. pancuronium) may cause flaccid paralysis (cf. MH: no effect)
— Therapy: dantrolene or bromocriptine (takes days)

* cf. pseudocholinesterase deficiency: specific for suxamethonium
‡ Also seen in L-DOPA 'drug holidays' in Parkinson's disease

OXYGENATION ANOMALIES

Anoxia survival times of various tissues
1 Hair and nails
— 1 week
2 Blood vessels
— 2 days
3 Muscle
— 1 h
4 Liver, kidney
— 15 min
5 Brain
— 3 min

Metabolic considerations in near-drowned patients
1 Fresh-water (hypotonic, hypervolemia) drowning
— Often leads to *mild* hypoxia only, due to surfactant inactivation and/or intravascular hemolysis
2 Salt-water (hypertonic) drowning
— Often causes *severe* hypoxia due to pulmonary edema
3 'Dry drowning'
— Death due to reflex laryngospasm without aspiration
4 Post-resuscitative course may be complicated by
— Aspiration pneumonia
— Acute tubular necrosis
— Disseminated intravascular coagulation
5 Prognosis post-resuscitation
— Hypothermia → better prognosis
— Neurologic signs → poor prognosis

Medical problems affecting underwater divers
1 Decompression sickness ('the bends')
— Symptom onset varies: 10 min → days
— Arteriovenous/lymphatic obstruction
— Tissue rupture
— Muscle fascial compartmental syndrome
2 Nitrogen narcosis ('rapture of the depths')
— Mimics drunkenness

— Occurs with air diving below 40 metres
3 Barotrauma
  — Face squeeze; facial nerve baroparesis
  — Dental or skin barotrauma
  — Gastric rupture

Symptoms and signs of high altitude cerebral edema
1 Headaches
2 Hallucinations, irrationality
3 Cerebellar ataxia
4 Papilledema and retinal hemorrhages

AROMATIC ABNORMALITIES

Gustatory/olfactory clues to diagnosis of metabolic disorders
1 Skin
  — Salty (cystic fibrosis)
  — Caramel (maple syrup urine disease)
  — Sweaty feet (isovaleric acidemia)
2 Urine
  — Rotting fish (trimethylaminuria)*
  — Mouse-like (phenylketonuria)

* Fish odor also detectable in breath, sweat, saliva, vaginal secretions

Anosmia: differential diagnosis
1 Post-traumatic
  — e.g. Skull fracture (commonest cause)
2 Frontal/olfactory groove meningioma
  → Asymptomatic unilateral loss
3 Inherited disease
  — Kallman's syndrome, Refsum's disease
4 Post-coryzal or chronic rhinitis; cadmium poisoning
5 Sjögren's syndrome, Paget's disease
6 CNS disease: Alzheimer's, Parkinson's

UNUSUAL DISORDERS

Diagnoses worth considering in obscure clinical presentations
1 Occult malignancy, esp. Ca lung/liver/kidney, lymphoma
2 Occult infection: tuberculosis, syphilis, infective endocarditis
3 Sarcoidosis
4 Polyarteritis nodosa
5 Iatrogenic
6 Functional
  — Alcoholism/narcotic addiction
  — Depression
  — Hysteria
  — Self-inflicted disease

Fibrosing syndromes in clinical medicine
1 Retroperitoneal fibrosis
2 Constrictive pericarditis
3 Sclerosing cholangitis
4 Riedel's thyroiditis
5 Peyronie's disease

6 Fibrosing alveolitis
7 Systemic sclerosis (scleroderma)

Clinical varieties of histiocytosis
1 Class I (Langerhans cell) histiocytosis*
  — Letterer–Siwe disease (→ infants)
    • Hepatosplenomegaly/lymphadenopathy
    • Cytopenias (marrow infiltration by H-X cells)
    • Lung infiltrates, recurrent pneumothoraces
  — Hand–Schüller–Christian disease (→ adolescents)
    • Skull lesions
    • Exophthalmos; ear discharge
    • Diabetes insipidus (in 30%)
  — Eosinophilic granuloma (→ adults)
    • Multiple lytic bony deposits (esp. in skull)
    • Malaise, weight loss, fever
    • Lung fibrosis
2 Class II histiocytosis
  — Hemophagocytic (non-Langerhans) syndromes
    • Sinus histiocytosis + massive adenopathy
3 Class III histiocytosis
  — Malignant histiocytosis
    • 'True histiocytic' lymphoma (celiac disease)
    • Histiocytic medullary reticulosis
    • Leukemias: AML (M4/M5), CMML

* = 'Histiocytosis X'; a group of histologically benign conditions (though clinical course may be lethal). Treatable with etoposide

CLINICAL PRESENTATIONS OF INHERITED DISEASE

Gaucher's (adult non-neuronopathic) disease: features
1 Occurs due to deficiency of β-glucosidase
2 Presents with
  — Hypersplenism ± massive splenomegaly
  — Bone pain due to
    • Infarcts/aseptic necrosis
    • Bone cysts (→ distal femur)
    • Vertebral collapse
    • Pathological fracture
  — Pingueculae; pigmentation
  — Pneumonia
3 Normal life expectancy
  — i.e. In adult (type III) disease
4 Best screening test
  — Serum acid phosphatase (tartrate-resistant)
5 Definitive diagnosis
  — Demonstration of Gaucher cells in marrow, liver or node (= PAS +ve cells, 'crumpled silk' cytoplasm*)
6 Treatable with IV recombinant enzyme (glucocerebrosidase) replacement, or else with substrate (glucocerebroside) depletion using glucosyltransferase inhibition

* NB: Gaucher cells may also be seen in CGL, myeloma, ITP

Clinical spectrum of mitochondrial disease
1 Progressive external ophthalmoplegia, incl. Kearns–Sayre syndrome
  — Ophthalmoplegia + retinitis pigmentosa + complete heart block + increased CSF protein

2 Hypermetabolic proximal myopathy
— e.g. Luft's: heat intolerance, fever, weakness
— May mimic thyrotoxicosis
3 'Ragged red fibre' syndrome
— Myopathy resembles facioscapulohumeral dystrophy
— Associated with myoclonic epilepsy, lactic acidosis
4 Cytochrome deficiencies
— e.g. Menke's ('kinky hair') syndrome

NB: Diseases of mitochondrial DNA are inherited via the maternal genome

Inborn abnormalities of connective tissue: features
1 Marfan's syndrome
— Autosomal dominant, variable penetrance
— Increasing frequency with paternal age
— 30% sporadic mutation rate
— Occurs due to fibrillin gene mutations
— Signs
• Armspan > height; scoliosis
• Joint hypermobility
• Arachnodactyly, 'wrist', 'thumb' signs
• High palate, iridodonesis
• Pectus deformity; MVP, AI
2 Osteogenesis imperfecta
— Occurs due to *qualitatively abnormal* (mutant) type I collagen
3 Homocystinuria (autosomal recessive)
— Some phenotypic similarity to Marfan's, but
• Atherothrombotic tendency
• Subclinical osteoporosis
• Downward lens dislocation
• 30% incidence of mental retardation
— Responds to
• Dietary methionine restriction
• Cystine supplements
• Pyridoxine (in 50%)
• Betaine
4 Pseudoxanthoma elasticum (dominant or recessive)
— Characterized by
• Flexural xanthoma-like lesions, lax skin
• Fundal angioid streaks
• Premature atherosclerosis ($\rightarrow$ hypothyroidism)
• Diagnostic calcium deposition on skin biopsy
— Occurs due to production of abnormal elastin
5 Ehlers–Danlos syndromes (dominant or recessive)
— Characterized by
• Joint hypermobility, recurrent dislocations
• Purpura
• 'Fish-mouth' scarring
• Diverticulosis, pneumothoraces
— Type IV
• GI bleeding, perforation, aneurysm rupture
• Occurs due to ↓ type III collagen
— Type VI
• Retinal detachment, corneal perforation
• Occurs due to ↓ lysyl hydroxylase
— Type VII
• Velvety skin, short stature
• Occurs due to ↓ procollagen protease
— Type VIII manifests as periodontitis
6 Disorders due to reduced lysyl oxidase activity
— Ehlers–Danlos type V (X-linked)

— Cutis laxa (X-linked)
• Emphysema, pulmonary hypertension
— Menke's 'kinky hair' syndrome
• Defective copper absorption

Laurence–Moon or Bardet–Biedl syndrome?
1 Features in common
— Mental retardation
— Hypogonadism
— Obesity
— Retinopathy
2 Additional features of Laurence–Moon syndrome
— Ataxia
— Spastic paraparesis
3 Additional features of Bardet–Biedl syndrome
— Polydactyly
— Renal abnormalities
• Persistent fetal lobulation
• Cystic dysplasia, clubbed calices
• Nephrogenic diabetes insipidus
• Aminoaciduria

INVESTIGATING METABOLIC DISORDERS

Acute respiratory acid-base changes
1 $PaCO_2$ 20 mmHg (2.5 kPa); plasma bicarbonate 20; pH 7.6
2 $PaCO_2$ 30 mmHg (4.0 kPa); plasma bicarbonate 22; pH 7.5
3 $PaCO_2$ 40 mmHg (6.0 kPa); plasma bicarbonate 24; pH 7.4
4 $PaCO_2$ 60 mmHg (8.0 kPa); plasma bicarbonate 26; pH 7.3
5 $PaCO_2$ 80 mmHg (10.0 kPa); plasma bicarbonate 28; pH 7.2

Causes of misleading results
1 (Pseudo)hyponatremia
— Dilutional
• High-grade paraproteinemia
• Chylomicronemia (ketoacidosis, hyperlipidemia)
• IV therapy: mannitol or parenteral fat emulsions
2 Spurious hyperkalemia
— Sample hemolysis
• (Leukemic) white cell count > 200 000/mL
• Difficult venepuncture
• Delay in processing specimen
3 Spurious hyperchloremia
— Bromism
4 Spurious hyperglycemia
— Venepuncture adjacent to dextrose infusion site
5 Spurious hypercalcemia
— Prolonged venous stasis
— Calcium binding by myeloma paraprotein (rare)
Spurious normocalcemia
— Hypoalbuminemia (esp. in cancer patients)
6 ↑ Triglycerides, ↑ gastrin, ↓ growth hormone
— Patient not fasted
7 Elevated CPK
— Recent intramuscular injection

8 Elevated acid phosphatase
— Recent rectal examination
9 Negative urinalysis for ketones
— Alcoholic ketoacidosis (leads to high β-hydroxybutyrate but normal acetone)

ELECTROLYTE DISORDERS AND THE ANION GAP

High-anion-gap metabolic acidosis*: common precipitants
1 Uremia
2 Ketoacidosis (diabetic or alcoholic)
3 Lactic acidosis (± dehydration, alcohol intoxication)
4 Overdose
— Aspirin
— Methanol, ethylene glycol
— Paraldehyde

* Anion gap = $Na^+ - Cl^- - HCO_3^-$; normal range = 8–12 mEq/L

Differential diagnosis of a low anion gap*
1 Hypoalbuminemia
2 Paraproteinemia
3 Electrolyte imbalance
— Hypercalcemia
— Hypermagnesemia
— Lithium intoxication

* May mask biochemical recognition of metabolic acidosis

Hyperchloremic (normal anion gap) acidosis: pathogeneses
1 Renal tubular acidosis
2 Gastrointestinal
— Diarrhea, esp. in neonates
— Pancreatic/biliary fistula
— Ureteroenterostomy ± obstructed ileal bladder/vesicocolic fistula
3 Iatrogenic
— Acetazolamide
— Colestyramine
— Parenteral nutrition with fructose, sorbitol

Normal anion gap acidosis with hyperkalemia*: causes
1 Treated diabetic ketoacidosis
2 Obstructive uropathy
3 Early uremic acidosis, esp. if due to medullary disease
4 Mineralocorticoid deficiency or insensitivity

* a.k.a. type 4 renal tubular acidosis

Lactic acidosis: antecedents and diagnosis
1 Type A
— Precipitated by *any* cause of severe tissue hypoxia
2 Type B
— Idiopathic onset in elderly debilitated patients
— Alcohol abuse and/or liver disease
— Uremia
— Some leukemias, myeloproliferative disorders
— Diabetes mellitus ± metformin ± ketoacidosis
3 Clinical
— Hyperventilation without dehydration*

4 Diagnosis requires exclusion of other causes of high-anion-gap acidosis ± demonstration of elevated plasma lactate

* cf. hyperosmolar coma (p. 89): vice versa

Clinical features of D-lactic acidosis
1 Occurs in:
— Short bowel syndrome
— Jejunoileal bypass
2 Increased frequency if
— Thiamine deficiency
— Renal tubular acidosis
— Large oral sugar load
3 Due to
— Increased colonic lactate load leads to hyperabsorption
— Selective failure to metabolize D-lactate isomer
4 Features
— Confusion, ataxia, nystagmus, stupor
— Mimics alcoholic inebriation
5 Treatment
— Bicarbonate infusion
— Thiamine (if deficient)
— Reduce colonic flora (and ?alkalinize gut)
• Oral vancomycin, neomycin, metronidazole

Examples of mixed metabolic acidosis
1 Normal plus high anion gap acidoses
— Renal tubular acidosis leading to nephrocalcinosis
— Diabetic with hyporeninemic hypoaldosteronism developing ketoacidosis
2 Mixed normal anion gap acidoses
— Acetazolamide therapy in patients with pre-existing renal tubular acidosis
3 Mixed high anion gap acidoses
— Alcoholic ketoacidosis complicated by lactic acidosis
— Methanol intoxication and lactic acidosis

Diagnostic significance of urinary chloride in metabolic alkalosis
1 *All* forms of metabolic alkalosis have low *serum* chloride
2 *Urinary* chloride is *normal* in some (*normovolemic*) metabolic alkaloses, e.g.
— Primary hyperaldosteronism
3 Urinary chloride *absent* in *hypovolemic* metabolic alkaloses
— Gastric losses (prolonged vomiting, suction)
— Following excessive use of diuretics
4 This is because the hypovolemic stimulus for ADH secretion *overrides* hypo-osmolar stimulus for ADH suppression
— i.e. Renal Na^+ (and Cl^-) are *conserved*
5 This leads to a *paradoxical aciduria* which persists until NaCl (volume) *and* KCl (electrolyte) replenishment is achieved
— i.e. Resolution of the alkalosis is *chloride-dependent*
6 Alkalosis may be treated if necessary with acetazolamide

Some causes of hypouricemia
1 Proximal renal tubular disease (e.g. Wilson's disease)
2 SIADH (e.g. acute interminent porphyria, Guillain–Barré)
3 Chronic liver disease
4 Carcinomatosis
5 Hereditary xanthinuria (xanthine oxidase deficiency)
6 Drug-induced: allopurinol, high-dose aspirin, NSAIDs, sulfinpyrazone, diflunisal, probenecid

Indications for serum magnesium estimation
1 Severe or intractable diarrhea and/or malabsorption, e.g.
 — Short bowel syndrome
 — Inflammatory bowel disease
2 Life-threatening alcohol withdrawal
3 Refractory cardiac arrhythmias (esp. ventricular) Unexplained digoxin toxicity
4 Apathetic thyrotoxicosis
5 Hypocalcemia and/or tetany unresponsive to calcium
6 Neuromuscular symptoms after cis-platinum or mannitol
7 Investigation of chronic fatigue

Clinically important causes of hypophosphatemia
1 Insulin treatment of diabetic ketoacidosis
2 Alcoholic withdrawal supported with dextrose infusions
3 Proximal renal tubular dysfunction
4 Following starvation or severe burns
5 Osteomalacia (unless associated with renal failure)
6 Iatrogenic
 — Hyperalimentation
 — Phosphate-binding antacids, hemodialysis
 — Paracetamol overdose ($\rightarrow \uparrow$ renal losses)

Manifestations of hypophosphatemia
1 Due to reduced erythrocyte 2,3-DPG (esp. in ketoacidosis)
 — Tissue hypoxia $\rightarrow$ ataxia, confusion, convulsions
2 Due to reduced intracellular ATP
 — Platelet dysfunction $\rightarrow$ bleeding
 — Hemolytic anemia, leukocyte dysfunction
3 Due to rhabdomyolysis (esp. in alcoholics)
 — Renal failure
 — Delayed hypercalcemia
 — Cardiomyopathy

HYPERCALCEMIA

Common causes of hypercalcemia
1 Hyperparathyroidism
2 Malignancy
 — Via production of PTHrP
 — Osteolytic bone metastases ± 'flare'

Steroid-suppressible hypercalcemia: differential diagnosis
1 Granulomatous diseases
 — Sarcoidosis
 — TB, histoplasmosis, leprosy

2 Vitamin D intoxication
3 Multiple myeloma

Differential diagnosis of hypercalcemia with detectable iPTH*
1 Hyperparathyroidism
 — Primary
 — Tertiary
 — Secondary, *if* overzealous phosphate-binding R_x
2 Immobilization
 — Urinary cAMP normal
3 Malignancy
 — Urinary cAMP often increased
 — iPTH normal; PTHrP* often increased
4 Pheochromocytoma
 — Part of MEN2 (Sipple's syndrome)
 — Catecholamine-stimulated PTH release‡

* iPTH = immunoreactive PTH; PTHrP = parathyroid hormone-related peptide
‡ Hence, hyperparathyroidism may reflect hyperplasia *or* adenoma

Steps in the diagnosis of primary hyperparathyroidism
1 $\uparrow$ Ca^{2+}; ± $\downarrow$ PO_4^{2-} (normalization may presage renal failure)
2 $\uparrow$ iPTH
 — Normal levels do not exclude the diagnosis*
 — The C-terminal fragment is generally assayed, though the N-terminal fragment confers activity
3 Elevated nephrogenous cAMP‡
4 Supportive (but not diagnostic) evidence
 — Phosphaturia (> hypercalciuria)
 — *Mild* $\uparrow$ serum alkaline phosphatase
 — Hyperchloremic acidosis with alkaline urine
 — No evidence of malignancy
5 Definitive diagnosis
 — Hyperplasia/adenoma confirmed at neck exploration
 — Resection followed by normalization of serum calcium

* Undetectable levels do
‡ Not suppressible with oral calcium tolerance test

Differential diagnosis of normocalcemic hypercalciuria
1 Idiopathic
2 Medullary sponge kidneys
3 Immobilization (esp. in Paget's disease)
4 Sarcoidosis
5 Acromegaly; Cushing's syndrome
6 (Mild) primary hyperparathyroidism*
7 Renal tubular acidosis
8 Iatrogenic
 — Corticosteroids
 — Furosemide (frusemide)

* Definitively diagnosed by elevated serum iPTH and/or urinary cAMP

Hypercalcemia: selected clinical aspects
1 Dehydration may arise due to any combination of
 — Vomiting
 — Reduced fluid intake (anorexia, obtundation)
 — Nephrogenic diabetes insipidus

2 Azotemia may supervene due to
   — Prerenal failure (i.e. secondary to dehydration)
   — (Acute) vasoconstriction, $\downarrow$ glomerular permeability
   — (Chronic) tubule vacuolization or nephrocalcinosis
3 Immobilization hypercalcemia (and hypercalciuria)
   — More frequent in patients with Paget's disease
   — Corticosteroids or phosphate R_x are contraindicated
4 Gut hyperabsorption contributes to hypercalcemia in
   — Sarcoidosis
   — 'Milk-alkali' syndrome
   — Primary hyperparathyroidism
5 Familial hypocalciuric ('benign familial') hypercalcemia*
   — Classically presents as failed neck exploration for hyperparathyroidism
   — Commonest hypercalcemia in patients < 10 years
6 Rhabdomyolysis hypercalcemia
   — May lead to initial hypocalcemia with azotemia
   — Hypercalcemia ensues during early renal recovery

* Caused by loss-of-function mutations affecting a calcium-sensing receptor

Metabolic consequences of traumatic rhabdomyolysis*
1 Hyperkalemia; hypercalcemia (see above)
2 Hypovolemic shock
3 Myoglobinuric renal failure (p. 318)
4 Cardiomyopathy
5 Disseminated intravascular coagulation

* 'Muscle crush syndrome'

VITAMIN D

Differential diagnosis of hypervitaminosis D
1 Intoxication with exogenous vitamin D
   — Renal failure
   — Hypoparathyroidism
   — Megadose ingestion
2 Granulomatous diseases
   — $\uparrow$ Extrarenal conversion of 25-OH-D to 1,25–$(OH)_2$D
   — Causes include sarcoidosis and lymphoma

Abnormal patterns of vitamin D metabolism in disease
1 Vitamin D intoxication
   — $\uparrow$ 25-Hydroxycholecalciferol (25-D_3)
   — Normal 1,25-D_3
2 Sarcoidosis
   — Normal 25-D_3
   — $\uparrow$ 1,25-D_3 (even in *anephric* patients)
3 Chronic renal failure
   — Normal 25-D_3
   — $\downarrow$ 1,25-D_3
   — $\uparrow$ 24,25-D_3
4 Rickets
   — Normal 1,25-D_3 (vitamin D-resistant rickets)
   — $\downarrow$ 1,25-D_3 (type I vitamin D-dependent rickets)
   — $\uparrow$ 1,25-D_3 (type II vitamin D-dependent rickets)

Differential diagnosis of abnormal vitamin D metabolism
1 $\uparrow$ 1,25-D_3
   — Primary hyperparathyroidism
   — Pregnancy
   — Sarcoidosis
2 $\downarrow$ 1,25-D_3
   — Malignancy-induced hypercalcemia
   — Post-menopausal osteoporosis
   — Chronic renal failure
3 $\uparrow$ 25-D_3
   — Vitamin D intoxication
   $\downarrow$ 25-D_3
   — Osteomalacia
   — Hypomagnesemia
   — Chronic liver disease (e.g. PBC)
   — Chronic peritoneal dialysis
   — Nephrotic syndrome
   — Phenytoin use*

* Stimulates vitamin D catabolism

DIAGNOSTIC ASPECTS OF METABOLIC BONE DISEASE

Clinical significance of elevated urinary hydroxyproline*
1 Paget's disease (often > 50× $\uparrow$)
2 Hereditary hyperphosphatasia (often > 50× $\uparrow$)
3 Hyperparathyroidism
4 Osteomalacia (*except* renal tubular type)
5 Thyrotoxicosis

* Indicates collagen breakdown; correlates with serum alkaline phosphatase

Features of pseudohypoparathyroidism
1 Features *not* found in 'idiopathic' hypoparathyroidism
   — Familial occurrence
     • X-linked dominant (maternal) transmission*
   — Physical examination
     • Short fourth and fifth metacarpals‡
     • No enamel hypoplasia or candidiasis
   — Laboratory
     • Normal or elevated serum iPTH
     • Subnormal increment of urinary phosphate and nephrogenous cAMP after PTH infusion
2 Features *not* found in pseudopseudohypoparathyroidism¶
   — Clinical
     • Associated endocrine abnormalities (e.g. hypothyroidism, amenorrhea)
   — Laboratory
     • Hypocalcemia, hypocalciuria, hyperphosphaturia
     • Normal or elevated serum iPTH
     • Subnormal increment of urinary phosphate and nephrogenous cAMP after PTH infusion
3 Signs more typical of pseudopseudohypoparathyroidism
   — Mental retardation, dwarfism, obesity
   — Subcutaneous calcification

4 Common features of pseudo- and pseudopseudo-variants
— Both may have Albright's osteodystrophy
— Both associated with G-protein (G_s) mutations
5 *All* may respond to pharmacological doses of calcitriol

* cf. idiopathic: familial (autoimmune) variety is autosomal recessive
‡ Part of Albright's osteodystrophy (cf. Turner's syndrome → short fourth metacarpal; Down's syndrome → short, curved middle phalanx of fifth finger, 'clinodactyly')
¶ Now classified as a pathogenetic subset of pseudohypoparathyroidism

Diagnostic considerations in osteomalacia
1 Pathogenetic factors
— Main source of vitamin D for most people is sunlight
— Elderly people with little sun exposure may become vitamin D deficient due to dietary malabsorption induced (say) by gastrectomy
2 Proximal myopathy
— May be a prominent presenting symptom
— Arises in part due to hypophosphatemia
— Arises in part due to vitamin D deficiency per se
3 Diagnosis
— Characteristic radiographic features
— Biochemical triad
• Hypocalcemia
• Hypophosphatemia
• Serum alkaline phosphatase
— Definitive
• Bone biopsy

RADIOGRAPHIC FEATURES OF BONE DISEASE

Radiologic stigmata of hyperparathyroidism
1 General
— Widespread osteopenia
2 Most specific sign
— Subperiosteal resorption of radial aspects of middle phalanges of second and third fingers
3 Other erosive/resorptive changes
— Resorption of distal phalangeal tufts
— 'Brown tumors'*
— 'Fleabitten' mandible
— 'Salt-and-pepper' skull
— Loss of (dental) lamina dura
— Distal clavicular erosions
4 Metastatic calcification
— Nephrocalcinosis, renal calculi
— Chondrocalcinosis
— Vascular calcification (secondary hyperparathyroidism)

* Bone cysts → phalanges, metacarpals, long bones

Classical spinal X-rays in metabolic bone disease
1 'Rugger-jersey' spine
— Renal osteodystrophy
— Osteopetrosis ('bone-within-bone')
2 'Ivory vertebrae'
— Paget's disease
— Hodgkin's disease

3 'Codfish' vertebrae
— Osteoporosis
— Osteomalacia
— Sickle-cell disease

Classical skull X-rays in bone disease
1 Osteoporosis circumscripta
— Paget's disease
2 'Raindrops' (many lytic lesions, no osteoblastic reaction)
— Myeloma
3 'Salt-and-pepper' skull
— Hyperparathyroidism
4 Wormian bones
— Osteogenesis imperfecta
5 'Hair-on-end' appearance
— Inherited anemias
6 'Punched-out' skull lesions
— Histiocytosis X
7 Enlarged frontal sinuses
— Acromegaly
8 Absent frontal sinuses
— Kartagener's syndrome
9 Hyperostosis frontalis interna
— Normal variant (esp. in women)

Other radiographic anomalies in bone disease
1 Rickets
— Widened epiphyseal plate with indistinct borders
— Splaying of bone ends (esp. wrists, knees)
— Deformities: tibial bowing, frontal bossing
2 Osteomalacia
— Pseudo-('Milkman's') fractures, Looser's zones*
3 Scurvy
— Sclerotic bone edge ('dense white line') at epiphysis
— No widening of epiphyseal plate (cf. rickets)
— Periosteal elevation due to hemorrhage (seen post-R_x)
4 Heavy metal poisoning
— Dense 'white line' at metaphysis (cf. scurvy)
5 Osteoid osteoma
— Densely sclerotic lesion surrounded by radiolucency
— Causes aspirin-sensitive bone pain in young patient
6 Osteopetrosis
— 'Erlenmeyer flask' deformity of metaphyses

* Affect pubic rami, proximal femurs, lateral scapulae, ribs

ISOTOPE BONE SCANNING

Possible indications for isotope bone scans
1 Suspected metastatic bone disease
2 Suspected (X-ray negative) fracture, esp.
— ? Stress fracture
— ? Sternal fracture
— ? Scaphoid fracture
3 Suspected aseptic necrosis
— Efficacy limited by non-specificity

4 Suspected sacroiliitis with non-diagnostic X-ray findings
   — Value in this context is controversial
5 Suspected periprosthetic infection (→ gallium scanning)
6 Paget's disease

Increased uptake on isotope bone scan?
1 New bone formation
   — Focal increase
     • Fracture*
     • Metastasis‡
   — Diffuse increase
     • Paget's disease
     • Hyperparathyroidism
     • Osteomalacia
2 Hyperemia
   — Infection¶
   — Trauma
3 Some primary tumors
   — Ewing's sarcoma
   — Osteosarcoma, neuroblastoma

* NB: Sacral and sternal lesions are often difficult to assess
‡ Solitary lesions and/or skull lesions can be difficult to interpret
¶ Osteomyelitis best diagnosed by bone scan ± ^{67}Ga or ^{111}In scan (esp. if prosthetic joint infection suspected)

Reduced uptake on isotope bone scan?
1 Avascular necrosis (incl. radiation osteonecrosis)
2 Multiple myeloma
3 'Eosinophilic granuloma'

NB: In patients with *pain*, normal uptake virtually excludes a bony origin

INVESTIGATION OF BONE METABOLISM

Diagnostic tests of bone density
1 X-ray
   — Singh index
2 Dual-energy X-ray absorptiometry (DXA)
   — e.g. Radial (or hip) bone mass
3 Iliac crest bone biopsy
   — Invasive; sampling error is a problem

Indications for densitometric bone monitoring
1 Premature menopause
2 Osteoporosis noted on X-ray
3 Vertebral deformity or fractures
4 Hyperparathyroidism, thyrotoxicosis, post-gastrectomy
5 Chronic steroid therapy (> 5 mg prednisone/day)
6 Assessment of anti-osteoporosis therapy

Markers of osteoblastic activity (new bone formation)
1 Isotope (^{99m}Tc-phosphate) bone scan
2 Serum alkaline phosphatase (esp. bone isoform)
3 Serum osteocalcin

Markers of osteoclastic activity (bone resorption)
1 Acid phosphatase (tartrate-resistant)
2 Urinary hydroxyproline*

3 Urinary pyridinium crosslinks/type I collagen β-crosslaps‡

* Utility reduced by non-specificity and insensitivity
‡ Used to monitor the efficacy of antiresorptive therapies in osteoporosis

INVESTIGATION OF GENETIC DISEASE

Biochemical screens available for inborn errors of metabolism
1 Benedict's test (copper reduction)
   — Galactosemia
2 DNP (dinitrophenylhydrazine) test
   — Maple syrup urine disease
3 Nitroprusside test
   — Homocystinuria
4 Alkaline silver reduction
   — Alkaptonuria (ochronosis)
5 Urinary colorimetry
   — Orotic aciduria

Presymptomatic disease identifiable by genetic linkage analysis
1 Huntington's chorea
2 Myotonic dystrophy
3 Duchenne muscular dystrophy
4 Neurofibromatosis (incl. acoustic variant)
5 Cystic fibrosis
6 α/β-thalassemias
7 Polycystic kidney disease
8 Familial adenomatous polyposis
9 Multiple endocrine neoplasia

Familial periodic fevers: the clinical spectrum
1 Autosomal dominant
   — Muckle-Wells syndrome
     • Mutations on chromosome 1q44
   — Familial Hibernian fever
     • Mutations of tumor necrosis factor receptor on 12p13
2 Autosomal recessive
   — Hyper-IgD syndrome
     • Mutations of mevalonate kinase gene on 12q24
   — Familial Mediterranean fever (see below)
     • Mutations of *Pyrin* gene (esp. exon 10) on 16p13

Familial Mediterranean fever (recurrent polyserositis): diagnosis
1 History
   — Ethnic origin, positive family history
   — Previous attacks ± failed exploratory laparotomy
   — Homozygous M694V *Pyrin* gene mutation* predicts amyloidosis
2 Acute episodes
   — Mild leukocytosis, ↑ ESR, ↑ fibrinogen during attacks
   — Rapid defervescence following attacks
3 Signs of chronicity
   — Proteinuria (if amyloidosis has supervened)

4 Important diagnostic exclusions
— Normal amylase; low C5a levels
— Normal microbiology (incl. joint fluid)
— Negative ANA and rheumatoid factor
5 Therapeutic normalization with colchicine
— Effective symptom prophylaxis
— Plasma dopamine β-hydroxylase (best test)

* At least one mutant allele detected in 80% of patients. Homozygosity predicts more severe disease

MANAGING METABOLIC DISEASE

Therapeutic priorities in metabolic derangements
1 Lactic acidosis
— Removal of underlying cause (e.g. alcohol)
— IV bicarbonate (esp. if methanol or ethylene glycol poisoning)
— Acidemia also treatable with 0.3M THAM (tromethamine: tris-hydroxymethyl aminomethane) acetate, pH 8.6 (watch for hypoglycemia or respiratory depression)
2 Alcoholic ketoacidosis
— Intravenous glucose, *plus*
— Intravenous thiamine
3 Diabetic ketoacidosis
— Insulin
— Fluid and electrolyte balance
4 Hyperosmolar (non-ketotic diabetic) coma
— IV fluids (use hypotonic saline unless hypotensive)
— Insulin (usually unnecessary long-term; cf. DKA)
5 Hypoglycemic coma
— Prevention
— Immediate therapeutic trial of IV dextrose (± naloxone) in any undiagnosed unconscious patient*
6 Myxedema coma
— Exclude hypothermia-/glycemia-/natremia-/-adrenal
— Low-dose IV T_3 with hydrocortisone

* If Wernicke–Korsakoff syndrome possible, give IV thiamine as well

Management approach to the hypothermic patient
1 Sinus rhythm, core temperature > 32°C
— Passive external rewarming
2 Sinus rhythm, core temperature < 32°C, *or* Arrhythmia, core temperature > 32°C
— Active core rewarming
• Heated humidified air via endotracheal tube
• Pleural or peritoneal lavage with heated (40–45°C) crystalloid or colloid fluid
3 Arrhythmia, core temperature < 32°C
— Extracorporeal core rewarming
• Cardiopulmonary bypass loop
• Extracorporeal venovenous rewarming
• Hemodialysis
— Bretylium 10 mg/kg for ventricular fibrillation

MANAGEMENT OF ELECTROLYTE ABNORMALITIES

Hypokalemia: when is prophylactic supplementation indicated?
1 Patients clinically hypovolemic due to gastrointestinal losses who are commencing resuscitation with IV fluids
2 Patients undergoing insulin and fluid replacement for diabetic ketoacidosis *unless* hyperkalemic *and*
— ECG changes of hyperkalemia *or*
— Biochemical evidence of prerenal failure *or*
— Known coexisting hyporeninemic hypoaldosteronism
3 Patients with anticipated large renal losses, e.g.
— Post-obstructive diuresis
— Sjögren's syndrome → post-partum
— Wilson's disease → renal tubular disease + cirrhosis
4 Patients commencing therapy with
— Loop diuretics
— Ticarcillin
— Amphotericin B
5 Patients stabilized on digoxin and commencing therapy with
— Thiazides
— Corticosteroids

An approach to acute hyperkalemia
1 Exclude diabetic ketoacidosis as a cause*
2 Check result on fresh specimen to exclude hemolysis artefact
3 Identify and remove precipitating cause if possible
4 Give 50 mL 50% dextrose IV, then soluble insulin (8–12 units)
5 Give 50 mL 8.4% sodium bicarbonate IV
6 Give 20 mL 10% calcium gluconate IV *if* ECG changes present
7 Give 15 g cation-exchange resin orally q 6 h, and 30 g PR q 12 h
8 Dialysis (esp. peritoneal) may be indicated

* Since hyperkalemia of insulin deficiency may be associated with total body potassium deficit (and hence require K^+ *supplements* with insulin)

Approach to management of severe hyponatremia*
1 Asymptomatic patient (e.g. on diuretics; normotensive; low plasma sodium found on routine testing)
— Discontinue diuretic
— Restrict water intake
— Encourage dietary salt intake until Na^+ normal
2 Minimally symptomatic patient, hypotensive, no CNS signs
— Restrict water intake
— IV normal saline to re-expand plasma volume
3 Symptomatic patient, CNS signs present (e.g. post-op)
— Restrict water intake
— Slow hypertonic (3%) saline infusion
— Calibrate rate to increase plasma Na^+ by a *maximum* of 1 mmol/h (25 mmol/48 h) until Na^+ > 125 mmol/L

— Too rapid infusion → central pontine myelinolysis
— Hypervolemic SIADH patients may require furosemide (frusemide)

* Plasma Na^+ < 110 mmol/L

Hazards of bicarbonate administration in metabolic acidosis
1 High sodium/osmotic load
2 Aggravation of tissue hypoxia ($\uparrow$ Hb affinity for oxygen)
3 Paradoxical fall in CSF pH, leading to hypoventilation

MEDICAL TECHNOLOGY

Potential indications for hyperbaric oxygen therapy
1 Decompression sickness ('the bends')
2 Air (arterial gas) embolism
3 Inhalational poisoning
— Carbon monoxide (if comatose)
— Smoke inhalation
— Hydrogen cyanide (adjunctive only)
4 Infections
— Gas gangrene (clostridial myonecrosis)
— Anaerobic sepsis with tissue necrosis
— Mucormycosis, actinomycosis
— Refractory chronic osteomyelitis
5 Impaired wound healing
— Radiation necrosis (esp. of bone)
— Severe thermal burns
— Diabetic wounds (if large vessels OK)
— Ischemic crush injury/compartment syndrome*
— Jeopardized skin flaps

* Must be treated immediately to be effective

Iatrogenic consequences of synthetic implantable devices
1 Infection, commonly affecting
— Prosthetic hip
— Cardiac valve replacement
— CSF shunts
— Soft contact lenses; lens implants
— Long-term vascular access catheters
— Indwelling urinary catheters
2 Thromboembolism, commonly affecting
— Vascular grafts
— Valve replacements
3 Specific valve problems
— Valve failure (acute incompetence)
— Valve thrombosis (acute stenosis)
— Hemolysis
4 Specific IUD problems
— Pelvic inflammatory disease, infertility
— Ectopic pregnancy; septic abortion
— Uterine perforation, peritonitis
— Actinomyces/fungal infections (with plastic IUDs)

NUTRITIONAL SUPPLEMENTATION

'Essential' amino acids*
1 Neutral (non-polar, uncharged)
— Valine, leucine, isoleucine
2 Polar uncharged
— Threonine
3 Strongly basic
— Lysine
4 Aromatic
— Histidine, phenylalanine, tryptophan
5 Sulfur-containing
— Methionine

* i.e. unable to be endogenously synthesized from precursors

Treatment approaches to morbid obesity
1 Dietary caloric restriction
— ± Psychotherapy, behavior modification, exercise
2 Anorexia-inducing drugs (controversial)
— Dexfenfluramine (for maximum of 12 weeks)
— Also improves peripheral insulin sensitivity
3 Surgery
— Jaw wiring
— Gastric stapling

Indications for hyperalimentation (parenteral nutrition)
1 Short bowel syndrome
2 Crohn's disease with severe malabsorption
3 Prolonged ileus
4 Pancreatic/intestinal fistula
5 Hypermetabolism (e.g. severe sepsis or burns)
6 Hyperemesis gravidarum (or other feeding difficulty)

Metabolic complications of total parenteral nutrition (TPN)
1 Hyperglycemia (may be aggravated by occult chromium deficiency) if insufficient insulin added to infusion
Hypoglycemia (most commonly due to kinking of dextrose infusion containing insulin, which continues to act)
Hyperosmolar coma (may be precipitated by sepsis)
2 Hypercalcemia (e.g. due to hypervitaminosis A or D)
Osteomalacia (in long-term TPN)
3 Hyperchloremic acidosis (prevent with acetate supplement)
Lactic acidosis (→ fructose infusions in neonates)
4 Hypophosphatemia (esp. during dextrose infusions)
Pseudohyponatremia (during infusion of fat emulsions)
Hypokalemia, hypomagnesemia, copper/zinc deficiency
5 Exfoliative dermatitis
— Due to $\uparrow$ vitamin A, $\downarrow$ zinc/fatty acids
6 Muscle wasting
— May be avoidable by glutamine supplementation
7 Liver disease
— Fatty infiltration
— Lymphocytic infiltration (+ transaminitis)

— Jaundice (± cholestasis, sepsis)
— Hyperammonemia (± encephalopathy)

VITAMIN THERAPY

Indications for high-dose vitamin supplements
1 Vitamins A, D, E, K
— Hereditary abetalipoproteinemia (Bassen–Kornzweig)
— Biliary atresia, ileal atresia
— Cystic fibrosis
2 Vitamin B_6
— Homocystinuria
— Idiopathic refractory sideroblastic anemia
— Renal oxalate stones
— Unexplained infantile convulsions
3 Vitamin B_{12}
— Transcobalamin II deficiency
— Juvenile pernicious anemia
— Homocystinuria
4 Folate
— Congenital megaloblastosis
5 Vitamin K
— Coagulopathy due to liver disease (esp. post-partum)

Toxicity of vitamin overdosage
1 Vitamin A
— Skin dryness, fissuring, hair loss
— Bone pain, hypercalcemia
— Raised intracranial pressure ('pseudotumor')
— Hepatic fibrosis
2 Vitamin B_3 (niacin)
— Pruritus, hair loss
— Peptic ulcer
— Abnormal liver function tests
3 Vitamin B_6 (pyridoxine)
— Sensory neuropathy
— Antagonism of L-DOPA
4 Vitamin C
— Renal oxalate stones
5 Vitamin D
— Hypercalcemia
— Hypertension
6 Vitamin E
— Warfarin potentiation ($\downarrow$ vitamin K absorption)
7 Vitamin K
— Hemolysis

Drug-induced vitamin deficiencies
1 Pyridoxine (B_6)
— Isoniazid (in slow acetylators)
— D-penicillamine
— Hydralazine; cycloserine; chloramphenicol; L-DOPA
— ?Oral contraceptives
2 Folate
— Colestyramine
— Phenytoin
— 'Antifolates': e.g. methotrexate, pyrimethamine
— Sulfasalazine (may 'unmask' mild deficiency)

3 B_{12}
— Chloramphenicol; long-term metformin, neomycin
4 B_1 (thiamine)
— Nitrofurantoin
B_2 (riboflavin)
— Thalidomide
5 Vitamin D
— *Long-term* phenytoin/phenobarbital (?hepatic induction $\rightarrow$ inactivation of 1,25-DHCC)
— Cadmium poisoning ('ouch-ouch' disease = malacia)
6 Vitamin K
— Warfarin
— Aspirin
— Megadose vitamin E

Disorders that may respond to pyridoxine
1 Homocystinuria
2 Primary hyperoxaluria
3 Idiopathic refractory sideroblastic anemia
4 Alcoholics developing neuropathy while taking isoniazid
5 Depression in women taking contraceptive pill
6 Vomiting in pregnant women
7 Convulsions of obscure cause in neonates
8 Premenstrual syndrome (see Ref. 17.7, p. 388)

MANAGEMENT OF METABOLIC BONE DISEASE

Hyperparathyroidism: indications for surgical management
1 Renal calculi *or* hypercalciuria (> 400 mg/24 h)
2 Renal impairment due to nephrocalcinosis
3 Recurrent peptic ulceration (exclude gastrinoma)
4 Reduction in height (vertebral osteopenia) or bone density
5 Recurrent pancreatitis
6 Recent onset of psychiatric symptoms
7 Severe or progressive radiological abnormalities*
8 High calcium (> 3.0 mmol/L) in patient from remote location

NB: Provided that surgical expertise is available, it may be best to operate if there is *any* doubt about the significance of symptoms
* e.g. osteitis fibrosa cystica with 2°/3° hyperparathyroidism in renal failure

Therapeutic modalities in post-menopausal osteoporosis
1 Hormone replacement therapy, esp. estrogens
2 Bisphosphonates (etidronate, alendronate, tiludronate)
3 Exercise*
4 Calcium citrate supplements (800 mg/day)
5 Subcutaneous or intranasal calcitonin
6 Vitamin D supplements (400–800 IU/day)

* Significance may relate to ovulatory effects rather than to activity alone

Bisphosphonates: mechanisms and indications
1 Drugs
   — Etidronate
   — Pamidronate
   — Alendronate
   — Clodronate
   — Tiludronate
2 Mechanism of action
   — Pyrophosphate analogs; bind hydroxyapatite
   — Inhibit osteoclast-mediated bone resorption
3 Indications
   — Paget's disease (alendronate*)
   — Hypercalcemia of malignancy (pamidronate)
   — Painful bone mets: myeloma, Ca breast
     (clodronate, pamidronate)
   — Vertebral osteoporosis (etidronate,
     alendronate)
4 Unlicensed indications
   — Hyperparathyroidism (1°, 2°, 3°)
   — Prevention of heterotopic ossification
5 Toxicity
   — Malacia, fractures (etidronate; inhibits
     mineralization)
   — Pill esophagitis (oral alendronate)

* Together with calcium supplements to prevent secondary hyperparathyroidism

Indications for medical therapy of Paget's disease
1 Bone pain
2 Bone deformity or joint complications
3 Neurologic sequelae
4 Prophylaxis if base of skull disease (risk of hearing loss), spinal disease (risk of neurologic compression), femora (risk of fracture)
5 Prior to elective orthopedic surgery (e.g. hip replacement) to reduce vascularity

Rationâle for vitamin D supplements in osteoporosis
1 Relative indications
   — Lack of sun exposure
   — Little physical activity
   — Low dietary vitamin D*
2 Oral vitamin D supplements suppress winter rise of PTH ($\rightarrow \downarrow$ bone density) due to reduced skin vitamin D synthesis
3 Antimyopathic effect of vitamin D supplements *may* also reduce falls in elderly independent of effects on bone density (unproven)

* Fatty fish/oils, liver, eggs, milk are the only substantive dietary sources

UNDERSTANDING METABOLIC DISEASE

Racial predispositions to disease
1 Ashkenazy Jews
   — Gaucher's
   — Tay–Sachs
   — Riley–Day
   — Niemann–Pick
   — Bassen–Kornzweig
   — Bloom's

Non-Ashkenazy (Sephardic) Jews
   — Familial Mediterranean fever (recurrent polyserositis)
2 African negro, Mediterranean littoral
   — Sickle-cell anemia
   — Thalassemias
   — Hb C
3 Lebanese
   — Hypercholesterolemia
   — Behçet's
4 Chinese
   — α-Thalassemia
   — Alactasia
5 Northern European caucasians
   — Idiopathic hemochromatosis
   — Phenylketonuria
   — Acute intermittent porphyria
   Swedes
   — Cystic fibrosis
   — Giant-cell arteritis
   — α_1-Antitrypsin deficiency
   — LCAT deficiency
   Finns
   — Imerslund's disease
   — *Diphyllobothrium latum* infestations
   — Mulibrey nanism ($\rightarrow$ pericarditis)
   — Congenital nephrosis
6 Eskimos (esp. Yupik)
   — Congenital adrenal hyperplasia
   — Pseudocholinesterase deficiency
   — Rapid acetylation status (close to 100%)
7 Other races
   Thais
   — Hb H disease (Hb Constant Spring $\rightarrow$ 2–5%)
   Pima Indians/Micronesians/Yemenite Jews
   — Type II (non-insulin-dependent) diabetes mellitus
   South Africans
   — Variegate porphyria
   Scottish
   — Peptic ulceration (acid hypersecretion)
   Quebecois
   — Tyrosinemia ($\rightarrow$ cirrhosis, renal tubular acidosis)

BODY WEIGHT HOMEOSTASIS

Role of leptin in body mass regulation
1 Leptin is a peptide hormone which acts as a satiety signal to the hypothalamus, and hence as an 'adipostatic hormone'
2 Mouse models of leptin deficiency exhibit an obese (*ob*) phenotype
3 The appetite-stimulating hormone, neuropeptide Y, is inhibited by leptin
4 Leptin also regulates the thyroid, reproductive and adrenal hormone systems
5 Obese humans tend to have high plasma leptin levels, indicating leptin resistance, and eliminating the possibility of treating obesity with leptin
6 Leptin gene mutations are rare in human obesity (unlike the mouse!)

Inducers and suppressors of leptin release
1 Inducers
— Feeding
— Obesity
— Insulin, glucocorticoids
2 Suppressors
— Fasting
— Thiazolidinediones (e.g. rosiglitazone)

Health benefits correlating with a 10% weight loss
1 30% fall in fasting serum glucose and triglycerides
2 30% improvement in exercise tolerance
3 20% fall in short-term mortality
4 10% reduction in plasma cholesterol
5 10 mmHg reduction in systolic blood pressure (20% in diastolic)

INHERITED DISEASES

Factors maintaining heterozygote mutation frequency
1 Duchenne muscular dystrophy
— New mutations
2 Hemoglobinopathies (e.g. sickle-cell anemia, thalassemias)
— Resistance to malaria
3 Cystic fibrosis
— Resistance to cholera toxin
4 Peptic ulcer diathesis, lipid storage diseases
— Resistance to TB
5 Congenital adrenal hyperplasia
— Resistance to *H. influenzae* #B
6 Idiopathic hemochromatosis
— Resistance to iron-deficiency anemia (in women)
7 Type I (insulin-dependent) diabetes mellitus
— Reduced miscarriages
8 Type II (non-insulin-dependent) diabetes mellitus
— Protects against starvation

Single-gene defects exhibiting autosomal dominant transmission
1 Familial hypercholesterolemia
2 Multiple polyposis
3 Neurofibromatosis
4 Tuberous sclerosis
5 Myotonic dystrophy
6 Huntington's chorea
7 Marfan's syndrome
8 Acute intermittent porphyria
9 Adult polycystic kidney disease

Single-gene defects exhibiting autosomal recessive transmission
1 Cystic fibrosis
2 β-Thalassemia
3 Sickle-cell anemia
4 Phenylketonuria
5 Galactosemia
6 Tay–Sachs disease
7 Infantile polycystic kidney disease

Single-gene defects exhibiting X-linked recessive transmission
1 Hemophilias A and B
2 Duchenne muscular dystrophy
3 Alport's syndrome
4 Lesch–Nyhan syndrome
5 Nephrogenic diabetes insipidus
6 Testicular feminization syndrome
7 G6PD deficiency

GENETIC COUNSELING

Referral for genetic counseling: potential indications
1 Suspected chromosomal abnormality
2 Diagnosed congenital and/or heritable abnormality
3 Abnormal mental or physical development
4 Abnormal sexual development
5 Unexplained infertility
6 Repeated abortions

Risk assessment in genetic counseling (general)
1 Risk of spontaneous abortion in established pregnancy
— 15%
2 Risk of married couple's infertility
— 10%
3 Risk of baby being born with physical or mental defect
— 2%
4 Risk of perinatal death or stillbirth
— 1%
5 Risk of death in infancy
— 0.5%

GENETIC DIAGNOSIS

Methods of localizing abnormal genes to specific chromosomes
1 Gene linkage (of a disease locus with a marker), e.g.
— Narcolepsy with HLA gene cluster
— Ataxia telangiectasia with polymorphic markers
2 Mutation-specific gene probes, e.g.
— Sickle-cell anemia
— α_1-Antitrypsin deficiency
— β-Thalassemias
— Phenylketonuria
— Cystic fibrosis

Dermatoglyphic stigmata of Down's syndrome
1 Distal axial triradius
— In 85%
2 Simian crease (single transverse palmar flexion crease)
— In 50%
3 Supernumerary ulnar loops

REVIEWING THE LITERATURE: METABOLIC AND NUTRITIONAL DISORDERS

9.1 Dumont L et al (2000) Efficacy and harm of pharmacological prevention of acute mountain sickness. Br Med J 321: 267–272

Systematic review of randomized placebo-controlled trials indicating that 67% of individuals ascending more than 4000 meters experience acute mountain sickness, and that both dexamethasone (8–16 mg) and acetazolamide (750 mg) are effective in prophylaxis.

9.2 Sidhu H et al (1998) Absence of *Oxalobacter formigenes* in cystic fibrosis patients: a risk factor for hyperoxaluria. Lancet 352: 1026–1029

Study of 43 children with cystic fibrosis (CF), showing that the known association of CF and hyperoxaluria (predisposing to urolithiasis and nephrocalcinosis) is associated with increased absorption of oxalate from the gut; and the latter is in turn associated with reduced gut colonization by the oxalate-metabolizing bacterium *O. formigenes* in CF patients.

9.3 Cochrane Injuries Group Albumin Reviewers (1998) Human albumin administration in critically ill patients. Br Med J 317: 235–240

Overview of 30 randomized albumin vs crystalloid studies in critically ill patients (e.g. burns, shock) which suggested that mortality may be increased by use of human albumin. The recommendation was that albumin should not be used in such patients outside a randomized trial setting.

9.4 Hosking D et al (1998) Prevention of bone loss with alendronate in postmenopausal women under 60 years of age. N Engl J Med 338: 485–492

Saag KG et al (1998) Alendronate for the prevention and treatment of glucocorticoid-induced osteoporosis. N Engl J Med 339: 292–299

Two randomized studies attesting to the antiosteoclastic efficacy of the bisphosphonate alendronate. The first study of 1174 women showed that alendronate arrested bone loss (though did not cause increased bone density) as well as hormone replacement, whereas the second study of 477 long-term steroid patients showed that alendronate increased bone density by 2.2% compared with the control group (a net gain of 1.2%).

9.5 Vestergaard P et al (2000) Cohort study of risk of fracture before and after surgery for primary hyperparathyroidism. Br Med J 321: 598–602

Study of 674 patients showing an increased frequency of fracture for up to 10 years prior to surgery. This increased risk returned to normal after parathyroidectomy.

9.6 Stevens J et al (1998) The effect of age on the association between body mass index and mortality. N Engl J Med 338: 1–7

Calle EE et al (1999) Body mass index and mortality in a prospective cohort of U.S. adults. N Engl J Med 341: 1097–1105

Two massive studies of body mass index (BMI: weight in kilograms divided by the square of the height in meters). The first study, lasting 12 years, of over 300 000 non-smoking individuals, showed increased all-cause mortality associated with increased BMI – every unit increase in BMI corresponded to a 10% relative increase in cardiovascular mortality risk – but this association was stronger for those individuals with raised BMI when young, and weaker for older individuals. The second study, of more than a million adults followed-up over 14 years, showed a synergistic increase in cardiac and cancer mortality in certain subgroups: smokers, males, and Caucasians.

9.7 Levine JA et al (1999) Role of nonexercise activity thermogenesis in resistance to fat gains in humans. Science 283: 212–215

Detailed study of 16 non-obese volunteers who were fed 1000 kcal/day in excess of weight maintenance needs for 8 weeks. This was associated with an increase in daily energy expenditure, two-thirds of which was accounted for by fidgeting (which the authors term non-exercise activity thermogenesis, or NEAT). Failure to activate NEAT in a subset of volunteers correlated with fat gain.

9.8 Homocysteine Lowering Trialists' Collaboration (1998) Lowering blood homocysteine with folic acid based supplements. Br Med J 316: 894–898

Unlike vitamins B_6 and B_{12}, this meta-analysis suggested that folate supplements reduce plasma homocysteine levels, especially in individuals with either high homocysteine levels or low folate levels. The hypothesis is raised that folate could reduce vascular disease.

9.9 Umeta M et al (2000) Zinc supplementation and stunted infants in Ethiopia. Lancet 355: 2021–2026

Randomized controlled study of 100 stunted Ethiopian infants, showing a benefit of zinc supplements in terms of catch-up growth, appetite, and reduced infective morbidity (such as anorexia). Hence, the benefits of zinc could relate in part to reduced infection.

9.10 James W et al (2000) Effect of sibutramine on weight maintenance after weight loss: a randomised trial. Lancet 356: 2119–2125

Two-year double-blind study of 605 obese patients, showing that the antidepressant drug sibutramine helped to improve weight in 80%, compared with 10% of placebo-treated patients.

CHAPTER 10

Neurology

Physical examination protocol 10.1 You are asked to examine the cranial nerves

6 CN V: muscles of mastication, trigeminal sensation
Motor: clench teeth (masseter, temporalis);
open mouth against resistance (pterygoids);
jaw deviates to weak side)
Sensory: ophthalmic/maxillary/mandibular
sensation/corneal reflex (distinguish efferent VII
limb)
jaw jerk (? hyperactive)

5 CN III, IV, VI: pupils and extraocular
movements; exophthalmos; enophthalmos
(Horner's); ptosis; lid retraction, lid lag
Pupils (CN III): turn out lights
equal? regular?
direct and consensual light reflex?
accommodation?
Extraocular movements:
diplopia? strabismus?
nystagmus?
fatiguability?

4 CN II: acuity, fields, fundi
Test acuity with glasses on:
Snellen's chart, newspaper,
count fingers; hand threat
Fields to confrontation:
visual inattention
map central scotoma
map enlarged blind spot
Fundi: ask to dilate pupils; turn
out lights; red reflex, cataract;
rubeosis iridis; optic disc retinal
vessels; venous pulsations;
macula ('look straight at the
light now')

3 Ask to examine olfaction
If request granted, test bilaterally (cortical
representation is ipsilateral)

2 General inspection:
craniotomy scar
ptosis, proptosis
facial weakness, hemiplegia
catheter

1 Introduce yourself (note speech in reply)
Position yourself opposite patient

7 CN VII: muscles of facial expression
facial asymmetry or general wasting
show teeth (if weak, ask to 'smile')
puff out cheeks; screw up eyes
frown; lift eyebrows
Ask to test taste
Ask to test lacrimation (Schirmer's test) if face
weak

8 CN VIII: auditory and vestibular function
Auditory: ticking watch, whispered numbers
(other ear occluded)
Weber's and Rinne's test
Vestibular: Hallpike maneuver, etc., if indicated

9 CN IX, X: pharyngeal function and sensation
Test palate elevates in midline ('Aaah': CN X);
moves away from paretic side
Ask to test gag reflex bilaterally (CN IX)
Speech: nasal (bulbar palsy), 'Donald Duck'
(pseudobulbar)
Bovine cough (recurrent laryngeal branch of CN X)

10 CN XI: trapezius and sternomastoids
shrug shoulders upwards against
resistance; rotate jaw against
resistance (rotating to right tests
left sternomastoid)

11 CN XII: tongue
wasting, fibrillation (lower motor neuron lesion)
stick tongue out (deviates to weak side)
rapid movements: side-to-side quickly 'la-la-la-
la-la-la-la'
percussion myotonia (if myotonic dystrophy
suspected)

12 If appropriate, ask to proceed further, e.g.:
auscultate carotids/orbits/skull/heart for bruit
take blood pressure; assess pulse regularity
look for absent abdominal reflexes (demyelination)
absent ankle jerks (tabes dorsalis)
extensor plantar responses
glycosuria

Physical examination protocol 10.2   You are asked to assess a patient who is having difficulty walking

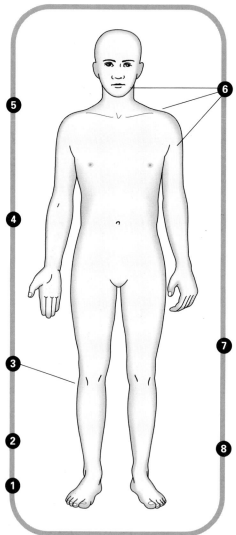

If predominant signs are upper
    motor neuron,
first:
elicit all deep tendon jerks to the
    level of the jaw, to determine
    the lesion level;
then examine:
abdominal reflexes; bladder size
Spine: examine for tenderness
mobility
deformity
bruit
Upper limbs:
fasciculations
pattern of weakness
hyperreflexia
reflex loss/inversion
Neck movements

6

If predominant signs are
cerebellar, proceed with cerebellar
examination

5

Examine lower limbs:
wasting, fasciculations
spasticity; clonus (ankle, patellar),
flaccidity
power (all muscle groups)
tendon jerks ± reinforcement;
Babinski sign
cerebellar examination
sensory examination, esp. if
sensory level suspected

4

Bulbar musculature
Tongue fibrillation
Fundi:
optic atrophy
papilledema

7

Observe gait:
standing (eyes open and closed)
walk and turn
heel-toe walking
walk on heels, on toes
characterize gait (e.g. 'wide-based',
'waddling') if unequivocal

3

Ask the patient to walk (if able)

2

Carotid/cranial bruits
Hypertension
Cardiac auscultation

8

Introduce yourself

1

Physical examination protocol 10.3   You are asked to examine a patient who has noticed wasting of the hand muscles

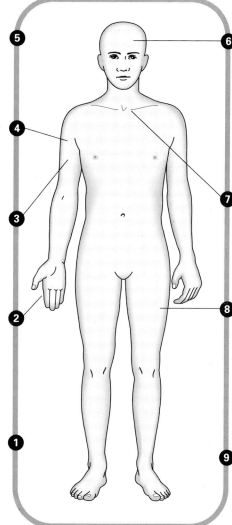

Sensory loss: test all modalities
Pattern: – 'glove' vs 'cape' vs
dermatomal (esp. T_1)
– thenar vs hypothenar
– dissociated
– 'cortical'

5

Muscle power – all groups (incl.
opponens/abductor pollicis brevis)
Reflexes (± reinforcement); finger
flexor
Tinel's sign

4

Muscle tenderness (biceps)
Muscle tone
Percussion myotonia (thenar
eminence) if indicated
Fatiguability on exercise

3

Inspection:
fasciculations
pattern of wasting –
generalized
upper limbs, incl. deltoids
unilateral vs bilateral
thenar vs hypothenar
interossei
burn marks (? syrinx)
clubbing, nicotine stains

2

Introduce yourself
Position the patient (sitting up)
Obtain adequate exposure

1

6

Frontal baldness
Ptosis ± Horner's
Heliotrope rash
Cataract
Fundi: papilledema
Jaw jerk
Bulbar musculature:
gag
speech (nasal, spastic)
tongue movements
tongue fibrillation

7

Cervical spine movements
Supraclavicular fossa:
'fullness', bruit

8   Examination of lower limbs

9

Further examination as dictated
by diagnostic suspicion:
e.g. chest (T_1 lesion)
heart (myotonic dystrophy)
parietal lobe:
unilateral wasting with cortical
sensory loss

Physical examination protocol 10.4 You are asked to examine the patient's cerebellar function

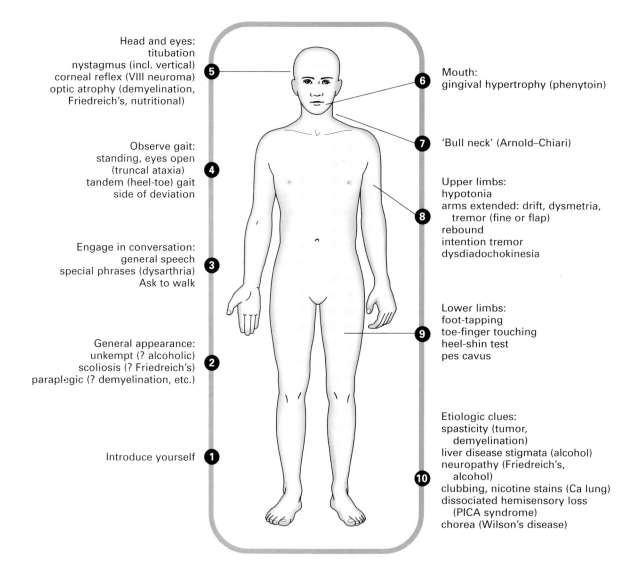

Head and eyes:
titubation
nystagmus (incl. vertical)
corneal reflex (VIII neuroma)
optic atrophy (demyelination,
Friedreich's, nutritional)
5

6 Mouth:
gingival hypertrophy (phenytoin)

7 'Bull neck' (Arnold–Chiari)

Observe gait:
standing, eyes open
(truncal ataxia)
tandem (heel-toe) gait
side of deviation
4

Upper limbs:
hypotonia
arms extended: drift, dysmetria,
tremor (fine or flap)
rebound
intention tremor
dysdiadochokinesia
8

Engage in conversation:
general speech
special phrases (dysarthria)
Ask to walk
3

Lower limbs:
foot-tapping
toe-finger touching
heel-shin test
pes cavus
9

General appearance:
unkempt (? alcoholic)
scoliosis (? Friedreich's)
paraplegic (? demyelination, etc.)
2

Introduce yourself **1**

Etiologic clues:
spasticity (tumor,
demyelination)
liver disease stigmata (alcohol)
neuropathy (Friedreich's,
alcohol)
clubbing, nicotine stains (Ca lung)
dissociated hemisensory loss
(PICA syndrome)
chorea (Wilson's disease)
10

Physical examination protocol 10.5 You are asked to examine a patient for signs of parkinsonism

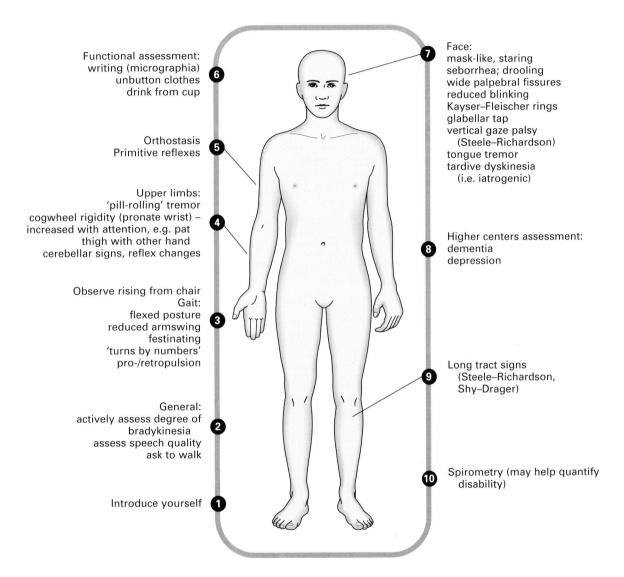

6 Functional assessment:
writing (micrographia)
unbutton clothes
drink from cup

5 Orthostasis
Primitive reflexes

4 Upper limbs:
'pill-rolling' tremor
cogwheel rigidity (pronate wrist) –
increased with attention, e.g. pat
thigh with other hand
cerebellar signs, reflex changes

3 Observe rising from chair
Gait:
flexed posture
reduced armswing
festinating
'turns by numbers'
pro-/retropulsion

2 General:
actively assess degree of
bradykinesia
assess speech quality
ask to walk

1 Introduce yourself

7 Face:
mask-like, staring
seborrhea; drooling
wide palpebral fissures
reduced blinking
Kayser–Fleischer rings
glabellar tap
vertical gaze palsy
(Steele–Richardson)
tongue tremor
tardive dyskinesia
(i.e. iatrogenic)

8 Higher centers assessment:
dementia
depression

9 Long tract signs
(Steele–Richardson,
Shy–Drager)

10 Spirometry (may help quantify
disability)

Diagnostic pathway 10.1   The patient has a speech defect. What do you make of it?

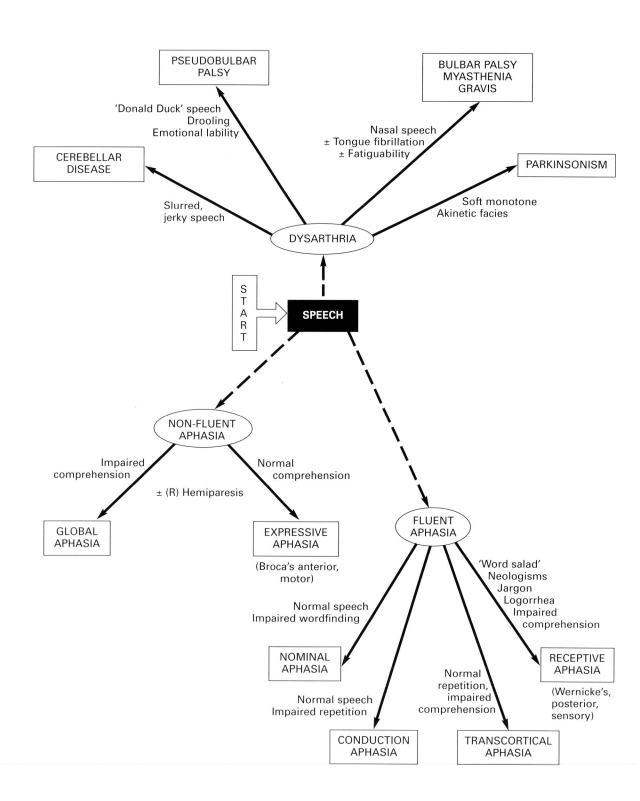

Diagnostic pathway 10.2   This patient is troubled by ptosis. Can you shed any light on the pathophysiology?

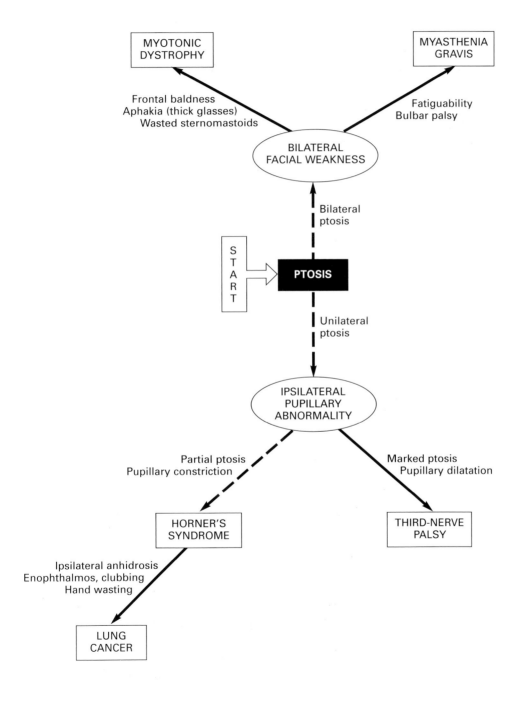

Diagnostic pathway 10.3   The patient is concerned about his legs. What do you think is the problem?

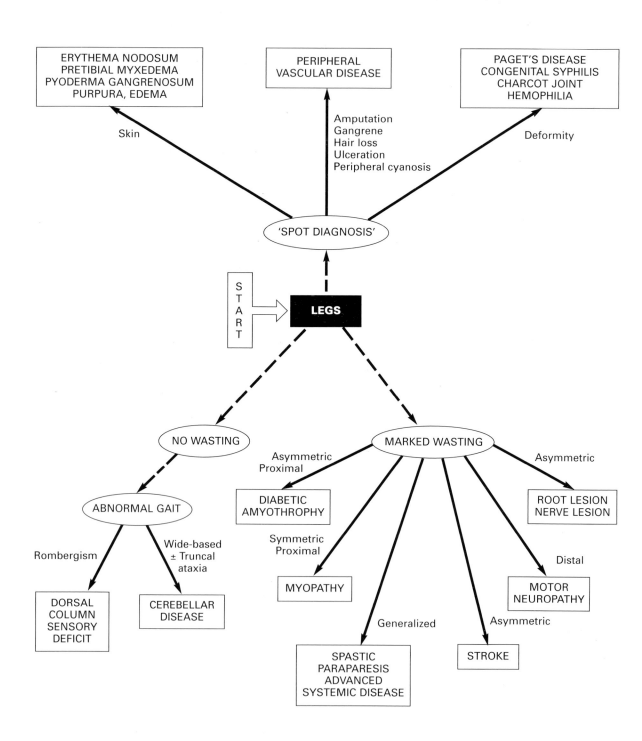

COMMON AND CLASSIC NEUROLOGIC DISORDERS

Common neurologic disorders in clinical practice
1 Headaches
2 Epilepsy
3 Vertigo

Classic neurologic disorders in clinical exams
1 Difficulty walking (e.g. due to spastic paraparesis)
2 Peripheral neuropathy
3 Ocular palsy

NEUROLOGIC EMERGENCIES

Differential diagnosis of thunderclap headache
1 Subarachnoid hemorrhage
2 Cerebral venous sinus thrombosis

Approach to management of status epilepticus
1 Initially: diazepam or lorazepam (slow IV)
2 At 10': phenytoin infusion 20 mg/kg @ 50 mg/min (+ ECG/plasma monitoring)
3 At 20': phenobarbital (IV) 20 mg/kg @ 50 mg/min
4 At 40': midazolam anesthesia (for 2 h)

CLINICAL ASSESSMENT OF NEUROLOGIC DISEASE

Clinical assessment of muscle weakness
1 Grade 1 — flicker of voluntary muscle activity*
2 Grade 2 — able to move with gravity eliminated
3 Grade 3 — able to move against gravity
4 Grade 4 — able to move against resistance
5 Grade 5 — normal power

* Paralysis = grade 0

Multiple CNS deficits: causes
1 Multiple sclerosis
Multifocal leukoencephalopathy
2 Multiple infarcts
3 Multiple metastases
Meningeal carcinomatosis
4 Meningovascular syphilis
5 Vasculitis (e.g. PAN)

Multiple cranial nerve palsies?
1 Malignancy
— Brainstem tumor (e.g. nasopharyngeal Ca → VI)
— Meningeal carcinomatosis
— Perineural tumor infiltration
2 Infection
— Basal meningitis (e.g. cryptococcal, tuberculous)
— Meningovascular syphilis (now rare)
— Herpes zoster
3 Sarcoidosis
— esp. VII; ± VIII, II
4 Vasculitis
— esp. Wegener's (→ VIII)
5 Paget's disease
— Usually causes hearing loss only
6 Hyperostosis cranialis interna (familial)
— Recurrent VII palsies ± I, II, VIII
7 Idiopathic
— Tolosa–Hunt syndrome
— Orbital pseudotumor
— Idiopathic cranial polyneuropathy

Differential diagnosis of transient focal signs
1 Migraine
2 Focal epilepsy*
3 Transient ischemic attack
4 Labyrinthine disorder
5 Hyperventilation

* With or without an underlying structural lesion (e.g. tumor, subdural); hence, symptom transience does not exclude a persistent lesion

Signs suggesting brainstem pathology
1 Conjugate gaze palsy/internuclear ophthalmoplegia
2 Vertical nystagmus
3 Opisthotonos and/or cerebellar signs
4 Crossed (cranial nerves vs long tract) signs
5 Deviation of eyes and head to paralysed side (cf. cortical)
6 Bilateral extensive deficit

Signs suggesting extracapsular (cortical) disease
1 Localized deficit
2 Dysphasia (cf. capsular lesion → pure dysarthria)
3 Hemianopia
4 Decreased proprioception/two-point discrimination
5 Apraxia
6 Obtundation

Clinical distinction between meningitis and encephalitis
1 Meningitis
— Conscious state unimpaired
— Meningism (including headache)
— Prominent fever
— ± Cranial nerve lesions (lower motor neuron)
2 Encephalitis
— Early impairment of consciousness (drowsiness, coma)
— Focal neurologic signs (upper motor neuron)
— Convulsions
— Associated hydrophobia (rabies)
— Associated temporal lobe epilepsy (HSV)

Assessment of neurologic function in the unconscious patient
1 Pupils
— Midbrain lesions
• Light reflex may be lost
• Hippus (fluctuation in pupil size)
• Ciliospinal reflex (dilatation on pinching neck)
— Pontine lesions
• Pinpoint pupils

— Lateral medullary lesions
  • Horner's syndrome
— Diffuse cerebral damage
  • Fixed dilated pupils (*not* diagnostic)
— Metabolic depression (e.g. overdose)
  • All brainstem reflexes lost *except* pupil light reflex
2 Reflexes
  — Corneal
    • Depressed in bilateral cerebral damage
  — Jaw jerk
    • Hyperactive in bilateral UMN lesions
  — Gag reflex
3 Conjugate gaze deviation (p. 261)
4 Caloric and oculocephalic testing (p. 262)
5 Spontaneous respiratory movements

Differential diagnosis of persistent olfactory impairment (anosmia)
1 Head injury → severance of olfactory nerve fibers (usually bilateral)
2 Frontal lobe tumor (ipsilateral)
3 Vitamin B_{12} deficiency
4 Alzheimer's disease, Parkinson's disease
5 Depression; hysteria
6 Nasal polyps, atrophic rhinitis

EPILEPSY

Features of fits
1 Absence (< 30 sec)
  — Staring, blinking ± automatisms*
  — Immediate return of consciousness
  — Characteristic EEG (p. 269)
2 Tonic–clonic (1–5 min)
  — Fall ± cry; cyanosis
  — ± Tongue-bite, incontinence
3 Myoclonic (1–5 sec)
  — Brief limb jerks
4 Complex partial ('psychomotor'; last minutes)
  — Déjà vu, jamais vu
  — Hallucinations (esp. olfactory, gustatory)
  — *Prominent* post-ictal confusion‡
5 Simple partial (focal; seconds → minutes)
  — EEG may be normal¶
  — *No* post-ictal confusion
  — Examples: an 'aura', Rolandic epilepsy
  — May generalize via Jacksonian march
  — ± *Painful* sensations (in *parietal lobe* origin)

* Chewing, lip smacking, finger-twiddling, etc.
‡ If *temporal lobe* in origin; *not* in frontal lobe variety
¶ Or there may be contralateral epileptiform discharges

Disorders mimicking epileptic seizures
1 Hyperventilation, agoraphobia, panic disorders
2 Cardiac arrhythmias (e.g. prolonged Q-T syndrome)
3 Migraine (with aura, or basilar artery variant)
4 Vasovagal syncope
5 Breath-holding episodes, night terrors (infants), narcolepsy
6 Non-epileptic myoclonus, tics, habit spasms

Features distinguishing syncope from seizure
1 Favoring syncopal disorder
  — Sweating and/or nausea prior to loss of consciousness
  — Pallor prior to or during loss of consciousness
  — Normal orientation following recovery of consciousness
2 Favoring seizure disorder
  — Duration of loss of consciousness > 5 min
  — Cyanosis or frothing at mouth during loss of consciousness
  — Tongue bitten during loss of consciousness
  — Muscle pain, somnolence or disorientation following recovery of consciousness

Common precipitants of status epilepticus
1 Subtherapeutic anticonvulsant levels
  — Poor compliance
  — Recent dose reduction
2 Metabolic derangement
  — Severe hyponatremia
  — Hepatic encephalopathy
  — Alcohol withdrawal
3 Inflammatory
  — Encephalitis
  — Cerebral vasculitis (e.g. SLE)
4 Head injury
5 Drug overdose
  — e.g. Theophylline, cocaine

CEREBROVASCULAR DISEASE: BACKGROUND

Clinical characterization of ischemic stroke
1 Mechanism
  — Large vessel atherothrombotic: 15%
  — (Cardio)embolic: 60%*
  — Lacunar/hypertensive: 25%
  — Vasculitis
  — Aneurysmal
2 Site
  — Internal carotid (atherothrombotic) stenosis: 10%‡
  — Middle cerebral
  — Anterior or posterior cerebral
  — Vertebrobasilar

* Atrial fibrillation is present in one-quarter of these
‡ i.e. accounts for two-thirds of atherothrombotic strokes

Symptoms suggesting carotid insufficiency
1 Amaurosis fugax
  — Complete or partial visual loss in *one* eye
2 Dysphasia
3 Unilateral limb weakness/paresthesiae *without* other (brainstem) features

Symptoms suggesting vertebrobasilar ischemia
1 Bilateral blindness
2 Other *bilateral* motor/sensory symptoms
3 Focal symptoms *plus* vertigo or diplopia

Clinical significance of transient ischemic attacks*
1 30% of patients will have only one episode
2 30% will continue to have TIAs alone

3 30% will have a completed stroke within 3 years
4 30% of the latter will do so within 3 months of
   presentation
5 30% of asymptomatic carotid bruits go on to TIA
   and/or CVA
6 30% of carotid-type TIAs will have normal
   arteriography

* The prognosis of transient monocular blindness is
approximately twice as good as for transient hemispheric attacks

Carotid-type TIAs: factors predictive of angiographic disease
1 Ipsilateral retinal emboli
2 Reduced superficial temporal and/or carotid artery
   pulse
3 Presence of forehead/scleral collaterals
4 Ipsilateral central retinal artery diastolic pressure
   < 20 mmHg
5 Ipsilateral carotid bruit, esp. if diastolic extension
   present; severe stenosis may → high-pitched,
   low-intensity bruit

Neurologic syndromes associated with hypertension
1 Lacunar infarcts
2 Intracranial hemorrhage
3 Hypertensive encephalopathy

Intracranial hemorrhage: classical site involvement
1 Aneurysms, amyloid angiopathy
   — Subarachnoid
2 Arteriovenous malformations
   — (Peri)ventricular, pons
3 Hypertension
   — Basal ganglia (putamen/caudate), thalamus
4 Warfarin
   — Cerebellar

PRESENTATIONS OF CEREBROVASCULAR DISEASE

Predispositions to intracerebral hemorrhage
1 Hypertension (50%)
2 Cerebral amyloid (15%)
3 Iatrogenic: warfarin, thrombolysis (10%)
4 Infarcts with secondary hemorrhage (10%)
5 Tumors (5–10%)
6 Vascular malformations (5%)
7 Vasculitis (1%)

Features suggestive of intracerebral hemorrhage
1 Gradual onset, smooth progression
2 Obtunded sensorium
3 Vomiting (95%), headache (50%)
4 Hypertension ± fundal stigmata/cardiomegaly
5 Diagnostic confirmation by CT

Signs suggestive of basal pontine hemorrhage
1 Rapid onset of decerebrate rigidity progressing to
   coma
2 Ophthalmoplegia with (classically) small reactive
   pupils
3 Abnormal oculocephalic and oculovestibular
   reflexes

4 Cheyne–Stokes/ataxic respiration
5 Sweating

Signs and symptoms of cerebellar hemorrhage
1 Subacute onset of occipital headache, vertigo and
   vomiting
2 Skew deviation of eyes; ocular bobbing (nystagmus
   unusual)
3 Paresis of gaze to affected side
4 Hemiparesis unusual (cf. putaminal/thalamic type)
5 Good recovery after prompt surgical evacuation

Clinical patterns of lacunar infarction
1 Pure motor hemiplegia
   — Pontine
   — Posterior limb of internal capsule
     • Associated with dysarthria
     • Typically affects upper limb > lower
2 Dysarthria–clumsy hand syndrome
   — Caused by pontine infarction
   — Associated with homolateral facial weakness
3 Pure hemisensory loss
   — Due to thalamic infarction (posterolateral
     nucleus)
4 Ipsilateral ataxia/crossed hemiparesis
   — Due to midbrain infarction
5 Dementia/incontinence/affective lability
   — Due to bipyramidal (pseudobulbar) palsy*

* Differential diagnosis = normal pressure hydrocephalus

Clinical deterioration following an apparently completed stroke?
1 Infarct extension
2 Hemorrhage into infarct
3 Further emboli
4 Worsening cerebral edema/vasospasm
5 Misdiagnosis (e.g. tumor/vasculitis)

Presentations of arteriovenous malformations
1 Epilepsy (45%)
2 Hemorrhage (40%; may mimic aseptic meningitis)
3 Headache (often migrainous: 15%)
4 Pseudotumor (neurologic deficit due to vascular
   'steal')
5 Apparent 'spontaneous' stroke
   — Age under 20
   — During 3rd trimester

Diagnostic considerations in the young patient with 'stroke'
1 Disseminated sclerosis
2 Cardiac disease
   — Arrhythmias (esp. atrial fibrillation)
   — Valvular disease (e.g. mitral stenosis, *not*
     prolapse)
   — Infective endocarditis
3 Vascular
   — Classical migraine
   — Arteriovenous malformation (AVM)*
   — Aneurysm
   — Vasculitis (e.g. SLE)
   — Severe hypertension
   — Hypercoagulable state (e.g.
     hyperhomocysteinemia)

4 Intracranial tumor
5 Infection
   — Encephalitis (e.g. HSV type 1)
   — Neurosyphilis
6 Post-ictal
7 Functional
   — Hyperventilation (may simulate TIA)
   — Hysteria

* Note that in hereditary hemorrhagic telangiectasia, most intracranial events arise secondary to paradoxical or septic emboli originating in pulmonary AVMs, rather than from intracranial AVMs

Clinical features of lateral medullary (PICA*) syndrome
1 Abrupt onset of vertigo and hiccups
2 Bilateral nystagmus
   — Maximal to side of lesion
   — Often varies with posture
3 *Contralateral* body anesthesia for pain and temperature
4 *Ipsilateral*
   — Facial anesthesia for pain and temperature
   — Palatal paresis
   — Taste loss
   — Horner's syndrome
   — Ataxia

* Posterior inferior cerebellar artery

LOCALIZING PATTERNS IN CEREBRAL DISEASE

Clinical manifestations of frontal lobe lesions
1 **A**nosmia — homolateral
  Ataxia — Brun's
  Aphasia — Broca's
  Apathy
  Amnesia
  Atrophy (optic)
2 Mass effects (headache*, papilledema, field defects, Foster–Kennedy)
3 Incontinence
4 Spastic paraparesis or contralateral UMN signs
5 Primitive reflexes (palmar–mental/grasp/snout/pout/suck)

* But note that 'cough headache' more often indicates a posterior fossa tumor

The aphasias: how to distinguish them
1 Broca's
   — Affected region: left frontal (inferoposterior)
   — Associated features: nil
   — Fluency: strained, 'effortful'
   — Repetition: impaired
   — Comprehension: intact
2 Wernicke's
   — Affected region: left temporal (superoposterior)
   — Associated features: euphoria, agitation
   — Fluency: abundant, melodic
   — Repetition: impaired
   — Comprehension: impaired
3 Global
   — Affected region: left perisylvian (large area)
   — Associated features: hemiplegia*

   — Fluency: absent
   — Repetition: impaired
   — Comprehension: impaired
4 Conduction
   — Affected region: left supramarginal gyrus‡
   — Associated features: ± right facial/arm weakness
   — Fluency: grossly normal
   — Repetition: impaired
   — Comprehension: intact
5 Transcortical (motor)
   — Affected region: left frontal¶
   — Associated features: nil
   — Fluency: non-fluent, 'explosive'
   — Repetition: intact
   — Comprehension: intact
6 Thalamic (atypical)
   — Affected region: anterolateral thalamus
   — Associated features: ± amnesia
   — Fluency: abundant, ± logorrhea
   — Repetition: intact
   — Comprehension: impaired

* Assuming single lesion; separate frontal and temporoparietal lesions can cause global aphasia without hemiplegia
‡ Or left auditory cortex plus insula
¶ Anterosuperior to Broca's area

Clinical manifestations of temporal lobe lesions
1 Superior quadrantanopia
2 Fluent aphasia (lesion in Wernicke's area)
3 Uncinate fits, depersonalization, micro-/macropsia,
4 Bilateral disease (rare)
   — Deafness
   — Severe amnesia
   — Kluver–Bucy syndrome

Clinical manifestations of parietal lobe lesions
1 Non-dominant lobe lesions
   — Dressing apraxia
   — Constructional apraxia (draw clock, house, 5-point star)
   — Anosognosia
2 Dominant lobe lesions
   — Ideomotor apraxia ('brush teeth, use saw, drink a cup')
   — Receptive dysphasia (in inferior lesions)
   — Gerstmann's
     • Alexia + acalculia
     • Finger agnosia
     • Left–right confusion
   — Agraphia (in posterior lesions)
3 Anterior lobe lesions
   — Astereognosis/graphesthesia
   — Sensory inattention
   — ↓ Proprioception/two-point discrimination
   — Focal sensory deficits
4 Posterior lobe lesions
   — Visual inattention, sensory inattention
   — Homonymous (albeit incongruous) hemianopia*
   — ↓ Opticokinetic nystagmus
5 Wasting (→ 'parietal lobe weakness')

* Or inferior quadrantanopia

Clinical manifestations of occipital lobe lesions
1 'Cortical' blindness, *or*
  Altitudinal hemianopia, *or*
  Congruous crossed hemianopia
2 Smooth pursuit defects, impaired opticokinetic nystagmus
3 Visual agnosia; visual hallucinations
4 Achromatopsia; prosopagnosia; topographical amnesia

Predominant lateralization of some cortical functions
1 Left cerebral cortex
  — Language
  — Mathematical ability
2 Right cerebral cortex
  — Spatioperceptual ability
  — Music appreciation

Classical localization of some CNS deficits
1 Mamillary bodies
  — Wernicke's
2 Amygdaloid bodies
  — Aggressive behavior
3 Hippocampus
  Ventromedial temporal lobe
  — Memory loss
4 Butterfly glioma of corpus callosum
  — Typically asymptomatic until advanced

Hemiplegia: cerebral or cervical cord lesion?
1 Cerebral
  — Facial weakness
  — Ipsilateral shoulder shrugging difficult
2 Low cervical cord lesions
  — No facial weakness
  — Ipsilateral shoulder shrugging normal (C1–5 trapezius innervation spared)

EXAMINING THE EYES

Clinical criteria for characterizing blindness
1 Complete blindness
  — Absent pupillary reactions
  — Absent opticokinetic nystagmus
2 Cortical blindness
  — Normal pupillary reactions (i.e. to light)
  — Absent opticokinetic nystagmus
3 Anton's syndrome
  — Cortical blindness (as above)
  — Blindness denied by patient*
4 Hysterical blindness
  — Normal pupillary reactions
  — Normal opticokinetic nystagmus
  — Blindness claimed by patient

* ? Due to destruction of visual association areas ± hallucinations, amnesia

Causes of painful visual loss
1 Optic neuritis
2 Acute glaucoma
3 Giant cell arteritis
4 Central retinal artery (CRA) occlusion*
5 Migraine

* Cause *par excellence* of amaurosis fugax

Classical patterns of visual field defect
1 Central field defects
  — Central scotoma
    • Macular pathology (e.g. demyelination)
  — Central arcuate scotoma
    • Early glaucoma
  — Pericentral scotoma (normal acuity)
    • Retinitis pigmentosa
    • Chloroquine retinopathy
  — Centrocecal scotoma (extends to involve blind spot)
    • Toxic optic neuritis (e.g. methanol, 'nutritional')
  — Congruous homonymous scotoma
    • Localized lesions of occipital cortex
2 Hemianopias
  — Bitemporal hemianopia
    • Chiasmal lesion, esp. pituitary tumor
  — Incongruous homonymous hemianopia
    • Optic tract lesion (rare)
  — Congruous homonymous hemianopia
    • Lesion of occipital lobe optic radiation
  — Homonymous hemianopia with macular sparing
    • Lesion of occipital cortex (usually vascular)
  — Bilateral homonymous hemianopia*
    • Small island of central vision
3 Quadrantanopias (usually due to tumors)
  — Superior
    • Lesion of temporal lobe optic radiation
  — Inferior
    • Lesion of parietal lobe optic radiation
4 Field defects in one eye only
  — Retinal detachment
  — Branch retinal vein occlusion
  — Ischemic optic neuropathy ($\rightarrow$ inferior defect)
  — Vasculitis
5 Concentric visual field constriction (tunnel vision)
  — Hysteria ('tubular' vision)
  — Migraine
  — Retinal disease
    • Advanced glaucoma or papilledema
    • 'Panretinal' laser photocoagulation‡
6 Other patterns of field defect
  — Enlarged blind spot
    • Early papilledema
  — Visual inattention
    • Lesion of posterior parietal lobe

* Due to bilateral posterior cerebral artery occlusion
‡ Causes peripheral field loss with normal acuity; cf. diabetic maculopathy impairs acuity with peripheral field sparing

Chiasmal lesions: clinical signs aiding localization
1 Posterior chiasm lesions
  — Due to suprasellar or third ventricle tumors
  — Typically involve macular fibers only
  — Manifest with central scotoma only
2 Anterosuperior chiasm lesions
  — Due to meningiomas (sphenoid ridge, frontal lobe) or aneurysms (anterior cerebral/ communicating)
  — Manifest with inferior temporal quadrant loss

3 Anteroinferior chiasm lesions
— Due to pituitary tumor, meningitis
— Involve maculopapillary bundle as well as chiasm
— Cause bitemporal hemianopia plus central scotoma
4 Posteroinferior chiasm lesions
— Due to pituitary tumors
— Initially cause bitemporal superior quadrantanopia
— May → optic atrophy, inferotemporal or nasal field loss

'Examine the eyes': important details
1 Position the patient in front of you (e.g. in chair, side of bed)
2 Inspection checklist
— Glasses (e.g. thick lenses, for aphakic patients)
— Ptosis (unilateral or bilateral)
— Proptosis (view orbits from all angles); ± pulsating
— Enophthalmos (esp. if pupil constricted), dry skin
— Rubeosis iridis; arcus senilis; band keratopathy
3 Visual acuity
— Test with patient's glasses on (newsprint, eye chart)
— Unilateral blindness? Exclude glass eye
4 Visual fields
— Test for visual inattention
— Map blind spot (and central scotoma, if present)
5 Fundoscopy
— Look for red reflex
— Characterize opacities (e.g. cataract)
— Indicate that you would like to dilate the pupils
— Comment on retinal vessels, venous pulsations, disc
— Inspect macula last ('look straight at the light now')
6 Extraocular movements
— Ask re diplopia in any direction
— Cover eyes sequentially when double image maximal (peripheral image is from the diseased eye)
— Is nystagmus present? Look for optic atrophy, dysarthria, bulbar palsy, cerebellar signs, etc.
— Is there fatiguability?
7 Pupils
— Check for regularity and circularity
— Turn off lights if possible to examine reactivity
— Test direct *and* consensual response to light in each eye
— Horner's syndrome? Check for ipsilateral facial anhidrosis (signifies lesion proximal to carotid bifurcation, e.g. in brachial plexus)
8 Palpate globes and temporal arteries for tenderness
9 Auscultate orbits (and skull if indicated)
10 Auscultate carotids if CVA suspected; ask to take BP, etc.

THE ABNORMAL FUNDUS

Papilledema: fundoscopic criteria
1 Loss of physiologic cup
2 Elevation of disc head (quantifiable in dioptres)
3 Blurring of disc margins
4 Distended non-pulsatile veins
5 Subhyaloid hemorrhages at disc margins

Differential diagnosis of optic disc swelling
1 Pseudopapilledema: benign anomalies, e.g.
— Drüsen of the disc (may → field defect)
— Hypermetropia
2 Papilledema
— Visual acuity: normal (unless long-standing disease)
— Visual field testing: enlarged blind spot
— Disc swelling usually bilateral (cf. papillitis)
3 Papillitis
— Subjective loss of brightness and color
— Pain on eye movement; tenderness on globe palpation
— Visual acuity: early, marked reduction
— Visual field testing: central scotoma (macular disease)
— Disc swelling usually unilateral (cf. papilledema)
— May progress to optic atrophy if long-standing
— Marcus–Gunn phenomenon (pp. 259–60)
4 Retrobular neuritis
— Similar to papillitis, but
  • *No* visible disc swelling
  • Temporal disc pallor may be the only sign
  • Commonest presentation of demyelination
5 Posterior uveitis
— Visual acuity only reduced if macular edema present
— Visual field testing usually normal
— Disc swelling may be unilateral or bilateral
— Cellular infiltrate visible in vitreous
6 Ischemic optic neuropathy
— Visual field testing → inferior altitudinal defect
— Disc swelling: pale, asymmetric
— Hypertensive vascular signs, else resembles papillitis

Disorders causing retinal arteriolar constriction
1 Malignant hypertension
2 Central retinal artery occlusion
3 Retinitis pigmentosa
4 Cinchonism

Disorders causing dilated retinal veins
1 Polycythemia, hyperviscosity
2 Central retinal vein (CRV) thrombosis
3 Increased intracranial pressure
4 CO_2 retention
5 Caroticocavernous fistula

Causes of angioid streaks (breaks in Bruch's membrane)
1 Paget's disease
2 Acromegaly
3 Pseudoxanthoma elasticum
4 Ehlers–Danlos syndrome
5 Hereditary hyperphosphatasia
6 Sickle-cell anemia

RETINOPATHY

Retinal hemorrhages: their morphologic significance
1 'Dot' hemorrhages
   — Microaneurysms in the posterior pole of the retina
   — Fundoscopic hallmark of diabetic retinopathy
2 'Blot' hemorrhages
   — Small hemorrhages deep in the posterior retinal pole
   — Vertical course of nerve fibers restricts spread here
   — Also characteristic of diabetic retinopathy
3 'Flame' hemorrhages
   — Rupture of superficial retinal capillary plexus
   — Track horizontally along superficial nerve fiber layer
   — Characteristic of grade III/IV hypertensive retinopathy
4 Preretinal ('subhyaloid') hemorrhages
   — Fluid level visible between retina and vitreous
   — Caused by new vessel rupture (e.g. proliferative diabetic retinopathy), or rapid rise in intracranial pressure (e.g. subarachnoid/intracerebral hemorrhage)
5 Subretinal hemorrhages
   — Greenish/brown appearance
   — Indicate choroidal pathology
6 Full-thickness hemorrhages
   — Widespread, dark, irregular appearance
   — Indicate retinal ischemia; predispose to new vessels

Retinopathy: hypertensive or diabetic?
1 Hypertensive
   — AV (arteriovenous) nipping*
   — Flame hemorrhages
   — Papilledema
2 Diabetic
   — Microaneurysms
   — Dot and blot hemorrhages
   — New vessel formation

* Not useful in assessing *severity* of hypertension

CLINICAL SIGNS IN THE ANTERIOR EYE

Clinical spectrum of corneal abnormalities
1 Stigmata of systemic disease
   — Arcus senilis (hyperlipidemia*)
   — Band keratopathy (hypercalcemia‡)
   — Crystals (cystinosis, myeloma)
   — Clouding (lipid storage disorders)
   — Kayser–Fleischer rings (Wilson's)
2 Corneal dystrophies¶
   — Fuchs' dystrophy (in elderly)
   — Lattice-type dystrophy
     • Localized amyloid
     • Finnish amyloidosis (p.179)
3 Post-keratitis scarring
   — Herpes simplex
   — Staphylococci, streptococci

   — *Pseudomonas* spp.
   — *Acanthamoeba* protozoal infections

* In young patients
‡ If long-standing
¶ Bilateral signs; usually autosomal dominant inheritance

Causes of a small pupil
1 Horner's syndrome
2 Neurosyphilis (Argyll Robertson pupils)
3 Myotonic dystrophy
4 Pontine lesions
5 Acute iritis
6 Opiates; organophosphate poisoning

Causes of a large pupil
1 Third nerve palsy (if due to compressive lesion)
2 Holmes–Adie syndrome
3 Midbrain lesions
4 Congenital syphilis
5 Trauma (local)
6 Anticholinergics, benzodiazepines, cocaine, mydriatics

Pupillary responses to mydriatics
1 Hyperactive (excessive mydriasis)
   — Holmes–Adie syndrome ('tonic' pupil; see below)
2 Hypoactive (sluggish response)
   — Myotonic dystrophy ('contratonic' pupil)
   — Argyll Robertson pupil
3 Autonomic neuropathy
   — *Hyperactive* dilatation to topical adrenaline (epinephrine)1:1000, indicating denervation hypersensitivity*
   — *Hypoactive* response to topical cocaine (2.5%) or hydroxyamphetamine, indicating depletion of endogenous noradrenaline (norepinephrine)

* Similarly, hyperactive constriction to 2.5% topical methacholine

Causes of Horner's syndrome
1 Pancoast tumor
2 Sympathectomy
3 Syringomyelia
4 Lateral medullary syndrome
5 Shy–Drager syndrome (may be alternating)

Double-barrelled eponymous pupillary anomalies
1 Holmes–Adie syndrome
   — 'Tonic pupil'; usually unilateral; commoner in women
   — Pupil reacts abnormally slowly to light*
   — Pupil reacts normally to accommodation
   — Pupil exhibits denervation hypersensitivity to mydriatics
   — Associated with hyporeflexia and peripheral anhidrosis
2 Argyll Robertson pupils
   — Small irregular pupils, frequently unequal
   — React to accommodation but not to light
   — Hallmark of neurosyphilis; rarely seen in diabetes
3 Marcus–Gunn phenomenon
   — Pupil constricts weakly to direct light, strongly to consensual illumination ('swinging light' test)

— Indicates relative afferent pupillary defect

--- Hallmark of optic neuritis (hence, of multiple sclerosis)

* But still constricts after prolonged exposure to bright light

Characteristic cataracts

1 'Snowflake'
   — Insulin-dependent diabetes (rare)
2 'Sunflower'
   — Wilson's disease (do not impair vision)
3 'Stellate' (punctate, radially distributed)
   — Hypoparathyroidism
4 'Scintillatory' (polychromatophilic, dustlike)
   — Myotonic dystrophy
5 Subcapsular posterior
   — Steroid-induced (dose- and duration-dependent)
   — Chronic uveitis (± steroid eyedrops)
   — Irradiation

OCULAR PALSIES

Clinical characterization of ptosis

1 Bilateral
   — Muscle disease (myasthenia; myotonic dystrophy)
2 Partial unilateral
   — Horner's syndrome*
   — Partial third nerve palsy
   — Congenital ptosis (commonest cause in healthy people)
3 Complete unilateral
   — Third nerve palsy

* 'Everything is smaller': ptosis, miosis, enophthalmos

Diplopia: signs favoring myopathic etiology

1 Bilateral ptosis or exophthalmos
2 Bifacial weakness (incl. orbicularis oculi)
3 Normal pupils; worsening of diplopia with fatigue
   — Myasthenia gravis

Syndromes with impaired vertical gaze

1 Parinaud's syndrome
2 Richardson–Steele (progressive supranuclear palsy)
3 Graves' disease
4 Thalamic hemorrhage

Rigidity with supranuclear ophthalmoparesis?

1 Progressive supranuclear palsy
2 Multisystem atrophy
3 Creutzfeldt–Jakob disease, Gerstmann–Sträussler disease
4 Machado–Joseph disease (spinocerebellar ataxia type 3)
5 Multiple infarcts or ganglionic degeneration

Painful ophthalmoplegic syndromes

1 Third nerve palsy
   — Posterior communicating artery aneurysm
   — Intracavernous internal carotid artery aneurysm
   — Diabetes mellitus*, ischemia*, vasculitis*
   — Migraine (esp. in children)

2 Sixth nerve palsy
   — Tolosa–Hunt syndrome
   — Gradenigo's syndrome
   — Nasopharyngeal carcinoma
   — Infraclinoid (extradural) carotid artery aneurysm
3 Total ophthalmoplegia (± proptosis)
   — Superior orbital fissure syndrome

* NB: Pupils may react normally due to separate blood supply of pupillary fibers

Varieties of nystagmus and their clinical significance

1 Physiologic (optokinetic) nystagmus
   — Reflex elicited by objects moving through fixed line of sight (e.g. looking out a train window)
   — Mediated by angular/supramarginal gyri in posterior parietal lobe (independent of vestibular nuclei)
   — Reduced (impaired) when looking at striped drum rotating *towards* side of destructive cerebral lesion
   — Provides evidence of sightedness in infants, retarded or aphasic patients, hysterics and malingerers
2 Rotary nystagmus
   — Usually due to *labyrinthine* lesions; hence, often accompanied by vertigo, deafness and/or tinnitus
   — Horizontal direction defined by fast (saccadic) phase
   — Maximal when eyes deviated in direction of fast phase
   — Saccadic correction is made by the paramedian pontine reticular formation (PPRF) on the 'fast' side (e.g. benign positional nystagmus, due to utricle pathology)
   — Fast phase towards dependent ear (e.g. clockwise rotation if left ear kept in dependent position)
   — Nystagmus exhibits *latency* (10–20 sec prior to onset after repositioning) and *adaptation* (lessening of nystagmus following repeated repositioning)
3 Pendular nystagmus (i.e. no 'fast' phase)
   — Difficulty fixating and/or maintaining gaze
   — Nystagmus evident even if gaze centered
   — Usually congenital or familial; also seen in acquired amblyopia, myopathies (esp. myasthenia) and pontine/cerebellar lesions affecting PPRF
4 Vertical nystagmus
   — Due to brainstem/cerebellar (not vestibular) pathology
   — In diffuse cerebellar lesions, nystagmus may occur on fixation in *any* direction
   — Upbeat nystagmus (fast phase up): lesions of pontine tegmentum or floor of fourth ventricle
   — Downbeat nystagmus: cerebellar atrophy, syrinx, brainstem ischemia, or lesion at foramen magnum (may be surgically treatable) such as tumor, Arnold–Chiari
5 'Ataxic' nystagmus
   — i.e. Internuclear ophthalmoplegia (brainstem lesion*)

— Horizontal nystagmus of abducting eye with paralysis of contralateral adductor
— (Almost) pathognomonic of multiple sclerosis
6 Ocular bobbing
— Indicates caudal pontine lesion
— Rapid downward movement of eyes, then slow return

* Lesion in medial longitudinal fasciculus

Lateralization of pathologic eye signs
1 Nystagmus
— Maximal looking away from side of vestibular lesion
— Maximal looking towards side of cerebellar lesion
2 Homonymous hemianopia
— Hemianopic field defect on the side *opposite* the cortical lesion (i.e. on the *same* side as the hemiplegic arm or leg) in hemispheric disease
3 Diplopia
— When looking in direction of maximal diplopia, the more peripheral image disappears when the *abnormal* eye is covered

Lateralization of abnormal conjugate gaze
1 Hemispheric stroke
— Eyes turned *towards* side of CVA (i.e. away from hemiplegic arm or leg)
2 Lateral pontine lesion
— Eyes turned *away* from side of brainstem disease (i.e. towards hemiplegic limb)
3 Epileptic seizure
— Eyes turned *away* from side of irritative cortical (i.e. hemispheric) epileptogenic focus
4 Caloric testing
— Eyes turned towards ear irrigated with ice-cold water in patients with *intact* brainstem and labyrinth

THE FACE IN NEUROLOGICAL DISEASE

Differential diagnosis of facial pain in trigeminal distribution
1 Trigeminal neuralgia
— Tends to occur in patients > 50 years
— Pain → maxillary and mandibular branches of CN V
2 Paratrigeminal neuralgia (Raeder's syndrome)
— May be caused by malignancy at skull base
— Pain in ophthalmic CN V; → orbit pain, Horner's
3 Post-herpetic neuralgia
— Tends to occur in elderly patients
— Pain → ophthalmic branch of CN V
4 Intracavernous internal carotid artery aneurysm
— May cause ophthalmoplegia, esp. CN III
— Pain/sensory loss → ophthalmic (± maxillary) CN V
5 Superior orbital fissure syndrome
— Often caused by tumor invasion; may cause proptosis
— Pain in ophthalmic CN V (± ophthalmoplegia)

6 Gradenigo's syndrome
— In petrous temporal lesions (e.g. chronic otitis media)
— Pain → CN V; associated CN VI palsy; now rare

Non-trigeminal patterns of facial pain
1 Ramsay–Hunt syndrome (geniculate neuralgia)
— Varicella-zoster of the geniculate ganglion of CN VII
— 'Otic zoster': ear pain, facial paralysis, vesicles in ear and/or ipsilateral fauces, ± involvement of CN VIII
2 Costen's syndrome
— Affects patients with jaw malocclusion
— Pain → temporomandibular region
3 Tolosa–Hunt syndrome
— Usually due to granulomatous angiitis or tumors
— Painful ophthalmoplegia (palsies of CN III, IV or VI)
4 Glossopharyngeal neuralgia
— Similar pain to trigeminal neuralgia; affects elderly
— Pain → CN IX, provoked by speaking or swallowing
5 Jaw claudication
— Usually due to giant-cell arteritis (elderly patients)
— Pain → jaw and/or tongue when eating or speaking

Clinical characterization of facial weakness
1 Unilateral upper motor neuron weakness (e.g. CVA)
— Upper face *spared* (bilateral innervation of frontalis and orbicularis oculi)
— No lower facial sagging (tone preserved)
— Facial paresis may disappear during emotion (mediated via extrapyramidal fibers)
— Often associated with ipsilateral hemiplegia
2 Unilateral lower motor neuron weakness (e.g. Bell's palsy)
— Upper face weak (loss of forehead wrinkling)
— Inability to voluntarily close eye (eye rolls up: Bell's sign) due to paralysis of orbicularis oculi → ectropion, conjunctivitis
— Lower facial sagging (± mild dysarthria)
— Slight droop of upper lip ('Cupid's bow')
— Progressively more proximal lesions
  • Loss of taste over ipsilateral anterior two-thirds tongue ± sensory loss in external auditory meatus (chorda tympani involvement)
  • Hyperacusis (involvement of nerve to stapedius)
  • Impaired or aberrant lacrimation during recovery (e.g. 'crocodile tears' while eating; due to greater petrosal nerve involvement)
— Involvement of neighboring cranial nerves
  • CN VI (e.g. brainstem lesion)
  • CN VIII (e.g. in Ramsay–Hunt syndrome)
  • CN V, VIII (e.g. cerebellopontine angle tumor)*
3 Myopathy (e.g. myotonic dystrophy)
— Symmetric facial wasting → long, haggard appearance
  • 'Transverse smile' (myotonic dystrophy)
  • 'Myasthenic snarl', 'jaw-supporting' (myasthenia gravis)

— Periorbital edema/heliotrope rash (polymyositis)
— Ptosis
  • May be asymmetric (i.e. albeit bilateral)
  • Absent in CN VII lesions
— Fatiguability
— Ophthalmoplegia‡
  • Usually asymmetric
  • Pupils normal (cf. CN III palsy)

* cf. CN VII palsy: more often due to surgery than tumor compression
‡ Complicates myasthenia gravis, *not* myasthenic syndrome or polymyositis

Facial presentations of systemic disease

1 Trigeminal neuralgia in a young patient
— Multiple sclerosis
— Cerebellopontine angle tumor
2 Bilateral lower motor neuron facial palsy
— Guillain–Barré syndrome
— Mikulicz syndrome (bilateral parotid infiltration, e.g. by sarcoidosis/tuberculosis/actinomycosis)
3 Facial neuromyopathy
— Myotonic dystrophy
— Facioscapulohumeral dystrophy
— Myasthenia gravis

DISORDERS AFFECTING THE LOWER CRANIAL NERVES

Characterizing and lateralizing hearing loss

1 Weber's test
— Lateralizes to deaf side
  • Conduction deafness (e.g. otosclerosis)
— Lateralizes to normal side
  • Nerve deafness (e.g. acoustic neuroma)
2 Rinne's test
— Bone > air conduction on affected side
  • Conduction deafness
— Air > bone conduction on both sides
  • Nerve deafness

Clinical evaluation of vestibular function

1 Caloric testing
— Tests integrity of one labyrinth at a time by slowly irrigating ear with hot (44°C) or cold (30°C) water
— Patient lies flat with head elevated 30–45° to make horizontal semicircular canal vertical
— Nystagmus induced exhibits one of two abnormalities
  • Canal paresis (weaker nystagmus on affected side)
  • Directional preponderance, i.e. longer duration of nystagmus on stimulation of one labyrinth
— Principal diagnostic uses
  • Ménière's disease
  • Acoustic neuroma
  • Unconscious patients: tests brainstem integrity
2 Oculocephalic testing
— Tests integrity of both labyrinths together by holding eyelids open and sharply rotating head to one side

— *Doll's-eye movements* are those in which eyes lag behind head, but slowly regain original position
— Doll's-eye movements indicate loss of hemispheric suppression but preservation of brainstem function

Distinction of acoustic neuroma from Ménière's disease

1 Discrete symptomatic episodes unusual
2 Vertigo uncommon; rarely occurs in isolation
3 May be associated with post-auricular/suboccipital pain, facial spasms, paresthesiae, or dysphonia/dysphagia
4 Physical signs may include limb ataxia, cranial nerve palsies (esp. V) or hemianesthesia/-paresis
5 Impaired oculovestibular (caloric) response
High frequency deafness with recruitment on audiometry
6 Radiology
— MRI: best test for cerebellopontine angle tumors
— SXR: widening of internal auditory meatus or erosion of petrous temporal (no longer routinely indicated)

Distinction of bulbar and pseudobulbar palsies

1 Bulbar palsy
— Affect: normal
— Swallowing: nasal regurgitation
— Speech: nasal
— Tongue: fasciculations
— Jaw jerk: normal/absent
2 Pseudobulbar palsy
— Affect: labile
— Swallowing: dysphagia
— Speech: 'Donald Duck'
— Tongue: small (spastic)
— Jaw jerk: increased

SPINAL CORD DISEASE: GENERAL

Clues to localizing a spinal cord lesion

1 Radicular pain (indicating myotome) and weakness
2 Pattern of reflex changes
3 Sensory level (indicating dermatome)
4 Spinal tenderness to percussion*
5 Vertebral bruit (indicating tumor/AVM)

* Esp. acute epidural abscess, malignancy

Clinical sequelae of spinal cord lesions

1 Vital signs
— Hypotension
— Poikilothermia
2 Sphincter dysfunction
— Incontinence
— Chronic UTI → amyloidosis
3 Autonomic dysfunction
— Paralytic ileus
— Excessive sweating below lesion level
4 Musculoskeletal
— Pressure sores
— Contractures

5 Immobilization
— Hypercalcemia, renal calculi, osteoporosis
— Venous thrombosis

NEUROLOGY OF THE UPPER SPINE

Cranial nerve signs of high cervical cord disease
1 Ipsilateral hemifacial dissociated sensory loss*
2 Horner's syndrome
3 Rarely: nystagmus, optic neuritis/atrophy

* = Isolated loss of pain and temperature sensation

Signs of craniocervical junction anomaly (e.g. Arnold–Chiari)
1 Occipital pain; facial sensory loss; ± Pagetoid appearance
2 Cerebellar signs (due to foraminal tonsillar herniation)
3 Downbeat nystagmus, esp. on lateral gaze
4 Finger deafferentation (esp. proprioception) pseudotremor
5 Bulbar palsy, spastic quadriparesis (may simulate MND)

Physical findings in cervical spondylosis
1 Limitation of neck movements
2 Absent tendon jerk(s) at level of lesion (root compression)
3 Increased tendon jerks below lesion (cord compression)
4 Inversion of reflexes
5 Dermatomal sensory loss in upper limbs
6 Dorsal column sensory loss in upper and lower limbs
7 Rombergism
8 Spastic paraparesis

Thoracic outlet syndrome: clinical features
1 Physical examination
— Supraclavicular 'fullness'/tenderness/bruit
— Dilated venous collaterals
— Arm pallor/cyanosis/edema
— Wasted interossei
— Sensory loss in C8–T1 distribution
2 Maneuvers
— Repetitive movements → arm claudication
— Arm abduction (to 90°) and external rotation lead to
• Symptoms
• Loss of radial pulse
• Reduction of systolic BP in arm by > 15 mmHg
3 Investigation
— Plain X-ray of thoracic outlet and cervical spine
— Apical lordotic chest X-ray views
— Cervical MRI
— Consider angiography (bilateral) if cervical rib present

C4 root lesions: clinical findings
1 Ipsilateral hemidiaphragmatic paralysis
2 C4 sensory loss (abutting T2 dermatome) at shoulder

C5 root lesions
1 Total loss of shoulder abduction
2 Axillary nerve involvement
— Weak elbow flexion
— Reduced biceps jerk
— Larger sensory loss (lateral arm) than circumflex nerve palsy
3 Supraspinatus wasting ± scapula winging

Differential diagnosis of painless neck weakness
1 Myasthenia gravis
2 Myotonic dystrophy
3 Polymyositis
4 Motor neuron disease

THE MOTOR SYSTEM

Distinguishing upper and lower motor neuron lesions
1 Upper motor neuron lesions
— Increased tone ± clonus
— Increased tendon reflexes
— Absent abdominal reflexes
— Extensor plantar response(s)
— 'Pyramidal' pattern of weakness (see below)
2 Lower motor neuron lesions
— Prominent wasting
— Fasciculation (in anterior horn cell disorders)
— Reduced tone
— Reflexes may be reduced or absent

Patterns of weakness in upper motor neuron lesions
1 Upper limb extensors, esp.
— Elbow and wrist extension
— Finger extension and abduction*
2 Lower limb flexors, esp.
— Hip and knee flexion
— Ankle dorsiflexion and eversion
3 Fine movements of fingers and feet (esp. in capsular lesions)

* But note 'myelopathy hand sign' due to pyramidal lesions of the cervical cord: passive abduction of the little finger occurs with the arms outstretched and supinated

Absent abdominal reflexes: differential diagnosis
1 Upper motor neuron lesions, esp.
— Multiple sclerosis
— General paresis of the insane (neurosyphilis)
— Spinal cord lesions above T7
2 Non-specific ('false-positives')
— Old age
— Gross obesity
— Multiparity

NB: Superficial abdominal reflexes usually *preserved* in motor neuron disease

Signs suggesting upper motor neuron lesions
1 Babinski sign
— Dorsiflexion of great toe and fanning of other digits on stroking lateral sole of foot
2 Oppenheim's sign
— Dorsiflexion of great toe on applying pressure while sliding thumb and forefinger down anterior tibia

3 Hoffman's sign
  — Adduction and flexion of all digits after passively flexing and releasing distal middle phalanx
4 Finger flexor
  — Adduction and flexion of all digits on tapping palmar surface of relaxed fingers with tendon hammer
5 Inverted supinator jerk and/or biceps jerks (often with increased triceps jerks)*
  — Caused by mechanical spread of reflex impulse through bone

NB: Exaggerated finger flexion indicates hypertonia rather than an upper motor neuron lesion *per se*
* Usually indicates cervical spondylosis (and is against diagnosis of motor neuron disease)

Fasciculations: differential diagnosis
1 Neurologic
  — Motor neuron disease (esp. in exams)
  — Acute phase of poliomyelitis
  — Localized fasciculations
    • Syringomyelia
    • Cervical spondylosis
    • Neuralgic amyotrophy
2 Metabolic
  — Thyrotoxicosis
  — Severe hyponatremia
3 Drugs
  — Clofibrate
  — Salbutamol (esp. IV)
  — Lithium (if toxic)

Clinical subtypes of motor neuron disease
1 Progressive bulbar palsy
  — Confined to brainstem-innervated muscles
2 Progressive muscular atrophy
  — Weakness, wasting, fasciculations prominent
3 Primary lateral sclerosis
  — Spasticity, hyperreflexia, extensor plantars prominent
4 Amyotrophic lateral sclerosis
  — Combined features of the above

THE SENSORY SYSTEM

Characteristic patterns of sensory loss
1 Symmetric 'glove-and-stocking' sensory loss to all modalities
  — Peripheral neuropathy
2 Dermatomal sensory loss
  — Nerve root lesion
3 Loss of proprioception/two-point discrimination/ vibration on one side of the body (ipsilateral to hemiparesis) associated with contralateral loss of pain and temperature
  — Brown–Séquard syndrome (classical but rare)
4 *Isolated* loss of pain and temperature* contralateral to hemiparesis
  — *Partial* Brown–Séquard syndrome due to anterior hemicord lesion
5 Bilateral loss of pain and temperature
  Normal proprioception/two-point discrimination‡

  — Syringomyelia
  — Anterior spinal artery thrombosis
6 Loss of proprioception/two-point discrimination/ vibration
  Loss of deep pain (e.g. in testes, Achilles' tendon)
  Patchy loss of pinprick sensation (e.g. along side of nose)
  — Tabes dorsalis

* Sensory level typically occurs 1–2 segments below lesion
‡ cf. *unilateral* dissociated sensory loss: high cervical cord lesion

Symptoms suggesting dorsal column pathology
1 Difficulty with fine movements ('clumsy')
2 Limb 'tightness' (as though bandaged)
3 'Cotton-wool' sensation over skin

Causes of reduced dorsal column function
1 Subacute combined degeneration
2 Cervical spondylosis
3 Friedreich's ataxia
4 Tabes dorsalis*

* cf. syringomyelia, anterior spinal artery thrombosis: *normal* dorsal column function is usual

TESTING NERVE ROOT INTEGRITY

Clinical assessment of nerve root integrity: reflex levels
1 Biceps/supinator jerk present
  — C6 intact*
2 Triceps jerk present
  — C7 intact
3 Finger flexor elicitable
  — C8 intact
4 Abdominal reflexes present
  — T7–12 intact
5 Cremasteric reflex present
  — L1–2 intact
6 Knee jerk present
  — L3–4 intact
7 Ankle jerk plantars present
  — S1 intact
8 Anal reflex present
  — S3–4 intact

* cf. inverted supinator jerk denotes C6 lesion; inverted biceps jerk (elbow flexion replaced by finger flexion) denotes C8–T1 lesion

Quick testing of nerve root integrity in the upper limb
1 C5: shoulder abduction (deltoid)
  — 'Make wings, keep them up, don't let me push down'
2 C6: elbow flexion (biceps) and wrist extension (extensor carpi radialis)
  — 'Pull me towards you'
3 C7: elbow extension (triceps)
  — 'Now push me away'
4 C8: finger flexion/hand grasp (long and short finger flexors)
  — 'Squeeze my fingers; try to break them'
5 T1: finger abduction (intrinsics)
  — 'Spread your fingers apart, don't let me push them in'

Quick testing of motor nerve root integrity in the lower limb
1 L1–3: hip flexion (iliopsoas)
   — 'Push up against my hand, keep it up'
2 L2–3: hip adduction (adductors)
   — 'Pull your knees together against my hands'
3 L3–4: knee extension (quadriceps)
   — 'Try to straighten your knee; kick out against my hand'
4 L4–5: ankle dorsiflexion (tibialis anterior)
   — 'Curl your ankle up, don't let me straighten it'
5 L5: great toe plantarflexion (extensor hallucis longus)
   — 'Push your big toe down into my hand'
6 L5–S1: knee flexion (hamstrings)
   — 'Pull your heel in towards you, don't let me pull it away'
7 S1: ankle plantarflexion (gastrocnemius)
   — 'Try to straighten your foot; don't let me bend it back'
8 S2–4: anal tone (anal sphincter)
   — 'Can you feel my finger on your bottom?'

NEUROLOGY OF THE UPPER LIMB

Clinical spectrum of radial nerve palsy
1 High axillary injury ('crutch palsy')
   — All supplied muscles paralysed
   — Paralysis includes triceps
     • Loss of elbow extension
     • Absent triceps jerk
   — Sensory deficit may extend to posterolateral upper arm and dorsal forearm/hand
2 Humeral midshaft injury ('Saturday night palsy')
   — Wrist- and finger-drop
   — Triceps spared, normal elbow extension and triceps jerk
   — Paralyses brachioradialis/supinator/forearm extensors
   — Sensory deficit limited to dorsum of hand
3 Posterior interosseous nerve injury (distal to supinator)
   — Loss of thumb/index extension
   — Loss of thumb abduction
   — Brachioradialis/supinator/forearm extensors spared
   — No sensory deficit

Small hand muscles affected by median nerve lesion 'LOAF'
1 **L**ateral two lumbricals
2 **O**pponens pollicis
3 **A**bductor pollicis brevis (best test of median nerve integrity)
4 **F**lexor pollicis brevis

Wasting of the small muscles of both hands
1 Disuse
   — Old age
   — Rheumatoid arthritis
2 Spinal cord disease
   — Syringomyelia
   — Motor neuron disease

3 Spinal cord compression
   — Cervical spondylosis
   — C8–TI tumor
4 Bilateral nerve root compression
   — Cervical spondylosis
   — Thoracic outlet syndrome
5 Peripheral neuropathy
   — Charcot–Marie–Tooth disease
   — Lead poisoning, acute intermittent porphyria

NB: Myotonic dystrophy causes prominent forearm wasting but characteristically *spares* the small hand muscles

Wasting of the small muscles of one hand
1 Ulnar nerve lesion
2 T1 nerve root lesion (e.g. bronchogenic carcinoma)

Differentiation of T1 root lesion from ulnar nerve palsy
1 No sensory deficit in the hand* in T1 root lesions
2 Dermatomal sensory loss in medial arm associated with T1 root lesions
3 Weakness of opponens pollicis/abductor pollicis brevis (supplied by median nerve; i.e. T1 lesion → all intrinsics) in T1 root lesions
4 In ulnar nerve lesions, weakness of thumb adduction is compensated for by intact median nerve innervation of flexor pollicis longus (Froment's sign)

* NB: Ulnar nerve lesion at *wrist* (rare) also produces no sensory loss

Differentiation of C8 root lesion from ulnar nerve palsy
1 Sensory loss involves the whole of the ring finger in C8 root lesions (but only the lateral half in ulnar nerve lesions)
2 Sensory loss extends to the medial forearm in C8 root lesions
3 Triceps jerk may be depressed in C8 root lesions

NEUROLOGIC SIGNS IN THE LOWER LIMB

Absent ankle jerks with extensor plantar responses
1 Coexisting lumbar and cervical spondylosis
2 Subacute combined degeneration
3 Friedreich's ataxia
4 Taboparesis
5 Motor neuron disease
6 Meningeal carcinomatosis
7 Diabetic amyotrophy
8 Conus medullaris lesion
9 Spinal shock

Clinical assessment of paraparesis
1 Cauda equina compression
   — Common
   — Gradual, unilateral onset
   — Pain occurs early
   — Sphincter dysfunction occurs late
   — Flaccid paralysis → wasted calves/absent knee jerks
2 Conus medullaris lesion
   — Uncommon
   — Sudden, bilateral onset

— Pain occurs late
— Sphincter dysfunction occurs early
— Spastic paraparesis → wasted quadriceps/upgoing toes
3 Parasagittal meningioma
— Rare
— Associated with papilledema
— Distal weakness often prominent
— Spastic paraparesis, extensor plantar response(s)

Clinical assessment of footdrop
1 Lateral popliteal nerve palsy
— Equinovarus deformity due to impaired eversion
— Variable sensory loss (usually none)
— Great toe: sensation/dorsiflexion usually normal
2 L5 root lesion
— Eversion unimpaired (cf. S1 root lesion)
— Dermatomal sensory loss (dorsum of foot)
— Great toe: sensation/dorsiflexion usually impaired
3 Charcot–Marie–Tooth disease
— Equinovarus deformity with pes cavus
— 'Inverted champagne bottle' appearance of limbs
— Mild glove-and-stocking sensory loss
— Bilateral signs; possible hand involvement

GAIT ABNORMALITIES

Diagnostic significance of abnormal posture
1 Rombergism (loss of balance with eyes closed)
— Proprioceptive deficit
2 Truncal ataxia (same with eyes open or closed)
— Cerebellar (flocculonodular lobe) disease
3 Simian posture
— Parkinsonism

Common pathologies underlying abnormal gait
1 Frontal gait apraxia
— Cerebrovascular disease
— Normal pressure hydrocephalus
2 Neurodegeneration
— Parkinsonism
— Encephalopathy (e.g. toxic)
3 Myelopathy
— Cervical spondylosis
4 Cerebellar disease
5 Sensory neuropathy

Clinical characterization of abnormal gait
1 Wide-based ('drunken') gait
— Cerebellar (vermis) disease
— Same gait with eyes open or closed
2 Stamping ('footslapping') gait; may also be wide-based
— Sensory (esp. dorsal column) ataxia
— Worse with eyes closed
— Associated with rombergism (e.g. in tabes dorsalis)

3 High-stepping ('equine') gait
— Footdrop (e.g. Charcot–Marie–Tooth disease)
4 Circumducting ('sticky') gait
— Hemiplegia
5 Scissors ('walking through mud') gait
— Spastic paraparesis
6 Waddling ('duck-like') gait
— Myopathy
7 Festinating gait (± pro-/retropulsion, turns-by-numbers)
— Parkinsonism
8 Marche à petits pas ('sputtering'/apraxic gait), 'magnetic foot'
— Pseudobulbar palsy
— Alzheimer's disease
— Normal pressure hydrocephalus

NB: In exams it is best to delay labelling the gait (if possible) until *after* the other signs have established the diagnosis!

PATTERNS OF PERIPHERAL NEUROPATHY

Important causes of hypertrophic (palpable) neuropathies
1 Charcot–Marie–Tooth disease
2 Acromegaly
3 Lepromatous leprosy
4 Amyloidosis

Predominantly motor neuropathies
1 Charcot–Marie–Tooth disease
2 Guillain–Barré syndrome
3 Acute intermittent (or variegate) porphyria
4 Diphtheria
5 Lead poisoning
6 Herpes zoster (common but usually subclinical)

Predominantly sensory neuropathies
1 Diabetes
2 Paraneoplastic
3 Nutritional (incl. B_{12}/folate deficiency, alcohol)
4 Uremia
5 Amyloid

Clinical detection of diabetic neuropathy
1 Claw toes and prominent metatarsal heads
2 Calluses on the soles of the feet
3 Impaired vibration perception*
4 Absent ankle jerks, reduced knee jerks
5 Reduced light touch and pinprick sensation
6 Associated signs of peripheral vascular disease

* Can rapidly screen for this in the diabetic clinic using biothesiometry

Frequently painful neuropathies
1 Diabetic amyotrophy
2 Nutritional
— Alcoholic neuropathy
— Beri-beri, Strachan's syndrome
3 Toxic
— Metronidazole
— Thallium poisoning
4 AIDS-related neuropathy

Cranial nerve involvement in peripheral neuropathy
1 Diphtheria (CN IX)
2 Guillain–Barré (CN VI, VII)
  Miller–Fisher variant (III, IV)
3 Sarcoidosis (CN VII)
4 Diabetes (CN III)

Nerves frequently involved in leprosy
1 Upper limb
  — Radial (and radial cutaneous)
  — Ulnar, median
2 Lower limb
  — Common peroneal
  — Posterior tibial
3 Head and neck
  — Facial
  — Preauricular

Drugs commonly associated with peripheral neuropathy
1 Vincristine, vindesine, taxol
2 Nitrofurantoin
3 Metronidazole
4 Perhexiline maleate
5 Gold
6 Isoniazid (B_6 deficiency), ethambutol
  Phenytoin (folate deficiency)

Guillain–Barré syndrome: diagnostic criteria
1 Major criteria
  — Progressive lower motor neuron limb weakness*
  — Areflexia
  — Maximal deficit induced within 4 weeks of onset
  — No other cause of neuropathy demonstrable
2 Minor criteria
  — Lack of fever
  — Symmetrical weakness with only mild sensory signs
  — ↑ CSF protein with normal cell count
  — Segmental demyelination pattern of nerve conduction
  — Peripheral nerve myelin antibodies detectable acutely
  — Successful trial of plasmapheresis within first week
3 Factors tending to *exclude* the diagnosis
  — Sensory level
  — Marked asymmetry of signs
  — Bladder or bowel dysfunction
  — Elevated CSF cell count (> 50/mm^3)

* Arms are also typically involved

AUTONOMIC NEUROPATHY

Principal causes of autonomic neuropathy
1 Diabetes mellitus
2 Uremia
3 Amyloidosis
4 Guillain–Barré syndrome
5 Liver disease ± alcoholism
6 Idiopathic (acquired): Shy–Drager syndrome
7 Idiopathic (congenital): Riley–Day syndrome

Presentations of autonomic neuropathy
1 Vital signs
  — Pulse
    • Fixed resting tachycardia (vagal paresis)
    • Postural tachycardia
  — Blood pressure*
    • Supine hypertension
    • Postural hypotension
2 Facial signs
  — 'Differential' gustatory sweating‡
  — Pupils: Horner's, anisocoria
3 Gastrointestinal
  — Epigastric pain (gastroparesis, esophageal reflux)
  — Nocturnal hyperdefecation; fecal incontinence
  — Chronic intestinal pseudo-obstruction, causing either
    • Constipation (usually), *or*
    • Diarrhea due to bacterial overgrowth
4 Pain unawareness
  — 'Silent' myocardial infarction
  — Loss of 'deep' pain (e.g. on compressing testis)
  — Loss of peripheral pain (small-fiber neuropathy)
5 Other functional losses
  — Hypoglycemic unawareness (e.g. in treated diabetics)
  — Stridor, apnea¶
  — Urinary retention, overflow incontinence (urgency)
  — Impotence (NB: rarely if ever presents in isolation) or ejaculatory failure

* Differential diagnosis: antihypertensive therapy
‡ Associated with *anhidrosis* affecting non-facial skin
¶ cf. oropharyngeal dysphagia or laryngeal abductor paresis: more suggestive of multiple system atrophy

Assessment of autonomic neuropathy
1 Heart rate variability (ECG R–R intervals), *and* Baroreflex sensitivity (blood pressure variability)
  — Posturing using tilt-table
  — Valsalva maneuver (4-phase response)
  — Isometric handgrip
  — Mental arithmetic (serial sevens)
  — Hands in iced water (for 90 sec)
  — Hyperventilation (for 30 sec)
  — Carotid sinus massage
  — Phenylephrine, nitroprusside
2 Pupillary responses
  — Intraocular adrenaline (epinephrine) 1:1000 → *no* dilatation normally, but dilates in autonomic neuropathy
  — Intraocular cocaine 2.5%: dilatation normally, but *not* in autonomic neuropathy
  — Intraocular methacholine 2.5% → *no* constriction normally, but constricts in autonomic neuropathy (reflecting parasympathetic denervation)
3 Sweat tests
  — Heat patient to cause 1°C rise in oral temperature
  — Give IM pilocarpine or intradermal methacholine
4 Bladder urodynamics (cystometry)

EVALUATING THE CENTRAL NERVOUS SYSTEM

Elevated CSF protein: differential diagnosis
1 Pyogenic meningitis
2 Meningeal carcinomatosis
3 Guillain–Barré syndrome
4 Froin's syndrome (spinal block)
5 Rare: alcoholism, amyloidosis, diabetes, acoustic neuroma

Paraneoplastic autoantibodies causing cerebellar ataxia
1 Anti-Yo
   — Caused by: ovarian cancer
2 Anti-VGCC (voltage-gated calcium channel)
   — Caused by: small cell lung cancer
   — Other features: Eaton–Lambert (myasthenic) syndrome
3 Anti-Hu
   — Caused by: small cell lung cancer
   — Other features: limbic encephalitis, sensory neuropathy
4 Anti-Tr
   — Caused by: Hodgkin's disease
5 Anti-Ri
   — Caused by: breast cancer
   — Other features: opsoclonus, myoclonus

Meningitis with negative CSF Gram-stain?
1 Partly treated pyogenic meningitis
2 Unusual organism (not detected by routine measures)
   — Tuberculous meningitis
   — Cryptococcal meningitis
   — Neurosyphilis
   — Leptospirosis, brucellosis
3 Viral, e.g.
   — HSV#2; polio
   — HIV*
4 Non-infectious causes
   — Vasculitis (esp. SLE)
   — Meningeal carcinomatosis
   — Sarcoidosis
   — Behçet's/Whipple's disease; Vogt–Koyanagi syndrome

* Usually with a secondary meningitic organism (bacterium, virus, etc.); biopsy may be required

Differential diagnosis of cerebral mass lesions in AIDS
1 Toxoplasma encephalitis
2 Primary CNS lymphoma
3 Progressive multifocal leukoencephalopathy

CSF examination after suspected subarachnoid hemorrhage
1 Macroscopic blood staining
   — Reducing red cell count with serial aliquots suggests a 'traumatic tap'
2 Xanthochromia
   — Supports diagnosis of subarachnoid bleed

— Insensitive test if macroscopic characterization relied upon (50% false-negative)
— Spectrophotometric assay (peak at 450 nm) is very sensitive

Relative contraindications to lumbar puncture*
1 Papilledema and/or severe uncontrolled hypertension
2 Coma or decerebrate
3 Status epilepticus
4 Focal signs (e.g. pupillary asymmetry)
5 Coagulopathy or widespread purpura

* e.g. suspected meningitis

Evoked responses: diagnostic utility
1 Visual evoked responses (VERs)
   — Multiple sclerosis: may be useful
     • Prior to firm diagnosis
     • Monitoring disease progress
   — Hemispheric disease, e.g.
     • 'Cortical' blindness vs hysteria
   — Retinal disease
   — Migraine (in children)
2 Brainstem auditory evoked responses (BAERs)
   — Suspected acoustic neuroma
   — Comatose patient
   — Hysterical deafness
   — Multiple sclerosis
3 Somatosensory evoked responses (SSERs)
   — Peripheral nerve vs spinal cord/root lesion
   — Multiple sclerosis

NB: Any of these electrophysiologic tests may be abnormal in HIV infection

ELECTROENCEPHALOGRAPHY (EEG)

Normal EEG patterns
1 Awake (eyes closed)
   — α waves (8–12 cps); over parieto-occipital region
2 Non-REM sleep
   — δ waves (0–3 cps)
3 REM sleep
   — β waves (> 13 cps); over frontal region
4 Hyperventilation
   — θ waves (4–7 cps)

Capabilities of the EEG
1 May diagnose epileptic activity
2 May confirm effect of metabolic disorder (e.g. liver failure)
3 May suggest focal pathology
4 May explain sleep disturbances and/or drop attacks
5 May help distinguish petit mal from temporal lobe epilepsy

Limitations of the EEG
1 Cannot exclude epilepsy
2 Cannot assess adequacy of antiepileptic treatment
3 Cannot exclude focal pathology
4 Cannot suggest structural nature of focal pathology

Principal indications for EEG
1 Diagnosis and management of epilepsy
2 Diagnosis of brain death
3 Unusual indications
   — Unexplained organic brain syndrome
   — Investigation of presenile dementia
   — Evaluation of birth asphyxia

Suggestive diagnostic EEG patterns
1 Hepatic encephalopathy
   — Triphasic waves (*not* in Wernicke's/DTs) $\pm$ δ waves
2 Barbiturate overdose
   — Excess fast-wave (β) activity
3 'α coma'
   — Follows infarction of midbrain tegmentum
4 Absence (petit mal) seizures
   — Characteristic 3 cps spike-and-wave pattern
5 HSV encephalitis, SSPE, Creutzfeldt–Jakob
   — Slow background repetitive sharp waves

The unconscious patient: utility of the EEG
1 Helps distinguish diffuse encephalopathy, e.g.
   — Myxedema ($\rightarrow$ diffuse slowing)
   — Dialysis dementia ($\rightarrow$ spike-and-wave pattern), *from*
2 Space-occupying lesions, e.g.
   — Frontal lobe tumor ($\rightarrow$ focal slowing) *or*
3 Other focal pathology, e.g.
   — HSV encephalitis ($\rightarrow$ temporal lobe slowing) *or*
4 Depressive pseudodementia ($\rightarrow$ normal EEG)

INVESTIGATING CEREBROVASCULAR DISEASE

Techniques available for assessing carotid disease
1 Direct tests
   — Angiography (incl. digital subtraction angiography)
   — 'Duplex scan': B-mode (real-time) + pulsed Doppler
2 Indirect tests
   — Ophthalmodynamometry
   — Oculoplethysmography
   — Periorbital directional Doppler ultrasonography
   — Radionuclide angiography

Which investigation to choose in carotid disease?
1 Angiograpy
   — Advantages
     • Reveals location and severity of disease
     • Still the 'gold standard' for pre-op diagnosis
   — Disadvantages
     • Invasive; may precipitate stroke
     • May fail to reveal intramural pathology
2 'Duplex scan'
   — Advantages
     • Non-invasive; useful to monitor known disease
     • May detect plaque hemorrhage or ulceration
     • Normal study may obviate need for angiography
   — Disadvantages
     • Abnormal? May still require pre-op angiography

3 Indirect tests (ophthalmic artery flow/pressure studies)
   — Advantages
     • Non-invasive
   — Disadvantages
     • Only reliably detect unilateral disease
     • Only reliably detect advanced (> 75% block) cases
     • Only reliably detect occlusive (not ulcerated) cases

Indications for carotid duplex scanning
1 Carotid artery signs
   — Hemiparesis, amaurosis, aphasia; *plus*
2 Good recovery, *plus*
3 Fit for carotid surgery

Indications for angiography in cerebrovascular disease
1 Operable patient *plus*
2 Symptoms suggesting carotid pathology, *or*
3 Subclavian steal syndrome

INVESTIGATING THE PERIPHERAL NERVOUS SYSTEM

Investigation of peripheral neuropathy
1 Qualitative tests
   — Nerve conduction studies
   — Nerve biopsy
2 Etiologic tests
   — Blood film, MCV
   — B_{12}, folate
   — GGT/urate (ethanol)
   — Fasting blood sugar level, HbA_{1c}, GTT
   — Paraprotein screen (see below)
   — Lead, mercury levels
   — Urinary porphobilinogen/δ-ALA
   — CSF protein and cell count
   — Carcinoma search (e.g. CXR) *only* if clinically indicated

Nerve conduction studies: diagnostic significance
1 General
   — Myopathy
     • Normal nerve conduction velocity
     • Reduced amplitude and duration of motor units
   — Neuropathy
     • Reduced nerve conduction velocity
     • Reduced number of motor units
2 Neuropathy: *segmental demyelination* (e.g. Guillain–Barré)
   — Marked slowing of conduction velocity
   — Amplitude may be normal
   — Early loss of reflexes and vibration sense
   — May $\rightarrow$ mononeuritis multiplex
   — Rapid recovery (often)
3 Neuropathy: *axonal degeneration* (e.g. nutritional deficiency)
   — Marked reduction of motor unit amplitude
   — Mild slowing of conduction velocity
   — Early onset of wasting
   — Incomplete recovery (usually)

4 Upper motor neuron lesion
— Normal evoked muscle potentials
— Low firing rate; slow to reach full interference pattern
— Unexpected 'H' reflexes

Indications for nerve biopsy
1 Prognostic clarification (see above) of neuropathies due to
— Axonal degeneration, or
— Segmental demyelination
2 Definitive diagnosis of neuropathies due to
— Polyarteritis/vasculitis
— Amyloidosis, sarcoidosis
— Leprosy
— Déjerine–Sottas disease

Paraprotein-associated peripheral neuropathies
1 Segmental demyelination: symmetric, progressive distal sensorimotor loss*
— Waldenstrom's macroglobulinemia
  • Paraprotein type: IgM-κ
  • Presentation: mucosal bleeding, visual blurring, encephalopathy
— Osteosclerotic myeloma
  • Paraprotein type: IgA-λ, IgG-λ
  • Presentation: POEMS syndrome, areflexia
2 Axonal degeneration: symmetric, distal, and often painful
— Myeloma (classical osteolytic)
  • Paraprotein type: high-titre (> 3 g/dL) IgM-κ/IgG-κ
  • Presentation: renal failure, hypercalcemia, amyloid
— Amyloidosis
  • Paraprotein type: IgA-λ, IgG-λ
  • Presentation: autonomic involvement, organomegaly
— Cryoglobulinemia
  • Paraprotein type: IgM, IgG
  • Presentation: purpura, leg ulcers, Raynaud's
— Lymphoma
  • Paraprotein type: IgM, IgG
  • Presentation: weight loss, fatigue, adenopathy

* Mimics chronic inflammatory demyelinating polyneuropathy

DIAGNOSTIC ASPECTS OF MUSCLE DISEASE

Muscle biopsy: diagnostic value
1 Polymyositis
2 Polyarteritis
3 Myotonic dystrophy
4 Trichinosis, toxoplasmosis
5 Metabolic muscle disease (e.g. glycogen storage) Special myopathies (e.g. mitochondrial)

Pathologic patterns in electromyography (EMG)
1 Polymyositis
— May cause *fibrillation* (brief low-amplitude action potentials due to denervation hypersensitivity), indicating pathology at the motor end-plate (i.e. in addition to the known muscle fiber pathology)
2 Myotonia
— *'Dive-bomber'* EMG (high-frequency action potentials)
3 Myasthenia gravis
— *Decremental* response to repetitive ('tetanic') stimuli
— Increased 'jitter'
4 Myasthenic (Eaton–Lambert) syndrome
— *Incremental* response to repetitive stimulation (= 'post-tetanic facilitation')

Myotonic dystrophy: recognition and diagnosis
1 General appearance
— Frontal alopecia
— Thick glasses (aphakia, cataracts)
— Facial abnormalities, hyperostosis frontalis interna
2 Affect
— Monotonous voice
— Somnolent; subnormal intellect
3 Pattern of weakness/wasting
— Myopathic facies
  • Ptosis, hanging jaw
  • Temporalis/sternomastoid wasting
— Weakness of neck flexion
— Distal limb weakness, wasted brachioradialis
4 Percussion myotonia
— Thenar eminence
— Forearm
— Quadriceps

Myotonic dystrophy: complications and management
1 Clinical complications
— Cardiac conduction defects; cardiomyopathy
— Hypoventilation; post-anesthetic respiratory failure
2 Biochemical complications
— Insulin resistance (impaired glucose tolerance)
— Gonadotrophin resistance (↑ FSH/LH, hypogonadism)
— Hypogammaglobulinemia
3 Management includes
— Family screening using FSH levels and/or EMG
— Drugs: quinine, phenytoin, procainamide

NEURORADIOLOGY

Intracranial calcification on skull X-ray
1 Oligodendroglioma, meningioma
— 20% calcify ('ball of calcium')
— May be associated with overlying bony hyperostosis
2 Craniopharyngioma, esp. in children
— 75% calcify
— May be intra- or suprasellar
3 Pineal gland
— Calcified in 60% adults, 10% children
— Midline shift may indicate intracranial mass lesion
4 Tuberous sclerosis
— Multiple discrete lesions → temporal lobes

5 Sturge–Weber syndrome
   — Subcortical 'tramline' calcification → parieto-occipital
   — Ipsilateral facial hemangioma, contralateral paresis
6 Infection
   — Toxoplasmosis
   — CMV; TB
7 Vascular
   — Aneurysm ('ring' calcification)
   — Angioma (spotty flecks of calcification)
   — Atheroma (curvilinear)
   — Chronic subdurals (outlined by calcification; rare)
8 Basal ganglia calcification
   — esp. Hypoparathyroidism
9 Cerebral calcifications and epilepsy
   — Celiac disease

Characteristic CT scan appearances
1 Normal pressure hydrocephalus
   — Large ventricles with minimal cortical atrophy
2 Benign intracranial hypertension
   — Small ventricles
3 Intracerebral abscess
   — Enhancing ring ± satellite edema

False-negative CT brainscans
1 Non-enhancing lesions < 1 cm diameter
2 Diffuse lesions (e.g. microgliomatosis)
3 Bilateral subdurals isodense with brain
4 Lesions near skull base or anterior optic pathways

Indications for CT brainscan after minor trauma*
1 Headache
2 Vomiting
3 Convulsion
4 Short-term amnesia
5 Any external evidence of head or neck trauma
6 Alcohol intoxication
7 Age > 60 years

* cf. major trauma: defined by loss of consciousness, confusion, or focal signs. CT is *always* indicated in such cases, whereas CT may *not* be mandatory in 'minor trauma' cases lacking the above features

Other neurologic indications for cerebral imaging
1 Focal neurologic signs
2 Adult-onset epilepsy
3 Presenile dementia

MAGNETIC RESONANCE IMAGING (MRI)

Advantages of magnetic resonance imaging over CT
1 No ionizing radiation with MRI*
2 MRI can provide imaging sections in *any* anatomic plane
3 Compact bone does not produce any signal with MRI, hence no artefacts, e.g. in posterior cranial fossa (cf. CT)

* MRI consists of radiofrequency radiation emitted within magnetic field → resonance of magnetic elements (e.g. H_2) in body

Suspected diagnoses where MRI is superior to CT
1 Brain tumor (esp. posterior fossa/brainstem)
2 Multiple sclerosis*
3 Pituitary tumors; hydrocephalus
4 Dementia‡ *or* movement disorders
5 Epilepsy
6 Lacunar TIAs
7 Craniocervical junction pathology (e.g. Arnold–Chiari)
8 Spinal cord/vertebral tumors, syrinxes
9 Disc disease, esp. herniation; torn knee meniscus
10 Contrast allergy

* Gadolinium highlights blood–brain barrier breakdown due to active perilesional inflammation
‡ e.g. pulvinar sign (bilateral high signals in posterior thalamus on T2 images) in variant CJD

Differential diagnosis of multifocal cerebral demyelination
1 Multiple sclerosis*
2 Hypertensive small vessel disease
3 Alzheimer's disease
4 Amyloid arteriopathy
5 Progressive multifocal leukoencephalopathy
6 HIV encephalitis
7 Vitamin B_{12} deficiency
8 Radiotherapy, chemotherapy, ciclosporin

* In patients presenting with localized symptoms (e.g. optic neuritis) MRI may be predictive of those who will progress to full-blown multiple sclerosis

Genetic syndromes causing MRI white matter lesions
1 Familial hemiplegic migraine (gene on chromosome 19)
2 CADASIL* (gene on chromosome 19)

* *C*erebral *a*utosomal *d*ominant *a*rteriopathy with *s*ubcortical *i*nfarcts and *l*eukoencephalopathy; manifests with multiple subcortical infarction (Binswanger's disease; sometimes without hypertension), migraine with aura, and depression

Conditions in which CT may be superior to MRI
1 Acute skull trauma
2 First 24 h of acute stroke (hemorrhagic or ischemic)
3 Cerebral aneurysm
4 Intracranial abscess
5 Headache

Contraindications to MRI
1 Cerebral aneurysm clips
2 Permanent pacemaker
3 Intraocular foreign bodies*
4 Shrapnel
5 Cochlear implants
6 Implanted infusion pumps
7 Pregnancy (esp. 1st trimester)

* Esp. if visible on X-ray

Artificial implants usually not contraindicating MRI
1 Dental fillings (non-magnetic)
2 Intrauterine devices
3 Prosthetic heart valves (most)
4 Orthopedic prostheses

CEREBROVASCULAR DISEASE

Management considerations in cerebrovascular disease
1 In symptomatic patients, the more severe the stenosis, the higher the risk of stroke, *but*
2 Many severe (even occlusive) stenoses are asymptomatic; if so, the risk of stroke is < 2%
3 Atheromatous carotid lesions may regress
4 Absence of a bruit is not a contraindication to angiographic assessment (severe stenoses may be inaudible)
5 Hypertension is the biggest risk factor for a cerebrovascular event; in patients with TIAs, reducing diastolic BP by 5–10 mmHg may reduce stroke risk by up to 40–50%

Important therapeutic negatives in cerebrovascular disease
1 Endarterectomy is *not* indicated for asymptomatic bruits
    — esp. If < 30% stenosis
2 High-dose steroids are of *no* benefit in cerebral infarction
3 Extracranial–intracranial bypass grafting is *not* of proven benefit to symptomatic patients with internal/carotid middle cerebral artery disease

Rationâle for aspirin prophylaxis in cardiovascular disease
1 Reduces morbidity and mortality of carotid TIAs in males
2 Reduces reinfarction (20%) and mortality (10%) following myocardial infarction
3 Reduces 'event rates' in unstable angina
4 Enhances coronary artery bypass graft patency
5 Helps prevent venous thrombosis after hip surgery in males
6 May retard progression of peripheral vascular disease

Indications for anticoagulation
1 TIAs associated with cardiac disease, e.g.
    — Mitral stenosis and/or atrial fibrillation
    — Post-infarct
2 Carotid-type TIAs
    — In a potentially operable patient prior to angiography
    — In a female unfit for surgery (or normal angiogram)
    — In a male unfit for surgery *and* unresponsive to aspirin
3 Vertebrobasilar insufficiency
    — In a female, *or*
    — In a male despite aspirin prophylaxis*
4 Relative need for anticoagulation is increased with
    — Recent onset (< 6/12) of TIAs
    — Increasing frequency or longer duration of attacks
    — Accumulating neurologic deficit with attacks

* Exception: subclavian steal syndrome may be surgically treated

Primary prevention of stroke: effective interventions
1 Treatment of hypertension*
    — 5 mmHg diastolic BP reduction lowers risk by 35–40%
2 Cessation of smoking
    — 5 years' cessation lowers risk by 35%
3 Statin treatment
    — 5 years' treatment prevents stroke in 10% of at-risk patients
4 Moderate alcohol consumption‡
    — Lower risk of ischemic stroke, higher risk of hemorrhagic stroke

* cf. acute phase of evolving stroke: no proven benefit of rapidly lowering high blood pressure
‡ Note that this is not actually recommended as an 'intervention' per se

Secondary prevention of stroke: effective interventions
1 Antiplatelet therapy
    — For patients who have incurred an ischemic stroke*
2 Warfarin
    — For stroke patients with non-valvular atrial fibrillation
    — For cardioembolic stroke patients with valvular heart disease
    — For cardioembolic stroke patients after myocardial infarction
3 Carotid endarterectomy
    — For patients with severe (> 70%) internal carotid stenosis linked to carotid TIAs
    — For patients with severe internal carotid stenosis linked to a non-disabling stroke

* Esp. within the last 48 h

SURGERY IN CEREBROVASCULAR DISEASE

Carotid endarterectomy: when should it be considered?
1 Logistic prerequisites
    — Fit patient with symptomatic carotid disease
    — Experienced vascular surgical team available*
2 Principal indication
    — > 70% stenosis (residual lumen < 2 mm) of cervical portion of internal carotid artery, *plus*
    — Symptoms
3 Other indications
    — Persistent symptoms of carotid stenosis (< 70%) despite appropriate medical therapy
    — Symptomatic carotid stenosis < 70% *plus* contraindication to aspirin/warfarin
4 Less definite indications
    — Ulcerated (potentially embologenic) carotid lesion
    — Clots (luminal filling defects) ± tight stenosis
    — Acute phase occlusion with mild/fluctuating deficit
    — Severely reduced post-stenotic blood flow, thus making complete occlusion likely

* 5% operative stroke rate

Scenarios precluding carotid endarterectomy
1 Stenosis too mild
2 Symptoms related to contralateral cerebral hemisphere
3 Established total carotid occlusion
4 Patient unfit for general anesthesia

SPASTICITY

Antispasticity drugs: therapeutic considerations
1 General
   — Drug therapy tends to be more effective in spasticity of spinal rather than intracranial origin
2 Diazepam
   — CNS GABA agonist
   — Dosage limited by sedation
3 Baclofen
   — CNS GABA agonist
   — May cause depression
   — Used intrathecally for reflex sympathetic dystrophy
4 Dantrolene
   — Peripheral effect on skeletal muscles; inhibits calcium release from sarcoplasmic reticulum
   — May exacerbate weakness (therefore less popular)
   — Occasionally associated with hepatotoxicity

Surgical measures in spasticity management
1 Neurolysis (or dorsal rhizotomy)
   — Phenol/alcohol injection into nerve or nerve root
2 Tenotomy
   — e.g. Hamstring, adductor, heel cord
3 Myotomy
   — e.g. Iliopsoas
4 Neurectomy
   — e.g. Obturator; pudendal (for detrusor instability)
5 Myelotomy
6 Cordectomy
   — A drastic measure for intractable symptoms (e.g. uncontrollable flexor/adductor spasms)

Therapeutic indications for botulinum toxin (type A)
1 Adult focal dystonias*
   — Blepharospasm
   — Spasmodic torticollis
   — Hemifacial spasm
   — Spasmodic dysphonia
   — Writer's cramp
2 Spasticity (e.g. cerebral palsy with spastic diplegia)
3 Strabismus
4 Achalasia (inject into LES)
5 Hyperhidrosis, esp. axillary
6 Cosmetic facial surgery (commonest use)

* Toxin is injected into dystonic muscles

ANTICONVULSANT THERAPY

Choosing an anticonvulsant for epileptic disorders
1 Localized seizures*
   — Drug of choice: carbamazepine
   — Other: vigabatrin, gabapentin, phenytoin, valproate, lamotrigine
2 Generalized seizures
   — Drug of choice: sodium valproate
   — Other: lamotrigine, topiramate, clobazam

* Incl. complex partial seizures, tonic–clonic seizures, focal epilepsy

Monotherapy vs 'add-on' antiepileptic drugs
1 First-line monotherapy
   — Valproate (generalized seizures)
   — Carbamazepine (partial seizures)
2 Second-line monotherapy
   — Phenytoin (now less used)
   — Lamotrigine (but limited track record as monotherapy as yet)
3 'Add-on' drugs (esp. used for partial epilepsy, though monotherapy preferable)
   — Vigabatrin
   — Gabapentin
   — Topiramate
   — Lamotrigine
   — Clobazam*

* Benzodiazepine used for *intermittent* back-up at times of high seizure incidence (e.g. menstruation, stress)

Epileptic disorders best treated by sodium valproate
1 Absence ('petit mal') seizures
   — Alternative: ethosuximide*
2 Tonic–clonic seizures associated with absence seizures
   — Alternative: lamotrigine‡
3 Myoclonic epilepsy
   — Alternatives: lamotrigine, clonazepam
4 Febrile convulsions (prophylaxis)
   — Alternatives: phenobarbital
5 Minor motor seizures (infantile spasms)
6 Lennox–Gastaut syndrome (epileptic encephalopathy)
   — Alternative: lamotrigine

* Fewer side-effects than valproate
‡ May cause hyponatremia, as can carbamazepine

Seizure subtypes worsened by specific anticonvulsants
1 Absence seizures and myoclonic epilepsy
   — Worsened by carbamazepine, phenytoin, vigabatrin
   — No benefit from phenobarbital, gabapentin
2 Tonic–clonic seizures
   — Worsened by ethosuximide

Distinguishing features of newer antiepileptics
1 Effective in idiopathic (generalized) epilepsies
   — Lamotrigine, topiramate
2 Highly potent
   — Topiramate, vigabatrin
3 Well tolerated (few side-effects)*
   — Gabapentin, lamotrigine

* cf. vigabatrin: may cause severe visual field defects, necessitating monitoring

Carbamazepine: indications and contraindications
1 Useful in
   — Complex partial seizures (drug of choice)
   — Tonic–clonic ('grand mal') seizures
   — Trigeminal neuralgia

2 *Not* indicated in
— Absence seizures
— Myoclonic epilepsy

Surgical treatment of epilepsy
1 Interventions
— Focal cortical resection: neocortical, anterior temporal, lesionectomy
— Cerebral hemispherectomy
— Corpus callosotomy
— Amygdalohippocampectomy
2 Ideal patient profile
— Refractory to drug therapy*, *and*
— Typical complex partial seizures, *and*
— Unilateral temporal lobe ictal onset; *or*
— Focal cerebral lesion, esp.
   • Hamartoma
   • Cavernous vascular malformation

* A prerequisite

MECHANISMS OF ANTICONVULSANT ACTION

Drugs acting as GABA agonists*
1 Valproate
2 Benzodiazepines
3 Barbiturates
4 Vigabatrin
5 Lamotrigine
6 Gabapentin; baclofen‡

* i.e. act by enhancing GABA-mediated CNS inhibition
‡ NB: May reduce seizure threshold

Anticonvulsants acting as membrane stabilizers
1 Phenytoin
— Increases membrane binding of calcium
2 Carbamazepine
— Structurally related to tricyclics*
3 Lamotrigine
— Blocks voltage–sensitive sodium channels, thus reducing release of glutamate

* i.e. *not* to benzodiazepines

Pharmacokinetics of anticonvulsant therapy
1 Phenytoin
— $t^{1/2} \approx 24$ h
— Time to plateau ≈ 5 days
— Once-daily dosage schedule is satisfactory
— Children may require up to double the usual adult maintenance dose due to ↑ liver metabolism
— Exhibits saturation kinetics (similar to aspirin, alcohol)
2 Phenobarbital
— $t^{1/2} \approx 100$ h
— Time to plateau $\approx 2–3$ weeks
— Once-daily dosage schedule is satisfactory
3 Carbamazepine
— $t^{1/2} \approx 12$ h
— Time to plateau ≈ 3 days (may take longer since *initial* $t^{1/2} \approx 36$ h; shortens due to autoinduction)
— Administered three times daily

4 Sodium valproate
— Plasma $t^{1/2} \approx$ h, but bears little relation to effect
— Administered twice- or thrice-daily

PROBLEMS WITH ANTICONVULSANT THERAPY

Indications for monitoring anticonvulsant plasma levels
1 Phenytoin therapy, esp. if
— Poor seizure control
— Suspected toxicity
— New drug added (e.g. valproate)
2 Carbamazepine therapy in initial stages
3 Renal or liver disease
4 Mentally retarded patients (if difficult to assess toxicity)
5 Suspected non-compliance

NB: For valproate, ethosuximide, or phenobarbital, 'therapeutic range' may need to be determined empirically on a patient-by-patient basis

Side-effects of phenytoin
1 Acute toxicity
— Occurs with IV use (or overdose)
   • Hypotension
   • Arrhythmias
   • CNS depression
2 Acute toxicity with oral use
— Dose-dependent; correlates with serum drug levels
   • Nystagmus → ataxia → drowsiness
3 Chronic toxicity with routine oral use
— Dose-dependent, but may occur at therapeutic levels
   • Vitamin D deficiency: osteomalacia, hypocalcemia
4 Idiosyncratic
— Not clearly dose-related
   • Nausea, vomiting, diarrhea
   • Skin rash
   • SLE; pseudolymphoma
5 Epilepsy-related
— More common in high-dose therapy
   • Worsening of absence seizures
   • Increased frequency of tonic–clonic seizures

Side-effects of other anticonvulsants
1 Sodium valproate
— Tremor (dose-dependent)
— Polycystic ovaries*, hyperandrogenism, amenorrhea
— Hair thinning (reversible), hair curling
— Increased appetite, weight gain; ankle edema
— Drowsiness (but less than most other anticonvulsants)
— Stupor, encephalopathy ± hyperammonemia
— Reye's-like hepatotoxicity (idiosyncratic)
   • Affects 1/10 000, esp. age < 3 years
   • Often preceded by increased seizure frequency
   • Potentially fatal
2 Carbamazepine
— Drowsiness (esp. if coadministered with phenytoin)

— SIADH with fluid retention (may → CCF in elderly)
— Anticholinergic effects (structurally resembles tricyclics)
— Leukopenia, agranulocytosis (rare)
3 Phenobarbital and congeners (e.g. primidone)
— Drowsiness/confusion, esp. in elderly
— Hyperactivity in children
— Megaloblastosis

* Affects 80% of women < 20 years taking valproate

Anticonvulsant interactions of clinical significance
1 Inducers of hepatic metabolism
— Carbamazepine, phenytoin, phenobarbital
• Dosage may need to be increased due to autoinduction of drug metabolism
• Starting any of these agents in a patient already stabilized on monotherapy (e.g. valproate) may lead to paradoxical initial deterioration
• May antagonize oral contraceptives*, steroids, quinidine, warfarin, and theophylline; toxicity of the latter may be precipitated by (say) carbamazepine withdrawal
2 Inhibitors of hepatic metabolism
— Sodium valproate
• Addition may precipitate *toxicity* of other anticonvulsants (e.g. phenobarbital, CMZ) which may in turn antagonize valproate
• Valproate may also precipitate phenytoin toxicity even in the absence of raised serum phenytoin levels, due to *plasma protein displacement* (i.e. ↑ free, not total, phenytoin)
— Isoniazid, another P_{450} inhibitor, may also precipitate phenytoin toxicity (esp. in slow acetylators)

* Hence, patients using oral contraception should use *valproate* if possible

Considerations in managing the pregnant epileptic
1 Anticonvulsant usage is associated with 6% incidence of teratogenesis (about 3-fold increased), esp.
— Phenytoin, phenobarbital
• Cleft palate, congenital heart disease
— Valproate, carbamazepine
• Spina bifida (1%), hypospadias
2 Always aim to use
— Monotherapy (where possible)
— Lowest possible dosage
3 Seizure control may deteriorate due to reduced drug concentration. If dosage is increased, toxicity may supervene in the puerperium unless levels are monitored
4 Antagonism of vitamin K-dependent coagulation factors by anticonvulsants, esp. barbiturates, may predispose to fetal or neonatal hemorrhage*
5 Phenytoin and phenobarbital may reduce folate levels, which may in turn predispose to neural tube defects. Hence, women on anticonvulsants should take folic acid‡ prior to conception and for the first 12 weeks of pregnancy

6 A small but significant increased incidence of congenital malformations is seen in the offspring of epileptics, incl.
— Epileptic mothers *not* receiving anticonvulsants
— Epileptic fathers (i.e. married to non-epileptic mothers)

* cf. hemorrhagic disease of the newborn: no bleeding until 24 h postpartum
‡ Precise dose is controversial, varying from 0.4–5 mg/day

Contraindications to surgical management of epilepsy
1 Absolute
— Inadequate trial of medical therapies
2 Relative
— Bilateral interictal epileptiform discharges on EEG
— Non-temporal lobe epilepsy
— Dominant lobe epilepsy

PARKINSON'S DISEASE

Drug therapy in Parkinson's disease
1 Mild disease (symptoms without disability):
— Anticholinergics (e.g. trihexyphenidyl (benzhexol), orphenadrine)
• Avoid in elderly patients (→ confusion)
• Best for controlling salivation, tremor
• Confer additive benefit to levodopa
— Selegiline (formerly, L-deprenyl)
• MAO-B inhibitor which may defer disability
• Prolongs dopamine action by blocking reuptake
• Delays need for L-DOPA by ~ 9 months
— Amantadine
• Weak non-specific dopamine receptor agonist
• Minimal toxicity: edema, livedo reticularis
• Amphetamine-like effect → insomnia, confusion
• Tolerance may be a problem
2 Moderately disabling disease
— L-DOPA
• Decarboxylated by neurons to dopamine
• Combined with peripheral decarboxylase inhibitor (e.g. carbidopa, benserazide)
• Mainstay of therapy for bradykinesia, rigidity
• Antagonized by phenothiazines (e.g. prescribed for levodopa-induced nausea) or pyridoxine
3 Advanced or refractory disability
— Dopamine agonists
• Bromocriptine*, pergolide, cabergoline, lisuride, ropinirole
• Prime indication: late failure of levodopa
• Longer duration of action than levodopa
• Expensive, toxic ('first-dose' reactions, psychosis)
— Catechol-*o*-methyltransferase inhibitors
• Entacapone
— Stereotactic surgery
• Rarely used; sole indication is incapacitating tremor (esp. unilateral) refractory to L-DOPA

* Bromocriptine is both a D2 receptor agonist and a D1 receptor antagonist, whereas pergolide is primarily a D2 agonist

Adjunctive measures in Parkinson's disease
1 Laxatives
   — esp. If on anticholinergics
2 Tricyclic antidepressants
   — Antidepressant + anticholinergic effects
3 β-blockers
   — esp. For tremor
4 Benzodiazepines
   — For myalgias
5 Counselling
   — esp. For sexual problems
6 Handwriting assistance

PROBLEMS IN MANAGING PARKINSON'S DISEASE

Correct diagnosis of Parkinson's disease?
1 Akinesia (always)
2 Lead-pipe rigidity (almost always)
3 Tremor*, esp. resting (usually)
4 Gait apraxia (usually)

* Coexisting tremor causes cogwheeling at the wrist

Physical signs suggesting secondary parkinsonism
1 Blepharospasm or downward gaze palsy
2 Jerky tremor or myoclonus
3 Symptomatic orthostasis
4 Lower body parkinsonism
5 Cerebellar signs
6 Pyramidal signs

Primary L-DOPA resistance in parkinsonism: factors to exclude
1 Non-compliance (± dementia, depression)
2 Coadministration of phenothiazines* or pyridoxine
3 Misdiagnosis

* Exception: domperidone (does *not* cross blood–brain barrier)

Differential diagnosis of atypical parkinsonism
1 Exclude curable causes
   — Wilson's disease
2 Richardson–Steele (progressive supranuclear palsy, PSP)
   — Associated downgaze palsy
   — Postural instability with falls
   — Axial rigidity with retained limb mobility
   — Early onset of dysarthria and dysphagia
3 Multiple system atrophy (MSA)*
   — Cerebellar signs (olivopontocerebellar atrophy)
   — Urogenital dysfunction
   — Pyramidal signs
   — Autonomic failure (Shy–Drager syndrome)

* Biochemically distinguishable from Parkinson's disease by failure of clonidine to raise serum growth hormone concentrations in MSA despite normal GH-releasing hormone rise

Symptom-driven antiparkinsonian therapy
1 Treatment of mild bradykinesia only
   — Amantadine (tremor may worsen)
2 Treatment of mild rigidity and bradykinesia
   — Anticholinergics
   — Selegiline

3 Treatment of moderate/severe rigidity, bradykinesia
   — L-DOPA (+ carbidopa)
   — L-DOPA + bromocriptine
4 Treatment of incapacitating tremor
   — β-blockers
   — Stereotactic surgery (see below)

Specific limitations of L-DOPA therapy
1 Episodic exacerbations of bradykinesia ('on-off' effect)
2 End-of-dose deterioration ('wearing-off' effect)
3 Dose-limiting effects
   — Confusion; nightmares
   — Depression, paranoid ideation
4 Dose-dependent toxicity
   — Vomiting (CNS effect and delayed gastric emptying)
   — Hypotension, orthostasis
   — Dyskinesias, blepharospasm, akathisia

The 'on-off' effect: therapeutic approaches
1 Add selegiline to L-DOPA
2 Substitute bromocriptine (or pergolide) for L-DOPA
3 L-DOPA 'drug holiday'

Surgical options in Parkinson's disease*
1 Tremor: thalamotomy
2 Dyskinesia: pallidotomy
3 Global symptoms: subthalamic nucleus lesioning
4 Neural grafting (e.g. transplantation of fetal substantia nigra)

* Lesioning *or* deep brain stimulation may be used

IATROGENIC NEUROLOGIC DISEASE

Neurologic sequelae of oral contraceptives
1 Migraine
2 Cerebral thrombosis/infarction
3 Hypertensive intracerebral hemorrhage
4 Subarachnoid hemorrhage
5 Dural sinus thrombosis
6 Chorea (Sydenham's); benign intracranial hypertension

Benign intracranial hypertension: iatrogenic causes
1 Tetracycline
2 Oral contraceptives, corticosteroids
3 Vitamin A
4 Nitrofurantoin; nalidixic acid; perhexiline

Varieties of drug-induced eye disease
1 Corneal microdeposits
   — Amiodarone (usually asymptomatic)
   — Chloroquine (reversible)
2 Cataracts
   — Steroids (incl. eyedrops)
   — Phenothiazines (usually asymptomatic)
3 Optic neuritis
   — Ethambutol
   — Chloramphenicol

4 Retinopathy
— Chloroquine ('bull's-eye' macula)
— Thioridazine (retinitis pigmentosa-like)
5 Stevens–Johnson syndrome
— e.g. Sulfonamides

HEADACHE TREATMENTS

Serotonin receptors in migraine pathophysiology
1 5-HT$_1$ receptors
— Inhibitory (cause vasoconstriction)
— Agonists used for acute attacks
2 5-HT$_2$ receptors
— Excitatory
— Antagonists used for prophylaxis

Drugs useful in treating acute migraine
1 Serotonin-1 (5-HT$_1$) receptor agonists
— Sumatriptan (most effective drug); also
zolmitriptan, naratriptan
• Oral (100 mg) or subcutaneous (6 mg)
• Unwanted effects include dizziness, nausea,
chest and throat pressure
2 Ergotamine*
• Oral, sublingual, suppository (2 mg)
• Subcutaneous dihydroergotamine (1 mg)
3 Dopamine antagonists
— IV metoclopramide 10 mg
— IV prochlorperazine, chlorpromazine
4 NSAIDs
— Aspirin (650 mg)
— Naproxen (750 mg)
— Mefenamic acid, diclofenac, ibuprofen

* Contraindicated in patients with vascular disease

Drugs useful in migraine prophylaxis
1 β-blockers
— Propranolol, metoprolol, atenolol, nadolol
2 Sodium valproate
3 Other
— Serotonin-2 (5-HT$_2$) receptor blockers:
methysergide*, pizotifen
— Tricyclics: amitriptyline

* May cause retroperitoneal, pleural or cardiac valvular
fibrosis

Therapeutic modalities in cluster headache
1 Lithium
2 Sumatriptan, ergotamine
3 Steroids
4 Oxygen

Sumatriptan: properties and problems
1 Properties
— Selective cerebral vasoconstrictor
— 60% relief after oral dose, 80% after SC dose
2 Problems
— 'Non-cardiac' chest pain
— Facial flushing/tingling (esp. after SC dose)
— Contraindicated in coronary atheroma/spasm
— Expense

UNDERSTANDING NEUROLOGICAL DISEASE

Heritable neurologic diseases involving trinucleotide repeats
1 Fragile X syndrome
2 Myotonic dystrophy
3 Huntington's disease
4 Spinocerebellar ataxia #2
5 Adult-onset spinal and bulbar muscular atrophy

Neurologic diseases associated with abnormal tau proteins
1 Alzheimer's disease (sporadic or familial)
2 Progressive supranuclear palsy (sporadic)
3 Pick's disease, frontotemporal dementia (sporadic
or familial)
4 Diffuse Lewy body disease, Lewy body dementia
(sporadic)

Neurologic diseases caused by abnormal prion proteins*
1 Kuru
2 Creutzfeldt–Jakob disease (CJD; various subtypes)
3 Fatal familial insomnia
4 Gerstmann–Sträussler–Schenker syndrome
5 Bovine spongiform encephalopathy (BSE)

* Transmissible spongiform encephalopathies

Pathogenesis of human spongiform encephalopathies
1 Kuru
— Only ever described in one New Guinea tribe
— Linked to cannibalism (i.e. orally transmissible)
2 Creutzfeldt–Jakob disease
— *Not* orally transmitted
— Vectors include pituitary extracts, corneal grafts,
contaminated brain electrodes
3 Gerstmann-Sträussler-Schenker syndrome (familial)
— Due to mutation of the protease-resistant prion
protein

Amine neurotransmitters in CNS disease
1 Excitatory
— Glutamate
— Aspartate
2 Inhibitory
— Glycine
— GABA (decarboxylation product of glutamate)

Viruses implicated in neurological syndromes
1 Bell's palsy (herpetic facial paralysis)
— Herpes simplex virus type 1
2 Ramsay–Hunt syndrome
— Varicella-zoster reactivation

Parkinson's disease vs Huntington's chorea: what's different?
1 Predominant site of neuronal loss in Parkinson's
— Pigmented nuclei: substantia nigra, locus ceruleus
Predominant site of neuronal loss in Huntington's
— Caudate nucleus (± frontal lobes, putamen)
2 Neurotransmitter loss in Parkinson's
— Dopamine
Neurotransmitter loss in Huntington's
— Acetylcholine (and GABA)

3 Pathophysiology of Parkinson's
   — Relative excess of acetylcholine → parkinsonism
   Pathophysiology of Huntington's
   — Relative excess of dopamine → chorea*
4 Dopamine receptor agonists (e.g. levodopa) in Parkinson's
   → Improvement of parkinsonism
   Dopamine receptor agonists in Huntington's
   → Exacerbation of chorea
5 Dopamine receptor antagonists‡ in Parkinson's
   → Exacerbation of parkinsonism
   Dopamine receptor antagonists in Huntington's
   → Improvement of chorea

* cf. *tardive dyskinesia*: due to striatal supersensitivity to dopamine
‡ e.g. phenothiazines

Movement disorders: predominant sites of pathology
1 Kernicterus
   — Caudate and lenticular nuclei
2 Neurodegeneration with brain iron accumulation, type I (neuroaxonal dystrophy)
   — Substantia nigra (zona reticulata)
3 Hemiballismus
   — Subthalamus (contralateral)
4 Wilson's disease
   — Putamen
   Kayser–Fleischer rings*
   — Descemet's membrane

* Absence of KFRs on slit-lamp examination reliably excludes Wilson's disease as a cause of neurologic, but not hepatic, dysfunction

Classical localization of selected intracranial pathologies
1 Herpes simplex encephalitis
   — Temporal lobes
2 Wernicke's encephalopathy
   — Mamillary bodies, mamillothalamic tracts
3 Pick's disease
   — Anterior frontal and temporal lobes
4 Sturge–Weber syndrome
   — Forehead hemangioma → occipital lobe involvement
   — Facial hemangioma → frontoparietal involvement
5 Tuberous sclerosis
   — Temporal lobe calcification

INTRACRANIAL VASCULAR COMPLICATIONS

Complications of severe concussive injuries in childhood*
1 Epilepsy
2 Personality change: impulsive behavior, poor temperament
3 Delinquency, criminality

* Defined by loss of consciousness exceeding 1 h

Predispositions to chronic subdural hematomata
1 Epilepsy
2 Alcoholism
3 Hemodialysis
4 Anticoagulant therapy
5 Poor socioeconomic status

Features of chronic subdurals
1 Headache occurs in 75%
2 History of head trauma in 50% (only)
3 Fluctuating level of consciousness in less than 25%

Predispositions to cerebral aneurysms
1 Aortic coarctation
2 Polycystic disease
3 Renal artery stenosis due to fibromuscular dysplasia
4 Essential hypertension
5 Ehlers–Danlos syndrome type IV
6 PAN/Wegener's/SBE

Sequelae of subarachnoid hemorrhage
1 Cerebral vasospasm
   — Severity lessened by early (oral) use of nimodipine
   — Nimodipine less useful for reversing delayed ischemia
2 Rebleeding
   — 40% rebleed within 12 months
   — 20% prove to have multiple aneurysms
3 Excessive catecholamine release (acute phase)
   — Hypertension
   — ECG abnormalities (e.g. T-wave inversion)
   — Glycosuria
4 Normal pressure hydrocephalus (long-term)

NEUROSYPHILIS

Clinical varieties of neurosyphilis
1 Meningovascular syphilis
   — Non-specific mental changes
   — Cranial nerve palsies
   — Argyll Robertson pupils, papilledema
   — Cerebral infarction, limb paresis
2 Tabes dorsalis
   — Symptoms: lightning pains, gastric crises, impotence
   — Argyll Robertson pupils, optic atrophy
   — Pseudoptosis (overactive frontalis)
   — Reduced vibration/proprioception/deep pain
   — Patchy loss of temperature/pinprick → nose, tibia
   — Charcot joints, trophic foot ulcers
   — Rombergism, stamping gait (sensory ataxia)
   — Hypotonia, hyporeflexia; flexor plantars
3 General paresis of the insane
   — Dementia, incontinence, fits
   — Argyll Robertson pupils
   — Dysarthria, tongue ('trombone') tremor
   — Upper motor neuron signs, incl. extensor plantars

NEUROLOGY AND THE AIDS PATIENT

Neurologic indications for HIV serology
1 Unexplained mental deterioration
   — Encephalitis
   — Encephalopathy
   — Dementia
2 Myelopathy (aseptic meningitis, transverse myelitis)
3 Inflammatory neuropathy

Central nervous system problems in the HIV patient

1 AIDS-dementia complex
   — Cognitive dysfunction affecting > 50% of advanced adult AIDS patients
   — Causes memory loss, ataxia, incontinence, mutism, snout reflex, quadriparesis
   — Reflects direct HIV infection of the brain
2 HIV encephalopathy
   — Developmental dysfunction affecting HIV-infected children
   — Causes delayed milestones and symmetrical motor deficits
3 Opportunistic CNS infection
   — e.g. Toxoplasmosis, cryptococcosis, JC virus
4 Vacuolar myelopathy (spinal cord lesions)
   — Bilateral leg weakness, incontinence
5 Atypical aseptic meningitis
   — May be recurrent, involve cranial nerves or long tracts
6 CNS lymphoma (EBV-induced)

Peripheral nervous system problems in the HIV patient

1 Distal (mainly sensory) polyneuropathy
   — Common in advanced AIDS
2 Inflammatory demyelinating (Guillain–Barré-like, mainly motor) polyneuropathy
   — Rare; may precede AIDS diagnosis
3 Viral reactivation
   — Shingles (VZ)
   — Bell's palsy (HSV-1)
   — Radiculopathy (CMV)
4 Nucleoside neurotoxicity
   — Occurs with zalcitabine, didanosine, stavudine, zidovudine
   — Idiosyncratic confusion, seizures
   — Dose-related ataxia/nystagmus
   — Symptoms may be precipitated by abrupt drug withdrawal

Differential of mononeuritis multiplex in the HIV patient

1 Inflammatory demyelinating polyneuropathy
2 CMV reactivation
3 Meningeal lymphomatosis

DEMYELINATING DISEASE

Diagnosis of multiple sclerosis

1 Clinical (best criterion)
   — At least 2 remitting episodes of at least 2 focal lesions
2 Evoked responses, esp. VERs (AERs, SSERs)
   — *Not* specific for MS (p. 268)
3 CSF EPG
   — Oligoclonal bands (cf. *not* in serum) in 90%
   — Also found in sarcoid, syphilis, SLE, etc; *not* routinely indicated
4 MRI (best test)
   — Plaques may appear typical (but not diagnostic) of MS
   — May reveal more extensive disease than suspected
   — Gadolinium enhancement suggests active disease
   — Can be false-negative, esp. in primary progressive MS

MRI correlations in multiple sclerosis

1 Positive detection of plaques in 98% of patients with *clinically convincing* MS; i.e. diagnostic role is purely supplementary to clinical evaluation
2 Gadolinium enhancement detects perivascular inflammation (*not* demyelination per se)
3 Enhancing and non-enhancing abnormalities change size rapidly; enhancing lesions last approximately 1 month
4 The incidence of new enhancing lesions far exceeds the number of clinical relapses
5 Standard MRI shows *poor* correlation with clinical deficit
6 Gadolinium-enhanced MRI is good for assessing treatment*

* e.g. showing that β-interferon reduces frequency of exacerbations

Predictors of poor prognosis in multiple sclerosis

1 Advanced age at onset
2 Presents with acute brainstem syndrome (simulating stroke)
3 Incomplete recovery (esp. weakness) from initial attack
4 Early onset of cerebellar ataxia
5 Early loss of mental acuity (may be associated with euphoria)

Common presentations of multiple sclerosis

1 CN II involvement
   — Retrobulbar neuritis
2 Brainstem involvement
   — Diplopia (CN VI or internuclear palsy)
   — Nystagmus, vertigo
3 Spinal cord involvement
   — Asymmetrical leg weakness and/or numbness

Classical presentations of multiple sclerosis

1 Facial presentations
   — Trigeminal neuralgia
   — Facial palsy (*upper* motor neuron type)
   — Facial myokymia (continuous rippling of one side)
2 'Useless hand' with proprioceptive loss only
   — DD$_x$: hysteria
3 Lhermitte's sign
   — 'Electric' pains on flexing neck*
4 Uhthoff's phenomenon
   — Worsening of weakness or vision with heat (e.g. hot bath or exercise)

* cf. paresthesiae induced by *extending* neck: suggests cervical spondylosis

Presentations suggesting alternative etiologic diagnoses

1 Peripheral neuropathy
2 Persistent loss of skin sensation
3 Epilepsy

Multiple sclerosis vs Friedreich's ataxia
1 Similarities
   — Optic atrophy
   — Nystagmus
   — Cerebellar signs
   — Extensor plantar responses
2 Factors favoring Friedreich's
   — Family history
   — Absent ankle jerks
   — Pes cavus/scoliosis
   — Cardiomegaly
3 Factors favoring multiple sclerosis
   — History of Lhermitte's or Uhthoff's phenomena
   — Trigeminal neuralgia (esp. bilateral)
   — Absent abdominal reflexes
   — Bladder enlargement
   — Brisk ankle jerks

Central pontine myelinolysis: features
1 Presentation
   — Quadriparesis, pseudobulbar palsy, cognitive impairment
2 Causes
   — Over-rapid correction of severe hyponatremia, esp. if also hypokalemic
   — Alcoholism
   — Hypoxia
3 Diagnosis
   — MRI

SPINAL DISEASE

Transverse myelitis: features
1 Presentation
   — Pain (e.g. interscapular) localizing to final sensory level
   — Lower limb paresthesiae, ascending weakness
   — Sphincter dysfunction
2 Established clinical deficit
   — Flaccid paralysis
   — Complete sensory loss (typically to thorax)
3 Investigations
   — CT/MRI usually normal
   — CSF may reveal non-specific pleocytosis, ↑ protein
   — VERs usually normal
4 Features associated with poor prognosis
   — Fulminant onset
   — Pain
   — Spinal shock

Common vertebral levels of various pathologies
1 Cervical cord
   — Syphilitic myelitis
   — Syringomyelia
2 Thoracic cord
   — Subacute combined degeneration
   — Anterior spinal artery thrombosis (~ T4)
   — Pott's disease
3 Thoracolumbar
   — Ependymoma; metastatic tumors
   — Transverse myelitis
4 Lumbosacral
   — Tabes dorsalis

Neurologic deficits in cervical spondylosis
1 Lateral disc protrusion
   — Root compression
2 Foraminal osteophytes
   — Root compression
3 Osteophytes
   — Vertebral artery insufficiency
4 Posterior disc protrusion
   — Cord compression
5 Posterior disc protrusion
   — Vascular myelopathy

Predispositions to kyphoscoliosis and/or pes cavus
1 Friedreich's ataxia
   Hereditary spastic paraplegia
2 Charcot–Marie–Tooth disease
3 Polio
4 Neurofibromatosis
5 Syringomyelia

Pes cavus and claw hands? Differential diagnosis
1 Reflexes depressed
   — Charcot–Marie–Tooth disease
2 Reflexes exaggerated
   — Syringomyelia

Associations of neurofibromatosis
1 Skin
   — Café-au-lait spots (> 5, > 1.5 cm diameter)
   — Axillary freckling
   — Melanoma
2 Neurogenic intracranial lesions
   — Optic glioma, cerebral glioma
   — Acoustic neuroma, meningioma
   — Ependymoma, malignant schwannoma
   — Syringomyelia
3 Vascular syndromes
   — Berry aneurysms
   — Aortic coarctation
   — Renal artery stenosis; pheochromocytoma
   — Mesenteric ischemia
4 Musculoskeletal
   — Limb deformities (tibial bowing, pes cavus)
   — Vertebral scalloping
5 Other associations
   — Pulmonary fibrosis
   — Diabetes insipidus
   — Hypospadias
   — Intellectual impairment

MOVEMENT DISORDERS

Patterns of cerebellar disease
1 Vermis involvement
   — Often due to alcoholism
   — Spinocerebellar tract connections involved
   — Signs
     • Wide-based gait (deviates to affected side)
     • Impaired tandem gait
     • Slurred speech
2 Flocculonodular lobe involvement
   — May be due to PICA syndrome/medulloblastoma
   — Vestibular connections involved

— Signs
  • Truncal ataxia (unable to sit/stand unsupported)
  • Nystagmus (may be vertical)
  • Titubation
3 Posterior lobe involvement
  — Cortical connections involved (many causes)
  — Signs
    • Hypotonia
    • Limb ataxia ('drift')
    • Dysmetria ('past-pointing')
    • Dysdiadochokinesis
    • Intention tremor

Periodic paralysis: classification
1 Hypokalemic
  — Familial, or
  — Associated thyrotoxicosis (esp. in oriental males), or
  — Associated with primary aldosteronism
  — Paralysis precipitated by
    • Carbohydrate meal ($\uparrow$ insulin $\rightarrow$ $\downarrow$ K$^+$)
    • Rest after exertion (duration: hours $\rightarrow$ days)
  — Prophylaxis with
    • Potassium supplements
    • Acetazolamide
    • Spironolactone
2 Normokalemic
  — Paramyotonia (von Eulenberg's disease)
  — Weakness and/or myotonia inducible by cold
  — Treat with tocainide
3 Hyperkalemic (Gamstorp's disease)
  — Often familial
  — Typically affects eye muscles (duration ~ 30 min)
  — Precipitated by cold weather
  — Responds to intravenous calcium gluconate

MYASTHENIA GRAVIS

Myasthenia gravis: classification
1 Ocular
  — Lowest AChRAb levels (25% are normal)
  — Unresponsive to thymectomy; responds to steroids
2 Thymoma
  — Highest AChRAb levels
  — Non-pathogenic striated muscle antibodies
3 'Thymitis' (age < 40 years)
  — Female > male
  — HLA-B$_8$DRw$_3$ commonly
  — Associated with other autoimmune disease
  — Negative striated muscle antibodies
  — Best response to thymectomy (80%)
4 'Thymitis' (age > 40 years)
  — Male > female
  — HLA-A$_3$B$_7$DRw$_2$ commonly
  — Low levels of AChRAb
  — Best response to corticosteroids
5 Don't confuse with non-immune 'congenital myasthenia'
  — Associated with consanguinity
  — Absent AChRAb
  — No response to thymectomy/plasmapheresis

Clinical signs in myasthenia gravis: special maneuvers
1 Sustained lateral/upward gaze
  — Ptosis
  — Diplopia
  — Ophthalmoplegia
2 Count to 50
  — Slurring of speech
3 Drink water
  — Regurgitation, dysphagia
4 Abduct one shoulder repeatedly
  — Then compare other side
5 Elevate limb for long period, assess power
  — Then note improvement with rest*

* cf. psychogenic fatigue: rest doesn't help

Investigating the patient with suspected myasthenia gravis
1 Edrophonium ('Tensilon') test
  — Pretreat with atropine to prevent bradycardia, nausea
  — Give 1 mg test dose prior to 5 mg test proper
  — False-negatives in up to 10% (e.g. due to wasting)
2 EMG
  — Post-tetanic inhibition (p. 270)
3 AChRAb:
  — 90% sensitivity (70% in ocular myasthenia)
  — False-positives
    • First-degree relatives
    • Myasthenics in remission
    • Rheumatoid patients on D-penicillamine

Approach to management of myasthenia gravis
1 Anticholinesterase therapy (losing popularity)
  — Commence with pyridostigmine 30 mg q.i.d
  — Beware of cholinergic crisis when increasing dosage
  — May test integrity of bulbar/respiratory muscle power by injecting edrophonium 2 mg IV
2 Corticosteroid therapy (1 mg/kg alternate days) if
  — Seriously ill before thymectomy
  — Insufficiently improved after thymectomy
  — Ocular myasthenia
  — Now often used as initial therapy
  — Anticholinesterase potentiation may precipitate initial deterioration; hence, start treatment as inpatient
3 Azathioprine: best results if
  — Patient > 40 years
  — Male sex
  — Long-standing disease (> 10 years)
  — Absent HLA-B$_8$DRw$_3$
  — High AChRAb levels
4 Thymectomy
  — 80% of patients without thymoma improve
  — Improvement may be delayed up to 5 years
  — Less effective for thymoma (but all the more necessary)
  — Thymoma may be managed with trans-sternal thymectomy and/or thymic irradiation
5 Plasma exchange
  — Consider in myasthenic crisis or prethymectomy

6 Unexpected deterioration? Exclude
— Thyrotoxicosis
— Pregnancy
— Sepsis
— Drugs
  • Quin(id)ine, procainamide; phenytoin
  • Propranolol; lidocaine (lignocaine)
  • Aminoglycosides
  • CNS depressants
  • D-penicillamine
  • Hypokalemia (e.g. due to diuretics)

REVIEWING THE LITERATURE: NEUROLOGY

10.1 Hankey GJ et al (2000) Thienopyridine derivatives versus aspirin for preventing stroke and other serious vascular events in high vascular risk patients. Cochrane Database Syst Rev 2: CD001246

Systematic review of ticlopidine and clopidogrel experience, showing modest superiority to aspirin in preventing stroke; less gastrointestinal upset and bleeding; but more skin rash and diarrhea. Ticlopidine can more often cause neutropenia or thrombotic thrombocytopenic purpura.

10.2 European Study Group on Interferon β-1b in Secondary Progressive MS (1998) Placebo-controlled multicentre randomised trial of interferon-β-1b in treatment of secondary progressive multiple sclerosis. Lancet 352: 1491–1497

Forbes RB et al (1999) Population based cost utility study of interferon beta-1b in secondary progressive multiple sclerosis. Br Med J 319: 1529–1533

Jacobs LD et al (2000) Intramuscular interferon beta-1a therapy initiated during a first demyelinating event in multiple sclerosis. N Engl J Med 343: 898–904

Three studies examining the use of interferon-β in multiple sclerosis. The first study of 358 patients with progressive MS confirmed a therapeutical (beneficial) effect, with a delay in time to progression of 9–12 months. The second study of 132 people cast doubt on the cost-utility of interferon-β in progressive MS, showing that it was necessary to treat 18 people to benefit one; cost per QALY was estimated as over one million pounds sterling. The third paper showed that treating the first presentation of a demyelinating event (e.g. optic neuritis) significantly reduced the development of MS over a 3-year follow-up.

10.3 Berger K et al (1999) Light-to-moderate alcohol consumption and the risk of stroke among US male physicians. N Engl J Med 341: 1557–1564

Thrift AG et al (1999) Risk of primary intracerebral haemorrhage associated with aspirin and non-steroidal anti-inflammatory drugs: case-control study. Br Med J 318: 759–764

White HD et al (2000) Pravastatin therapy and the risk of stroke. N Engl J Med 343: 317–326

Three studies about the relationship of stroke incidence to putative risk factors. The first showed that drinking as little as one unit of alcohol per week is associated with a lower risk of stroke; the benefit appeared dose-dependent up to a maximum intake of one unit per day. The second study of 331 cases and an equal number of controls reported no increase in hemorrhagic stroke with aspirin (including low-dose) and other NSAIDs. The third study assessed the effect of pravastatin in 9014 patients with ischemic heart

disease and hypercholesterolemia on the incidence of ischemic stroke; a mild (20%) reduction in incidence was observed in association with pravastatin.

10.4 Kwiatkowski TG et al (1999) Effects of tissue plasminogen activator for acute ischemic stroke at one year. N Engl J Med 340: 1781–1787

Randomized study of 624 ischemic stroke patients, showing a sustained 30% reduction in post-stroke disability in those who received tPA within 3 hours of stroke onset.

10.5 International Study of Unruptured Intracranial Aneurysms Investigators (1998) Unruptured intracranial aneurysms – risk of rupture. N Engl J Med 339: 1725–1723

Mixed retrospective and prospective study of 2621 aneurysm patients: individuals with aneurysms less than 10 mm diameter were prone to rupture in patients with a past history of subarachnoid hemorrhage from a different aneurysm (722 patients). In patients without such a history (i.e. presenting for the first time with a solitary unruptured aneurysm), however, the risk associated with aneurysms less than 10 mm diameter was so low as to preclude surgical intervention.

10.6 European Carotid Surgery Trialists' Collaborative Group (1998) Randomised trial of endarterectomy for recently symptomatic carotid stenosis: final results of the MRC European Carotid Surgery Trial (ECST). Lancet 351: 1379–1387

Barnett H et al (1998) Benefit of carotid endarterectomy in patients with symptomatic moderate or severe stenosis. N Engl J Med 339: 1415–1425

Inzitari D et al (2000) The causes and risk of stroke in patients with asymptomatic internal-carotid-artery stenosis. N Engl J Med 342: 1693–1700

Three studies analyzing surgical treatment of carotid artery disease. The first randomized study compared 669 operated patients with 442 unoperated patients in multiple centers over 14 years; a benefit of surgery (11.6% absolute risk reduction for the first 3 years after surgery) was apparent in patients with symptomatic stenoses of greater than 80%. The second study showed a smaller (7%) absolute benefit in patients with moderate (50–70%) stenosis, but no benefit in patients with < 50% stenosis; benefit was greater in males, patients with hemispheric symptoms, and patients with recent strokes. The final study was a 10-year retrospective analysis of 1820 patients with asymptomatic stenoses; 45% of strokes in these patients appeared due to non-carotid causes (cardioembolism or lacunes), supporting the case against endarterectomy in asymptomatic patients.

10.7 Ben-Shlomo Y et al (1998) Investigation into excess mortality seen with combined levodopa and selegiline treatment in patients with early, mild Parkinson's disease. Br Med J 316: 1191–1196

Fine J et al (2000) Long-term follow-up of unilateral pallidotomy in advanced Parkinson's disease. N Engl J Med 342: 1708–1714

Two studies analyzing outcomes following treatment for Parkinson's disease. The first study reviewed the outcome of 624 patients, from which a subgroup of 120 had died; the analysis supported the impression that coprescription of L-DOPA and selegiline was associated with excess mortality, and cautioned against use of this combination in either newly diagnosed patients, or in advanced disease associated with hypotension or confusion. The second study followed a cohort of 40 unilateral pallidotomy patients, and confirmed significant improvements in contralateral symptoms, particularly dyskinesia (which symptom remained improved when antiparkinsonian drugs were prescribed).

10.8 Kivipelto M et al (2001) Midlife vascular risk factors and Alzheimer's disease in later life: longitudinal population-based study. Br Med J 322: 1447–1451

In this prospective study with average follow-up of 21 years, hypertension and hypercholesterolemia in midlife were predictive of presenile dementia.

10.9 Karnath H et al (2001) Spatial awareness is a function of the temporal not the posterior parietal lobe. Nature 411: 950–952

Study showing that the right superior temporal cortex is actually responsible for spatial awareness in humans; this area lies contralateral to the language cortex.

10.10 Kotani N et al (2000) Intrathecal methylprednisolone for intractable postherpetic neuralgia. N Engl J Med 343: 1514–1519

Randomized study of 277 Japanese postherpetic neuralgia patients, showing efficacy paralleling declines in CSF interleukin-8 levels, as well as good tolerability.

CHAPTER 11

Palliative care, rehabilitation and gerontology

Physical examination protocol 11.1   You are asked to assess the current clinical status of a patient who has recently ceased treatment for progressive malignant disease

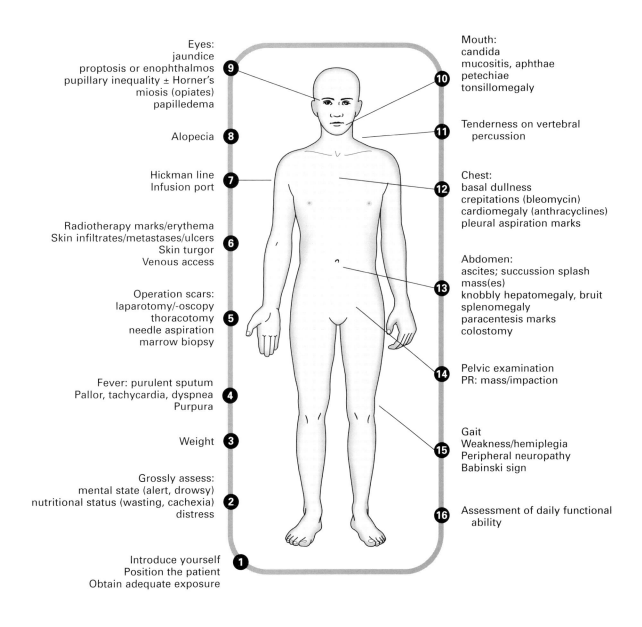

Eyes:
jaundice
proptosis or enophthalmos
pupillary inequality ± Horner's
miosis (opiates)
papilledema
9

Alopecia **8**

Hickman line
Infusion port **7**

Radiotherapy marks/erythema
Skin infiltrates/metastases/ulcers
Skin turgor
Venous access **6**

Operation scars:
laparotomy/-oscopy
thoracotomy
needle aspiration
marrow biopsy **5**

Fever: purulent sputum
Pallor, tachycardia, dyspnea
Purpura **4**

Weight **3**

Grossly assess:
mental state (alert, drowsy)
nutritional status (wasting, cachexia)
distress **2**

Introduce yourself
Position the patient
Obtain adequate exposure **1**

10 Mouth:
candida
mucositis, aphthae
petechiae
tonsillomegaly

11 Tenderness on vertebral
percussion

12 Chest:
basal dullness
crepitations (bleomycin)
cardiomegaly (anthracyclines)
pleural aspiration marks

13 Abdomen:
ascites; succussion splash
mass(es)
knobbly hepatomegaly, bruit
splenomegaly
paracentesis marks
colostomy

14 Pelvic examination
PR: mass/impaction

15 Gait
Weakness/hemiplegia
Peripheral neuropathy
Babinski sign

16 Assessment of daily functional
ability

COMMON AND CLASSIC PALLIATIVE PROBLEMS

Common palliative or rehabilitative problems in clinical practice
1 Pain control and/or analgesic side-effects
2 Terminal counselling, placement and care
3 Incontinence

Classic palliative or rehabilitative problems in clinical exams
1 Stroke-induced paralysis and/or dysphasia/dysarthria
2 Management of refractory or progressive local disease or wounds
3 Aspiration pneumonitis

EMERGENCIES IN PALLIATIVE CARE

Diagnosis of brain death
1 Sufficient cause
   — Exclude hypothermia/sedative overdose/myxedema
2 No response to noxious stimuli except spinal reflexes
3 Fixed pupils
4 Loss of oculovestibular and oculocephalic reflexes
5 Absent gag/corneal/cough reflexes
6 No spontaneous respiratory movements after ventilator disconnected and patient observed for 5 min with oxygen supplied via tracheal catheter

CLINICAL ASSESSMENT OF THE PALLIATIVE PATIENT

Patient performance status
1 Grade 0: asymptomatic
2 Grade 1: symptomatic, fully ambulant
3 Grade 2: symptomatic, ambulant > 50% waking hours
4 Grade 3: symptomatic, in bed > 50% waking hours
5 Grade 4: symptomatic, confined to bed

Differential diagnosis of confusion in the cancer patient
1 Metabolic
   — Hypercalcemia
      • With bone metastases (e.g. Ca breast, myeloma)
      • Humorally mediated (e.g. in SCC lung)
   — Hyponatremia (SIADH; e.g. in small cell lung cancer)
   — Hyperviscosity (esp. in IgM dysproteinemias)
2 Septic, esp.
   — Pneumonia
   — Cryptococcal meningitis
   — Progressive multifocal leukoencephalopathy
3 Hypoxic, esp.
   — Pulmonary emboli

4 Iatrogenic
   — Opiates
   — Steroids
   — Procarbazine, L-asparaginase
   — Ifosfamide encephalopathy (may be fatal)
5 Tumor-related
   — Paraneoplastic encephalopathy/dementia
   — Cerebral metastases

Differential diagnosis of vomiting in the cancer patient
1 Iatrogenic
   — Chemotherapy and/or anticipatory
   — Other drugs (e.g. opiates)
2 Gastrointestinal obstruction
   — Primary gastrointestinal tumors (e.g. linitis plastica)
   — Peritoneal seedlings (e.g. Ca ovary, lobular Ca breast)
3 Raised intracranial pressure due to intracranial metastases
   — Cerebral edema
   — Ventricular obstruction
4 Hypercalcemia

INVESTIGATIONS IN PALLIATIVE CARE:

DIAGNOSING DISORDERS OF CONSCIOUS STATE

Distinguishing features of conscious state disorders
1 Locked-in syndrome
   — Self-awareness and cerebral metabolism may be normal
   — Able to move eyes vertically and blink voluntarily
   — Can perceive pain
   — Respiratory function normal
   — Sleep/wake cycle normal
   — Brainstem function impaired
   — EEG: may be normal
2 Persistent vegetative state (PVS)
   — Self-awareness and cerebral metabolism impaired
   — No purposeful movements
   — No pain perception
   — Respiratory function normal
   — Sleep/wake cycle normal
   — Brainstem function variable
   — EEG: slow α, δ, or θ activity
3 Coma
   — Self-awareness and cerebral metabolism impaired
   — No purposeful movements
   — No pain perception
   — Respiratory function impaired
   — Sleep/wake cycle absent
   — Brainstem function variable
   — EEG: polymorphic δ or θ activity
4 Brain death
   — Self-awareness and cerebral metabolism severely impaired
   — No purposeful movements

— No pain perception
— Respiratory function absent
— Sleep/wake cycle absent
— Brainstem function absent
— EEG: θ activity or electrocerebral silence

Imaging sequence in stroke patients
1 To distinguish hemorrhage from infarct, tumor, subdural
— CT brainscan*
2 To assess carotid patency in patients who have recovered well from hemispheric TIA or minor stroke
— Carotid ultrasound
3 To exclude cardiogenic source of emboli *if* carotid ultrasound normal *or* brainstem TIA/stroke + known cardiac disease
— Cardiac echo
4 To evaluate extracranial and intracranial vessels if carotid ultrasound shows ≥ 50% stenosis and/or ulceration
— Intra-arterial digital subtraction angiography
5 To clarify infarct mechanism and prognosis in patients whose initial CT was normal
— Follow-up non-enhanced CT at 10 days

* Non-enhanced unless tumor figures strongly in differential diagnosis

Indications for CT brainscan in the stroke patient
1 Diagnostic uncertainty
— Young patient
— No history available
— Gradual/progressive onset of signs (?tumor/subdural)
— Atypical clinical course (esp. rapid deterioration)
2 Suspected intracranial hemorrhage
— Cerebellar hemorrhage (surgically evacuable)
• Acute onset of ataxia
• 'Stroke somewhere, stroke nowhere'*
— Subarachnoid hemorrhage‡
— Recent history of anticoagulant therapy¶
— Planned anticoagulant therapy¶

* i.e. no localizing signs
‡ CT = investigation of choice
¶ Incl. antiplatelet and thrombolytic therapy

RADIOLOGIC ABNORMALITIES IN NEOPLASTIC DISEASE

Pulmonary infiltrates in the cancer patient
1 Infiltration (by tumor)
— Lymphangitis carcinomatosa (esp. in breast cancer)
— Lymphoma, bronchioloalveolar cell carcinoma
2 Infection (opportunistic)
— Neutropenic: esp. Gram-negative pneumonia
— Immunosuppressed: CMV, *Pneumocystis,* fungi
3 Infarction (pulmonary)
— Thromboembolism
4 Collapse/consolidation (hypostatic)
— Obstructing primary tumor

5 Aspiration
— Intrinsic/extrinsic esophageal obstruction by tumor
— Cytotoxic-induced emesis in a sedated patient (rare)
6 Iatrogenic
— Radiation pneumonitis or fibrosis
— Cytotoxic-induced lung disease (e.g. bleomycin, gemcitabine, methotrexate)

Osteolytic lesions in the cancer patient
1 Focal lesions
— Myeloma
— Metastatic renal cell carcinoma
— Other metastatic carcinoma, esp.
• Ca breast
• Ca lung
• Ca thyroid
— Primary bone tumors
2 Generalized osteopenia
— Myeloma
— Old age ± immobilization
— Prolonged steroid therapy

Osteosclerotic lesions in the cancer patient*
1 Metastatic prostate cancer
2 Metastatic breast cancer
— De novo mixed lytic/blastic
— Treatment → lytic healing → sclerosis
3 'Ivory vertebrae' or patchy sclerosis
— Hodgkin's disease
— Myelofibrosis
— Coincidental Paget's disease

* Rarely associated with hypercalcemia; cf. osteolytic lesions

HEMOSTATIC DISORDERS

Pathogenesis of secondary bleeding tendencies
1 Liver disease
— Reduced synthesis of clotting factors
2 Renal disease
— Reduced platelet function
3 Lymphoproliferative or autoimmune disease
— Coagulation factor inhibitors
4 Amyloid
— Factor X deficiency, vessel infiltration
5 Sepsis, carcinomatosis
— DIC

MANAGING PALLIATIVE CARE

Common fallacies in palliative management
1 A dire prognosis justifies toxic treatment even if therapeutic benefit is unproven
2 Disease responsiveness to a given therapy ustifies treatment even if quality-of-life benefit unproven
3 Lack of toxicity justifies treatment even if cost-effectiveness is unproven

Opportunities for surgical palliation of malignant disease

1 Colostomy, gastrojejunostomy or feeding gastrostomy for neoplastic gastrointestinal obstruction
2 Placement of intraluminal silastic (e.g. Celestin) or infant feeding tube in esophageal obstruction
3 Percutaneous insertion of biliary drainage catheter following transhepatic cholangiography for extrahepatic obstruction
4 Nephrostomy drainage, or passage of ureteric stent(s), for malignant ureteric obstruction
5 Creation of tracheostomy for obstructing laryngeal carcinoma
6 Insertion of Hickman's catheter or implantable infusion port
7 LeVeen shunt for intractable malignant ascites
8 Prophylactic pinning of impending pathological fracture
9 Ventriculoatrial or peritoneal shunt for hydrocephalus
10 Resection of (apparently) solitary metastasis (e.g. in germ-cell tumors, osteosarcoma, hepatic spread of bowel cancer)

Approach to intestinal obstruction in palliative care

1 Commence nasogastric suction and intravenous fluids
2 If obstruction does not resolve following supportive measures, surgical palliation should be considered
3 Plain abdominal films may help establish the obstructive site
4 Small bowel intubation may resolve incomplete obstructions
5 Right transverse colostomy relieves large bowel obstruction, and can be done under local anesthesia if necessary

Malignant complications responsive to palliative radiotherapy

1 Painful bone metastases (local or hemibody irradiation)
2 Refractory lymphomas (e.g. whole-body irradiation)
3 Neoplastic skin ulceration/fungation
4 Obstructed hollow viscus (esp. trachea, esophagus, vena cava)
5 Neural compression (cerebral, spinal cord, nerve)
6 Uncontrolled tumor bleeding (e.g. hemoptysis, hematuria)

Palliative efficacy of corticosteroids in malignant disease

1 Intracranial tumor with edema + raised intracranial pressure
2 Nerve (incl. spinal cord) compression, esp. preradiotherapy
3 Acute inflammation following radiotherapy (e.g. radiation proctitis (steroid enemas), non-candidal esophagitis)
4 Dyspnea due to lymphangitis carcinomatosa
5 Hypercalcemia (in myeloma)
6 Antiemetic prophylaxis
7 Appetite stimulation
8 Antitumor effect (e.g. in B cell malignancies)

Principles of treating refractory pain in malignant disease

1 Adequate (large) doses
2 Regular rather than p.r.n. administration
3 Oral route if possible
4 Single rather than multiple drugs
5 Hospital admission for severe pain control
6 Narcotic infusions via pump for relief of refractory pain

Indications for parenteral/rectal analgesia

1 Rapid effect desired
2 Inability to swallow (dysphagia, cachexia)
3 Persistent vomiting or bowel obstruction
4 Intractable pain despite optimal regular oral dosing
5 In the last few hours of life

Suboptimal narcotic analgesics for malignant pain

1 Propoxyphene, pentazocine, oral pethidine
   — Weak agonists which may precipitate dysphoria (i.e. simulate withdrawal) in opiate-dependent patients
2 Dextromoramide (Palfium)
   — Short (2 h) duration of action
   — Rapid development of tolerance
3 Methadone (Physeptone)
   — Long (18–36 h) half-life $\rightarrow \uparrow$ risk of toxicity

Clinical guidelines for use of narcotic analgesics

1 Approximate oral equivalents for 30 mg oral morphine q 4 h
   — 400 mg propoxyphene q 6 h
   — 200 mg codeine phosphate q 4 h
   — 150 mg dihydrocodeine q 4 h
   — 30 mg hydrocodone q 4 h
   — 20 mg methadone q 8 h
   — 20 mg oxycodone q 4 h
2 Fentanyl transdermal patches
   – Deliver 50 μgh for 72 h each. In general, the equipotent microgram per hour dose approximates 50% of the required daily milligram dose of oral morphine
3 Morphine
   — Oral:parenteral bioavailability ratio is about 1:3, though patient dosage requirements vary markedly. Hence, 10 mg IV q 4 h approximates 30 mg q 4 h.
   — No advantage from using oral diamorphine (heroin)
4 Nausea, if it occurs, usually settles after 72 h of opiate use
5 Constipation is invariable and should be prevented by routine laxative administration: prevent with bisacodyl at night, or b.d. senna; treat established opiate-induced obstipation with lactulose q 6 h and/or phosphate enemas
6 Addiction (cf. tolerance) is rarely a problem in malignant pain, nor is respiratory depression

Oral analgesic regimens for cancer-associated pain

1 Mild
   — Paracetamol 1 g q 4 h
   — Aspirin 600 mg q 4 h (or other NSAID)

2 Moderate
— Dihydrocodeine 30–60 mg q 4 h (constipating), or
— Buprenorphine 0.2–0.4 mg q 6–8 h sublingually (emetic)
3 Severe
— Morphine 5–200 mg q 3–4 h

Specific indications for adjuvant non-narcotic drug therapy
1 Bone pain
— NSAIDs (e.g. 400 mg ibuprofen q 8 h)
— Pamidronate 90 mg infusion q 4 weeks, or daily oral clodronate
— Radiostrontium (^{89}Sr) 4 mCi IV q 3 months
2 Nerve compression
— Cord compression: dexamethasone 10 mg IV q 6 h
— Pain without neuro deficit: dexamethasone 4 mg q 8 h p.o.
3 Neuropathic/-algic pain
— Amitriptyline 50 mg at night
— Carbamazepine 200 mg q 6–12 h
— Clonazepam 0.5–1.0 mg q 8 h
— Mexiletine 150 mg q 8 h
— Bupivacaine 0.25%, 5 mL/h epidurally
4 Muscle spasm
— Baclofen 10–20 mg q 8–12 h
— Diazepam 5 mg q 8 h
5 Neoplastic ulcer
— Antibiotics (e.g. metronidazole)
6 Insomnia/depression
— Tricyclics, hydroxyzine
7 Bowel obstruction
— Octreotide
8 Opiate constipation
— Lactulose
9 Opiate antiemesis
— Haloperidol
10 Opiate sedation
— Amphetamines

Neurosurgical approaches to intractable pain in cancer patients
1 Phenol nerve block
— e.g. Celiac axis (Ca pancreas)
2 Dorsal rhizotomy
— For pain in trunk, neck, perineum
3 Percutaneous cordotomy
— For unilateral pain below C5 dermatome
4 Thalamotomy
— For 'central' pain
5 Epidural anesthesia

UNDERSTANDING PALLIATIVE CARE

Opioid receptors mediating opiate function and toxicity
1 μ (mu) receptors
— Mediate analgesia and respiratory depression
— Also mediate euphoria and dependence
— Best agonists: morphine, diamorphine
— Partial agonist: buprenorphine
— Weak affinity: dextropropoxyphene
— Partial antagonist: pentazocine
— Full antagonist: naloxone
2 κ (kappa) receptors
— Mediate spinal analgesia
— Also mediate miosis and sedation
— Partial agonists: pentazocine, nalbuphine
3 δ (delta) receptors
— Responsible for constipation, nausea
— Also → respiratory depression, euphoria
— (Dihydro)codeine activates these receptors; some is metabolized to morphine → μ receptors (analgesia)

Predispositions to lung infections in the elderly
1 Increased frequency of aspiration
— Impaired epiglottic and esophageal function
— Impaired cough reflex
— Impaired mucociliary clearance
— Impaired level of consciousness
2 Comorbid conditions favoring infection
— Diabetes mellitus
— Malnutrition, uremia, etc.
3 Nosocomial transmission
— Mini-epidemics (esp. influenza) in nursing homes

REVIEWING THE LITERATURE: PALLIATIVE CARE

11.1 Robinson SM et al (1998) Psychological effect of witnessed resuscitation on bereaved relatives. Lancet 352: 614–617

Observational study of 25 patients undergoing emergency room resuscitation, 13 of which were witnessed by relatives. No adverse psychological effects were noted in the group who witnessed resuscitation.

11.2 Li Wan Po A et al (1997) Systematic overview of co-proxamol to assess analgesic effects of addition of dextropropoxyphene to paracetamol. Br Med J 315: 1565–1571

Overview of 26 randomized studies, concluding that there was little objective evidence to justify an extra analgesic benefit of propoxyphene.

11.3 Allan L et al (2001) Randomized crossover trial of transdermal fentanyl and sustained release oral morphine for treating chronic non-cancer pain. Br Med J 322: 1154–1158

Study of 256 patients in 35 centers, showing better pain relief, less constipation and improved quality of life with transdermal fentanyl than with SR oral morphine.

11.4 Johnson RE et al (2000) A comparison of levomethadyl acetate, buprenorphine, and methadone for opioid dependence. N Engl J Med 343: 1290–1297

Randomized study of 220 opioid-dependent patients, showing poorer efficacy of low-dose methadone in promoting abstinence.

11.5 Kendall JM et al (2001) Multicentre randomized controlled trial of nasal diamorphine for analgesia in children and teenagers with clinical fractures. Br Med J 322: 261–265

Multicenter randomized study of 404 children with a clinical limb fracture, showing markedly better analgesia from inhaled diamorphine spray than from intramuscular morphine.

11.6 Baker D et al (2000) Cannabinoids control spasticity and tremor in a multiple sclerosis model. Nature 404: 84–87

Description of Biozzie ABH mouse model in which cannabinoids (including THC) improved tremor and spasticity, raising therapeutic hopes for this approach in human disease.

CHAPTER 12

Pharmacology and toxicology

Physical examination protocol 12.1   You are asked to examine a patient known to be a drug addict

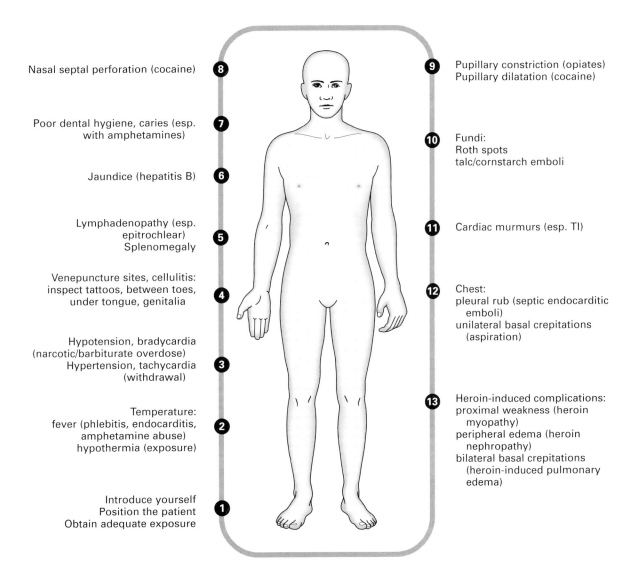

Nasal septal perforation (cocaine) — **8**

Poor dental hygiene, caries (esp. with amphetamines) — **7**

Jaundice (hepatitis B) — **6**

Lymphadenopathy (esp. epitrochlear) Splenomegaly — **5**

Venepuncture sites, cellulitis: inspect tattoos, between toes, under tongue, genitalia — **4**

Hypotension, bradycardia (narcotic/barbiturate overdose) Hypertension, tachycardia (withdrawal) — **3**

Temperature: fever (phlebitis, endocarditis, amphetamine abuse) hypothermia (exposure) — **2**

Introduce yourself Position the patient Obtain adequate exposure — **1**

9 — Pupillary constriction (opiates) Pupillary dilatation (cocaine)

10 — Fundi: Roth spots talc/cornstarch emboli

11 — Cardiac murmurs (esp. TI)

12 — Chest: pleural rub (septic endocarditic emboli) unilateral basal crepitations (aspiration)

13 — Heroin-induced complications: proximal weakness (heroin myopathy) peripheral edema (heroin nephropathy) bilateral basal crepitations (heroin-induced pulmonary edema)

COMMON AND CLASSIC TOXICOLOGIC PROBLEMS

Common pharmacologic or toxicologic disorders in clinical practice
1 Alcoholism
2 Drug treatment failure due to noncompliance
3 Drug-induced side-effect (e.g. urticaria)

Classic pharmacologic or toxicologic disorders in clinical exams
1 Chronic heavy metal poisoning
2 Digoxin toxicity
3 Teratogenic congenital malformation

PHARMACOLOGIC AND TOXICOLOGIC EMERGENCIES

Acute medical emergencies: parenteral adult treatment
1 Acute psychotic agitation
   — Haloperidol (5 mg/mL) 1 mL IMI *or* chlorpromazine 25 mg IMI
2 Severe non-psychotic anxiety refractory to conservative measures
   — Diazepam 10 mg slow IV (or IM if unable to cannulate)
3 Bradycardia and/or hypotension due to myocardial infarct
   — Atropine (600 µg/mL) 0.5 mL IV under cardiac monitoring
4 Acute meningococcal meningitis
   — Benzylpenicillin 1200 mg slow IV
5 Severe pneumonia in chronic lung patient
   — Amoxicillin 500 mg slow IV
6 Acute pulmonary edema
   — Morphine 5 mg slow IVI; furosemide (frusemide) 20–40 mg IV over 5–10 min
7 Acute severe asthma
   — Hydrocortisone 200 mg over 1 min (plus other measures)
8 Narcotic overdose
   — Naloxone 2 mg IV (repeat every 3 min until responsive)

CLINICAL ASSESSMENT OF THE POISONED PATIENT

HEAVY METAL INTOXICATION

Clinical stigmata of mercury poisoning
1 Tremor ('hatter's shakes') → tongue, eyelids, legs
2 Erethism: irritability, easy embarrassment
3 Salivation, gingivitis, pharyngeal pain, bloody diarrhea
4 Nephrosis, renal tubular dysfunction (often reversible)
5 'Pink disease' (acrodynia) – skin hypersensitivity in infants exposed to topical mercury solutions (10% mortality)

Features of lead poisoning: acute vs chronic toxicity
1 Acute poisoning
   — Commoner in children
   Chronic poisoning
   — Commoner in adults
2 Musculoskeletal effects
   — Acute: arthralgias
   — Chronic: 'saturnine' gout
3 Renal effects
   — Acute: renal tubular dysfunction
   — Chronic: gouty nephropathy
4 Hematologic effects
   — Acute: hemolytic anemia, basophilic stippling
   — Chronic: basophilic stippling, hemolytic anemia
5 Gastrointestinal effects
   — Acute: colicky abdominal pain precipitated by alcohol and relieved by palpation or IV calcium
   — Chronic: constipation, gingival 'blue line' (adults), premature tooth loss (children)
6 Neurologic effects
   — Acute: headache, ataxia, fits, encephalopathy
   — Chronic: peripheral neuropathy (predominantly motor), psychiatric sequelae

Reversibility of complications in heavy metal poisoning
1 Lead poisoning
   — Chelation can reverse the GI and blood effects
   — R_x does *not* reverse the neurologic or renal sequelae
2 Wilson's disease (copper overload)
   — Penicillamine can reverse renal tubular dysfunction
   — R_x does *not* reverse end-stage liver/neurologic disease
3 Hemochromatosis (iron overload)
   — Phlebotomy may *prevent* all sequelae, incl. cardiac
   — Phlebotomy *prolongs life* in symptomatic patients
   — Phlebotomy is *not* effective in *reversing* established
     • Hypogonadotropic hypogonadism
     • Diabetes mellitus
     • Arthropathy
   — Phlebotomy does *not* reduce *hepatoma risk* in established *cirrhosis*

TOXIC OVERDOSE SYNDROMES

Clinical features of sympathomimetic overdose*
1 Paranoia, delusions
2 Tachycardia, hypertension, arrhythmias
3 Fever, sweating, piloerection
4 Mydriasis
5 Hyperreflexia
6 Stroke (esp. with cocaine), seizures

* e.g. due to cocaine, amphetamines (incl. 'ice'), theophylline, (pseudo)ephedrine, caffeine

Clinical features of anticholinergic overdose*
1 Tachycardia
2 Dry, flushed skin; mumbling speech

3 Mydriasis
4 Decreased bowel sounds
5 Urinary retention
6 Delirium, seizures

* e.g. due to tricyclics, antispasmodics, antihistamines, antiparkinsonian drugs, amantadine, mydriatics, certain plants

Clinical features of cholinergic overdose*
1 Salivation, lacrimation, fasciculation
2 Miosis
3 Weakness, sweating
4 Abdominal cramps, vomiting
5 Incontinence (urinary and fecal)
6 Pulmonary edema, confusion, fits

* e.g. organophosphate overdose, neostigmine, edrophonium

Clinical features of sedative/opiate/alcohol overdose
1 Hypotension, hypothermia, bradycardia
2 Respiratory depression, pulmonary edema
3 Miosis
4 Decreased bowel sounds
5 Needle marks
6 Coma

Clinical features of triazolam* overdosage
1 Hyperexcitability, behavioral disinhibition
2 Diurnal anxiety and confusion
3 Rebound insomnia, somnambulism
4 Excessive daytime sedation

* A benzodiazepine; common brand name is 'Halcion'

Odoriferous diagnosis of substance intoxication
1 Breath
   — Rotten apples (salicylism)
   — Bitter almonds (cyanide intoxication)
   — Mothballs (naphthalene)
   — Wintergreen (methylsalicylate)
   — Pears (paraldehyde, chloral hydrate)
   — Acetone (isopropyl alcohol)
2 Vomitus
   — Garlic (arsenic poisoning, organophosphates)

DRUG ABUSE

Complications of cocaine abuse
1 Agitation
2 Tachycardia, hypertension, fever
3 Priapism
4 Rhabdomyolysis ± acute renal failure
5 Inhalational sequelae
   — (CSF) rhinorrhea
   — Sinusitis, bronchitis, pneumonitis
   — Pneumothorax (-mediastinum, -pericardium)
6 Obstetric sequelae
   — Placental abruption
   — Fetal abortion
   — Prematurity
7 Infarctions
   — Myocardial
   — Bowel, skin
   — Cerebral

8 Other cardiovascular sequelae
   — Aortic dissection
   — Subarachnoid hemorrhage
   — Arrhythmias

Specific complications of parenteral drug abuse
1 Infective endocarditis
2 Chronic hepatitis; tetanus, botulism
3 AIDS
4 Osteomyelitis, septic arthritis, cellulitis
5 Thrombophlebitis; arteriovenous aneurysms
6 Pulmonary septic emboli/infarction
7 Renal failure

Symptoms and signs of narcotic withdrawal
1 Irritability, tremulousness, panic
2 Yawning
3 Runny nose, watery eyes
4 Chills, sweating, cramps, nausea ('cold turkey')

Drugs abused by athletes
1 Anabolic steroids
2 Erythropoietin*
3 Growth hormone
4 β-agonists (e.g. to induce bronchodilatation)
   β-blockers (e.g. to reduce tremor in snooker)
5 Diuretics
6 Narcotics, amphetamines, cocaine, caffeine

* Autologous transfusion (blood doping) is also used, and is harder to detect

INVESTIGATING DRUG THERAPY

General reasons for checking plasma drug levels
1 Low toxic:therapeutic ratio
2 Substantial interpatient variability in drug metabolism
3 Efficacy difficult to monitor on clinical grounds

Specific indications for measuring drug levels
1 Life-threatening overdose
   — Paracetamol (if urine screen +ve)
   — Tricyclics, salicylate (peak levels occur late due to delayed gastric emptying)
   — Methanol, salicylate (↑↑ levels → early hemodialysis)
2 Routine regular dose calibration
   — Aminoglycosides
   — Lithium
   — Digoxin
   — Anticonvulsants: phenytoin, carbamazepine
3 Initial calculation of maintenance dosage (esp. in cardiac, renal or liver failure)
   — Quinidine, procainamide, disopyramide, lidocaine (lignocaine)
   — Theophylline
4 High probability of drug interaction, e.g.
   — Adding quinidine to maintenance digoxin therapy
   — Adding valproate to maintenance phenytoin
5 Treatment failure
   — esp. Suspected non-compliance

Laboratory diagnosis of lead poisoning
1 ↑ Blood lead (esp. in children)
2 ↑ Urinary coproporphyrin III (good screening test)
3 ↑ Urine and serum ALA
4 ↑ Urine lead (EDTA mobilization)
5 ↑ Serum iron and red cell protoporphyrin
  (→ ineffective erythropoiesis)

PHARMACOGENETICS

Genetic polymorphisms determining drug toxicity
1 Pseudocholinesterase deficiency (autosomal recessive)
  — Causes suxamethonium (succinylcholine) sensitivity
  — Leads to prolonged apnea post-anesthesia
2 Malignant hyperthermia (autosomal dominant)
  — Hypercatabolic response to anesthetic agents, esp. halothane, suxamethonium; ± MAOIs, tricyclics
3 Favism (G6PD deficiency; X-linked dominant)
  — Manifests as hemolysis
  — Caused by primaquine, sulfonamides, nitrofurantoin
4 Acute intermittent porphyria (autosomal dominant)
  — Causes abdominal pain (acute), neuropathy (chronic)
  — Precipitated by many drugs, esp. barbiturates, alcohol
5 Steroid-induced glaucoma (autosomal recessive)
  — Precipitated by topical (or long-term systemic) steroids
  — Occurs in about 5% of the population
6 Slow acetylation (autosomal recessive)
  — Generally manifests as drug toxicity
  Rapid acetylation (autosomal recessive)
  — Generally manisfests as drug insensitivity
7 Sulfonylurea flushing (autosomal dominant)
  — Precipitated by chlorpropamide or tolbutamide
  — Occurs in about 30% of Caucasians
8 Warfarin resistance (autosomal dominant)
  — Rare

METABOLIC POLYMORPHISMS

Rationâle for determining the acetylation phenotype*
1 Isoniazid
  — Slow acetylators
    • ↑ Peripheral neuropathy (B$_6$-responsive)
    • ↑ Iatrogenic SLE
    • ↑ Phenytoin/carbamazepine toxicity
    • ↑ Rifampicin-induced hepatotoxicity
  — Rapid acetylators
    • Failure of once-weekly TB therapy
    • ↑ Isoniazid-induced hepatitis
2 Sulfasalazine
  — Slow acetylators
    • ↑ Toxicity from sulfapyridine moiety, esp. headaches, leukopenia
    • ↑ Hemolysis in G6PD-deficient patients

3 Hydralazine
  — Slow acetylators
    • ↑ Iatrogenic SLE, esp. in females
  — Rapid acetylators
    • Failure of antihypertensive therapy
4 Procainamide
  — Slow acetylators
    • ↑ Iatrogenic SLE
5 Dapsone
  — Slow acetylators
    • ↑ Hemolysis in G6PD-deficient patients
  — Rapid acetylators
    • Failure of therapy for dermatitis herpetiformis
* 50% of the population are slow acetylators

Diseases associated with slow acetylation phenotype
1 Gilbert's syndrome
2 Sjögren's syndrome
3 Arylamine-induced bladder cancer

Clinical sequelae of 'poor' debrisoquine oxidation phenotype*
1 Excessive hypotension with
  — Debrisoquine
  — Propranolol, metoprolol, timolol
2 Lactic acidosis with metformin
3 Neuropathy/hepatotoxicity with perhexiline
4 Agranulocytosis with captopril
5 Confusion with nortriptyline (+ other anticholinergic effects)
* 50% of the population are poor metabolizers of debrisoquine
– i.e. they have homozygous monoxygenase deficiency

MANAGING DRUG THERAPY

APPROACH TO THE POISONED PATIENT

When to consider dialysis?
1 Methanol intoxication
2 Severe salicylate intoxication
3 Lithium poisoning (if plasma level > 5 mmol/L)
4 CCl_4 (within 48 h of ingestion)

Other treatment options in life-threatening overdosage
1 Forced alkaline diuresis (urine pH → 7.5–8.5)
  — (Pheno)barbital
  — Salicylate
2 Forced acid diuresis (urine pH → 5.5–6.5)
  — Quin(id)ine
  — Amphetamine, phencyclidine
3 Charcoal hemoperfusion
  — Theophylline (if plasma level > 60 mg/L)
  — Barbiturates, methaqualone
  — Paraquat

Clinical use of oral activated charcoal ('gastrointestinal dialysis')
1 Technically simpler than hemoperfusion or dialysis
2 Suitable for use in district hospitals or remote locations
3 Most effective for weakly acidic drugs with small V_D

Drugs effectively eliminated by repeated oral charcoal

1 Phenobarbital, carbamazepine
2 Salicylate, quinine
3 Theophylline, aminophylline
4 Dapsone
5 Digoxin
6 Paraquat

Paracetamol* overdose: principles of management

1 Gastric lavage ± charcoal adsorption, if
   — Ingestion of 10 g paracetamol within last 4 h, *or*
   — Time and/or quantity of ingested dose unknown
2 Specific therapy (if overdose taken within last 16 h)
   — Best guide: paracetamol level > 4 h post-ingestion
   — If above reference level for toxicity, infuse *N*-acetylcysteine according to nomogram‡
   — Therapy indicated if overdose taken within last 24 h; may require continuation until 72 h post-ingestion
3 If *N*-acetylcysteine unavailable, use oral methionine¶
4 Prothrombin time and transaminases should be monitored closely (may rise within 12 h of overdose)
5 In patients at risk of hepatic necrosis (esp. if massive overdose and/or late presentation), give 5% dextrose infusion to obviate risk of hypoglycemia
6 Liver transplant may be considered in otherwise fatal cases

* Called acetaminophen in the USA
‡ e.g. 150 mg/kg over 15 min, then 50 mg/kg over 4 h, then 100 mg/kg over 16 h
¶ Another glutathione precursor

Specific antidotes to inhaled or ingested poisons

1 Carbon monoxide (CO)
   — 100% oxygen (if carboxy-Hb > 30%)
   — *Hyperbaric* (2 atm/200 kPa) if unconscious
2 Cyanide (CN⁻)*
   — 100% oxygen ± sodium bicarbonate IV, *plus*
   — Dicobalt EDTA IV, *or*
   — Sodium nitrite then sodium thiosulphate IV, *or*
   — Amyl nitrite inhaled every 5 min, *or*
   — Hydroxocobalamin IV (in mild cases)‡
3 Organophosphate insecticides (cholinesterase inhibitors)
   — IV atropine every 10 min (to keep heart rate > 60)
   — Pralidoxime (PAM) slow IVI hourly
4 Ethylene glycol or methanol
   — Gastric lavage, *plus*
   — 50 g ethanol IV loading dose, *plus*
   — IV 4-methylpyrazole, *or*
   — 5% ethanol IV + forced alkaline diuresis + hemodialysis

NB: Gastric lavage contraindicated following ingestion of paraffin, kerosene, or petrol (due to risk of aspiration pneumonitis)
* Cyanide intoxication may occur secondary to smoke inhalation
‡ e.g. due to prolonged sodium nitroprusside therapy (p. 47)

Antidotes to metal or elemental poisoning

1 Lead (Pb; 'plumbism')
   — Calcium disodium EDTA slow IV b.d. + dimercaprol
   — Intramuscular administration is less hazardous in children at risk of encephalopathy
   — Oral or intragastric administration is *contraindicated*
2 Iron (Fe; presents with GI bleeding or hepatic necrosis)
   — Desferrioxamine (DFO) ± charcoal adsorption (by gastric lavage; then leave in stomach; then deep IM DFO loading dose; then *slow* infusion)*
3 Mercury (Hg), arsenic (As), gold (Au)
   — Dimercaptosuccinic acid, penicillamine
   — Dimercaprol (BAL) by deep IM injection (traditional)
4 Zinc (Zn; → 'metal-fume fever')
   — D-Penicillamine p.o.
   — Also used in Pb, Hg, As, Au, Cu poisoning
   — Dimercaprol (BAL)
5 Thallium (used in rodenticides)
   — Prussian (Berlin) blue via nasogastric tube
   — Also used in Fe, CN⁻ poisoning
6 Bromism (Br)
   — Saline infusion
   — Also helpful in lithium poisoning

* NB: DFO should *not* be used in patients receiving vitamin C due to risk of cardiac damage. Also infusions longer than 24 h may cause excess free radicals leading to shock lung (ARDS); hence, keep them short

Antidotes to drug overdoses

1 Benzodiazepines
   — Flumazenil (0.2 mg over 30 sec)
2 Calcium channel blockers
   — Calcium (1 g over 5 min IV with ECG monitor)
3 Anticholinergics
   — IV neostigmine over 60 sec using ECG monitor
4 Tricyclics
   — Bicarbonate (1 mmol/kg IV for arrhythmias)
   — Neostigmine IV for anticholinergic effects
5 Isoniazid
   — Pyridoxine (5 g slow IVI)
6 β-blockers
   — Glucagon (5 mg IVI)
7 Digoxin
   — Fab fragments (for arrhythmias)
8 Nitrates
   — Methylene blue (if MetHb > 30%)
9 Warfarin
   — Vitamin K (note risk of anaphylaxis)

SALICYLISM

Salicylate overdose: therapeutic options

1 Mild poisoning (salicylate level < 500 mg/L)
   — Fluid and electrolyte balance alone
2 Moderate (level < 500 mg/L + acidosis; or < 750 mg/L alone)
   — Forced alkaline diuresis, *or*
   — Oral activated charcoal

3 Severe (< 750 mg/L + renal impairment; < 900 mg/L alone)
 — Charcoal hemoperfusion, *or*
 — Hemodialysis

Metabolic complications of salicylate overdosage
1 Fever, sweating
 — Due to uncoupling of oxidative phosphorylation
2 Confusion
 — Due to neuroglycopenia, esp. in adults
3 Epigastric discomfort, vomiting
 — Due to delayed gastric emptying
4 Tachypnea (primary respiratory alkalosis)
 — Due to direct respiratory center stimulation ($\rightarrow$ adults)
5 Primary metabolic acidosis ($\rightarrow$ children)
 — Due to multifactorial pathogenesis, incl. lactic acidosis
6 Prerenal failure
 — Due to dehydration, renal vasoconstriction
7 Hypo- or hyperglycemia
 Hypo- or hypernatremia
8 Pulmonary edema and/or hypokalemia
 — esp. If forced alkaline diuresis
9 Gastrointestinal bleeding
 — *Unusual* despite gastric irritation, platelet dysfunction and/or hypoprothrombinemia

CLINICAL PHARMACOKINETICS

Drugs exhibiting saturation kinetics
1 Phenytoin
2 Salicylate
3 Alcohol

Important clinical contexts for drug interaction
1 Where dose and response are critically balanced
 — Anticoagulants
 — Oral hypoglycemics
2 Where major toxicity may supervene
 — Cytotoxics
 — Digoxin
 — Theophylline
 — Aminoglycosides
 — Lithium
3 Where loss of effect may be catastrophic
 — Antiarrhythmics (e.g. quinidine)
 — Anticonvulsants (e.g. valproate)
 — Corticosteroids (e.g. in temporal arteritis)
 — Oral contraceptives
4 Where indications for interacting drugs may be similar
 — Digoxin and loop diuretics ($\downarrow$ K$^+$ $\rightarrow$ $\uparrow\uparrow$ digoxin toxicity)
 — Digoxin and quinidine, amiodarone ($\uparrow$ plasma digoxin)
 — Captopril and potassium-sparing diuretics ($\uparrow\uparrow$ K$^+$)
 — β-blockers and acetazolamide (acidosis may $\rightarrow$ CCF)
 — β-blockers and clonidine ($\uparrow$ risk of clonidine 'rebound')
 — Cimetidine and antacids ($\downarrow$ cimetidine absorption)

 — Azathioprine/6MP + allopurinol (4-fold potentiation)
 — Ketoconazole + ciclosporin ($\uparrow$ ciclosporin nephrotoxicity)
 — Tranylcypromine + clomipramine (hypertensive crisis)

Drugs interacting adversely with alcohol
1 Disulfiram
2 Metronidazole
3 Chlorpropamide
4 Procarbazine
5 Ketoconazole, cefamandole, griseofulvin
6 Verapamil

Drugs often prescribed in slow-release formulations
1 Theophylline
2 Lithium
3 Morphine
4 Carbamazepine
5 L-DOPA

Pharmacologic vs idiosyncratic drug reactions
1 Pharmacological examples
 — Digoxin toxicity (pharmacokinetic)
 — CCF due to indometacin-induced sodium retention (pharmacodynamic)
 — Gastric bleeding due to aspirin (pharmaceutical)
2 Idiosyncratic examples
 — Eosinophilia–myalgia syndrome due to L-tryptophan
 — Halothane hepatitis
 — Penicillin-induced anaphylaxis

PHARMACOKINETIC FACTORS IN ELDERLY PATIENTS

Physiologic alterations affecting drug metabolism in elderly
1 Impaired renal excretion
2 Impaired hepatic metabolism
3 Impaired (oral) drug absorption
 — e.g. Due to achlorhydria
4 Altered drug distribution
 — Cardiac failure, dehydration
 — $\uparrow$ Fat, $\downarrow$ lean body mass
 — $\uparrow$ α_1-acid glycoprotein, $\downarrow$ albumin

Considerations in prescribing specific drugs for elderly patients
1 Reduced renal clearance
 — e.g. Digoxin, lithium, cimetidine, clopropamide, aminoglycosides
2 Reduced hepatic metabolism
 — e.g. Tricyclics, clomethiazole, propranolol, nifedipine
3 Reduced volume of distribution (V$_D$; for water-soluble drugs)
 — e.g. Ethanol, digoxin, cimetidine
4 Reduced sensitivity
 — e.g. Some antihypertensives
5 Increased sensitivity
 — e.g. Benzodiazepines, warfarin, opioids, some diuretics

DRUG TOXICITY

Approximate incidences of some adverse drug reactions

1 Retroperitoneal fibrosis due to methysergide
   — 1 in 250 patient years
2 Pseudomembranous colitis due to clindamycin
   — 1 in 5000 patient years
3 Aplastic anemia due to chloramphenicol
   — 1 in 6000 patient years
   Aplastic anemia due to phenylbutazone
   — 1 in 10 000 patient years
4 Thrombotic complications of oral contraceptives
   Hepatitis due to halothane
   Vaginal carcinoma due to maternal diethylstilbestrol
   — 1 in 10 000 patient years*

* Though this frequency appears roughly doubled in patients taking third-generation oral contraceptives, i.e. those containing either gestodene or desogestrel as the progestogen component

Iatrogenic causes of gingival hypertrophy

1 Phenytoin
2 Ciclosporin
3 Nifedipine

Iatrogenic causes of priapism

1 Antihypertensives (esp. α-blockers)
   — Labetalol, hydralazine, prazosin, guanethidine
2 Phenothiazines
   — Chlorpromazine, fluphenazine
3 Cocaine

Associations of Reye's syndrome*

1 Aspirin ingestion
2 Influenza B

* Acute hypoglycemia, liver infiltration, coma in children

VENOMS AND TOXINS

Some venoms and toxins of clinical significance

1 Botulinum toxin (p. 273)
   — Used in some neurologic disorders
2 Hirudin (from leeches)
   — Anticlotting agent
3 Venoms used in coagulation testing
   — Batroxobin ('Reptilase')
   — 'Stypven' (detects lupus anticoagulant)

UNDERSTANDING DRUG THERAPY

CLINICAL PHARMACOLOGY

Drugs referred to differently in USA and UK: a selection

1 Acetaminophen (US), paracetamol (UK)
2 Epinephrine (US), adrenaline (UK)
3 Furosemide (US), frusemide (UK)
4 Lidocaine (US), lignocaine (UK)

Drugs derived from plants

1 Quinine (cinchona)
2 Aspirin
3 Digoxin (foxglove)
4 Morphine (opium poppy)
5 Curare
6 Nifedipine
7 Vincristine, etoposide, paclitaxel

Pharmacokinetics: principles underlying clinical practice

1 For a given dosage, the plasma level of any drug is inversely proportional to its volume of distribution (V_D)
2 The *loading dose* of any drug is directly proportional to its V_D
   The *maintenance dose* of any drug is directly proportional to its clearance
3 Drugs with low V_D (i.e. high concentration in plasma relative to tissues) tend to be heavily protein-bound
   The lower the V_D of a given drug, the more readily it is removed by dialysis
4 The steady-state plasma level of any drug is achieved following regular administration for a period approximating 3–5 half-lives of the drug
5 Biliary excretion tends to be of minor pharmacokinetic significance; enterohepatic recirculation will occur until hepatic metabolism produces polar drug metabolites able to be renally excreted

Clinical significance of plasma protein binding

1 Drug interactions due to displacement from plasma protein binding sites tend to be transient and of minor clinical significance
2 Changes in protein binding may greatly affect assayed *total* plasma concentrations of drug
3 If assay for *free* drug not available, *salivary* concentrations of phenytoin, isoniazid or theophylline may be used
4 Protein-bound drug molecules do not undergo glomerular filtration
   Ionized drug molecules may undergo active tubular secretion irrespective of plasma protein binding status
   Non-ionized (non-polar, liposoluble) drugs undergo passive renal tubular reabsorption and then hepatic metabolism
5 Acidic drugs tend to be highly protein-bound

Examples of significant alterations in plasma protein binding

1 Precipitation of kernicterus by sulfonamides displacing bilirubin
2 Precipitation of mucositis by aspirin displacing methotrexate (hence increasing free methotrexate levels)
3 Precipitation of hypoglycemia by phenylbutazone displacing tolbutamide
4 Precipitation of hemorrhage by clofibrate displacing warfarin
5 Precipitation of phenytoin toxicity by uremia, hepatic failure, or concomitant valproate administration

6 Antagonism of lidocaine (lignocaine)/propranolol/
disopyramide effect due to major increases in
α_1-acid glycoprotein (an acute phase reactant
elevated in burns, trauma, surgery, etc.)

CHARACTERISTICS OF DRUG STRUCTURE AND FUNCTION

Polar vs non-polar drugs: the clinical distinction
1 Polar (ionized, water-soluble) drugs typically
exhibit
— Heavy plasma protein binding
— Low V_D
— Long plasma $t^{1/2}$
— Low CNS penetration and toxicity
— Acidic pK_a
— Predominant renal excretion (via active tubular
secretion without glomerular filtration)
— Examples: warfarin, furosemide (frusemide)
2 Non-polar (un-ionized, lipophilic) drugs typically
exhibit
— Little plasma protein binding
— Large V_D
— Short plasma $t^{1/2}$
— High CNS penetration and toxicity
— Basic pK_a
— Predominant hepatic metabolism (via
glomerular filtration and passive renal tubular
reabsorption)
— Examples: propranolol, nortriptyline

Acidic vs basic drugs
1 Acidic
— 'ates': salicylate, clofibrate, valproate,
barbiturate
— 'ins': warfarin, phenytoin, penicillins,
cephalosporins*
— 'ides': furosemide (frusemide), thiazides,
sulfonamides, chlorpropamide, probenecid,
most NSAIDs‡
2 Basic
— 'ines': chlorpromazine, imipramine, nortriptyline,
morphine, quinidine, cimetidine¶
— 'ols': propranolol, ethambutol, dipyridamole
— other: verapamil, trimethoprim, diazepam

* NB: *Prazosin* is basic
‡ NB: *Procainamide, amiloride* are basic
¶ NB: *Theophylline* is acidic

Drugs yielding active hepatic metabolites responsible for efficacy
1 Aspirin ($\rightarrow$ paracetamol); phenylbutazone
2 Carbamazepine; diazepam
3 Verapamil; enalapril; lidocaine (lignocaine);
procainamide
4 Carbimazole ($\rightarrow$ methimazole)
5 Amitriptyline; imipramine; chloral hydrate;
L-DOPA
6 Cyclophosphamide; azathioprine ($\rightarrow$ 6MP)
Prednisone ($\rightarrow$ prednisolone)

Drugs yielding hepatic metabolites responsible for toxicity
1 Isoniazid ($\rightarrow$ acetylhydrazine, esp. in fast acetylators)
2 Methanol ($\rightarrow$ formaldehyde)
3 Clofibrate, procainamide
4 Cyclophosphamide (acrolein metabolites $\rightarrow$ bladder
toxicity)
5 Alcohol ($\rightarrow$ acetaldehyde)

Drugs excreted by the kidney
1 β-blockers — atenolol
2 Antibiotics — penicillins, cephalosporins,
aminoglycosides, tetracycline
3 Diuretics — furosemide (frusemide),
chlorothiazide
4 Cardiac drugs — digoxin, procainamide
5 CNS drugs — lithium
6 Hypoglycemics — chlorpropamide, metformin
7 Analgesics — aspirin (in overdosage only)
8 Other — cimetidine, ranitidine

MECHANISMS OF DRUG ACTION

Enzymes inhibited by drug therapy
1 Xanthine oxidase — allopurinol
2 Na^+/K^+-ATPase (cardiac) — digoxin
Na^+/K^+-ATPase (loop of Henle) — furosemide
(frusemide)
3 H^+/K^+-ATPase (gastric) — omeprazole
4 Angiotensin-converting enzyme (ACE) — captopril,
enalapril
5 Prostaglandin synthetase — aspirin
6 Monoamine oxidase — phenelzine, moclobemide
7 Carbonic anhydrase — acetazolamide
8 DOPA decarboxylase — carbidopa
9 DNA topoisomerase II (human) — VP-16 (etoposide)
DNA topo II (bacterial) — nalidixic acid, ciprofloxacin
10 Acetylcholinesterase — neostigmine

Adrenergic receptors involved in drug action
1 α_1-adrenergic (post-synaptic) receptors
— Antagonist: prazosin
2 α_2-adrenergic (brainstem) receptors
— Agonist: clonidine
3 β_1-adrenergic receptors
— Agonist: dopamine
— Antagonist: metoprolol, atenolol
4 β_2-adrenergic receptors
— Agonist: salbutamol

Other receptors involved in drug action
1 Endorphin receptors
— Agonist: morphine
— Antagonist: naloxone (IV), naltrexone (oral)
2 Aldosterone receptors
— Antagonist: spironolactone
3 Histamine receptors
— H_1 antagonists: chlorphenamine, terfenadine
— H_2 antagonists: ranitidine, famotidine
4 Dopamine (CNS) receptors
— Agonist: bromocriptine
— Antagonist: chlorpromazine

5 Serotonin (5HT) receptors
— 5HT1A receptor partial agonist: buspirone
— 5HT2 receptor antagonist: nefazodone,
clozapine, risperidone
— 5HT3 receptor antagonist: ondansetron,
granisetron
— Selective serotonin reuptake inhibitors:
fluoxetine etc.
6 GABA receptors
— GABA receptor agonist*: benzodiazepines,
barbiturates, valproate, vigabatrin, gabapentin,
lamotrigine, acamprosate, baclofen

* Because GABA is a CNS-inhibitory neurotransmitter,
treatment with *agonists* causes CNS *inhibition*

DRUG METABOLISM BY HEPATIC MICROSOMAL ENZYMES

Drugs commonly inhibiting cytochrome P_{450}
1 Alcohol
— Acute binge
2 Antibiotics
— Isoniazid
— Erythromycin
— Sulfonamides
— Metronidazole
— Chloramphenicol
3 Anticonvulsants
— Valproate
4 Other drugs*
— Cimetidine
— Allopurinol
— Chlorpromazine, imipramine
— Propranolol, metoprolol
— Dextropropoxyphene
— Disulfiram

* Note that > 1 g/day of *paracetamol/acetaminophen* can also
significantly potentiate warfarin therapy to the point of
toxicity

Drugs commonly inducing cytochrome P_{450}
1 Alcohol
— Chronic ingestion
2 Antibiotics
— Rifampicin
3 Anticonvulsants
— Phenytoin
— Carbamazepine
— Phenobarbital, primidone
4 Other
— Aminoglutethimide
— Spironolactone
— Griseofulvin
— Cigarette smoking

Drugs undergoing major hepatic metabolism
1 β-blockers
— Propranolol, labetalol, metoprolol, oxprenolol
β_2-agonists
— Salbutamol, terbutaline
2 Antibiotics
— Rifampicin, erythromycin

3 Diuretics
— Spironolactone
4 Cardiac drugs
— Nitrates, verapamil, nifedipine, lidocaine
(lignocaine), prazosin
5 CNS drugs
— Clomethiazole, tricyclics, phenothiazines,
benzodiazepines, barbiturates, L-DOPA
6 Oral hypoglycemics
— Glibenclamide, tolbutamide
7 Analgesics
— Paracetamol, pethidine, pentazocine
— Aspirin

PROSTAGLANDINS

Physiological actions of prostaglandins
1 PGI_2 (prostacyclin), PGE_1 (→ ↑ intracellular cAMP)
— Prevents calcium influx
— Relaxes vascular smooth muscle (i.e.
vasodilates)
— ↓ Platelet aggregation
2 PGE_2
— Mediates edema in inflammation
— Mediates furosemide (frusemide) effect: inhibits
renal tubule ADH
— Induces bronchodilatation
3 PGE_{2a}
— Abortifacient
— Induces bronchoconstriction
4 TXA_2 (thromboxane A_2)
— Induces vasoconstriction (incl. pulmonary
arterial)
— ↑ Platelet aggregation
— Implicated in primary pulmonary hypertension,
respiratory distress syndrome, and renal
vasoconstriction with proteinuria

Drugs interacting with prostaglandins
1 Cyclooxygenase inhibitors
— Include aspirin and other NSAIDs
— Do *not* inhibit lipo-oxygenase; hence
arachidonate metabolism is redirected away
from prostaglandin synthesis and towards
leukotriene synthesis (incl. the
bronchoconstrictor SRS-A)
— Latter mechanism may → aspirin-induced
asthma
2 Phospholipase A_2 inhibitors
— Include high-dose steroids, hydroxychloroquine
— Block both prostaglandin and leukotriene
synthesis
3 Selective TXA_2 synthetase inhibitors
— e.g. Dazoxiben (investigational)

DRUGS AND THE REPRODUCTIVE SYSTEM

Drugs contraindicated in pregnant women
1 Alcohol, nicotine, narcotics
2 Antithyroid drugs (esp. [131]I); sulfonylureas

3 Drugs predisposing to kernicterus
— Sulfonamides
— Aspirin
— Vitamin K
4 Vasoactive drugs
— Ergotamine, propranolol (placental insufficiency)
— ACE inhibitors ($\rightarrow$ fetal death)
— Guanethidine (meconium ileus)
5 Antibiotics
— Tetracyclines (dental staining, enamel hypoplasia)
— Chloramphenicol ('grey syndrome': cardiovascular collapse in newborns)
— Aminoglycosides (esp. streptomycin): deafness
— Sulfonamides (fetal abnormalities in 1st trimester; kernicterus in late pregnancy)

Recognized teratogens
1 Warfarin ('koala bear' facies, Dandy–Walker syndrome)
2 Phenytoin (digital hypoplasia), valproate (spina bifida), phenobarbital (cleft palate), carbamazepine (neural tube, limb, cardiac)
3 Lithium (Ebstein's anomaly; cretinism)
4 ACE inhibitors (renal tubular dysgenesis)
5 Antithyroid drugs (fetal goiter)
6 Misoprostol (Moebius syndrome)
7 NSAIDs (ductus arteriosus constriction*, necrotizing enterocolitis)
8 Thalidomide (phocomelia), tetracycline (teeth and bone anomalies)
9 Ergometrine (Poland anomaly)
10 Cytotoxics (esp. methotrexate, alkylators): CNS malformations
11 Steroid hormones (DES $\rightarrow$ vaginal carcinoma in adolescent female progeny; androgens, cardiac/esophageal defects; danazol, masculinization; low-dose prednisone probably safe)
12 Alcohol (acetaldehyde metabolite $\rightarrow$ 'fetal alcohol syndrome')
13 Isotretinoin (13-cis-retinoic acid), etretinate: numerous defects
High-dose vitamin D or vitamin A
14 Radioisotopes, esp. ^{131}I
Live vaccines

* This effect used therapeutically in the puerperium for patent ductus

Diseases in which thalidomide may be useful*
1 Neoplastic disorders
— Myeloma
— Myelodysplastic syndrome
— Kaposi's sarcoma in AIDS
— Glioblastoma multiforme
— Renal cell carcinoma
2 Gastrointestinal disease
— Crohn's disease with fistulae or mucocutaneous symptoms
— HIV-associated aphthous or esophageal ulcers
— Mucocutaneous ulcers in Behçet's disease

3 Skin disease
— Erythema nodosum leprosum (major indication)
— Chronic graft versus host disease

* Ensure no pregnancy

Drugs contraindicated in breast-feeding mothers
1 Antibiotics
— Chloramphenicol, clindamycin, tetracycline
— (Safer choice: penicillins, cephalosporins, macrolides)
2 Vitamins
— Etretinate, high-dose vitamin A or D
3 Analgesics/anti-inflammatories
— Aspirin (esp. high-dose), indometacin, gold salts, penicillamine, methotrexate, ciclosporin, azathioprine, ergotamine, oxycodone
— (Safer choice: paracetamol, ibuprofen, mefenamic acid, loratadine, sumatriptan)
4 Psychotropics
— Lithium, fluoxetine, doxepin; diazepam, alprazolam
— (Safer choice: sertraline, most tricyclics)
5 Anticonvulsants
— Phenobarbital, primidone, ethosuximide
— (Safer choice: carbamazepine, valproate)
6 Cardiac
— Amiodarone, atropine, atenolol, nadolol, sotalol, methyldopa
— (Safer choice: propranolol, labetalol)

Antihypertensives in pregnancy
1 First trimester
— Try to avoid all
2 Second trimester
— Avoid ACE inhibitors and β-blockers
— Safer alternatives: methyldopa, nifedipine, clonidine
3 Third trimester
— Avoid ACE inhibitors and diuretics
— Safer alternatives: labetalol, nifedipine, methyldopa

Relatively safe drugs in pregnancy
1 Digoxin
2 Heparin (does not cross placenta)*
3 Insulin, thyroxine
4 Antibiotics
— Penicillins, cephalosporins, erythromycin, ethambutol; INH (plus pyridoxine, nystatin
5 Inhaled salbutamol (avoid theophylline)

* Heparin does not appear teratogenic, but is associated with increased antepartum hemorrhage, prematurity and stillbirth, and may contribute to maternal and fetal bone demineralization

Influences on drug metabolism in pregnancy
1 ↑ Glomerular filtration rate
— ↑ Clearance of digoxin, lithium
2 ↑ Hepatic microsomal (P_{450}) enzyme activity
— ↑ Anticonvulsant metabolism
3 ↑ Volume of distribution (e.g. for flucloxacillin)
4 ↓ Plasma protein binding (e.g. aspirin, phenytoin)
5 ↓ Gastric emptying

REVIEWING THE LITERATURE: PHARMACOLOGY AND TOXICOLOGY

12.1 Mocarelli P et al (2000) Paternal concentrations of dioxin and sex ratio of offspring. Lancet 355: 1858–1863

Serum dioxin measurements were taken from 500+ men and women who parented 600+ children over a 20–year period. Paternal exposure was associated with a lower proportion of male births.

12.2 Guthrie E et al (2001) Randomized controlled trial of brief psychological intervention after deliberate self-poisoning. Br Med J 323: 135–138

Randomized trial of 119 attempted suicides, showing that suicidal ideation and behavior were reduced in those who received four counselling sessions at home after discharge.

12.3 Hawton K et al (2001) Effects of legislation restricting pack sizes of paracetamol and salicylate on self poisoning in the United Kingdom. Br Med J 322: 1203–1207

Reduction of packet size was associated with a 20–50% reduction in overdoses, and a two-thirds reduction in associated liver transplants.

12.4 Rogan WJ et al (2001) The effect of chelation therapy with succimer on neuropsychological development in children exposed to lead. N Engl J Med 344: 1421–1426

Effective chelation therapy did not improve cognition or behavior.

12.5 Brent J et al (2001) Fomepizole for the treatment of methanol poisoning. N Engl J Med 344: 424–429

Study of 11 consecutively methanol-poisoned patients, nine of whom survived after treatment with fomepizole (4-methylpyrazole), and alcohol dehydrogenase inhibitor; this being an alternative to the traditionally toxic treatment with ethanol.

12.6 Heckmann M et al (2001) Botulinum toxin A for axillary hyperhidrosis. N Engl J Med 344: 488–493

Of 136 patients with excessive sweating who received intradermal botulinum toxin A (Botox™), 98% felt better.

12.7 Zornberg GL, Jick H (2000) Antipsychotic drug use and risk of first-time idiopathic venous thromboembolism. Lancet 356: 1219–1223

A seven-fold increase in thrombosis was found in this case-control study of patients receiving antipsychotic medication.

12.8 Taguchi A et al (2001) Selective postoperative inhibition of gastrointestinal opioid receptors. N Engl J Med 345: 935–940

An opioid blocker that does not cross the blood–brain barrier was found to accelerate postoperative bowel recovery; similar drugs can prevent morphine-induced constipation.

12.9 Kontiokari T et al (2001) Randomised trial of cranberry-lingonberry juice and Lactobacillus GG drink for the prevention of urinary tract infections in women. Br Med J 322: 1571–1573

Three-arm randomized study of 150 women, showing a preventive benefit of cranberry juice on UTIs.

CHAPTER 13

Psychiatry and addiction

Physical examination protocol 13.1 You are told to begin by asking the patient a few questions

4 Test repetition (articulation, reading, writing, short-term memory)
Say, 'British constitution'
'Royal Irish Constabulary'
'baby hippopotamus'
'la-la-la-la-la-la-la'
Tell me all the boys' names you can
Name all the days of the week, starting with Wednesday and going backwards
Repeat, 'The one thing a nation must have to be rich and great is a large secure supply of wood' (Babcock sentence)
Read (from printed sheet), 'The war broke out last December'
Write, 'The rain in Spain'

5 Commands (comprehension):
Clap your hands
Make a fist
Close the book
Shake your head
Written commands:
Touch your nose
Pick up the pen
Stick out your tongue
Tap your foot

3 General questions (to test hearing, phonation, orientation, short- and long-term memory (e.g. in dementia, confabulation):
Can you hear me all right?
How are you today?
Is it okay if I ask you a few questions?
What's your full name and address?
Do you know the name of this hospital?
What is today's date (month and year)?
What year did World War II end?
Who's the Prime Minister at the moment?
What did you have for breakfast today?
Are you right or left handed?

6 Name objects (wordfinding):
Point to a chair (table/window)
Show me your index finger
Nod your head if you recognize this ...
Is it a ...? or a .....?
Close your eyes and put out your hand ... what's that? (key, pen)

7 Further examination as indicated:
pupils; fundi
extraocular movements
primitive reflexes
chronic liver disease
gait
peripheral neuropathy
plantar reflexes

2 General inspection:
apathy; emotional lability
hemiplegia, facial weakness, catheter

1 Introduce yourself
Shake hands (look for intention tremor)

COMMON AND CLASSIC PSYCHIATRIC PROBLEMS

Common psychiatric or addictive problems in clinical practice
1 Depression
2 Anxiety disorders
3 Schizophrenia

Classic psychiatric or addictive problems in clinical exams
1 Complications of opiate addiction
   — e.g. infective endocarditis, hepatitis, phlebitis
2 Tardive dyskinesia
3 Dementia

PSYCHIATRIC EMERGENCIES

Suicide: risk factors
1 Male sex, age > 60, living alone*
2 Unemployed or financially insecure
3 Recent adverse event

* Or for *attempted* suicide, females < 30 living alone

CLINICAL ASSESSMENT OF THE PSYCHIATRIC PATIENT

HIGHER CEREBRAL DYSFUNCTION

Common presentations of organic brain syndromes
1 Impaired consciousness (esp. acute pathologies)
2 Impaired short-term memory (esp. chronic pathologies)
3 Disorientation
4 Disinhibition
5 Visual hallucinations

Signs favoring organic (rather than affective) psychosis
1 Positive suck/pout reflex
2 Positive palmar–mental reflex
3 Positive (tonic) grasp reflex

Psychiatric disease with thyroid dysfunction?
1 Hypothyroidism*
   — Depression
   — (Pseudo)dementia
   — Coma
2 Thyrotoxicosis
   — Delirium

* May arise *secondary* to lithium therapy of MDP; alternatively, 'rapid-cycling' MDP patients often develop hypothyroidism which deteriorates symptomatically with antidepressants; carbamazepine or T_4 may be useful

Psychiatric presentations of Parkinson's disease
1 Frontal–subcortical cognitive dysfunction (affects 70%)
   — May improve with levodopa

2 Frank dementia (affects 10%)*
   — Secondary (reversible) causes require exclusion
3 Depression
   — May be prevented by good control of motor symptoms
   — Alternatively, may *mask* motor benefit of levodopa
   — Tricyclics, ECT may improve mood *and* motor function
4 Psychosis (usually drug-induced)
   — Withdraw anticholinergics
   — Reduce dose of levodopa, bromocriptine

* NB: Alzheimer's patients develop parkinsonism in about 60%

Common causes of confusion in elderly patients
1 Hypoxemia (any cause)
2 Sepsis (e.g. UTI, pneumonia)
3 Depression
4 Drugs (e.g. digoxin, indometacin, cimetidine, L-DOPA)
5 Dementia (diagnosis of exclusion)

DEMENTIA

Quick verbal screen for dementia
1 'Tell me your name, address and telephone number'
2 'Repeat the words: inscrutable, elucidate, indigo'
3 'Tell me all the different flowers you can think of'
4 'Name these parts of my face' (pointing)
5 'Show me how you cut a piece of wood with a saw'
6 'Walk around the chair to the door, then touch the table'
7 'Draw a clock face showing the time at 4:30'
8 'What's the difference between a river and an ocean?'
9 'Tell me the days of the week backwards'

Prerequisites for the diagnosis of dementia
1 Acquired memory defect
2 Associated non-memory cognitive defect* interfering with normal social or work abilities, e.g.
   — Dysphasia
   — Visuospatial impairment
3 Arousal state normal

* Severity of cognitive impairment tends to be *underestimated* (or not recognized at all: anosognosia) by demented patients, unlike in depression

Differential diagnosis of dementia* in the AIDS patient
1 Primary cerebral HIV infection
   — Basal ganglia; tends to spare cortex
2 Secondary cerebral infection
   — Cerebral toxoplasmosis or cryptococcosis
   — Herpes simplex encephalitis
   — JC virus (progressive multifocal leukoencephalopathy)
3 Cerebral neoplasm
   — Cerebral lymphoma
   — Cerebral Kaposi's

* Affects 50% of patients dying with AIDS

Disorders causing dementia and gait disturbance
1 Normal pressure hydrocephalus
2 Vascular
   — Multi-infarct dementia/pseudobulbar palsy
   — Binswanger's encephalopathy
3 Parkinson's disease
4 Progressive supranuclear palsy (Richardson–Steele syndrome)

NORMAL PRESSURE HYDROCEPHALUS

Clinical features of normal pressure hydrocephalus
1 Gait apraxia (most consistent feature; absent in Alzheimer's)
2 Dementia
3 Incontinence (usually a late feature)
4 Signs: extensor plantar responses, suck/grasp reflexes

Predispositions to normal pressure hydrocephalus
1 Subarachnoid hemorrhage
2 Meningitis, esp. if chronic
3 Paget's disease

Diagnostic confirmation of normal pressure hydrocephalus
1 CT brainscan
   — Marked ventricular enlargement
   — Minimal cortical atrophy
2 Lumbar puncture
   — Symptomatic improvement after CSF sampling
   — Pressure monitoring: intermittent high-pressure waves
3 Clinical response to ventricular shunting

ALZHEIMER'S DISEASE

Clinical significance of Alzheimer's disease
1 Accounts for up to 75% of dementias
2 Responsible for up to 50% of nursing home admissions

Clinical features of Alzheimer's disease
1 Early stage
   — Mild memory impairment
   — Anomia
   — Impaired calculation
   — Reduced insight and judgment
   — EEG, and PET scan: often abnormal
2 Intermediate stage
   — Severe amnesia
   — Agitation
   — Impaired language function
   — Delusions
3 Advanced stage
   — Mute
   — Bedfast
   — Extrapyramidal deficit
   — CT: cerebral atrophy
   — EEG: frank slowing

Features suggesting dementias other than Alzheimer's
1 *Sudden* onset
2 *Early* onset of
   — Gait disturbance
   — Seizures
3 *Focal* neurologic signs

Key disorders to exclude prior to diagnosing Alzheimer's*
1 Depression
2 Drug toxicity
   — Alcohol, sedatives
   — L-DOPA
   — Antihypertensives

* NB: Definitive diagnosis is only possible by brain biopsy (which is rarely indicated; hence, this is a clinical diagnosis)

AFFECTIVE DISORDERS

Potentially misleading presentations of depression
1 Anorexia, weight loss
2 Fatigue
3 Constipation
4 Loss of libido
5 Amenorrhea
6 Sleep disturbance

Features of seasonal affective disorder (SAD)
1 Winter
   — Hypersomnia, fatigue*
   — Increased appetite (esp. carbohydrate craving)
2 Summer
   — Well (unipolar SAD)
   — Mania or hypomania (bipolar SAD)

* May improve with bright morning light (phototherapy) during winter

Differential diagnosis of hypersexuality
1 Manic phase of manic-depressive psychosis (MDP)
2 Huntington's chorea
3 Kleine–Levin syndrome

ALCOHOLISM

Confusion in the alcoholic patient: differential diagnosis
1 Acute intoxication
2 Delirium tremens (48–72 h post-withdrawal)
3 Hypoglycemia (6–36 h post-binge)
4 Head injury → subdural hematoma
5 Post-ictal
6 Wernicke–Korsakoff syndrome
7 Ketoacidosis or lactic acidosis
8 Hepatic encephalopathy
9 Sepsis (e.g. *Klebsiella* pneumonia, aspiration pneumonia)
10 Unusual neurological syndromes
    — Central pontine myelinolysis
    — Marchiafava–Bignami disease*

* Callosal demyelination; rarely diagnosed pre-mortem

Neuropsychiatric manifestations of alcoholism
1 Epilepsy; may complicate
  — Acute alcohol intoxication
  — Chronic heavy alcohol ingestion
  — Alcohol withdrawal
  — Subdural hematoma
2 Withdrawal-related
  — Tremulousness
  — Agitation
  — Delirium tremens
3 Toxic neuronal degeneration
  — Cerebral atrophy ± dementia
  — Cerebral atrophy
  — Central pontine myelinolysis (typically precipitated by use of hypertonic saline or lactulose)
  — Callosal demyelination (Marchiafava–Bignami)
4 Nutrition-related (hypovitaminemic)
  — Wernicke's encephalopathy
  — Korsakoff's psychosis
  — Pellagra
  — Neuropathy (typically painful)
  — 'Tobacco-alcohol' amblyopia

The confused alcoholic: DT's rather than encephalopathy?
1 Severe agitation
2 Gross tremulousness without asterixis
3 Autonomic overactivity (sweats, fever, miosis, ↑HR/BP)
4 Visual hallucinations
5 EEG: *no* triphasic waves
6 Improvement with sedation*

* NB: This is *not* a diagnostic test

Features of Korsakoff's (alcohol amnesia) syndrome
1 Loss of past memories
2 Inability to form new memories
3 Loss of insight
4 Confabulation*
5 Apathy
6 Limited response to thiamine‡

* *Not* invariable; may disappear with disease progression. 'Provoked' confabulation may also occur in Alzheimer's and other dementias
‡ cf. Wernicke's; Korsakoffian neuropathology tends to be far more severe, hence only 25% respond completely (50% partial)

Statistical associations of alcohol ingestion
1 75% of suicides and deaths from fire
2 50% of murders and car accidents
3 35% of divorces and child abuse cases
4 20% of hospital admissions and drownings

ANXIETY STATES

Clinical spectrum of primary anxiety disorders
1 Phobia: agoraphobia, social phobia, other
2 Panic disorder, generalized anxiety disorder
3 Obsessive–compulsive disorder

4 Stress reaction: acute stress reaction, post-traumatic disorder
5 Mixed anxiety and depression
6 Conversion (hysteria)

Differential diagnosis of recurrent acute anxiety attacks
1 Primary
  — Anxiety neurosis
  — Agoraphobia
  — Panic attacks causing hyperventilation syndrome
2 Thyrotoxicosis
3 Pheochromocytoma, insulinoma
4 Temporal lobe epilepsy
5 Paroxysmal supraventricular tachycardia, *or* Recurrent pulmonary emboli
6 Drugs
  — Excessive caffeine, nicotine, amphetamine, cocaine
  — Drug withdrawal (esp. alcohol, opiates, sedatives)

Presentations of functional anxiety states
1 Panic attacks: sweating, palpitations
  Headaches
  — May simulate
    • Pheochromocytoma
    • Insulinoma
2 Presyncopal episodes, visual disturbance
  Paresthesiae, tetany
  — May simulate
    • Epilepsy
    • TIAs
3 Fatigue, breathlessness, tremulousness
  Atypical chest pain
  — May mimic
    • Thyrotoxicosis
    • Pulmonary emboli
    • Mitral valve prolapse
4 Poor concentration
  Sleep disturbance
  — May simulate
    • Intracranial tumor
    • Sleep apnea
    • Hepatic failure
5 Feelings of unreality; fear of madness
  Difficulty swallowing
  — May simulate
    • Schizophrenia
    • Hysteria
    • Aerophagy
    • Agoraphobia

Medical complaints often associated with anxiety disorder
1 Irritable bowel syndrome
2 Atypical angina
3 Migraine
4 Dyspepsia
5 Chronic back pain
6 Asthma

Diagnosis of hyperventilation syndrome
1 High index of suspicion
2 Relief of symptoms following use of rebreathing bag

3 Reproduction of symptoms by forced voluntary overbreathing (best test)

NB: Measuring the $PaCO_2$ during an attack is *not* a reliable test

'Funny turns': features favoring epilepsy
1 Clouding of consciousness
2 Prodromal irritability; premonitory stereotyped 'aura'
3 *Witnessed* absence or transiently impaired consciousness
   Regular, stereotyped tonic–clonic activity
   Tongue-bite, cyanosis or incontinence
4 Post-ictal paresis or confusion but *no* retrograde amnesia*
5 Abnormal EEG during attack

* cf. hysterical fugue

HYSTERIA

Clinical spectrum of somatoform disorders
1 Hysteria
2 Psychogenic pain
3 Hypochondriasis
4 Münchausen's syndrome
5 Dermatitis artefacta
6 Compensation neurosis

Manifestations of hysteria
1 Conversion or dissociative symptoms, e.g.
   — Paralysis
   — Pseudoseizures
   — Sensory disturbance
   — Abnormal gait
2 Symptoms associated with
   — *Belle indifference*
   — Secondary gain
3 Briquet's (familial) syndrome
   — Multiple recurrent somatic complaints
4 Ganser syndrome
   — Amnesia, pseudodementia
   — Fugue state, hallucinations
   — Absurd answers, abrupt termination
5 Multiple personality
6 Mass hysteria

ANOREXIA NERVOSA

Physical findings in the patient with anorexia nervosa
1 Vital signs
   — Bradycardia
   — Hypotension
   — Hypothermia
2 Musculoskeletal
   — Marked weight loss
   — Myopathy (nutritional)
   — Weakness (hypokalemic)
3 Cardiovascular
   — Pallor (normochromic anemia)
   — Peripheral cyanosis
   — Arrhythmias

4 Skin
   — Carotenemia
   — Excessive lanugo hair
   — Edema (secondary hyperaldosteronism)
5 Gastrointestinal
   — Parotidomegaly
   — Rectal prolapse
6 Hypothermia

NB: Secondary sexual development is *normal* in anorexia nervosa

Investigating anorexia nervosa: potential abnormalities
1 Elevated plasma urea
2 Abnormal LFTs
3 'Sick euthyroid'
4 Elevated growth hormone, reduced somatomedin C
5 Multifollicular cystic ovaries on pelvic ultrasound

Complications of anorexia nervosa other than amenorrhea
1 Dental caries
2 Gastric dilatation or atrophy
3 Constipation, cathartic colon
4 Renal calculi
5 Osteoporosis

INVESTIGATING PSYCHIATRIC DISORDERS

INVESTIGATION OF DEMENTIA

Investigation of the patient with presenile dementia
1 Looking to exclude reversible organic etiologies
   — CT brainscan (see below)
   — Thyroid function tests/TSH
   — Vitamin B_{12} (B_1, B_6) assay
   — VDRL
2 HIV serology (in 'at-risk' patients)
3 Drugs
4 Depression

Prerequisites for CT scanning in dementia
1 Presenile onset
2 Less than 2 years' duration
3 Mild to moderate in severity
4 Patient fit for neurosurgery if indicated

Reversible pathologies excluded by CT scanning
1 Space-occupying intracerebral lesion (tumor, abscess)*
2 Subdural hematoma
3 Normal pressure hydrocephalus

NB: *Unilateral* cerebral abnormalities usually do not affect conscious state
* e.g. subfrontal meningioma

Neuroreceptor radioligand brain imaging modalities
1 ^{123}I-labeled
   — MIBG: Norepinephrine receptor
   — Iodobenzamide: Dopamine D2 receptor
   — Iomazenil: Benzodiazepine receptor
   — Iododexetemide: Muscarinic ACh receptor
   — Epibatidine: Nicotinic ACh receptor

2 ^{18}F-labeled
— Fluoro-trifluperazine: Serotonin (5HT1) receptor
— Setoperone: Serotonin (5HT2) receptor
— Fluoro-carazolol: β-adrenergic receptor
— Fluoro-DOPA: Dopamine transporter
3 ^{111}In-labeled
— Octreotide: Somatostatin receptor
4 ^{11}C-labeled
— Carfentanil: μ-opioid receptor

THE ABNORMAL BRAIN BIOPSY

Definitive histological confirmation of Alzheimer's disease
1 Cerebral amyloid (A4) angiopathy, *plus*
2 Neuritic β-amyloid plaques*, *and/or*
3 Neurofibrillary tangles*

* Correlate quantitatively with dementia severity

Dementia: neurofibrillary tangles in autopsied brain?
1 Alzheimer's disease
2 Post-encephalitic parkinsonism*
3 Dementia pugilistica ('punch-drunk' syndrome)
4 Creutzfeldt–Jakob disease
5 SSPE

* cf. sporadic Parkinson's disease → Lewy bodies

MANAGING PSYCHIATRIC DISEASE

IATROGENIC ORGANIC BRAIN SYNDROMES

Drugs commonly causing confusion in the elderly
1 Digoxin (may also → fatigue, euphoria)
2 Propranolol (also → nightmares, insomnia); methyldopa
3 Indometacin (also → vertigo, headache)
4 Cimetidine (esp. in renal or hepatic insufficiency)
5 Amantadine, L-DOPA (esp. if used with anticholinergics)
6 Sedative-hypnotics, tricyclics, phenothiazines; alcohol

Psychiatric side-effects of steroid therapy
1 Commoner in
— High-dose treatment
— Prolonged duration of treatment
— Patient with psychiatric history
2 Commonest symptom
— Euphoria*
3 Frank psychosis
— Affects about 5%

* cf. primary Cushing's disease → depression

ACETYLCHOLINESTERASE INHIBITORS

Acetylcholinesterase inhibitors of value in Alzheimer's disease
1 Tacrine*
2 Donepezil
3 Rivastigmine

* Tetrahydro-9-acridinamine-monohydrochloride

Pros and cons of antiacetylcholinesterase therapy for Alzheimer's
1 Side-effects
— Hepatotoxicity*
— Nausea, diarrhea
2 Efficacy
— Cognitive benefits are mild‡
— Course of disease is unchanged
— Prolongs CNS cholinergic activity, thus reversing one of the key neurotransmitter defects in Alzheimer's

* Must monitor ALT; withdraw drug if ALT > 3× normal
‡ Benefits about 20% of patients with mild to moderate disease

ANTIPSYCHOTIC DRUG THERAPY

Clinical spectrum of lithium toxicity (level > 1.5 mmol/L)*
1 CNS toxicity
— Lethargy → drowsiness → seizures → coma
2 Gastrointestinal toxicity
— Nausea, vomiting, diarrhea
3 Cerebellar toxicity
— Tremulousness; dysarthria; ataxia
4 Renal toxicity
— Polyuria, polydipsia (nephrogenic diabetes insipidus)
— Affects 30% but usually subclinical; may → renal failure
5 Thyroid toxicity
— Goiter, hypothyroidism
6 Cardiovascular
— ECG → T-wave flattening/inversion
— Cardiovascular collapse in massive overdose

* Lower plasma levels may cause toxicity, esp. in *sodium-depleted* patients (e.g. on diuretics) or in *dehydration* due to vomiting, diarrhea or polyuria

Drug classes used to treat endogenous depression
1 'First-generation' antidepressants
— Tricyclic antidepressants: e.g. amitriptyline, imipramine, dosulepin
— Tetracyclic antidepressants: e.g. mianserin
— Monoamine uptake inhibitors (MAOIs): e.g. phenelzine, moclobemide
2 'Second-generation' antidepressants
— Selective serotonin reuptake inhibitors (SSRIs): e.g. fluoxetine (Prozac), paroxetine, sertraline, citalopram, fluvoxamine
3 'Third-generation' antidepressants
— Nefazodone: a mixed SSRI and 5-HT$_2$ receptor blocker

— Venlafaxine: a mixed SSRI and norepinephrine reuptake inhibitor
— Mirtazapine: a norepinephrine-specific serotonergic antidepressant*
— Lofepramine: a newer, improved tricyclic with lower toxicity

*α_2 adrenergic receptor antagonist, *and* 5-HT$_2$ and 5-HT$_3$ receptor antagonist

Clinical pharmacology of mianserin
1 Tetracyclic structure bears no similarity to tricyclics
2 Fewer arrhythmogenic and anticholinergic side-effects
3 Safer in overdose: an advantage in treating suicidal patients
4 Agranulocytosis (1:5000) and aplasia limit enthusiasm

Disadvantages of tricyclic antidepressants
1 Sedation
2 Postural hypotension and falls*
3 Anticholinergic effects limit compliance
4 Often fatal in overdose‡

* Also seen with SSRIs; see Ref. 13.8
‡ Lofepramine appears safer

MONOAMINE OXIDASE INHIBITORS

Pharmacologic classification of MAOIs
1 Irreversible MAOIs
— Phenelzine, tranylcypromine (antidepressants)
— Isoniazid
2 Selective MAO-B inhibitors*
— Selegiline
3 Reversible (and selective) MAO-A inhibitors
— Moclobemide

* No 'cheese effect' (tyramine-induced hypertensive crisis)

Important interactions with MAOIs
1 (Tyr)amine-rich foods (flavor often enhanced by age)
— Mature cheese
— Yeast extracts (e.g. Marmite, packet soups)
— Soya bean, broad bean pods
— Pickled herring
— Alcoholic (or dealcoholized) drinks, esp. red wine
2 Drugs
— Pethidine (may be lethal)
— Tricyclics, levodopa, terbutaline
— Amine-containing drugs, esp. cold remedies*
— SSRIs (e.g. fluoxetine‡; see below)

* Contain (pseudo)ephedrine, phenylpropanolamine
‡ cf. paroxetine: short half-life, hence can start MAOI after 2 weeks

Life-threatening MAOI interactions
1 Pseudopheochromocytoma
— Seen with SSRIs *or* drugs listed above
— Noradrenaline-mediated paroxysmal hypertension
— Other symptoms: confusion, sweating, abdominal pain

2 Serotonin syndrome (see below)
— Seen with SSRIs *or* serotoninergic tricyclics*
— Consists of CNS irritability, seizures, myoclonus
3 Management implications of these interactions
— Lethal combination; SSRIs must *never* be co-prescribed, even when 'selective' MAOIs used
— Cease MAOI 2 weeks before starting SSRI
— Cease fluoxetine ≥ 5 weeks before starting MAOI

* e.g. clomipramine, amitriptyline

Management of MAOI-induced hypertensive crisis
1 IV phentolamine 5–10 mg
2 IV chlorpromazine 25 mg

SELECTIVE SEROTONIN REUPTAKE INHIBITORS (SSRIs)

Advantages of SSRIs over tricyclic antidepressants
1 Less muscarinic receptor blockade
— Fewer anticholinergic side-effects
2 No membrane-stabilizing effects on the heart
— Fewer arrhythmias, lower suicide risk (i.e. safer)
3 Less sedation
4 Less weight gain
5 Effective for obsessive–compulsive symptoms

Side-effects of SSRIs
1 CNS hyperstimulation
— Insomnia, 'nervy' sensation, tremor, headache
— ?Aggressive behavior, ?precipitation of mania
2 Gastrointestinal toxicity (more so than tricyclics)
— Weight loss*
— Nausea, diarrhea, abdominal discomfort
3 Sexual problems
— Reduced libido
— Delayed ejaculation
4 General malaise ± cognitive impairment
5 Sweating
6 Hyponatremia

* Or, less often, weight gain

Major drug interactions with SSRIs
1 SSRI potentiation (esp. CNS excitation)
— MAOIs
— Lithium
— Selegiline*
— Sumatriptan
2 Potentiation of interacting drug
— Tricyclics (cardiotoxicity)
— Warfarin (hemorrhage)

* Esp. if using fluoxetine

ANTISCHIZOPHRENIC DRUG THERAPY

Drugs used in schizophrenia
1 Conventional strategies
— Dopamine-blocking neuroleptics
• Phenothiazines (e.g. chlorpromazine)
• Butyrophenones (e.g. haloperidol)

2 Refractory cases ('atypical' neuroleptics)
— Clozapine
• 5-HT$_2$ receptor blocker; a very potent antipsychotic
• Minimal extrapyramidal toxicity
• Lowest risk for inducing tardive dyskinesias
• Agranulocytosis occurs in 0.5%; hence, monitor blood count *weekly*
• May cause troublesome hypotension
• Dose-dependent seizure induction
— Risperidone, sulpiride
• Catecholamine*/5-HT$_2$ receptor blockers
• Low incidence of extrapyramidal toxicity
• Cholinergic rebound may occur when converting from older drugs
• May cause major increase in prolactin levels
• Minimal sedation (cf. clozapine); good for apathetic patients
— Olanzapine
• Good option if extrapyramidal toxicity is a problem
• Transaminitis may occur
— Sertindole
• Increased QT interval is a hazard (2% incidence)
• ECG monitoring is required; limits utility

* Incl. dopamine D$_2$ receptors

NEUROLEPTIC SIDE-EFFECTS

Distinguishing features of drug-induced movement disorders
1 Neuroleptic-induced pseudoparkinsonism
— Usually appears after several months of therapy
— Commoner in high dosage and in *elderly* patients, esp. if demented
— May remit with continued treatment, respond to conventional antiparkinsonian therapy, or persist despite total drug withdrawal
— May be indistinguishable from Parkinson's disease
— Occurs in 20–30% of treated patients
— Treat with anticholinergics
2 Neuroleptic-induced acute dystonic reactions
— Usually occur within 24 h of (usually initial) dosage; occasionally precipitated by drug withdrawal
— May be due to metoclopramide*
— Commoner in *men* than women, *young* > old
— Occurs within 48 h of administration; duration variable
— May be preceded by akathisia, grimacing, hyperreflexia
— May → oculogyric crisis, opisthotonus, trismus/torticollis
— Responsive to IV benzatropine, diphenhydramine
— Affects approximately 2% of treated patients
3 Neuroleptic-induced tardive dyskinesia
— Insidious onset; may be unmasked after dose reduction
— Affects 30% after 4 years' therapy‡

— Commoner in *women* than men, *elderly* > young
— Probably reflects dopamine receptor hypersensitivity
— *No* subjective patient distress; disappears during sleep
— 40% remit after drug ceased; 60% persist or worsen
— Treat with tetrabenazine (also used in Huntington's)
— Continued treatment with offending drug does *not* increase severity of dyskinesia, but *does* reduce likelihood of remission (disorder not progressive)

* cf. *rarely* causes parkinsonism or tardive dyskinesia; avoid in children
‡ But *may* occur as early as 3 months

Neuroleptic drug toxicity: major associations
1 Sedation
— Chlorpromazine; risperidone, clozapine, thioridazine
2 Hypotension
— Chlorpromazine; clozapine
3 Extrapyramidal effects
— Haloperidol, pimozide; chlorpromazine; fluphenazine, trifluoperazine
4 Anticholinergic effects
— Clozapine, thioridazine; chlorpromazine

Clinical features of tardive dyskinesia
1 Orofacial dyskinesia: hyperkinesis of cheeks/tongue/mouth
— 'Fly-catcher's tongue'
— 'Bon-bon' sign
— Rumination, pouting
2 Glottal dyskinesia
— Grunting
3 Blepharospasm, increased blink frequency
4 Torticollis
5 Upper limbs
— 'Piano-playing' fingers
— Choreiform or ballistic movements
— Shoulder shrugging
6 Lower limbs
— Foot-tapping
— Great toe dorsiflexion

Differential diagnosis of tardive dyskinesia
1 Huntington's disease
Wilson's disease
— Patients may be receiving phenothiazines for psychiatric disorder, but develop extrapyramidal symptoms de novo
2 Gilles de la Tourette's syndrome
— Grimacing and profanities in children
— Important to diagnose, since treatable with haloperidol

Features of neuroleptic malignant syndrome*
1 Clinical signs
— Fever
— Rigidity
— Autonomic dysfunction

- Fluctuations of heart rate, blood pressure
- Sphincter disturbance
- Sweating, salivation
— Clouding of consciousness
2 Diagnosis
— Grossly elevated plasma CPK ± renal failure
— Leukocytosis
3 Therapy
— Dantrolene
— Bromocriptine
4 Outcome
— Up to 50% die

* = Malignant hyperthermia

TREATMENT OF ANXIETY STATES

Drugs of choice for treating anxiety*
1 Panic disorder
— Alprazolam; sertraline, paroxetine
2 Social phobia
— Moclobemide, paroxetine
3 Generalized anxiety
— Buspirone‡, venlafaxine
4 Stage fright
— Propranolol
5 Post-traumatic stress disorder
— Sertraline
6 Bulimia nervosa
— Fluoxetine
7 Obsessive–compulsive disorder
— SSRIs (e.g. fluvoxamine, fluoxetine)
8 Premenstrual dysphoric syndrome
— Sertraline

* NB: Cognitive–behavior therapy is often the most critical intervention
‡ A 5-HT$_{1A}$ receptor partial agonist

DRUGS USED IN ADDICTION

Drugs used to control opiate withdrawal symptoms
1 Naltrexone*
2 Methadone
3 Buprenorphine
4 Lofexidine
5 Fluoxetine, fluvoxamine

* For *either* accelerated detoxification *or* as relapse prevention

Drugs used to control alcohol withdrawal symptoms
1 Benzodiazepines
2 β-blockers
3 Clomethiazole

Drugs used to promote alcohol abstinence
1 Disulfiram (an aldehyde dehydrogenase inhibitor)
2 Acamprosate* (a GABA agonist)
3 Citalopram (an SSRI)

4 Naltrexone (oral opioid antagonist)

* Calcium acetyl homotaurinate, which resembles the inhibitory neurotransmitter GABA. This drug needs to be administered together with counselling.

CANNABINOIDS

Side effects of cannabis use
1 Anxiety, panic
Paranoia; visual hallucinations
Predisposition to schizophrenia in chronic users
2 Tachycardia
Supine hypertension with postural hypotension
3 Bronchitis, emphysema
4 'Amotivational syndrome'

Potential therapeutic scenarios for cannabinoid use
1 Nausea (e.g. prior to cancer chemotherapy)
2 Glaucoma
3 Spasticity

ELECTROCONVULSIVE THERAPY (ECT)

Indications for ECT
1 Severe depression in patients resistant to tri-/tetracyclics
2 Severe depression complicated by dehydration or weight loss
3 Depression associated with suicidal ideation or delusions
4 Drug-resistant mania
5 Puerperal psychosis (treatment of choice)

Contraindications to ECT
1 Increased intracranial pressure
2 Known cerebral aneurysm
3 Past history of
— Cerebrovascular disease
— Myocardial infarction
— Aortic aneurysm
4 Unfit for general anesthesia

PSYCHOSURGERY

Potential indications for psychosurgery
1 Cingulotomy
— Refractory incapacitating obsessional neurosis
2 Ventromedial frontal lobe surgery
— No longer used for schizophrenia
— Occasionally still used for severe refractory depression
3 Temporal lobectomy, callosal sectioning, commissurotomy
— Drug-resistant epilepsy

UNDERSTANDING PSYCHIATRIC DISEASE

Spectrum of self-inflicted diseases
1 Münchausen syndrome
2 Diuretic and/or laxative abuse*
3 Factitious fever
4 Factitious hypoglycemia
5 Thyrotoxicosis factitia
6 Dermatitis artefacta

* Results in symptomatic hypokalemia, nephropathy

NEUROTRANSMITTER ABNORMALITIES

Neurotransmitter abnormalities in schizophrenia
1 ↓ Somatostatin
2 ↓ CCK } — In the hippocampus

Neurotransmitter abnormalities in Huntington's chorea
1 Preservation of *aspiny* neurons in caudate
   — ↑ Somatostatin
   — ↑ Dopamine
2 Depletion of striatal *spiny* neurons
   — ↓ GABA
   — ↓ Substance P
   — ↓ Metenkephalin
   — ↓ Acetylcholine

PATHOGENESIS OF ALZHEIMER'S DISEASE

Neurotransmitter abnormalities in Alzheimer's disease
1 ↓ Acetylcholine (neuronal degeneration in nucleus basalis)
2 ↓ Somatostatin (cortical degeneration of *aspiny* neurons)
3 ↓ Noradrenaline (neuronal degeneration in locus ceruleus)
4 ↓ Dopamine (neuronal degeneration in ventral tegmentum)
5 ↓ Serotonin (degeneration of raphé nucleus)

Role of the ApoE4 allele in Alzheimer's disease
1 Predisposes to *early onset* of the disease
2 Genotyping can improve diagnostic accuracy in patients who are already clinically considered to have signs of the disease
3 Negative predictive value is *poor**

* i.e. negativity for the allele is diagnostically *unhelpful*

REVIEWING THE LITERATURE: PSYCHIATRY

13.1 Keller MB et al (2000) A comparison of nefazodone, the cognitive behavioral analysis system of psychotherapy, and their combination for the treatment of depression. N Engl J Med 342: 1462–1470

Therapeutic benefit was seen using either antidepressants or psychotherapy, but the depression improved most when both were used together.

13.2 Berger SP et al (1996) Haloperidol antagonism of cue-elicited cocaine craving. Lancet 347: 504–508

Randomized study of 20 cocaine addicts, showing that pretreatment with haloperidol reduced drug craving.

13.3 Itzhaki RF et al (1997) Herpes simplex virus type 1 in brain and risk of Alzheimer's disease. Lancet 349: 241–244

Controversial autopsy study of Alzheimer patients showing that the ApoE4 genotype was associated not only with Alzheimer's, but also with a four-fold increased risk of cold sores (suggesting a possible pathogenetic link with HSV1).

13.4 Bookheimer SY et al (2000)Patterns of brain activation in people at risk of Alzheimer's disease. N Engl J Med 343: 450–456

Study of 30 neurologically normal individuals, half of whom expressed ApoE4 allele, and half of whom expressed ApoE3. Functional MRI revealed greater brain activation in the at-risk (ApoE4-positive) subgroup, suggesting that such activation may play a pathogenetic role.

13.5 Doll R et al (2000) Smoking and dementia in male British doctors: prospective study. Br Med J 320: 1097–1102

Ott A et al (1998) Smoking and risk of dementia and Alzheimer's disease in a population-based cohort study: the Rotterdam Study. Lancet 351: 1840–1843

Two studies contradicting earlier reports of a reciprocal association between smoking and dementia. The former study showed no significant effect, whereas the latter found a doubling of dementia risk in smokers, *unless* (unexpectedly) they were ApoE4-positive.

13.6 Rosler A et al (1998) Treatment of men with paraphilia with a long-acting analogue of gonadotropin-releasing hormone. N Engl J Med 338: 416–422

Treatment of 25 pedophiliacs with monthly injections of a GnRH agonist reduced libido and caused impotence, suggesting a possible effective 'treatment' for their deviation.

13.7 Forette F et al (1998) Prevention of dementia in randomized double-blind placebo-controlled Systolic Hypertension in Europe trial. Lancet 352: 1347–1351

Randomized study of over 2000 elderly hypertensives, showing that antihypertensive treatment lowered the frequency of dementia.

13.8 Liu B et al (1998) Use of selective serotonin-reuptake inhibitors or tricyclic antidepressants and risk of hip fractures in elderly people. Lancet 351: 1303–1307

Case-control study of over 8000 patients, showing that exposure to either SSRIs or tricyclics increased the risk of hip fracture.

13.9 Hurt RD et al (1997) A comparison of sustained-release bupropion and placebo for smoking cessation. N Engl J Med 337: 1195–1202

Double-blind placebo-controlled study of 615 smokers showing efficacy of bupropion in facilitating smoking cessation and preventing weight gain, albeit with about a quarter having relapsed within a year.

13.10 Liu RS et al (2000) Association between brain size and abstinence from alcohol. Lancet 355: 1969–1971

Serial measurements confirmed an increase in cerebral, cerebellar and hippocampal volume following abstinence from alcohol, indicating that the well-known alcohol-induced brain shrinkage is at least partially reversible.

13.11 Glassman AH et al (2001) Smoking cessation and the course of major depression. Lancet 357: 1929–1932

Prospective study of 100 smokers with a depressive history, showing that those trying to kick the smoking habit had a much higher incidence of recurrent depression.

CHAPTER 14

Renal and urologic disease

Physical examination protocol 14.1   You are asked to examine a patient for signs of renal disease

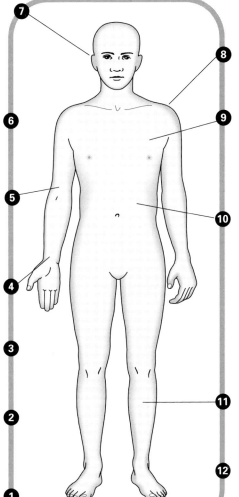

Eyes:
band keratopathy
cataract (diabetes, steroids)

Fundus:
hypertension, diabetes

Ears:
deafness (Alport's)

Face:
butterfly rash; mouse-like

Mouth:
ammoniacal fetor

Hydration:
skin turgor; JVP
eyeball pressure

Skin:
pallor, purpura, pigment
'urea frost'
scratch marks
tophi, xanthomata
vasculitic lesions
'half-and-half' nails

Fistula/external shunt in situ
(with bruit and/or thrill) – if
absent, assess vascular access

Hypertension, orthostasis
Fever, tachycardia
Sputum – hemoptysis

General:
level of consciousness
Cushingoid stigmata
hiccups, twitching
flapping tremor

Introduce yourself
Position the patient
Obtain adequate exposure

Proximal weakness (↓ Vit D,
steroid myopathy)

Chest:
pericardial rub
basal crepitations
sacral edema
vertebral tenderness

Abdomen:
transplant scar(s)
Tenchkoff catheter
ballottable kidney(s)
hepatosplenomegaly
(e.g. PCK, amyloid)
loin tenderness
bladder distension
epigastric/graft bruit
left-sided varicocele
PR: enlarged prostate

Edema
Peripheral pulses
Neuropathy

Urinalysis and microscopy

COMMON AND CLASSIC RENAL/UROLOGIC PROBLEMS

Common renal and urologic problems in clinical practice
1 Acute urinary retention
2 Incontinence
3 Acute renal failure

Classic renal and urologic problems in clinical exams
1 Polycystic kidneys
2 Renal transplant (± cushingoid)
3 Chronic renal failure

RENAL AND UROLOGIC EMERGENCIES

Urological emergencies: assessment and approach
1 Acute retention
 — Catheterization
2 Ureteric obstruction
 — Stent(s) or percutaneous nephrostomy
3 Hemorrhagic cystitis
 — Alum irrigation
4 Priapism (p. 380)

CLINICAL ASSESSMENT OF RENAL DISEASE

The abdominal mass: why do you think it's a kidney?
1 Able to get above it
2 Moves little with respiration
3 Bimanually ballottable
4 Resonant on percussing above

Clinical assessment of hydration status
1 Vital signs
 — Heart rate, blood pressure
 — Marked orthostatic response if dehydrated
2 Weight loss
 — Mildly dehydrated: < 3%
 — Profoundly dehydrated: > 10%
3 Skin turgor/elasticity
 — Test over tibiae, scapulae, sternum
 — Reduction implies at least moderate dehydration
 Eyeball pressure
4 CNS signs
 — Confusion (may reflect severe dehydration)
5 Urine output
 — Less than 30 mL/h suggests hypovolemia
6 Signs of fluid overload
 — Tachycardia, tachypnea
 — Elevated JVP
 — S_3, gallop
 — Aortic incompetent murmur (e.g. if dialysis overdue)
 — Pulmonary and/or peripheral edema

RENAL FAILURE

Minimal diagnostic criteria for acute renal failure
1 Oliguria (< 500 mL/day)

2 Rising serum creatinine, urea, phosphate and potassium
3 Declining serum calcium and bicarbonate

Features indicating chronicity of renal failure
1 Band keratopathy
2 Peripheral neuropathy
3 Bilaterally shrunken kidneys on plain abdominal film or IVP
4 CXR: annular calcification of mitral/aortic valve(s)
5 Renal osteodystrophy on X-ray and biopsy

Potentially reversible precipitants of renal failure
1 Vascular
 — Prolonged hypotension (e.g. dehydration, shock, CCF)
 — Malignant hypertension
 — Vasculitis (esp. Goodpasture's syndrome)
 — Renal vein thrombosis
2 Obstruction (exclude with ultrasound)
 — Prostatomegaly
 — Bladder atony (e.g. in diabetic autonomic neuropathy)
 — Calculi
 — Idiopathic retroperitoneal fibrosis
 — Tumor infiltration (e.g. Ca bladder → ureteric orifices)
3 Infection*
 — Pyelonephritis (? secondary to subacute obstruction)
 — Septicemia → acute tubular necrosis
 — Glomerulonephritis (see below)
 — Genitourinary TB → upper tract obstruction
 — Amyloidosis (e.g. due to chronic UTI in paraplegic)
4 Metabolic derangement
 — Acute hyperuricemia (e.g. tumor lysis syndrome)
 — Hypercalcemia
 — Chronic hypokalemia (laxative abuse, Conn's)
 — Heavy metal poisoning
5 Iatrogenic
 — Radiographic contrast examination‡, esp. IVP
 — Drug toxicity (e.g. NSAIDs, aminoglycosides)

* Esp. in patients with single kidneys or pre-existing renal impairment
‡ Renal failure of this etiology may be avoided by prehydration together with prophylactic oral administration of the antioxidant acetylcysteine

Renal failure due to glomerulonephritis?
1 Intrinsic renal disease
 — Normal serum complement
 • IgA nephropathy (commonest nephritis)
 — Low serum complement
 • Acute (post-infectious) GN
 • Membranoproliferative GN
2 Systemic disease
 — Normal serum complement
 • PAN, Wegener's (ANCA-positive)
 • Anti-GBM disease (Goodpasture's)
 • Henoch-Schönlein purpura
 — Low serum complement
 • SLE
 • SBE
 • *Staphylococcus albus*: 'shunt nephritis'

Clinical evolution of renal dysfunction
1 Reduced renal reserve (creatinine clearance 60–100 mL/min)
   — Asymptomatic
2 Renal insufficiency (creatinine clearance 30–60 mL/min)
   — Nocturia; leg cramps
   — Hypertension
   — Hyperuricemia: elevated blood urea nitrogen
3 Renal failure (creatinine clearance 15–30 mL/min)
   — Nausea, anorexia, diarrhea
   — Edema; infections; occult bleeding, mouth ulcers
   — Phosphate retention; metabolic acidosis
   — Anemia (exception: polycystic disease)
4 Uremia (creatinine clearance < 15 mL/min)
   — Lethargy, irritability ($\rightarrow$ fits, coma)
   — Pruritus, hiccups, flapping tremor
   — Pericarditis; pulmonary edema
   — Bone pain
   — Hyperkalemia
   — Hypocalcemia, $\uparrow$ alkaline phosphatase

Common indicators of inadequate dialysis
1 Nausea, vomiting, anorexia, diarrhea
2 Weakness, weight loss, poor functional capacity, obtundation
3 Fluid retention, ascites, hypertension
4 Neuropathy
5 Pericarditis
6 Persistent anemia resistant to erythropoietin

RENAL DISORDERS IN MULTISYSTEM DISEASE

Renal failure with hemoptysis: differential diagnosis
1 Goodpasture's syndrome
   Wegener's granulomatosis
   Henoch-Schönlein purpura
   PAN, SLE, cryoglobulinemia
2 Renal vein thrombosis with pulmonary embolism
3 Acute renal failure with pulmonary edema
4 Right-sided infective endocarditis with septic pulmonary emboli and immune-complex nephritis
5 Infection: tuberculosis, Legionnaires' disease, HIV

Renal disease with jaundice: differential diagnosis
1 Hemolytic–uremic syndrome
2 Hepatorenal failure (hepatic nephropathy)
3 Leptospirosis (Weil's disease)
4 Hepatitis B with nephrotic syndrome
5 Alcoholic cirrhosis with IgA nephropathy
6 Polycystic disease with congenital hepatic fibrosis
7 Stauffer's syndrome: renal cell carcinoma with non-metastatic hepatic dysfunction (e.g. cholestasis)
8 Toxic: CCl_4, methoxyflurane

Hepatorenal failure: clinical features
1 Occurs in advanced liver failure
2 Precipitated by
   — Diuretics, paracentesis
   — Portocaval shunt
   — Biliary contrast radiography

3 Characterized by
   — Oliguria
   — Normal urinary sediment
   — Urinary sodium < 5 mmol/L
4 No improvement following IV volume repletion*
5 Transplanted kidneys work well in host with normal liver

* cf. prerenal failure

Diagnostic significance of skin lesions in renal failure
1 Impetigo, erythema nodosum
   — Suggest post-streptococcal glomerulonephritis
2 Purpura
   — Amyloid ('pinch'; post-proctoscopic periorbital type)
   — Vasculitis (palpable)
   — Henoch-Schönlein ($\rightarrow$ thigh, buttock)
   — Cryoglobulinemia (± ulceration, gangrene)
3 Inherited nephropathies
   — Scrotal angiokeratomata (Fabry's disease)
   — Carotenemic pigmentation (Balkan nephropathy)
   — Hypoplastic nails (nail–patella syndrome)
   — Adenoma sebaceum, ash-leaf macules (tuberous sclerosis; angiomyolipomata $\rightarrow$ massive hematuria)

SYMPTOMS AND SIGNS OF RENAL DISEASE

Renal disease with small kidney(s) size
1 Chronic glomerulonephritis
   — Symmetrically smooth
2 Chronic pyelonephritis
   — Asymmetrically scarred
   — Cortical scars opposite dilated calices, esp. upper poles
3 Medullary cystic disease
4 Post-obstructive atrophy
5 Renovascular insufficiency
6 Late stage of many diseases causing large kidneys initially

Renal disease with bilateral renal enlargement
1 Polycystic disease
2 Medullary sponge kidneys
3 Obstructive uropathy (bilateral hydronephrosis)
4 Acute nephropathies
   — Acute glomerulonephritis
   — Acute interstitial nephritis
   — Acute tubular necrosis
   — Acute urate nephropathy
5 Other
   — Amyloidosis
   — Renal vein thrombosis (± nephrosis, amyloid)
   — Insulin-dependent diabetes
   — Acromegaly (renal function typically normal)
   — Radiation nephritis

Common features of interstitial nephritis
1 Fever, arthralgias, rash
2 Renal failure with microhematuria ± polyuria/pyuria
3 Eosinophilia (esp. if drug-induced), eosinophiluria > 5%

4 Abnormal liver function tests
5 Radiographically enlarged kidneys

Differential diagnosis of loin pain
1 Calculus; sloughed papilla
2 Pyelonephritis; perinephric abscess
3 Acute glomerulonephritis (esp. proliferative)
4 Vesicoureteric reflux
5 Hemorrhage into cyst; infected cyst
6 Segmental infarction (sickle-cell disease, embolism)

Nocturia: diagnostic significance
1 Prostatism
2 Edematous states
3 Salt-losing nephropathies, e.g.
— Analgesic nephropathy
— Medullary sponge kidneys
— Sickle cell disease
4 Polyuric states, e.g.
— Diabetes mellitus/insipidus
— Primary polydipsia
— Post-ATN
5 Bladder pathology
— Tumor, fibrosis, infection
— Loss of reflex inhibition (e.g. multiple sclerosis)
— Vesicoureteric reflux ('double micturition' in children)

INVESTIGATING RENAL DISEASE

URINARY ABNORMALITIES

Highly diagnostic features on urine microscopy
1 Red cell casts (acute glomerulonephritis)
2 Doubly-refractile oval fat bodies (nephrotic syndrome)

Urinary stigmata of glomerular disease
1 Red cell casts
2 Heavy proteinuria (> 2 g/day)
3 Pleomorphic red cells on phase-contrast microscopy

Clinically important causes of 'sterile pyuria'
1 Inadequately treated urinary tract infection
2 Genitourinary TB, or other fastidious organism, e.g.
— *Strep. morbillorum/agalactiae/milleri*
— *Corynebacteria,* lactobacilli
3 Inflammatory non-infective disease
— Papillary necrosis (esp. analgesic nephropathy)*
— Calculi (renal or bladder)
— Interstitial nephritis/polycystic disease (light pyuria)
4 Lower tract inflammation
— Prostatitis
— Chemical cystitis (e.g. due to cyclophosphamide)
5 Dysuria–pyuria ('urethral') syndrome
— Pathogenic bacteriuria < 10^5 organisms/mL
— Bacterial urethritis (e.g. chlamydial)
— Periurethral herpes simplex

6 'False pyuria' (i.e. nil on suprapubic tap)
— Primary vaginal infection, poor specimen collection
— e.g. *Gardnerella vaginalis, Candida albicans, Trichomonas*

* Can be reliably diagnosed by CT scanning without contrast

Urinary tract infection: factors favoring pyelonephritis
1 Clinical
— Loin pain/tenderness, fever, tachycardia, rigors
2 Urine microscopy
— White blood cell casts
3 Blood
— Leukocytosis ± positive blood cultures
4 IVP
— Poor excretion of contrast on affected side
5 Therapy
— Failure of appropriate single-dose antibiotics

Iatrogenic causes of reddish urine*
1 Drug excretion products
— Rifampicin
— Metronidazole
— Sulfasalazine
— Doxorubicin
— Desferrioxamine
2 Drug toxicity
— Drugs inducing acute intermittent porphyria
— Drugs inducing rhabdomyolysis (e.g. clofibrate, heroin)
— Drugs inducing hematuria (e.g. warfarin, urokinase)

* But note that eating beetroot may also cause red urine in 15% of individuals

Myoglobinuria: precipitants and laboratory features
1 Causes
— Muscle crush injury
— Hyperthermia (e.g. malignant) ± convulsions
— Polymyositis
— McArdle's syndrome
— Meyer–Betz (familial) disease
— Haff disease
— Drugs: acute alcoholic binge; heroin; 'angel dust' (phencyclidine, PCP); clofibrate
2 Features
— Acute oliguric renal failure with red urine
— Urinalysis 'heme +', but no red cells on microscopy
— Serum clear*
— Initial hypocalcemia → 'rebound' hypercalcemia
— ↑ Serum potassium, phosphate, urate

* Myoglobin does not bind haptoglobin and is thus renally cleared immediately; cf. intravascular hemolysis

Crystalluria: differential diagnosis
1 Cystinuria (autosomal recessive)
2 Xanthinuria (hereditary *or* allopurinol-induced)
3 Orotic aciduria (hereditary)
4 Uricosuria (acquired, hereditary or drug-induced)
5 APRT* deficiency (→ 2,8-dihydroxyadenine urolithiasis)

6 Hyperoxaluria
  — Autosomal recessive (pyridoxine-responsive)
  — Ileal disease‡ (e.g. Crohn's, resection)
  — Toxic: ethylene glycol ingestion, methoxyflurane
7 Drugs
  — Sulfadiazine, nitrofurantoin
  — Acetazolamide, triamterene
  — Aciclovir; 5-FC

* Adenine phosphoribosyltransferase
‡ Calculous tendency partly due to *hypocitruria* → alkaline urine

PROTEINURIA

Clinical sequelae of heavy proteinuria
1 Edema
2 Weakness (muscle catabolism ± diuretic-induced ↑ K^+)
3 Frothy urine
4 Postural hypotension
5 Thromboembolism (incl. renal vein thrombosis)
6 Hypercholesterolemia (xanthomata, vascular disease)

Laboratory characterization of proteinuria
1 *Selective* (glomerular) proteinuria is characterized by urinary losses of albumin and/or transferrin primarily
2 *Non-selective* proteinuria leads to loss of IgG; *selectivity* may therefore be quantified by urinary albumin:IgG ratio
3 Similarly, *tubular* proteinuria may be confirmed by the urinary β_2 microglobulin:albumin ratio
4 Low IgG:transferrin (albumin) ratios predict steroid responsiveness in nephrotic syndrome (e.g. 'minimal lesion' with selective proteinuria)
5 *Microalbuminuria* is excessive urinary protein excretion which is persistently less than that detectable by conventional dipstick testing

Clinical significance of microalbuminuria
1 Defined as overnight urinary albumin excretion in the range 20–200 g/min
2 Predicts impending nephropathy in diabetes mellitus
3 Correlates with hypertension in diabetics and in the general population
4 Predicts morbidity and death from cardiovascular causes in both diabetics and the general population

Characteristics of benign orthostatic proteinuria
1 Non-selective
2 Benign sediment
3 < 1 g/day
4 Typical diurnal fluctuation
5 No increase with time

Diagnostic utility of proteinuria in renal failure
1 Trace or undetectable proteinuria
  — Pre- or post-renal failure
2 Mild-to-moderate proteinuria
  — Acute interstitial nephritis*
  — Ischemia or nephrotoxicity

3 Moderate-to-severe proteinuria
  — Acute glomerulonephritis‡

* With white cell (incl. eosinophil) casts
‡ With red cell casts

NEPHROTIC SYNDROME

Laboratory manifestations of the nephrotic syndrome
1 ↓ Albumin
2 ↓ Transferrin
  → Iron-resistant hypochromic anemia
3 ↓ IgG, ↑ α_2 globulins
  → Hypogammaglobulinemia
4 ↓ 25-hydroxyvitamin D (due to urinary losses)
  → Secondary reduction in 1,25 dihydroxyvitamin D
5 ↑ Cholesterol*
  → Accelerated atherosclerosis

NB: GFR may be overestimated by creatinine clearance. Reduced GFR (reflecting hypovolemia rather than renal damage) is more accurately measured using ^{51}Cr-EDTA clearance
* Occurs due to increased synthesis of LDL apoprotein B; treat with statins

Prothrombotic changes in nephrosis*
1 ↓ Plasma volume
2 ↑ Fibrinogen, ↓ plasminogen
3 ↑ Factor V, VIII
4 ↓ AT-III
5 ↑ Platelet factor IV and ADP
6 Thrombocytosis

* e.g. predisposing to renal vein thrombosis

Prognostic variables in the nephrotic syndrome
1 Clinical features portending poor prognosis
  — Oliguria; hematuria
  — Hypertension
  — Purpura
2 Results portending poor prognosis
  — Non-selective proteinuria
  — Hypocomplementemia
3 Etiologic significance of steroid-resistance in minimal change disease
  — Hodgkin's disease
  — Amyloid
  — Focal sclerosis (i.e. biopsy sampling error)
4 Indications for alkylator therapy in minimal change disease
  — At least two relapses after initial response to steroids

GLOMERULAR DISEASE

Investigation of unexplained glomerular disease
1 Urinalysis: blood, protein, glucose, nitrites
2 Careful microscopic examination of freshly voided urine
3 Urine screen for opiate derivatives
4 Serum albumin and 24-h urine protein

5 Infection screen
  — ASO titre, HBsAg, VDRL
  — Thick/thin film (if history of travel/malarial exposure)
  — Blood cultures
    • Infective endocarditis
    • 'Shunt' (*S. albus*) nephritis
    • Pneumococcal peritonitis
    • Brucellosis, leptospirosis
6 CXR
  — Sarcoid
  — Malignancy
7 Immunologic screen
  — ANA, rheumatoid factor; C_3, C_4
  — Cryoglobulins
  — Anti-GBM
  — EPG/IEPG/urinary BJP (± marrow pending result)
8 Rectal biopsy
  — Congo red
9 Renal biopsy
  — Light microscopy
  — Immunofluorescence, Congo red
  — Electron microscopy

NB: A low *carbamylated hemoglobin* measurement may indicate acute rather than chronic renal failure, thus clarifying desirability of urgent intervention

Spectrum of renal pathology in diabetes
1 Renal enlargement (in early insulin-dependent diabetes)
  Osmotic polyuria
2 Diffuse glomerulosclerosis
  Nodular glomerulosclerosis (Kimmelstiel–Wilson lesion)*
3 Glycogen deposition in tubules (Armanni–Ebstein lesion)
4 Interstitial nephritis
  Pyelonephritis, papillary necrosis
  Recurrent urinary tract infections
5 Hyporeninemic hypoaldosteronism ($\uparrow K^+$, $\uparrow Cl^-$)

* Suggests insulin-dependent diabetes

WHO grading of renal pathology in SLE
1 Normal light microscopic appearances
  Positive mesangial immunofluorescence
2 Mesangial changes only
3 Focal proliferative glomerulonephritis
4 Diffuse proliferative glomerulonephritis
5 Membranous glomerulonephritis
6 Advanced sclerosis*

* Important diagnosis, since absent inflammation contraindicates treatment

Electron microscopy of renal disease
1 Minimal lesion nephrosis
  — Epithelial podocyte fusion
2 Fanconi syndrome, congenital nephrosis
  — 'Swan-neck' deformity, dilatation of proximal tubule
3 Alport's syndrome
  — Splitting of lamina densa and lamina propria of glomerular basement membrane*

4 Medullary cystic disease
  — Cystic dilatation at corticomedullary junction
5 Medullary sponge kidneys, infantile polycystic kidneys
  — Dilatation of collecting ducts‡

* Similar to chronic rejection
‡ cf. adult polycystic kidneys – abnormality involves entire nephron

IMMUNOPATHOLOGY OF THE NEPHRON

Secondary causes of minimal change nephropathy
1 Lymphomas/leukemias, esp. Hodgkin's disease
2 Drugs (e.g. NSAIDs, gold, lithium)

Secondary causes of membranous nephropathy
1 Paraneoplastic
2 Autoimmune disease, esp. SLE
3 Sarcoidosis
4 Infections
  — Hepatitis B/C, syphilis
  — *Plasmodium malariae**
5 Drugs
  — Gold, penicillamine
  — Captopril (esp. high-dose)
  — NSAIDs (reversible)

* Cure of malaria will *not* necessarily lead to resolution of the nephropathy

Secondary causes of focal sclerosing glomerulonephritis
1 Heroin, or other illicit injectable drugs
2 HIV infection
3 Malignancy
4 Morbid obesity
5 Lithium therapy

Immunofluorescence of glomerular disease
1 Helpful in diagnosing early membranous nephropathy
  — Diffuse IgG ± C_3
2 Distinguishes
  — Minimal change disease (IF-)
  — Mesangial nephropathy (+IgM, weak +C_3)
3 Focal sclerosis
  — +IgM, +C_3
4 Mesangiocapillary GN
  — Bright C_3 staining
  — Modest Ig/C_{1q} staining
5 SLE
  — Heavy IgG, A, M deposits
  — +C_{1q}, C_3
  — +ANA → 5–10% (pathognomonic)
6 IgA nephropathy/HSP
  — Mesangial IgA + C_3 ± IgM/G, but *without* C_{1q} (cf. SLE)
7 Goodpasture's (associated with circulating anti-GBM)
  — *Linear* IgG in kidney, lung (rarely → SLE, rejection)
8 Post-infectious (e.g. post-strep)
  — 'Lumpy-bumpy' electron-dense deposits with +C_3

Complement levels in glomerulonephritis
1 Reduced ($\downarrow C_3$)
  — Post-infectious (SBE, 'shunt', post-strep)
  — SLE; cryoglobulinemia
  — Mesangiocapillary type I and (esp.) II
    • May be low even with quiescent nephritis
    • C_3-nephritic factor may be detectable in type II
2 Normal
  — Minimal lesion
  — IgA nephropathy
  — Goodpasture's syndrome; rapidly progressive GN
  — PAN, HSP, Wegener's
  — Membranous

Associations of IgA nephropathy
1 Cirrhosis
2 Celiac disease
3 Tuberculosis
4 Seronegative arthritis

INVESTIGATING RENAL FAILURE

Diagnostic approach to unexplained acute renal failure
1 Clinical
  — Hypovolemia (favors prerenal cause)
  — Fluid overload (favors renal/post-renal cause)
2 Urine microscopy/urinalysis/MSU
  — Helps exclude glomerulonephritis, UTI
3 Renal ultrasound
  — Excludes postrenal obstruction
4 Blood cultures, coagulation screen
  — Helps exclude septicemia, DIC
5 Renal biopsy ± high-dose IVP
  — Confirms or refutes diagnosis of glomerulonephritis

Disproportionate elevation of blood urea vs creatinine
1 Increased catabolism: trauma, infection, fever
2 Dehydration (loss of water and sodium): nephrosis, CCF
3 Gastrointestinal hemorrhage (with volume loss)
4 High protein intake
5 Drugs: tetracycline, corticosteroids, ciclosporin

Disproportionate reduction of blood urea vs creatinine
1 Liver disease
2 Pregnancy (expanded plasma volume)
3 Starvation
4 Selective increase of creatinine (muscle trauma, cimetidine)

Acute renal failure: 'prerenal' or renal origin?
1 Prerenal
  — Urinary sodium < 20 mmol/L
  — Urinary osmolality > 500 mosm/L
  — Urine:plasma osmolality > 1.5
  — Urine:plasma creatinine concentration > 40
2 Renal (e.g. acute tubular necrosis)
  — Urinary sodium > 40 mmol/L
  — Urinary osmolality < 400 mosm/L
  — Urine:plasma osmolality < 1.1
  — Urine:plasma creatinine concentration < 20

Drugs that can trigger acute renal failure
1 Prerenal (reduced renal perfusion)
  — NSAIDs
  — ACE inhibitors (e.g. in renal artery stenosis)
  — Radiocontrast agents
2 Tubular toxicity
  — Aminoglycosides
  — Cisplatin
  — Ciclosporin, tacrolimus
  — Amphotericin B
3 Hypersensitivity interstitial nephritis
  — Penicillins, cephalosporins; ciprofloxacin, rifampicin, sulfonamides
  — NSAIDs, allopurinol
  — Cimetidine, phenytoin
  — Furosemide (frusemide), thiazides
4 Intratubular drug precipitation (*see also* tumor lysis syndrome)
  — Sulfonamides, aciclovir
  — Methotrexate
5 Rhabdomyolysis
  — Fibrates, statins
6 Hemolytic uremic syndrome
  — Mitomycin
  — Quinine
  — Ciclosporin, tacrolimus

RENAL BIOPSY

Indications for renal biopsy
1 Hematuria with proteinuria
2 Hematuria with negative cystoscopy and IVP
3 Proteinuria > 1 g/day, esp. with renal impairment
4 Nephrotic syndrome in adults
5 Acute renal failure (esp. oliguric/nephritic type) following exclusion of pre- and post-renal causes
6 Chronic renal failure* with radiographically normal kidneys
7 Renal vasculitis (before and during therapy)
8 Malfunctioning transplant kidney

* But *not* end-stage, irreversible renal failure

Renal biopsy: complications and contraindications
1 Complications
  — Persistent gross hematuria
  — Pain ('clot colic', perinephric hematoma)
  — Hypotension (transient), brady-/tachycardia
  — Intrarenal AV fistula
  — Urinoma, urinary fistula
  — Hypertension (chronic)
2 Contraindications
  — Inadequate immunofluorescence/electron microscopy
  — Coagulopathy; $\downarrow$ platelet number and/or function
  — Bilaterally small kidneys on IVP
  — Diastolic BP > 120 mmHg
  — Solitary (functioning) kidney
  — Diabetic glomerulosclerosis clinically suspected
  — Established uremia

TUBULAR DISORDERS

Indicators of proximal tubular dysfunction
1 Glycosuria (i.e. without hyperglycemia)
2 Phosphaturia
3 Uricosuria
4 Aminoaciduria

Indicators of distal tubular dysfunction
1 Urinary concentration defect
 — Screen: overnight urine < 700 mosm/L is abnormal
 — Water deprivation test: < 900 mosm/L is abnormal
 — DDAVP stimulation: < 800 mosm/L is abnormal
2 Urinary acidification defect: ammonium chloride test
 — pH > 5.0 is abnormal

Pathological spectrum of renal tubular dysfunction*
1 Defective tubular responsiveness to hormones
 — Nephrogenic diabetes insipidus (XR; distal tubular dysfunction)
 — Bartter's syndrome (AR, distal)
 — Liddle's syndrome (AD, distal)
 — Pseudohypoparathyroidism (XD, proximal)
 — Hypophosphatemic rickets (XD, proximal)
2 Primary tubular defects (± intestinal transport defects)
 — 'Renal' glycosuria (AD, proximal)
 — Hartnup disease (AR, proximal)
 — Cystinuria (AR, proximal)‡
 — Cystinosis (AR, proximal; → uremia, childhood death)
 — Fanconi's (AR, proximal)¶
 — Renal tubular acidosis type I (AD, distal)
3 Secondary tubular transport defects
 — Distal tubule defects
  • Liver disease
  • Medullary sponge kidneys
  • Infantile polycystic disease
  • Amphotericin B
  • Ciclosporin toxicity
  • Lithium
 — Proximal tubule defects
  • Wilson's disease; heavy metal poisoning
  • Medullary cystic disease
  • Fanconi's syndrome; cystinosis
  • Acetazolamide use
 — Distal and/or proximal defects
  • Myeloma
  • Sjögren's syndrome, other autoimmune disorders
  • Renal transplant rejection
  • Long-standing hypercalciuria/-emia or hypokalemia
  • Obstructive uropathy
  • Analgesic nephropathy, chronic pyelonephritis

* X = X-linked, A = autosomal, R = recessive, D = dominant
‡ Recurrent calculi due to cystine loss, though ornithine, arginine and lysine – 'COAL' – are also lost
¶ Aminoaciduria, glycosuria, phosphaturia, natriuria, hypercalciuria, uricosuria, 'tubular' proteinuria

Renal tubular acidosis: clinical presentations in adults
1 Weakness (hypokalemia)
2 Bone pain (osteomalacia)
3 Constipation
4 Renal calculi
 — Calcium phosphate (± nephrocalcinosis)
 — Struvite (due to associated hypocitruria)
5 Renal failure

When to suspect renal tubular acidosis (RTA)
1 General
 — High urine pH relative to plasma pH *and*
 — Negative urine culture
2 Distal and proximal RTA
 — Hyperchloremic hypokalemic acidosis ($\uparrow$ Cl^-, $\downarrow$ HCO_3^-)
 — Normal anion gap (i.e. $Na^+ - Cl^- - HCO_3^- = 8-12$)
 — Symptomatic hypokalemia
3 Distal RTA (acidification defect)
 — Urine pH > 5.4 following oral acid load*
 — Nephrocalcinosis, calculi
4 Proximal RTA (bicarbonate-wasting)
 — Urine pH < 5.4 after oral acid load
 — Hypouricemia and hypophosphatemia
 — ± Fanconi's syndrome
5 RTA type 4
 — Hyporeninemic hypoaldosteronism
 — Urine pH < 5.4 after oral acid load
 — Occurs in elderly diabetics or obstructive uropathy
 — Causes *hyperkalemia* and acid urine

* Ammonium chloride 100 mg/kg

Possible constituents of 'tubular proteinuria'
1 'Physiological'
 — Tamm–Horsfall protein
 — β_2 microglobulin
 — IgA
2 Pathological
 — Myoglobin
 — Lysozyme
 — Bence-Jones protein

How to distinguish urinary concentrating defects
1 Water deprivation*/DDAVP → > 1000 mosm/L
 — Normal
2 Water deprivation/DDAVP → *no* increase
 — Nephrogenic diabetes insipidus
3 Water deprivation → no increase
 DDAVP → *major* increase
 — Pituitary diabetes insipidus
4 Water deprivation/DDAVP → *submaximal* increase
 — Long-standing primary polydipsia

* i.e. for 12 h; plasma osmolality should be ~ 295 mosm/kg

DISORDERS OF WATER METABOLISM

Primary polydipsia: its clinical significance
1 80% of primary polydipsia patients are schizophrenic

2 Commonest presentation of primary polydipsia is fitting

3 10% of primary polydipsics die within 2 years of diagnosis

Features of nephrogenic diabetes insipidus

1 The diagnosis may be effectively *excluded* if any voided urine specimen has an osmolality exceeding 600 mosm/L or specific gravity exceeding 1.015. Conversely, if an overnight voided specimen has an osmolality less than 350 mosm/L, a water-deprivation test may be indicated

2 Distinction from 'central' diabetes insipidus may be made if concentration defect persists after bilateral intranasal instillation of 20 g DDAVP

3 Primary polydipsia tends to be associated with a low plasma osmolality (~ 275 mosm/L) whereas diabetes insipidus is associated with higher readings (~ 295 mosm/L). In long-standing primary polydipsia, however, definitive distinction from nephrogenic diabetes insipidus may not be possible on the basis of osmolalities alone

4 Nephrogenic diabetes insipidus may occur as an X-linked recessive (XR) disorder or, more commonly, as a manifestation of other disorders including sickle-cell disease/trait, obstructive uropathy, chronic hypercalcemia/hypokalemia, or drugs (e.g. lithium)

5 Potentially useful management options include
— Treatment of underlying cause
— Thiazides (or ethacrynic acid) ± dietary salt restriction

NB: Chlorpropamide, which is of potential benefit in incomplete central diabetes insipidus, is *ineffective* in nephrogenic diabetes insipidus

Drug-induced disturbances of water metabolism

1 SIADH
— Chlorpropamide
— Carbamazepine
— Amitriptyline

2 Nephrogenic diabetes insipidus
— Lithium
— Demeclocycline
— Amphotericin B

Diagnosis of inappropriate ADH secretion

1 Plasma osmolality* < 275 mosm/L

2 Urinary osmolality inappropriately high‡ (see below)

3 Urinary sodium > 20 mmol/L

* Plasma osmolality = BUN + glucose + 2 × Na^+
‡ *Normal* waterloading causing urine flow of 10 mL/min should cause urine osmolality ~ 100 mosm/kg and serum osmolality ~ 280 mosm/kg

Inappropriate ADH secretion: features

1 Remains a diagnosis of exclusion
— Measurement of plasma ADH is *not* useful

2 Not characterized by significant edema, weight gain or hypertension despite hypervolemia*

3 Development of symptoms may be more dependent on *rate* of decline of serum sodium than on absolute level‡

4 Unlike other hyponatremias (see below), may also cause
— Hypouricemia
— ↓ Albumin
— ↓ Creatinine/BUN
— ↓ Hematocrit

5 Important differential diagnoses of ↓ Na^+
— Myxedema (ADH-independent ↓ free water clearance)
— Addison's disease (but associated with ↑ K^+)
— Chlorpropamide (→ ↑ ADH secretion *and* sensitivity)

6 Therapeutic options include
— Treatment of underlying cause
— Water restriction ± furosemide (frusemide) ± ↑ dietary NaCl
— Demeclocycline (or lithium)
— V_2-receptor (renal tubular ADH receptor) antagonists
— Hypertonic saline (a desperation measure)

* NB: Elderly patients may develop cardiac failure
‡ Urinary osmolalities need only be *inappropriately* elevated for the diagnosis to be entertained; e.g. a urinary osmolality of 250 mosm/L would be consistent with SIADH in association with an identical plasma value (provided that urinary Na^+ also elevated)

RENAL RADIOLOGY

Intravenous pyelography: predispositions to renal failure*

1 Myeloma

2 Diabetes (controversial)

3 Old age (esp. if hypovolemic, e.g. nephrotic) Infants (esp. if dehydrated, since unable to concentrate urine)

* NB: May be prevented by avoiding routine preparatory dehydration

Retrograde pyelography: causes of 'spidery infundibula'

1 Polycystic kidneys

2 Intrarenal space-occupying lesion (e.g. tumor)

3 Renal vein thrombosis

Pelviureteric junction translucency: differential diagnosis

1 **C**arcinoma (TCC)

2 **C**lot

3 **C**alculus (radiolucent; p. 329)

4 **C**rystals (p. 318)

Differential diagnosis of papillary necrosis

1 Analgesic abuse

2 Diabetes mellitus

3 Sickle-cell disease

4 Tuberculosis

Common congenital renal abnormalities* seen on IVP

1 Duplex collecting systems
— Commoner in females
— Upper pole ureter → lower bladder (and vice versa)
— Lower pole ureter is prone to vesicoureteric reflux

2 Horseshoe kidney
— Fused lower poles
3 Pelvic (ectopic) kidney
— May interfere with parturition
— May simulate a pathological pelvic mass
4 Crossed renal ectopia
— Ectopic kidney lies directly below orthotopic partner
— Fusion may occur
— Collecting system of ectopic kidney crosses midline to enter bladder on correct side

* All may predispose to infection, obstruction, and calculi

Rationâle of isotope renal scans
1 ^{131}Iodo-hippuran scan
— 80% excreted by renal tubular secretion
— Helps assess effective renal plasma flow (RPF) and, thereby, functional status of renal homograft
— Renography may be useful in follow-up of (diagnosed) obstructive uropathy and/or assessment of pelviureteric junction obstruction
2 ^{99m}Tc-DTPA or ^{51}Cr-EDTA (inulin analog) scans
— Help assess renal perfusion (varies with GFR)
— *Dynamic* (vascular phase) studies
  • Useful for checking post-transplant anastomosis
  • Gross hypoperfusion in a non-functioning graft favors rejection over tubular necrosis
  • Also useful in assessment of suspected renovascular trauma
— *Static* (parenchymal phase) studies may be useful in
  • Assessing renal cortical function in severe renal failure (more sensitive than IVP)
  • Evaluating suspected intrarenal trauma
3 ^{66}Gallium scan
— Helpful in excluding graft infection, usually in conjunction with ultrasound or transplant biopsy

MANAGING RENAL DISEASE

THERAPY OF RENAL FAILURE

Immediate management priorities in acute renal failure
1 To treat life-threatening hyperkalemia and/or pulmonary edema
2 To establish the nature, hence reversibility, of renal disorder

Treatments of proven efficacy in acute renal failure
1 Diuretics (furosemide [frusemide], mannitol)
— ↑ Urine flow and GFR
— Useful in ischemic or toxic renal failure
2 Alkalinization (bicarbonate)
— ↓ Renal failure if used early
— Useful in renal failure due to toxins, urate, rhabdomyolysis
3 Chelators (EDTA, penicillamine, etc.)
— ↓ Renal failure if used early
— Useful in renal failure due to heavy metal poisoning

4 Antidotes (*N*-acetylcysteine, calcium folinate [calcium leucovorin], ethylene glycol, etc.)
— ↓ Renal failure if used early
— Useful in renal failure due to metabolic toxins
5 Intermittent hemodialysis (via external shunt) or peritoneal dialysis
— Supportive treatment for patients without multiorgan failure
6 Continuous arteriovenous hemofiltration
— Supportive treatment, esp. for patients with multiorgan failure

Therapeutic considerations in end-stage chronic renal failure
1 Exclude reversible factors contributing to azotemia
2 Treat hypertension
3 Reduce protein intake if symptomatically uremic*
4 Administer bicarbonate (unless sodium restricted), phosphate binders and/or vitamin D analogs as needed
5 Manage anemia
— Treat symptoms with erythropoietin
— Ensure regular blood transfusion if transplantation feasible
6 Modify drug intake for degree of azotemia
7 Realistically assess age, general condition, mental capacity and overall prognosis prior to definitive intervention
8 Assess patient suitability for chronic ambulatory peritoneal dialysis (CAPD) or hemodialysis
— Will the patient cope?
— How adequate is vascular access?
— When would a fistula be created?
— How is the patient's cardiovascular stability?
9 Document HBsAg status
10 Determine age and number of siblings, and document degree of 'matching' between patient and siblings with respect to
— ABO compatibility (essential)
— HLA (B and DR: 'cytotoxic' crossmatch) compatibility
— MLC compatibility‡

* Also assists in controlling acidosis and hyperkalemia
‡ Helps distinguish relative suitability of similar HLA matches

Erythropoietin-resistant anemia in chronic renal failure?
1 Coexisting iron deficiency
— Treat with oral iron *plus* vitamin C to aid absorption
2 Subclinical aluminum intoxication
— Treat with desferrioxamine
3 Inadequate dialysis
— Increase urea reduction ratio > 70%
4 Concomitant secondary hyperparathyroidism
— Routine benefit of treatment not established
5 Chronic infection or inflammation
— e.g. Chronic sinusitis
6 Malnutrition
— Suspect if hypoalbuminemic

Treating the complications of chronic renal failure
1 Anemia
— Folate, multivitamins
— Ferrous sulfate

— Erythropoietin
— Dialysis
2 Acidosis
— Sodium bicarbonate
— Dialysis
3 Hyperuricemia
— Allopurinol
4 Renal bone disease
— Phosphate binders (aluminium hydroxide)
— Vitamin D (calcitriol*) or analogs (dihydrotachysterol)
— Calcium carbonate or acetate, high-calcium dialysate
— Parathyroidectomy

* *Unless* serum phosphate > 225 mmol/L

ERYTHROPOIETIN

Specific indications for erythropoietin in renal failure
1 Transfusion often required
— e.g. > 6 times per year
— Risk of iron overload, hepatitis C
2 Symptoms due to recurrent anemia
— Angina, CCF
— Reduced quality of life (any cause)
3 Absolute level of hemoglobin
— Consistently < 8 g/dL

Differential diagnosis of erythropoietin-resistant anemia
1 Iron deficiency* (e.g. menorrhagia, occult GI bleeding)
2 Inadequate dialysis
3 Aluminum toxicity‡
4 Marrow fibrosis due to secondary hyperparathyroidism
5 Occult infection (esp. bacterial) or other inflammation
6 Occult hemopoietic insufficiency (e.g. myeloma, thalassemia)
7 Treatment with ACE inhibitors
8 Non-compliance with self-administered injections

* Responds to iron dextran infusion (diagnostic test)
‡ Diagnose by bone biopsy. R_x: desferrioxamine, reduce aluminum exposure

Side-effects of erythropoietin treatment
1 Injection site pain, 'flu-like syndrome
2 Rapid changes in hematocrit
— Exacerbation of hypertension
— Headaches, seizures
— Thrombosis of shunts or fistulae
3 Hyperkalemia

PRESCRIBING IN RENAL DISEASE

Drugs competing for renal excretion: clinical significance
1 Probenecid
— Reduces tubular secretion of penicillin (aspirin, indometacin, AZT) → potentiation
2 Quinidine, verapamil, spironolactone
— Decrease tubular secretion of digoxin → toxicity

3 Thiazides, furosemide (frusemide)
— Increase lithium reabsorption → toxicity
4 Aspirin
— Reduces tubular secretion of methotrexate → toxicity

'Safe' drugs in chronic renal failure
1 Antihypertensives — β-blockers
2 Antiarrhythmics — Disopyramide
3 Antibiotics — Amoxicillin, co-trimoxazole, cefalexin, doxycycline
4 Analgesics — Paracetamol (low-dose)
5 Gastrointestinal — Cimetidine, metoclopramide
6 Hypnotic — Temazepam

Popular antihypertensives in chronic renal disease
1 Furosemide (frusemide)
— Used in preference to thiazides* once renal function falls to < 50% normal
2 β-blockers
— esp. metoprolol
3 Calcium antagonists
— Efficacy maintained as GFR falls
— Nifedipine may increase microalbuminuria
4 ACE inhibitors
— Oppose high-renin hypertension‡, hence very effective
— Toxicity (e.g. captopril neutropenia) worse in uremia
— Appear to reduce proteinuria and slow renal disease

* Exception: the thiazide-like drug metolazone potentiates furosemide (frusemide) in refractory hypervolemia
‡ May catastrophically reduce GFR and thus precipitate acute renal failure if inadvertently used in patients with bilateral renal artery stenosis

Principles of corticosteroid use in renal disease
1 Renal biopsy precedes steroid use in adult renal disease
2 Steroids may lead to rapid resolution of
— Minimal lesion nephrosis (esp. in children)
— Acute interstitial nephritis
— Mesangial proliferative glomerulonephritis
— Idiopathic retroperitoneal fibrosis (exclude TB first)
3 Steroids usually need to be combined with other drugs in
— RPGN (including Goodpasture's)
— PAN
— Multiple relapses of minimal-lesion nephrosis
4 Steroids may help membranous nephropathy if used early
5 Steroids are rarely useful in sclerodermatous nephropathy

DIURETICS

Mechanisms of diuretic action
1 Acetazolamide
— Carbonic anhydrase inhibitor
— ↓ Proximal tubular transport of NaCl/bicarbonate

— *Ineffective* if serum bicarbonate < 20 mEq/L
— Toxicity: hyperchloremic acidosis due to 'bicarbonate wasting' (p. 322); nephrocalcinosis if long-standing
— Useful short-term treatment of edema, esp. if pregnant, premenstrual, or with metabolic alkalosis
— Also useful in urate nephropathy, and in salicylism (i.e. as part of forced alkaline diuresis)
2 Mannitol
— Acts by delivering osmotic load to proximal tubule
— Used in head trauma etc.
3 Furosemide (frusemide)
— Blocks Cl⁻ pump (thick ascending limb, loop of Henle)
→ Blocks countercurrent multiplier system
→ Blocks water reabsorption from collecting system
— Also increases renal cortical perfusion
— Systemic venodilator (acts acutely in heart failure)
— Effective at low clearances
4 Thiazides
— Act on thin ascending limb (cortical diluting segment) of distal tubule → block active sodium reabsorption
— *Reduce* renal perfusion
— Also useful in proximal renal tubular acidosis
— *Not* effective at clearance < 20 mL/min
5 Potassium-sparing diuretics
— Triamterene → ↓ permeability of distal tubule/collecting ducts
— Amiloride → ↓ sodium/H_2O reabsorption, ↓ K^+ loss (mainly used as diuretic for patients on digoxin)
— Spironolactone: inhibits aldosterone action on distal tubule and collecting ducts; antiandrogenic side-effects (mainly used for cirrhotics with ascites)

Opposing indications for furosemide (frusemide) and thiazides
1 SIADH
— Furosemide (frusemide) (+ sodium supplements)
Nephrogenic diabetes insipidus
— Thiazides (+ sodium restriction)
2 Hypercalcemia
— Furosemide (frusemide)
Idiopathic hypercalciuria
— Thiazides

Clinically significant diuretic side-effects in elderly patients
1 Commoner with potassium-sparing diuretics
— Hyperkalemia (esp. in renal impairment)
— Hyponatremia (symptomatic in up to 20%)
— Precipitation of prerenal failure
2 Commoner with thiazides/furosemide (frusemide)
— Hypokalemia (esp. significant in patients on digoxin)
— Precipitation of gout (esp. in females)
— Precipitation of clinical diabetes
— Precipitation of incontinence

DRUG TOXICITY IN RENAL DISEASE

Nephrotoxicity of non-steroidal anti-inflammatory drugs*
1 Electrolyte disturbances
— Sodium retention (edema)
— Hyponatremia ± SIADH
— Hyperkalemia, esp. in diabetics (↓ renin release)
2 Acute renal failure in volume-contracted patients due to antagonism of prostaglandin-mediated renal arteriolar vasodilatation (reversible)
3 Acute tubular necrosis
4 Interstitial nephritis with proteinuria (drug hypersensitivity)
5 Papillary necrosis (due to medullary ischemia)
6 Minimal change nephrosis (indometacin, naproxen)
7 Nephrotic syndrome due to membranous nephropathy (reversible)
8 Antagonism of antihypertensive therapy (e.g. furosemide [frusemide], ACE inhibitors) by indometacin

* *Including* COX-2 inhibitors such as rofecoxib.

Patient subsets at increased risk of NSAID nephrotoxicity*
1 Elderly
2 Pre-existing renal impairment
3 Volume contraction
— Diuretics
— Cardiac failure
— Cirrhosis, nephrosis
— Perioperative
4 Hypertension
5 Diabetes
6 Concomitant aspirin use

* *Paracetamol should be the analgesic of choice for intermittent use in all such individuals.*

Spectrum of antibiotic-induced nephrotoxicity
1 Antianabolic effect (→ ↑ BUN)
— Tetracyclines (exception: doxycycline)
2 Interstitial nephritis
— Penicillins (esp. methicillin)
— Cephalosporins, sulfonamides
— Rifampicin (esp. intermittent)
3 Hypokalemic alkalosis
— Penicillins (esp. ticarcillin)
4 Proximal tubular necrosis
— Aminoglycosides potentiated by furosemide (frusemide)
Distal tubular necrosis
— Amphotericin B
5 Nephrogenic diabetes insipidus
— Demethylchlortetracycline (demeclocycline)
6 Crystalluria (→ collecting duct obstruction)
— Sulfadiazine (for nocardiosis)
— Nitrofurantoin
— 5-FC, aciclovir

Accumulation of toxic drug metabolites in chronic renal failure?
1 Allopurinol
2 Digoxin
3 Methyldopa, metoprolol

4 Clofibrate
5 Opiates; propoxyphene

ALTERING DRUG REGIMENS IN RENAL DISEASE

Modification of drug therapy in renal failure
1 Avoid due to toxicity
 — K+-sparing diuretics (esp. in elderly or diabetics)
 — ACE inhibitors
  → Life-threatening hyperkalemia
 — Tetracyclines (except doxycycline)
  → Worsen azotemia
 — Nitrofurantoin
  → Neuropathy; also ineffective
 — Chloramphenicol
  → Accumulate myelotoxic inactive metabolites
 — Lithium carbonate
  → Toxicity potentiated by diuretic therapy
 — Metformin
  → Lactic acidosis
 — Clofibrate
  → Toxic myopathy
 — Methotrexate
2 Avoid due to ineffectiveness
 — Thiazides
 — Nalidixic acid
3 Major dose reduction required*
 — Digoxin, procainamide
 — Cimetidine; amantadine
 — Vancomycin; aminoglycosides; amphotericin B
 — Penicillin G, ampicillin, ticarcillin
 — Sulfonamides, cephalosporins
 — 5-Flucytosine (→ crystalluria)
 — Ethambutol (→ optic neuritis)
4 *No* dose reduction usually required
 — Digitoxin; furosemide (frusemide) (but beware of ototoxicity)
 — Prazosin, minoxidil, hydralazine
 — Tolbutamide, glibenclamide
 — Prednisone, azathioprine, heparin
 — Doxycycline
 — Flucloxacillin, erythromycin, fusidic acid
 — Isoniazid, rifampicin
 — Griseofulvin, miconazole, ketoconazole, clotrimazole

NB: A rare example in which dosage may require *increase* in renal failure is that of phenytoin: ↓ plasma protein binding of phenytoin in renal failure → ↑ free drug → ↑ liver metabolism; renal excretion of phenytoin is insignificant
* i.e. according to nomogram or serum level

Drugs requiring repeat dosage following dialysis*
1 After *either* peritoneal dialysis or hemodialysis
 — Aminoglycosides
 — Ticarcillin
 — Cefuroxime, cephalothin
 — Isoniazid, ethambutol
 — 5-FC
 — Methyldopa
 — Aspirin
2 After hemodialysis only
 — Penicillins
 — Cephalosporins

 — Metronidazole, trimethoprim
 — Aciclovir
 — Allopurinol
 — Paracetamol
 — Azathioprine, cyclophosphamide, prednisone (prednisolone)
 — Captopril, metoprolol, minoxidil, nadolol
* cf. heavily *protein-bound* drugs – *not* dialysable

HEMODIALYSIS

Indications for dialysis in renal failure
1 Symptomatic uremia (despite conservative management)
2 Fluid overload (diuretic-resistant)
3 Refractory hyperkalemia (after diet, resins, bicarbonate)
4 Unacceptable decline in quality of life, esp. if due to long-term complication (e.g. neuropathy, pericarditis)

Biochemical consequences of a hemodialysis treatment
1 Reduction in
 — Plasma creatinine/BUN
 — Plasma potassium
 — Plasma phosphate
 — Plasma osmolality
2 Increase in
 — Plasma bicarbonate/pH
 — Plasma sodium
 — Plasma calcium

Conditions with poor prognosis when treated by hemodialysis
1 Diabetes mellitus
2 Amyloidosis
3 Scleroderma
4 SLE
5 Hypertensive nephrosclerosis

Acute complications of hemodialysis
1 Hypotension
2 Arrhythmias (± digoxin toxicity)
3 Cramps; nausea; headaches; fever*
4 Air embolism (due to IV bags with airways)
5 Exsanguination (due to external shunts)
6 Disequilibrium syndrome
 — Headaches, hypertension, confusion, fitting
 — Occurs during first few dialyses due to rapid reduction of extracellular osmolarity → cerebral edema
* e.g. due to *Staph.* bacteremias, or microcystin contamination of dialysate

Chronic complications of hemodialysis
1 Accelerated atherosclerosis*
2 Hepatitis B
3 Sexual dysfunction, infertility, depression
4 Wernicke's syndrome; central pontine myelinolysis
5 Vascular
 — Fistula thrombosis or endarteritis
 — Hemorrhage (subdural, pericarditis, stroke, GI bleeding)

6 Dialysis dementia (due to cerebral aluminum overload)
7 Arthropathy (amyloidosis)
8 Nephrogenic ascites (indicates *dire* prognosis unless transplanted or switched to CAPD)

* 60% die from myocardial/cerebral infarction

ALTERNATIVES TO HEMODIALYSIS

Relative indications for chronic ambulatory peritoneal dialysis (CAPD) in end-stage renal failure
1 Unsuitability for hemodialysis
   — Extremes of age
   — Cardiovascular instability
   — Inadequate vascular access
   — Heparin contraindicated (e.g. in pericarditis)
   — Geographical remoteness
   — Religious conviction (Jehovah's Witness)
2 Symptomatic progression while on hemodialysis
3 Diabetic retinopathy
4 Scleroderma

NB: CAPD precluded by previous laparotomy ($\rightarrow$ adhesions)

Problems encountered in CAPD patients
1 Peritonitis (esp. due to *S. albus*; Gram-negatives may indicate visceral perforation by catheter); loculated ascites
2 Catheter blockage
3 Hyperglycemia, hypertriglyceridemia
   $\rightarrow$ Obesity, accelerated atheroma, worsening of diabetic control (necessitating intraperitoneal insulin)
4 Protein and amino acid depletion
5 Basal atelectasis, pleural effusions
6 Hernias; ileus (constipation)

Advantages of CAPD over hemodialysis
1 Early benefits
   — Better blood pressure control
   — Higher Hb
   — Less muscle wasting and weight loss
   — Less acidosis
   — No dialysis disequilibrium
2 Long-term benefits
   — Loss of pigmentation
   — Return of menstruation
   — Improved calcium/phosphate balance

RENAL TRANSPLANTATION

Specific indications for transplantation
1 Severe renal osteodystrophy
2 Inability to cope with dialysis, esp. in young patient

Contraindications to transplantation
1 Lack of compatible kidney donor
2 Advanced age or debility
3 Chronic infection (TB, HBV, bronchiectasis, osteomyelitis)

4 Malignancy
5 Peptic ulceration
6 Primary disease known to recur in grafts

Differential diagnosis of post-transplant hypertension
1 Fluid overload
2 Chronic rejection
3 Stenosis of donor renal artery
4 Iatrogenic
   — Ciclosporin (i.e. *independent* of nephrotoxicity)
   — Steroids
5 Renin production from remnant kidneys (rare)

Features of ciclosporin nephrotoxicity
1 Acute toxicity
   — $\downarrow$ GFR/renal blood flow
2 Chronic toxicity
   — Interstitial fibrosis, tubular atrophy
3 Toxicity may be potentiated by other drugs
   — esp. Ketoconazole

Graft complications related to surgery in renal transplantation
1 Ureteric obstruction
2 Lymphocele
3 Renal vein thrombosis
4 Renal artery stenosis

Prolonged post-transplant oliguria; differential diagnosis
1 Acute rejection
2 Acute tubular necrosis
3 Arterial (anastomotic) stenosis* or thrombosis
4 Ureteric obstruction (lymphocele, hematoma ischemia)
5 Ciclosporin nephrotoxicity
6 Sepsis (e.g. CMV, UTI)

* May be non-invasively detected by magnetic resonance angiography

Management of prolonged post-transplant oliguria if rejection suspected
1 Exclude vascular and ureteric obstruction
2 Transplant biopsy: is rejection confirmed?
3 If not, measure intrarenal pressure manometrically using 25 G needle (abnormally elevated in rejection)
4 If diagnosis still in doubt, decrease ciclosporin dose
5 If no improvement in serum creatinine within 48 h of CSA reduction, proceed with therapeutic trial of steroids or azathioprine (i.e. as for confirmed graft rejection)

Features of cytomegalovirus graft infection
1 Manifests with post-transplant azotemia and/or oliguria
2 Most severe infections occur in seronegative patients receiving grafts from seropositive donors (a relative contraindication to matching)
3 Other mechanisms of infection include reactivation in seropositive hosts (occurs in 90%, mild) and transmission by granulocyte transfusions
4 Biopsy reveals diffuse glomerular lesions with minimal interstitial inflammatory response (cf. rejection)

5 The helper: suppressor (CD4:CD8) T cell ratio in peripheral blood is generally lower in CMV graft infection than in rejection, but this is inconsistently affected by the immunosuppressive regimen

Clinical stigmata of graft rejection
1 Hyperacute
   — May occur within minutes
   — Irreversible; graft nephrectomy mandatory
2 Acute
   — May occur at *any* time
   — Graft swelling, tenderness, fever
   — Oliguria, azotemia
   — ↓ Urinary sodium
   — Active urine sediment
   — May respond to immunosuppression
3 Chronic
   — Occurs after months to years
   — Inexorable, irreversible decline in GFR
   — May manifest as interstitial nephritis or proliferative glomerulonephritis

Late problems following renal transplantation
1 Recurrent glomerulonephritis (contraindicates further attempts at transplantation; see below)
2 Reflux nephropathy
3 Avascular necrosis of bone (usually head of femur) Other steroid-related morbidity (e.g. cataracts)
4 Infections
5 Malignancy
   — Non-Hodgkin's lymphoma (incl. cerebral)
   — Skin BCC or SCC (incl. vulva, perineum)
   — SCC cervix (in situ)
   — Hepatobiliary carcinoma
   — Kaposi's sarcoma

Renal biopsy patterns classically recurring in transplants
1 Dense deposit disease*
2 Focal sclerosis and hyalinosis
   — e.g. Due to reflux, heroin or analgesic abuse
3 Oxalosis, cystinosis, amyloidosis
4 Severe diabetic glomerulosclerosis
5 Vasculitis
   — Anti-GBM disease (Goodpasture's syndrome)
   — Cryoglobulinemia
6 IgA nephropathy

* Mesangiocapillary glomerulonephritis type II

Graft biopsy in transplant rejection: implications for therapy
1 Acute rejection refractory to steroids
   — Biopsy → cellular infiltrate
     • Increase the steroids
   — Biopsy → intimal proliferation
     • Organize graft nephrectomy
2 Chronic rejection provisionally diagnosed
   — Biopsy → recurrence of original disease process
     • Abandon graft (further transplant *contraindicated*)
   — Biopsy → confirmation of chronic rejection
     • Prepare for dialysis (± retransplantation)

RENAL CALCULI

Radiological appearances predicting stone composition
1 Opaque stones
   — Calcium oxalate
   — Calcium phosphate
   — Struvite ('infection' stones, 'triple phosphate': magnesium ammonium phosphate, MAP), esp. if large staghorn
2 Semiopaque
   — Cystine
3 Lucent
   — Urate
   — Xanthine
   — Orotic acid
   — 2,8 dihydroxyadenine*

* Responsive to allopurinol prophylaxis

Determining the etiology of renal calculi
1 Family history
   — Cystinuria, xanthinuria, hyperoxaluria
   — Gout
   — Multiple endocrine neoplasia (→ 1° HPT)
2 Medication history
   — Megadose vitamin therapy
   — Milk–alkali syndrome
   — Acetazolamide (→ alkaline urine → urea-splitting bugs)
   — Probenecid
3 Strain urine for passed stone fragments
   — Quantitative chemical analysis: calcium, magnesium, ammonium, phosphate, oxalate, carbonate, urate
   — Qualitative chemical analysis (cystine)
   — Bacteriological analysis, esp. for *Proteus* spp.
4 Urine specimen analysis
   — pH
   — Microscopy
   — Culture (esp. for urea-splitting organisms*)
   — Sodium nitroprusside test (for cystine)
   — Crystal counts (cystine, struvite) in fresh sample
5 Quantitative 24-h urine analysis
   — Volume
   — Oxalate
   — Calcium, phosphate, urate
   — Cystine (if qualitative tests positive)
   — cAMP (if hyperparathyroidism suspected)
6 Plasma biochemistry
   — Calcium, bicarbonate
   — Urate (abnormally low? exclude xanthinuria)
   — Creatinine
   — iPTH (if calcium elevated)
7 IVP
   — Polycystic kidneys
   — Medullary sponge kidneys
   — Duplex collecting system

* *Proteus mirabilis, Pseudomonas aeruginosa, Klebsiella* spp.

Stone composition as a pointer to pathogenesis
1 Uric acid
   — Hyperuricosuria (± hyperuricemia)

2 Struvite, carbonate apatite
— Infection with urease-splitting organisms
3 Cystine
— Cystinuria
4 Calcium oxalate
— Primary hyperoxaluria
— Enteric hyperoxaluria (e.g. ileal resection)
5 Calcium phosphate *or* calcium oxalate
— Hypercalciuria (see below)
— Hyperuricosuria
— Primary hyperparathyroidism
— Hypocitraturia (e.g. distal RTA) → ↓ urinary pH

Varieties of hypercalciuria
1 Absorptive hypercalciuria (intestinal hyperabsorption)
— Normal serum calcium, *normal* serum PTH
— Treat with sodium cellulose phosphate (binds gut calcium)
2 Resorptive hypercalciuria (primary hyperparathyroidism)
— Raised *or* normal serum calcium, *high* serum PTH
3 Renal hypercalciuria (renal leak)
— Normal serum calcium, *high* serum PTH
— Treat with thiazides (→ ↑ renal calcium absorption)

Children with renal stones: diagnoses to exclude
1 Cystinuria
2 Distal RTA (calcium phosphate stones)
3 Hereditary hyperoxaluria
4 Medullary sponge kidneys (calcium oxalate stones in adolescents)

Preventive management of recurrent renal calculi
1 All stone types
— High fluid intake
— Low-salt diet
— Avoid high-protein diet
2 Calcium oxalate stones (50%)
— Thiazides
— Allopurinol
— Low-oxalate diet *or* potassium citrate
— Pyridoxine (*if* hereditary hyperoxaluria)
— Colestyramine (*if* ileal disease present)
3 Calcium phosphate stones (25%)
— Thiazides (→ ↓ urinary calcium)
— Potassium citrate (→ ↑ urinary pH, ↓ urinary calcium)
— Cellulose phosphate (binds calcium in gut)
— Low-calcium diet (*if* hypercalciuria is diet-dependent)
4 Struvite stones (15%)
— Surgery *or* extracorporeal shock wave lithotripsy (ESWL)
— Antibiotics plus acetohydroxamic acid (a urease inhibitor)
— Urinary acidification (pH < 5.5)
— Percutaneous nephrostomy with lavage chemolysis
5 Urate stones (5–10%)
— Allopurinol
— Potassium citrate
— Low purine diet

6 Cystine stones (0.5–3%)
— Aggressive hydration (3–5 L/day)
— Chelation: tiopronin or D-penicillamine
— Potassium citrate

IMMEDIATE THERAPY OF RENAL CALCULI

Ablative approaches to renal stone removal
1 Stones < 4 mm diameter
— Expectant (70% chance of spontaneous passage)
2 Upper ureteric stones
— Extracorporeal shockwave lithotripsy (see below)
3 Middle or lower ureteric stones
— Ureteroscopy
4 Failure of above methods
— Open ureterolithotomy (virtually obsolete)

Prerequisites for ureteroscopic* removal of ureteric stones
1 Stone diameter < 5 mm, *and*
2 Stone situated < 5 cm from ureteric orifice, *and*
3 Stone impacted < 5 weeks' duration

* i.e. using Dormia basket

Potential indications for surgical management of renal stones
1 Symptoms
2 Obstruction
3 Infection

EXTRACORPOREAL SHOCK WAVE LITHOTRIPSY (ESWL)

Factors favoring use of ESWL
1 Stones < 2 cm diameter
2 Renal pelvis or upper ureteric stones
3 Opaque stones* (most types), incl.
— Calcium oxalate dihydrate
— Calcium phosphate
— Struvite

* Tend to fragment well

Relative contraindications to ESWL
1 Large (> 3 cm diameter) staghorn stones*
2 Stone(s) in lower third of ureter‡
3 Risk of precipitating renal failure
— Obstruction preventing passage of fragments
— Simultaneous treatment of bilateral stones
4 Stone composition (if known)
— Radiolucent stones, esp. urate
• May be dissolved by alkalinization
• Catheterization or contrast required for fluoroscopic localization
— Some opaque stones
• Cystine¶ (may dissolve with penicillamine/H_2O)
• Calcium oxalate monohydrate¶
5 Pregnancy, bleeding diathesis

* Best treated by percutaneous nephrolithotomy; for staghorns, ESWL can be combined with surgery. *All* residual struvite must be removed to eliminate infective nidus
‡ Best treated by ureteroscopy
¶ Tend not to break up into fine (< 4 mm) fragments

Complications of ESWL
1 Renal colic
2 Perirenal hematoma*
3 Newly acquired hypertension
4 Pancreatitis (rare)

* Bowel hematomas have also been reported

MASSIVE BLADDER HEMORRHAGE

Precipitants of massive bladder hemorrhage
1 Trauma
2 Bladder tumors (esp. post-radiotherapy)
3 Long-term cyclophosphamide therapy (hemorrhagic cystitis)
4 Amyloidosis

Management modalities in massive bladder hemorrhage
1 Intravesical vasopressin
  — Works only for as long as infusion continued
2 Intravesical alum irrigation
  — Precipitates mucosal protein; no toxicity (cf. formalin)
3 Helmstein balloon compression
  — May cause fibrosis (similar to formalin instillation)
4 Arterial embolization
  — Effective measure in trauma cases
5 Supravesical urinary diversion
  — For intractable bleeding
6 Emergency cystectomy
  — For life-threatening hemorrhage resistant to above measures

Genitourinary morbidity of long-term cyclophosphamide
1 Hemorrhagic cystitis (preventable by hydration and MESNA)
2 Bladder telangiectasia and/or fibrosis
3 Azoospermia, amenorrhea
4 Inappropriate ADH secretion
5 Transitional cell carcinoma of the bladder

UNDERSTANDING RENAL DISEASE

COMPLICATIONS OF RENAL DISEASE

Major pathogenetic mechanisms of anemia in renal failure
1 ↓ Erythropoietin secretion
2 ↓ Utilization of iron (anemia of chronic disease) due to ? 'uremic toxins'
3 ↓ Production of glutathione by pentose phosphate pathway leading to shortened erythrocyte survival (hemolysis)
4 Marrow fibrosis due to secondary hyperparathyroidism

5 Occult blood loss due to
  — Impaired platelet function
  — Heparinization during hemodialysis
  — Loss of blood and folate during hemodialysis
  — Surreptitious ongoing aspirin ingestion
6 Diagnostic phlebotomies

Mechanisms of impotence in chronic renal failure
1 Depression
2 Reduced serum testosterone
3 Hyperprolactinemia
4 Autonomic neuropathy
5 Antihypertensive medications

Renal disorders which often deteriorate in pregnancy
1 Pyelonephritis
2 Reflux nephropathy
3 IgA nephropathy
4 Scleroderma, PAN, Wegener's
5 Renal artery stenosis

Psychiatric etiologies in chronic renal failure
1 Uremia
2 Water intoxication
3 Rapid electrolyte shifts
4 Dialysis disequilibrium syndrome (?cerebral edema)
5 Dialysis dementia (?aluminum-induced)

Manifestations of disturbed calcium homeostasis in renal disease
1 Proximal myopathy (vitamin D deficiency)
2 Hyperparathyroidism: bone pain and deformity
3 Osteopenia
4 Osteomalacia: bone pain, deformity, pathological fracture
5 Avascular necrosis of the femoral head (in transplants)
6 Extraskeletal calcification
  — Band keratopathy
  — Pruritus
  — Vascular calcification
  — Periarticular soft tissues

RENAL OSTEODYSTROPHY

Pathogenesis of renal bone disease
1 Nephron loss → ↓ GFR
  → Phosphate retention
2 Nephron loss → ↓ dihydroxylated vitamin D (25-HCC)
  — ↓ 1,25-DHCC → osteomalacia
3 Skeletal PTH resistance + phosphate retention + ↓ 1,25-DHCC
  → ↓ Ionized serum calcium (Ca^{2+})
4 ↓ Ca^{2+} → ↑ PTH
  — Secondary hyperparathyroidism
  — Osteosclerosis and/or osteitis fibrosa cystica
5 Dialysate
  — Aluminum* → osteomalacia
  — Heparin → osteoporosis
6 Anorexia
  → Dietary deficiencies

* NB: Aluminum also present in oral phosphate binders

Radiographic features of renal osteodystrophy
1 90% of biopsy-proven cases exhibit radiological abnormalities
2 50% have vascular calcification
3 50% have 'rugger-jersey' spine
4 25% have subperiosteal lesions

Factors predicting incidence and severity of osteomalacia
1 Duration of dialysis (cf. transplant: osteomalacia *rare*)
2 Bone aluminum content

Approach to management of renal osteodystrophy
1 GFR < 30 mL/min
— Prophylactic calcium (5 g/day $CaCO_3$ = 2 g/day Ca^{2+})
2 Development of significant hyperphosphatemia
— Add oral phosphate binders
3 Indications for oral 1,25-DHCC/dihydrotachysterol
— Development of hypocalcemia
— Development of myopathy and/or bone pain
— Radiographic erosions or fractures
— Elevation of serum alkaline phosphatase
4 Tertiary (or severe secondary) hyperparathyroidism
— Regular calcitriol (1,25-DHCC) *infusions*
— Subtotal parathyroidectomy
5 Use aluminum-free dialysate when dialysing

INCONTINENCE

Urinary incontinence: important physical signs
1 Fever, cachexia; foul urine
— Urinary tract infection
2 Suprapubic tenderness
Bladder enlargement to percussion
— Retention with overflow
3 Pelvic and rectal examination
— Tumors, fistulae, uterine prolapse
4 ↓ Anal sphincter tone
↓ Bulbocavernosus reflex
Perianal anesthesia ± fecal incontinence
— Cauda equina syndrome
5 Pyramidal signs + sensory level
— Cord compression
6 Peripheral neuropathy; optic atrophy
Postural hypotension
— Autonomic neuropathy
7 Gait apraxia, dementia; primitive reflexes
— Normal pressure hydrocephalus
8 Urinalysis (glycosuria, hematuria, nitrites)

Medical management of urinary incontinence
1 Stress incontinence
— Phenylpropanolamine
— Systemic or topical estrogens if post-menopausal
2 Urge incontinence (detrusor instability)*
— Oxybutynin, propantheline
— Imipramine
— Intranasal desmopressin

3 Overflow incontinence
— Bethanechol (may exacerbate symptoms in elderly)
4 Functional (e.g. dementia)
— No specific drug therapy

* Best response to treatment

Other measures in treating urinary incontinence
1 Pelvic floor exercises
Bladder retraining
Biofeedback
2 Pessary
Penile clamp
Intermittent catheterization
3 Surgical repair (for stress incontinence)
Electrical sphincter stimulation
Artificial sphincters

THERAPY OF BENIGN PROSTATIC HYPERPLASIA

Medical therapies in prostatism
1 α-blockers ($\to \uparrow$ flow by relaxing prostatic smooth muscle)
— Uroselective: Alfuzosin, tamsulosin (less hypotension)
— Non-selective: Terazosin, doxazosin, indoramin
2 Drugs that may shrink benign prostatic hypertrophy (BPH)
— Finasteride (5-α-reductase inhibitor*)
— Flutamide (non-steroidal antiandrogen)
3 Antispasmodics (for frequency due to detrusor instability)
— Oxybutinin

* 5-α-reductase converts testosterone to the active dihydrotestosterone (DHT); hence, finasteride reduces libido and causes impotence and gynecomastia. In terms of efficacy, it is also inferior to α-blockers for BPH management

Absolute indications for transurethral resection of the prostate (TURP)
1 Acute urinary retention
2 Chronic urinary retention with renal impairment*
3 Recurrent urinary tract infections or hematuria
4 Bladder stones or diverticula

* i.e. obstructive uropathy

Morbidity of transurethral resection of the prostate
1 Retrograde ejaculation (60%)
2 Impotence (5%)
3 Incontinence (5%)
4 Hemorrhage (10% require transfusion)
5 Urethral stricture (5%)

RENAL CYSTIC DISEASE

Clinical spectrum of renal cystic disease
1 Medullary sponge kidneys (sporadic inheritance)
— Manifests with stones or UTI in adults
— Normal life expectancy

2 Medullary cystic disease (adult type = AD)
— Causes renal failure and osteodystrophy in childhood
— Associated with liver fibrosis and retinitis pigmentosa
3 Infantile polycystic disease (AR)
— Causes renal failure in childhood
— Associated with liver fibrosis and portal hypertension
4 Adult polycystic disease (AD)
— Causes renal failure in middle life
— Associated with cysts in liver, pancreas, spleen, lungs

Features of medullary sponge kidneys
1 Asymmetrically enlarged kidneys
2 Probably underdiagnosed (as idiopathic hypercalciuria) in calcium stone-formers; IVP → 'grapelike clusters'
3 Presents between 10 and 40 years of age (bimodal) 60% get calculi; usually oxalate*
4 30% get
— Hematuria
— Urinary tract infections
— Papillary necrosis/nephrocalcinosis
5 Does not usually lead to uremia; may be totally asymptomatic
6 Instrumentation should be avoided if possible

* *S. albus* infections may cause struvite stones

Features of medullary cystic disease
1 Asymmetrically shrunken kidneys
2 Histology similar to chronic interstitial nephritis
3 Hypertension rare
4 Urinalysis typically normal
5 No calcification on IVP
6 Progresses inexorably to uremia via proximal RTA (p. 322) and/or salt-losing nephropathy

ADULT POLYCYSTIC KIDNEY DISEASE

Polycystic kidney disease: features
1 Episodic loin pain
— Cyst hemorrhage
— Cyst torsion
— Clot colic
— Calculi
2 Hematuria ± nocturia, mild proteinuria
3 Hypertension
4 Urinary tract infections
5 Anemia (normochromic *or* hypochromic) *or* polycythemia

Associations of polycystic kidney disease
1 Extrarenal cysts
— Liver (30%)
— Spleen, pancreas
2 Saccular aneurysms, esp. cerebral (10%)
— Present with subarachnoid hemorrhage
3 Gastrointestinal manifestations
— Colonic diverticulosis
— Herniae

4 Cardiac valve disease
— Aortic root dilatation, aortic incompetence
— Mitral valve prolapse, mitral incompetence
5 Rare associations
— Myotonic dystrophy
— Hereditary spherocytosis
— Peutz–Jeghers syndrome

Principles of managing adult polycystic disease
1 Prompt treatment of hypertension or urinary tract infection*
2 Non-nephrotoxic analgesics for recurrent flank pain
3 Transplant work-up (if azotemia supervenes)
4 Genetic counselling‡
5 Rarely, cyst puncture or nephrectomy may be indicated

* Infected cysts are best treated with co-trimoxazole
‡ Normal IVP ± ultrasound at age 20 makes future polycystic disease unlikely

MISCELLANEOUS RENAL DISORDERS

Pathogenetic mechanisms implicated in 'heroin nephropathy'
1 Nephritis due to contaminants (e.g. lead)
— Typically focal sclerosing glomerulonephritis
2 Immune-complex mediated nephritis
— Heroin acting as a hapten
3 Post-infective
— Staphylococcal bacteremias
— Hepatitis B
4 Myoglobinuric nephropathy
— Due to associated rhabdomyolysis

Clinical spectrum of analgesic-related disease
1 General
— Psychiatric disorder; passive aggression; headaches
— Premature aging; pigmentation
— Dementia
2 Anemia
— Normochromic (often disproportionate to azotemia)
— Hypochromic (occult gastric bleeding)
— Megaloblastic (post-gastrectomy)
3 Gastrointestinal symptoms
— Dyspepsia, esophagitis
— Gastric ulcer
4 Cardiovascular associations
— Hypertension (± renovascular component)
— Ischemic heart disease
5 Renal complications
— Sterile pyuria; hemoproteinuria
— Salt-losing nephropathy, nocturia
— Nephrogenic diabetes insipidus
— Renal tubular acidosis
— Renal colic
— Osteomalacia
— Ureteric strictures
— Frequent UTI (esp. *Proteus*)
— Chronic renal failure
6 Malignancy
— Transitional cell carcinoma of renal pelvis

Spectrum of heredofamilial renal disease

1 Alport's syndrome (AD)
   — Females are mildly affected; no nerve deafness
   — Associated with
     • Lens abnormalities
     • Platelet dysfunction
     • Hyperprolinemia, cerebral malfunction
   — Does *not* recur after transplantation
2 Fabry's disease (AR; galactosidase A deficiency)
   — Affected females have isolated renal impairment
   — Associated (in affected males) with
     • 'Bathing trunk' punctate spots (angiokeratomas)
     • Corneal dystrophy
     • Ischemic heart disease
     • Acroparesthesiae
3 Nail–patella syndrome (AD)
   — Often presents with nephrotic syndrome
   — 'Moth-eaten' glomerular basement membrane
   — Associated stigmata
     • Dystrophic nails, esp. thumb and index
     • Absent patellae
     • Absent iliac horns on plain pelvic X-ray
4 Cystinosis (AR)
   — Lysosomal storage disease → intracellular cystine excess
     • Fanconi's syndrome, renal failure ~ age 10
     • Dysphagia in adulthood (esophageal dysfunction)
   — Oral mercaptamine depletes cystine and arrests disease

Retroperitoneal fibrosis: associations and features

1 Etiologic associations (NB: usually idiopathic)
   — Methysergide, dexamfetamine, ergotamine, methyldopa
   — Carcinoma, carcinoids
   — Crohn's disease, Raynaud's disease
   — Connective tissue disorders, autoimmune diseases
   — Middle-aged males; HLA-B27
2 Clinical associations
   — Mediastinal fibrosis (→ aortic/caval involvement)
   — Sclerosing cholangitis
   — Fibrosing alveolitis
   — Riedel's thyroiditis
   — Peyronie's disease
   — Pseudotumor oculi
   — Coronary arterial fibrosis
   — Constrictive pericarditis
3 Pathologic features
   — Periaortic inflammation: mononuclear infiltration commencing in lower abdomen/mediastinum
   — Ureters fibrosed, but lumen *not* occluded
4 Radiographic features (IVP)
   — Medial deviation of lower two-thirds of both ureters
5 Therapeutic features
   — May respond to corticosteroids and/or mycophenolate mofetil, *but*
   — Genitourinary TB must first be *actively* excluded

NB: *Sclerosing peritonitis* due to practolol or carcinoid syndrome is a distinct entity

REVIEWING THE LITERATURE: RENAL AND UROLOGIC DISEASE

14.1 Vincenti F et al (1998) Interleukin-2 receptor blockade with daclizumab to prevent acute rejection in renal transplantation. N Engl J Med 338: 161–165

Randomized double-blind placebo-controlled study of 260 patients, showing that the 126 who were given daclizumab incurred fewer rejection episodes.

14.2 Hateboer N et al (1999) Comparison of phenotypes of polycystic kidney disease types 1 and 2. Lancet 353: 103–107

Comparative study of 333 PKD1 and 291 PKD2 patients, confirming the milder phenotype. PKD2 patients presented with renal failure 20 years older than PKD1 patients, on average, and the mean life expectancy was 16 years greater.

14.3 Hooton TM et al (2000) A prospective study of asymptomatic bacteriuria in sexually active young women. N Engl J Med 343: 992–997

This study found 5% of sexually active women aged 18 to 40 had asymptomatic bacteriuria. Infection was usually transient and remained asymptomatic, but in 8% of cases a symptomatic infection supervened within a week (compared with 1% in those without asymptomatic infection). Contraceptive use of diaphragm and spermicide correlated with asymptomatic infection.

14.4 Goldstein I et al (1998) Oral sildenafil in the treatment of erectile dysfunction. N Engl J Med 338: 1397–1404

Placebo-controlled study of 532 men, confirming the efficacy of the now-famous drug for improving male sexual performance. Success rates improved from 22 to 69% of attempts, while the number of successful attempts per month also increased from 1.5 to 5.9. Headache, flushing and dyspepsia were common.

14.5 Walma EP et al (1997) Withdrawal of long term diuretic medication in elderly patients: a double blind randomized trial. Br Med J 315: 464–468

In this placebo-controlled study of 202 long-term diuretic-dependent patients, most became symptomatic (e.g. from hypertensive heart failure) on discontinuing therapy.

14.6 Besarab A et al (1998) The effects of normal as compared with low hematocrit values in patients with cardiac disease who are receiving hemodialysis and epoetin. N Engl J Med 339: 584–590

Argiles A et al (1998) Seasonal changes in blood pressure in patients with end-stage renal disease treated with hemodialysis. N Engl J Med 339: 1364–1370

Two studies documenting variables affecting the blood pressure and associated morbidity in renal dialysis patients. The former study involved a randomized prospective assessment of erythropoietin treatment in a cohort of 1233 dialysis patients with congestive heart failure or ischemic heart disease; this showed increased mortality in treated patients, indicating an adverse effect of normalizing the hematocrit. The second study showed that French dialysis patients have higher blood pressures in the winter, and lower in the summer.

14.7 Nickeleit V et al (2000) Testing for polyomavirus type BK DNA in plasma to identify renal allograft recipients with viral nephropathy. N Engl J Med 342: 1309–1315

Study showing that plasma testing for BK viral DNA using PCR is reasonably sensitive and specific for the diagnosis of viral interstitial nephritis, which arises secondary to reactivation of either BK virus or its related JC polyomavirus in immunosuppressed transplant patients.

14.8 Ligtenberg G et al (1999) Reduction of sympathetic hyperactivity by enalapril in patients with chronic renal failure. N Engl J Med 340: 1321–1328

Study of sympathetic nerve activity in 14 patients, showing that sympathetic nerve overactivity contributes to hypertension in renal failure, but that this is effectively reversed by ACE inhibitor treatment.

14.9 Brenner BM et al (2001) Effects of losartan on renal and cardiovascular outcomes in patients with type 2 diabetes and nephropathy. N Engl J Med 345: 861–869

Randomized double-blind study of the angiotensin II receptor antagonist, losartan, in 686 patients, showing reduction of proteinuria with few side effects, but no improvement in survival; as with ACE inhibitors, the benefits appeared to be in excess of the blood pressure reduction.

14.10 Eriksson U et al (2001) Comparison of effects of amphotericin B deoxycholate infused over 4 or 24 hours: randomized controlled trial. Br Med J 322: 579–582

Randomized study of 80 refractory febrile neutropenics, showing less nephrotoxicity and mortality in the amphotericin prolonged-infusion arm.

CHAPTER 15

Respiratory disease

Physical examination protocol 15.1 You are asked to examine the respiratory system

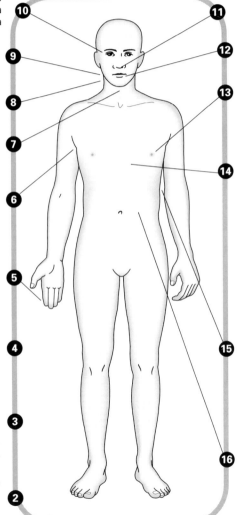

Eyes:
Horner's syndrome
xerophthalmia
papilledema

Ask to cough (? 'bovine')
Say 'ee' (? hoarse)

Jugular venous pressure:
elevation
'ventricularization' (TI)

Trachea:
position
tug

Lymphadenopathy:
epitrochlear
axillary
posterior cervical

Hands:
nicotine stains
clubbing, peripheral cyanosis
wasting of small muscles
wrist/metacarpal tenderness
flapping tremor

Vital signs:
fever
pulse rate, ?bounding quality
BP, paradox (? palpable)

General:
respiratory distress
accessory muscle use
stridor, audible wheeze
central cyanosis; eczema
chest deformity
thoracotomy/-acentesis scar

Inspect sputum cup
(?copious/foul/purulent/
bloodstained/frothy)

Nose:
lupus pernio
polyps, granulomata

Mouth, tongue:
central cyanosis

Breast lumps, gynecomastia

Examine anterior thorax:
chest expansion
vocal fremitus
pulmonary arterial impulse
right ventricular heave
apex beat (incl. dextrocardia)
percussion (incl. clavicles and
liver dullness)
breath sounds (and post-tussive)
P_s intensity; S_3
Pemberton's sign

Sit forward and repeat above
Palpate anterior cervical and
supraclavicular nodes
Feel for sacral edema
Demonstrate
aegophony/whispering
pectoriloquy if indicated
Forced expiratory time (> 5 sec
→ probable obstruction)
Pain's test (single-breath
counting) (< 20 → probable
restriction)

Abdomen: liver ptosis
liver enlargement
splenomegaly; urinalysis
Ask to view CXR if appropriate

Introduce yourself
Position the patient
Obtain adequate exposure

Diagnostic pathway 15.1   The patient is breathless. Why do you think that might be?

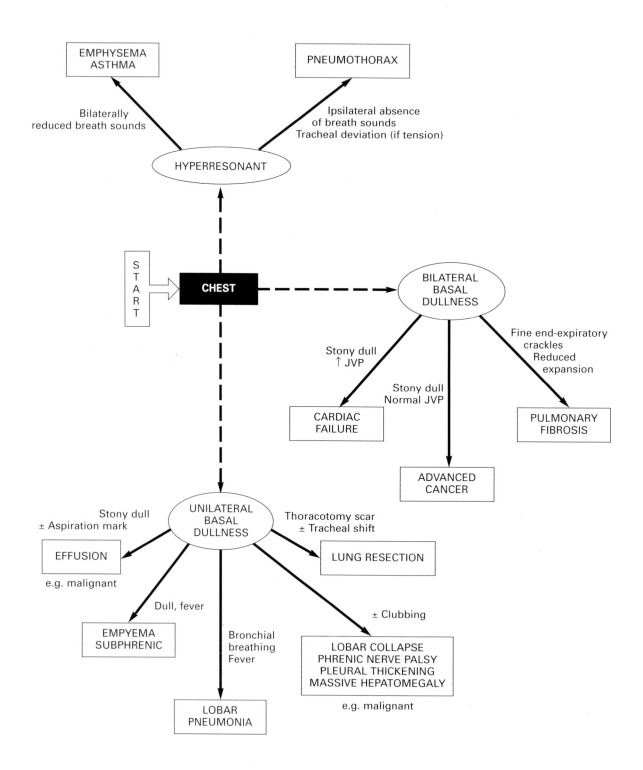

COMMON AND CLASSIC RESPIRATORY PROBLEMS

Common respiratory problems in clinical practice
1 Asthma
2 Emphysema and/or chronic bronchitis
3 Acute bronchitis

Classic respiratory problems in clinical exams
1 Pleural effusion ± metastatic neoplasm
2 Lobar consolidation ± primary endobronchial neoplasm
3 Cor pulmonale

RESPIRATORY EMERGENCIES

Don't be misled: indicators of lifethreatening asthma
1 Sleepy patient (i.e. looks not distressed, but actually exhausted)
2 No audible bronchospasm (i.e. silent chest; implies PEFR < 35%)

Therapeutic options in hemoptysis
1 Conservative measures
— Transfusion
— Cough suppressant
— Avoid chest percussion
— Treat any associated coagulopathy
2 Additional measures if hemoptysis severe
— Intubation with large bore endotracheal tube
— Bronchoscopy to localize and control bleeding
3 Definitive measures (if endobronchial lesion located)
— Laser therapy
— Radiotherapy (for neoplastic bleeding)
— Bronchial artery embolization
— Surgery and lobectomy

CLINICAL ASSESSMENT OF THE RESPIRATORY PATIENT

DYSPNEA

Grading of exertional dyspnea by clinical history: MRC criteria
1 Grade I
— Breathless hurrying on level ground or walking uphill
2 Grade II
— Breathless walking flat with people of one's own age
3 Grade III
— Breathless enough to stop walking at one's own pace

Dyspnea: typical rates of onset
1 Maximal within seconds
— Pneumothorax
— Pulmonary embolism*

2 Maximal within hours
— Asthma
— Hypersensitivity pneumonitis
— Pneumonia
— Cardiac failure
— Hemorrhage
3 Maximal within days to months
— Progressive anemia (any cause)
— Progression of restrictive lung disease
— Exacerbation of obstructive airways disease
— Enlarging pleural effusion(s)
— Primary or secondary malignancy

* Symptoms will worsen, perhaps gradually, with subsequent emboli; hence, small emboli may *not* be associated with rapid symptom onset

'Blue bloater' or 'pink puffer'? Features favoring the latter*
1 Severe subjective dyspnea
2 Scanty sputum, few infections
3 CXR: hyperlucent lungs, 'thin' heart
4 $PaCO_2 < 40$ mmHg
$PaO_2 > 60$ mmHg
5 Hematocrit not elevated
6 No signs of pulmonary hypertension or cor pulmonale

* i.e. features suggesting dominant emphysema rather than chronic bronchitis

Relationship of dyspnea to exercise training*
1 The commonest factor limiting exercise tolerance is muscle deconditioning
2 Blood lactate accumulation restricts the rate of oxygen consumption
3 Elevating the hemoglobin concentration improves tissue oxygen delivery
4 Training can increase peripheral tissue oxygen extraction by up to 30%

* In individuals with normal lung function

PRESENTATIONS OF RESPIRATORY DISEASE

Differential diagnosis of recurrent hemoptysis
1 Bronchiectasis
2 Bronchial adenoma
3 Mitral stenosis; recurrent left ventricular failure
4 Recurrent pulmonary embolism with infarction
5 Telangiectasia (arteriovenous malformation)

Predispositions to recurrent lower respiratory tract infections
1 Hypogammaglobulinemia
2 Ciliary dysfunction
— Cystic fibrosis
— Immotile cilia syndrome
— Pulmonary alveolar proteinosis
— Bronchiectasis
3 Autoimmune disease
— Sjögren's syndrome
— Relapsing polychondritis
4 Esophageal disease
— Achalasia

— Scleroderma
— Riley–Day syndrome
— Pharyngeal pouch
5 Cardiovascular disease
— Atrial septal defect
— Mitral stenosis
— Pulmonary emboli

Lifestyle clues to unusual lung infections
1 Bird fanciers
— Psittacosis
2 Abattoir or farm workers
— Brucellosis
— Q fever (*Coxiella burnetii*)
3 Florists, gardeners
— Sporotrichosis (from rose thorns)
4 Camping enthusiasts
— Tularemia
5 Wool classers, leather workers
— Anthrax

Diagnostic considerations in slow-resolving pneumonia
1 Wrong antibiotics
2 Multiple or unusual organisms
3 Immunosuppressed patient (e.g. myeloma, AIDS)
4 Empyema/abscess formation
5 Recurrent aspiration (e.g. sinus disease)
6 Endobronchial neoplasm
7 Misdiagnosis: lymphoma, alveolar cell carcinoma

Differential diagnosis of unexplained pleuritic pain
1 **P**leurodynia (Bornholm's disease, epidemic myalgia)
2 **P**neumonia
3 **P**neumothorax
4 **P**ulmonary infarction
5 **P**ericarditis
6 (Sub)**p**hrenic abscess
7 **P**ancreatitis
8 **P**athologic rib fracture
9 **P**leural disease, esp. mesothelioma
10 **P**ost-herpetic neuralgia

Churg–Strauss syndrome: when to think of it
1 Late-onset asthma
2 Systemic vasculitis
3 Eosinophilia
4 Peripheral neuropathy
5 Transient pulmonary infiltrates or cardiomegaly
6 Microscopic hematuria
7 Antimyeloperoxidase pANCA
8 Refractory symptoms requiring steroids

CLINICAL SIGNS OF RESPIRATORY DISEASE

Diagnostic clues from sputum examination
1 Copious, purulent, pungent
— Bronchiectasis, lung abscess
2 Copious, pink, frothy
— Acute left ventricular failure
3 Copious, clear, watery
— Alveolar cell carcinoma
4 Rubbery brown plugs
— Allergic bronchopulmonary aspergillosis
5 'Anchovy sauce'
— Amebic abscess
6 Melanoptysis (jet-black fibrotic particles)
— Pneumoconiosis with progressive massive fibrosis
7 'Blood oyster' (blood within mucopurulent sputum)
— TB, primary lung cancer
8 Rusty staining of mucoid sputum
— Early pneumococcal pneumonia
9 Stones (lithopsis)
— Broncholithiasis

Clinical components of clubbing
1 Soft tissue swelling
2 Loss of nailfold angle (> 150°)
3 Exaggerated curvature of long axis of nail
4 Increased nailbed fluctuation ('boggy') on pressure
5 May be associated with wrist metacarpal tenderness (HPO)

Differential diagnosis of basal crackles with clubbing
1 Bronchiectasis
— Coarse crackles (may be unilateral)
2 Asbestosis; idiopathic pulmonary fibrosis
— Bibasilar fine end-inspiratory crackles

Differential diagnosis of basal dullness
1 'Stony' dullness
— Pleural effusion
2 'Non-stony' dullness
— Loss of aeration (consolidation, abscess)
— Loss of lung volume (collapse, severe fibrosis)

Examination of the patient with bronchiectasis
1 Copious purulent sputum (foul-smelling? anaerobic)
2 Clubbing, coarse crackles
3 Nasal discharge and/or polyps
4 Dextrocardia
5 Hepatosplenomegaly; enlarged kidneys
— Indicative of secondary (reactive) amyloidosis

Causes of hepatomegaly in respiratory disease
1 Chronic venous congestion
— In cor pulmonale
2 Metastatic liver disease
— In lung cancer
3 Spurious (ptosed liver)
— In emphysema

Chronic cough with normal CXR?
1 Smoking
2 ACE inhibitor treatment
3 Post-nasal drip syndrome
4 Gastroesophageal reflux disease

Peripheral edema: pathogenesis in respiratory disease
1 Right ventricular failure
2 Sequelae of chronic systemic venous congestion
— 'Cardiac cirrhosis'

— Protein-losing enteropathy
— Nephrosis
3 Membranous nephropathy (paraneoplastic)
4 Yellow nail syndrome (lymphedema)
5 Fluid retention due to corticosteroid administration

OBSTRUCTIVE SLEEP APNEA

Sleep apnea: presenting complaints*
1 Snoring (in obstructive variety)
  Nocturnal choking and/or panic attacks
  Hypnagogic hallucinations; nightmares
2 Disorientation after waking
  Excessive daytime somnolence
3 Morning headaches (CO_2 retention‡)
4 Depression, personality change
5 Impotence; nocturnal enuresis; reduced libido
6 Related to etiology (e.g. myxedema, acromegaly)
7 Motor vehicle accidents
8 Weight gain

* NB: Partner's history important (may present with spouse complaint)
* Associated with $\geq$ 4% decrease in oxyhemoglobin saturation

Complications of sleep apnea
1 Systemic hypertension*
  — Present in 70%
2 Left ventricular disease
  — Left ventricular hypertrophy
  — Dilated cardiomyopathy
3 Ischemic heart disease
  — Myocardial infarction
  — Nocturnal cardiac arrhythmias (incl. bradycardia)
  — Unexpected death during sleep
4 Secondary cardiovascular sequelae
  — Pulmonary hypertension
  — Cor pulmonale (40%)
  — Polycythemia
5 Respiratory sequelae
  — Impaired (diurnal) pulmonary function (70%)
  — Respiratory failure

* Due to increased sympathetic activity

INVESTIGATING RESPIRATORY DISEASE

Electrophoretographic clues in respiratory diagnosis
1 α_1 pallor
  — Emphysema due to α_1AT deficiency
2 Hypogammaglobulinemia
  — May underlie chronic bronchiectasis and sinus disease
3 Polyclonal gammopathy
  — Sarcoidosis (inter alia)

Diagnosis of α_1-antitrypsin deficiency
1 Family history of emphysema or childhood liver disease*
2 Emphysema in a young patient (< 40 years) or non-smoker‡

3 *Basal* hyperlucency on CXR
4 Panacinar (panlobular) emphysema on lung biopsy
5 α_1 pallor on electrophoresis;
  $\downarrow$ α_1AT levels on quantitative assay

* Neonatal hepatitis $\pm$ infantile cirrhosis
‡ Rarely may present with mesangiocapillary glomerulonephritis

Sputum microscopy in atopic asthma: features
1 Eosinophils
2 Charcot–Leyden crystals (eosinophil derivatives)
3 Creola bodies (clumps of bronchiolar epithelial cells)
4 Curschmann's spirals (bronchiolar casts)

Differential diagnosis of pulmonary eosinophilia*
1 Allergic bronchopulmonary aspergillosis (ABPA; p. 353)
2 Vasculitis
  — PAN
  — Churg–Strauss syndrome
3 Hypereosinophilic syndrome
4 Tropical eosinophilia
  — Filariasis
5 Löffler's syndrome (in temperate zones)
  — Helminth infestation
6 Drug reactions

* Lung infiltrates on CXR and eosinophil count > 0.5×10^9/L

TESTING LUNG FUNCTION

Lung function tests: typical disease panerns
1 Obstructive airways disease
  — $\downarrow$ FEV_1, *and*
  — $\downarrow$ FEV_1/FVC
2 Restrictive lung disease
  — $\downarrow$ TLC, *and*
  — $\downarrow$ FVC

Lung function monitors in large airway disease
1 FEV_1 (FEV_1 /VC)
2 PEFR (peak expiratory flow rate)
3 Airways resistance

Lung function monitors in small airway disease
1 Maximal mid-expiratory flow rate (MMFR), *or* FEF 25–75% (forced expiratory flow)
2 Flow-volume curves
  — 'Scoop' in expiratory curve

Severity of chronic obstructive airways disease
1 FEV_1 < 60–80% predicted: mild
2 FEV_1 < 40–60% predicted: moderate
3 FEV_1 < 40% predicted: severe

Post-bronchodilator reversibility of obstruction
1 Increase in FEV_1 > 200 mL (absolute) or > 15% (relative) implies reversibility
2 Lesser improvements do *not* necessarily preclude a therapeutic trial of bronchodilators or steroids, however, if clinical suspicion of 'asthma' remains

ARTERIAL BLOOD GAS ANALYSIS

Diagnostic scenarios for arterial blood gas measurement
1 Suspected sedative overdose
2 Suspected CO_2 narcosis in 'blue bloater'
3 Suspected pulmonary embolism
4 Assessment of severe asthma
5 Suspected surreptitious vomiting*

* Associated with metabolic alkalosis

Clues to the interpretation of arterial blood gases
1 ↓ PaO_2 normalizing on 100% oxygen; > PaO_2
   — Alveolar hypoventilation (overdose, Guillain–Barré)
2 ↓ PaO_2 normalizing on 100% oxygen; normal or low $PaCO_2$
   — V/Q mismatch*
3 ↓ PaO_2 not correcting with 100% oxygen; normal $PaCO_2$
   — Shunting (intrapulmonary or intracardiac)
4 Normal or slightly reduced PaO_2; ↓↓ PaO_2 on exercise, normalizing with 100% oxygen; normal or low $PaCO_2$
   — Diffusion defect (rare)
   — Altitude
5 PaO_2 < 60 mmHg, $PaCO_2$ > 45 mmHg
   — Inadvertent venous (non-arterial) blood sample

* NB: Severe mismatching may cause ↑ $PaCO_2$

Significance of increased alveolar-arterial (A-a) oxygen gradient*
1 Ventilation/perfusion mismatching, e.g.
   — Airways obstruction
   — Pulmonary embolism
2 Shunt
   — Intrapulmonary (e.g. ARDS, pulmonary edema)
   — Intracardiac (e.g. Eisenmenger's syndrome)
3 Diffusion defect‡

* PaO_2/R, where R = 0.8 normally; normal A-a gradient < 15 mmHg
‡ Only minor contribution to pathophysiology of fibrotic and emphysematous lung disease; V/Q mismatch is more important

Tissue hypoxia with normal cardiorespiratory capacity
1 Hypoxemia despite normal A-a gradient
   — Alveolar hypoventilation
   — ↓ FiO_2 (e.g. altitude)
2 Normal PaO_2 with increased oxyhemoglobin affinity
   — Massive stored blood transfusion (↑ citrate → ↓ 2,3-DPG)
   — Bicarbonate administration in ketoacidosis
   — Profound hypothermia/acidemia/hypophosphatemia – myxedema
   — High-affinity Hb (e.g. Köln, Chesapeake)
   — Carbon monoxide poisoning
3 Cyanide intoxication
4 Hyperviscosity
5 Anemia

Acid–base disturbances in respiratory disease
1 Acute respiratory acidosis (ventilatory failure)
   — 10 mmHg ↑ $PaCO_2$ → 1 mEq/L ↑ HCO_3^- (tissue buffer)
2 Chronic respiratory acidosis (incl. 'acute-on-chronic' exacerbations, e.g. of chronic bronchitis)
   — 10 mmHg ↑ $PaCO_2$ → 3 mEq/L ↑ HCO_3^- (↑ renal reabsorption of HCO_3^- and ↑ acid excretion)
   — High base excess
3 Acute respiratory alkalosis (e.g. secondary to ketoacidosis)
   — 10 mmHg ↓ $PaCO_2$ → 2 mEq/L ↑ HCO_3^-
4 Chronic respiratory alkalosis (e.g. 'pink puffer')
   — 10 mmHg ↓ $PaCO_2$ → 5 mEq/L ↓ HCO_3^-
   — Rarely does bicarbonate level drop to < 15 mmol/L

Clinical manifestations of carbon dioxide retention
1 $PaCO_2$ > 80 mmHg
   — Progressive impairment of consciousness
   — Central cyanosis seen at rest if HbO_2 saturation < 85%
2 Neurological
   — Flapping tremor
   — Hyporeflexia; muscle twitching
   — Headache
3 Vascular
   — Hypertension
   — Bounding pulse
   — Warm extremities (cf. peripheral cyanosis), sweating
   — Edema, tender pulsatile liver if cor pulmonale present
4 Ocular
   — Miosis
   — Retinal vein distension
   — Papilledema
5 $PaCO_2$ > 120 mmHg
   — Extensor plantar responses
   — Coma

Clinical significance of central cyanosis
1 Alveolar hypoventilation (type II respiratory failure)
   — e.g. Sedative overdose
2 Right-to-left shunting
   — i.e. ↑ FiO_2 fails to cause ↑ PaO_2
3 Mechanical
   — Superior vena caval obstruction
4 Normal PaO_2
   — Polycythemia vera
   — Low-affinity Hb (e.g. Kansas, Hammersmith)
5 Severe V/Q mismatching (type I respiratory failure)
   — e.g. Massive pulmonary embolism

SERUM ANGIOTENSIN-CONVERTING ENZYME (ACE)

Differential diagnosis of elevated ACE with lung infiltrates
1 Dust diseases (antigenic reactions)
   — Asbestosis
   — Silicosis
   — Berylliosis

2 Infections
 — Miliary TB
 — Coccidioidomycosis, histoplasmosis
3 Hypersensitivity pneumonitis
4 Either ARDS (p. 354) or AIDS
5 Primary biliary cirrhosis
6 Lymphoma, malignant histiocytosis

Differential diagnosis of elevated ACE without lung infiltrates

1 Young age
2 Thyrotoxicosis
3 Diabetes mellitus
4 Dysproteinemia: myeloma, amyloidosis
5 Whipple's disease
6 Gaucher's disease

RESTRICTIVE LUNG DISEASE

Lung function monitors in restrictive lung disease

1 Post-exercise A-a (alveolar-arterial oxygen) gradient, *or*
 HbO_2 desaturation
2 DL_{CO}
3 Static compliance
4 VC, TLC (e.g. in myasthenia gravis)

Additional disease monitors in pulmonary fibrosis

1 Cellularity of bronchoalveolar lavage (see below)
2 ^{67}Gallium scanning (macrophage uptake; semiquantitative)
3 Transbronchial biopsy (restricted to initial diagnosis)

Conditions affecting measurement of diffusing capacity

1 ↑ DL_{CO}
 — Alveolar hemorrhage (Hb sequestered in alveolae)
  • Goodpasture's syndrome (if *recent* bleed)
  • Idiopathic pulmonary hemosiderosis
  • Mitral stenosis
 — Acute asthma (hyperinflation)
 — Physiological
  • High-output states: exercise, altitude
  • Supine position
 — Polycythemia
2 ↓ DL_{CO}
 — Pulmonary fibrosis (restrictive lung disease), e.g.
  • Asbestosis
  • Sarcoidosis
  • Connective tissue diseases, PAN
  • Idiopathic (cryptogenic fibrosing alveolitis)
 — Severe V/Q mismatching
  • Emphysema
  • Pulmonary embolism
  • Pneumonectomy
 — Smoking (↑ carboxyhemoglobin)
 — Anemia*

* NB: May complicate alveolar hemorrhagic states

BRONCHOALVEOLAR LAVAGE (BAL)

Indications for bronchoalveolar lavage

1 Diagnostic (saline) lavage
 — Opportunistic infections
 — Alveolar hemorrhagic syndromes
 — Alveolar proteinosis
 — Dust diseases (e.g. asbestosis)
 — Histiocytosis X
2 Prognostic lavage
 — Pulmonary fibrosis
 — Sarcoidosis
 — Hypersensitivity pneumonitis
 — ARDS
 — Drug-induced lung disease
3 Therapeutic (heparin/acetylcysteine) lavage
 — Pulmonary alveolar proteinosis
 — Cystic fibrosis/bronchiectasis
 — Asthma with mucus plugging

Normal composition of BAL fluid

1 Total leukocyte count
 — Non-smokers: $5–10 \times 10^6$/L
 — Smokers: $20–50 \times 10^6$/L
2 Leukocyte differential
 — Macrophages
  • 80–90% (non-smokers)
  • 95% (smokers)
 — Lymphocytes
  • 5–15% (non-smokers)
  • 1–10% (smokers)
 — Neutrophils
  • 0–2% (non-smokers)
  • 2–5% (smokers)
 — Eosinophils: < 1%
3 T cell subsets
 — Helpers* (T_H, $CD4^+$) ~ 50%
 — Suppressors (T_S, $CD8^+$) ~ 30%
 — Killers ~ 5–10%
 — B cells, plasma cells ~ 5–10%
 — Null cells ~ 5%

* cf. bronchoalveolar T_{H2} lymphocytes: normal number, but functionally activated in atopic asthma

Infections able to be diagnosed by BAL

1 *Pneumocystis carinii*
 — Gomon's silver stain (and culture)
2 *Legionella* spp., HSV, influenza, adenovirus
 — Direct fluorescence assay, and culture
3 *Mycoplasma* spp., *Nocardia* spp., *Mycobacteria* spp.
 — (Modified) acid-fast stain and culture
4 *Toxoplasma gondii*
 — Histopathology (+ serum titres)
 Fungi (e.g. histoplasma, candida, aspergillus)
 — Cytology
5 CMV
 — PCR, antigen assay, shell-virus culture
6 Bacterial organisms (e.g. Gram-negatives, *Staphylococcus aureus*)
 — Gram stain, and culture

Lymphocytosis vs granulocytosis on BAL?

1 Predominant lymphocytosis
   — Sarcoidosis (unless chronic)
   — Hypersensitivity pneumonitis
   — Berylliosis, silicosis
   — Tuberculosis
   — Sjögren's syndrome
   — Drug-induced lung disease
2 Predominant granulocytosis
   — Idiopathic pulmonary fibrosis*
   — ARDS
   — Bacterial infection
   — Asbestosis
   — Scleroderma, rheumatoid arthritis

* More responsive subtypes may be associated with lymphocytosis (see below)

BAL cell counts in disease

1 Smokers
   — Overall increase in cellularity (up to 5-fold)
   — Reduced number of activated T cells
   — Reduced function of macrophages and lymphocytes
2 Idiopathic pulmonary fibrosis
   — Increased neutrophils (5–50%) in active disease
   — Worse if > 10% neutrophils (esp. if + ^{67}Ga scan)
   — Prognosis better *if* lymphocytosis (> 25%) present
3 Sarcoidosis
   — Lymphocytosis (up to 40%)
   — May be predictive of steroid-responsiveness
   — Marked excess of T_H cells* indicates poor prognosis
   — Neutrophil excess associated with advanced disease
4 Hypersensitivity pneumonitis
   — Lymphocytosis (cf. pulmonary fibrosis)
5 Histiocytosis X
   — Histiocytosis X cells (containing 'X bodies')
   — Cholesterol-laden macrophages ('foam cells')
6 Eosinophilic pneumonia
   — Eosinophils
7 Drug-induced lung disease
   — Lymphocytosis, macrophages
8 Chronic lipoid pneumonia
   — Fat globules in macrophages
9 Asbestosis
   — Ferruginous bodies
10 Alveolar proteinosis
   — PAS-positive alveolar cell lipoprotein

* cf. peripheral blood: lymphopenia, relative excess of suppressor T cells

Therapeutic significance of BAL counts in pulmonary fibrosis

1 Lymphocytosis
   — Better response to steroids
2 Neutrophil/eosinophil granulocytosis
   — Worse response to steroids
   — Better response to cyclophosphamide

Indications for bronchoscopy

1 Rigid (under general anesthesia)
   — Removal of foreign body
   — Therapeutic bronchoscopy (e.g. stenting, laser)
2 Fiberoptic
   — CXR suggesting primary endobronchial neoplasm
   — Hemoptysis and/or positive sputum cytology
   — Assessment of stridor or localized wheeze
   — Unexplained diffuse lung disease or CXR opacities
   — Diagnosis of suspected opportunistic (e.g. invasive fungal) infection, esp. if immunosuppressed

Contraindications to bronchoscopy

1 Severe hypoxemia (any cause, esp. respiratory)
2 Severe asthma
3 Severe pulmonary hypertension
4 Severe hemoptysis
5 Cardiovascular instability (e.g. recent infarct)
6 Hepatitis B, HIV infection, or untreated TB
7 Unavailability of experienced bronchoscopist

Contraindications to transbronchial lung biopsy

1 Coagulopathy
2 Uremia
3 PEEP
4 Severe pulmonary hypertension

NB: SVC obstruction is *not* generally regarded as a contraindication to bronchoscopic biopsy

Diagnostic significance of lung granulomata

1 Infection
   — Caseating
     • Tuberculosis
     • Some atypical mycobacteria
   — Non-caseating
     • Histoplasmosis, other fungi
2 Hypersensitivity
   — Sarcoidosis
   — Hypersensitivity pneumonitis
   — Chronic berylliosis
3 Vasculitis
   — Wegener's granulomatosis
   — Churg–Strauss syndrome*
4 Neoplasm
   — Histiocytosis X
   — Lymphomatoid granulomatosis

* Associated with peri- or extravascular granulomata

Diagnostic aspects of pleural effusions

1 Transudate (< 30 g/L protein; often bilateral)*
   — Cardiac failure, constrictive pericarditis
   — Cirrhosis, nephrosis
   — Myxedema

— Meigs' syndrome
2 Uniformly bloodstained effusion
   — Metastatic carcinoma (i.e. to pleura)
   — Pulmonary infarction
3 Chylous effusion (positive Sudan III stain)
   — Trauma (esp. endoscopy or surgery)
   — Lymphomas
   — Filariasis
   — Nephrosis, cirrhosis (uncommon)
4 Pseudochylous effusions (due to cholesterol; Sudan III negative)
   — TB
   — Rheumatoid arthritis

* Hence, transudate and/or edema suggest that local pathology is *unlikely*

Diagnostic characteristics of empyema (> parapneumonic effusion)
1 Thickened pleura on CT
2 Pleural fluid
   — Turbid
   — pH < 7.2
   — LDH > 1000 U/L
   — Glucose < 40 mg/dL*

* Low glucose is also seen in rheumatoid effusions

Differential diagnosis of high amylase in pleural fluid
1 Pancreatitis
   — Left > right effusion
   — Pancreatic amylase isoenzyme
2 Esophageal rupture
   — Right > left effusion
   — Salivary amylase isoenzyme
   — pH < 6.0

Possible indications for pleural biopsy
1 Suspected tuberculosis (biopsy should be cultured)
2 Suspected malignant pleural effusion; cytology negative
3 Suspected granulomatous disorder

RADIOGRAPHIC DIAGNOSIS OF LUNG DISEASE

Upper zone CXR infiltrates: differential diagnosis
1 Infection
   — Tuberculosis
   — Aspergillosis
   — *Klebsiella* pneumonia
2 Fibrosis
   — Silicosis
   — Radiation fibrosis
   — Ankylosing spondylitis
   — Hypersensitivity pneumonitis (long-standing)
3 Histiocytosis X

Lower zone CXR infiltrates: differential diagnosis
1 Idiopathic pulmonary fibrosis*
2 Pulmonary fibrosis due to connective tissue disease
3 Asbestosis
4 Cytotoxic-induced lung disease

5 Pulmonary hemosiderosis
6 Aspiration
7 Hypersensitivity pneumonitis (acute)

* a.k.a. cryptogenic fibrosing alveolitis

Radiographic localization of mediastinal masses
1 Superior mediastinum
   — Thymoma
   — Retrosternal thyroid
   — Zenker's diverticulum
2 Anterior
   — Teratoma
   — Thyroid
   — Thymoma
3 Posterior
   — Neurogenic tumors (and other paravertebral masses)
   — Bochdalek diaphragmatic hernia (cf. Morgagni)
   — Achalasia, hiatus hernia (may also be in middle)
4 Any mediastinal compartment
   — Aortic aneurysm (usually middle)
   — Lymphoma, teratoma (usually anterior)
   — Metastatic carcinoma (usually middle)

Indications for special CXR projections
1 (Lateral) decubitus
   — Suspected small pleural effusion, esp. if subpulmonic
2 Expiratory
   — Suspected pneumothorax
   — Suspected bronchial occlusion (? inhaled foreign body)
3 Erect
   — Suspected perforation of abdominal hollow viscus
4 Penetrated PA
   — Suspected left atrial enlargement
   — Suspected left lower lobe collapse
5 Oblique
   — Visualization of pleural plaques
   — Suspected rib fracture(s)
6 Apical lordotic
   — Visualization of lesions in lung apex

Differential diagnosis of unilateral hemithorax transradiancy
1 Pneumothorax
2 Mastectomy
3 Pulmonary embolism
4 Emphysematous bullae
5 Macleod's syndrome, Swyer–James

Significance of the apparently elevated hemidiaphragm
1 Phrenic nerve palsy
2 Segmental/lobar collapse ($\rightarrow$ tracheal deviation) or resection
3 Subpulmonic effusion (decubitus film $\rightarrow$ diagnosis)
4 Subphrenic collection
5 Massive hepatomegaly
6 Diaphragmatic rupture (e.g. post-traumatic) or dysfunction (e.g. herpes zoster affecting C4 nerve root)

Interstitial vs alveolar infiltrates
1 Interstitial ('honeycombing', e.g. sarcoidosis)
   — 'Ground glass' appearance (e.g. asbestosis, berylliosis)
   — Reticular appearance (e.g. pulmonary fibrosis)
   — Nodular (e.g. histoplasmosis, pneumoconiosis)
2 Alveolar (e.g. pulmonary edema, pneumonia)
   — Fluffy opacities
   — Air bronchograms
   — Lobar or segmental distribution
   — Rapid evolution

Clinically important causes of 'honeycomb lung'
1 Idiopathic pulmonary fibrosis
2 Granulomatous lung diseases
   — Sarcoidosis
   — Histiocytosis X
   — Hypersensitivity pneumonitis (long-standing)
3 Vasculitis
   — Scleroderma
   — Rheumatoid arthritis (± effusion)
4 Dust diseases
   — Organic dusts
     • Hypersensitivity pneumonitis
   — Inorganic dusts
     • Pneumoconiosis; silicosis; berylliosis
     • Asbestosis (± 'holly-leaf' pleural plaques)
5 Neoplasia
   — Lymphangitis carcinomatosa
   — Alveolar cell carcinoma

Clinically important causes of bilateral hilar adenopathy
1 Sarcoidosis
   — Typically symmetrical lymphadenopathy
   — Patient usually looks well
2 Lymphoma
   — Typically asymmetrical lymphadenopathy
   — Patient often looks ill
3 Unusual causes
   — TB, fungal infections
   — Carcinomatosis

Differential diagnosis of hilar calcification
1 TB
2 Silicosis ('egg-shell' appearance)
3 Histoplasmosis

Disseminated interstitial nodules: differential diagnosis
1 Previous varicella pneumonia, esp. if adult-onset
2 Histoplasmosis; hydatid disease
3 Miliary TB
4 Mitral stenosis
   — Microlithiasis due to 2° pulmonary hemosiderosis
5 Malignancy
   — Metastases (basal predominance with variable size of nodules)
6 Sarcoidosis
7 Silicosis

Causes of pulmonary cavitation
1 Infection
   — TB

— Anaerobes (± aspiration)
— *Klebsiella pneumoniae*, *S. aureus*
— Invasive aspergillosis, nocardiosis, actinomycosis, histoplasmosis, coccidioidomycosis, blastomycosis
— Amebiasis
2 Pulmonary infarction
   — Septic emboli
   — Bland emboli (with secondary infection)
3 Primary lung cancer, esp. squamous
4 Wegener's granulomatosis
5 Rheumatoid nodule

Radiographic pointers to bacterial diagnosis of pneumonia
1 Lobar consolidation with pleural effusion
   — Pneumococcus
2 'Bulging' fissure
   — *Klebsiella* (classical)
   — Pneumococcus (common)
3 Periosteal reaction
   — *Actinomyces* spp.
4 Right lower lobe involved
   — Aspiration

Investigation of bronchiectasis
1 CXR
   — 'Tramline' bronchial thickening
   — Dextrocardia (Kartagener's)
2 High-resolution lung CT (gold standard)
3 Bronchoscopy
   — For focal bronchiectasis, *or*
   — To rule out local lesions (e.g. foreign body)
4 Etiology
   — Sweat test, immunoglobulins (in children)
   — Nasal biopsy for electron microscopy (immotile cilia)
   — AFBs; *Aspergillus* precipitins/skin test
5 Complications
   — Sputum culture (for *S. aureus*, *Pseudomonas aeruginosa*)
   — Protein electrophoresis; biopsy (for amyloid)

Radiographic features of miscellaneous disorders
1 Asbestosis
   — Calcified pleural plaques (esp. diaphragmatic)
   — Bibasilar interstitial fibrosis (lower lobe predominance)
   — 'Shaggy' pericardial silhouette
2 Pulmonary infarction
   — Can be normal
   — Linear atelectasis
   — (Small) pleural effusion(s)
   — Wedge-shaped peripheral lesion(s), apex towards hilum (Hampton's harp)
   — Elevated hemidiaphragm (if collapse)
   — Enlarged pulmonary artery
3 Emphysema
   — Hyperinflation (DD$_x$ = asthma)
     • Hyperlucent lungfields ('black lungs')
     • 'Flat' low hemidiaphragms
     • Visible 11th rib
     • Long tubular heart shadow
   — Bullae

— Pulmonary artery > 2 cm (pulmonary hypertension)

Potential indications for high-resolution chest CT
1 Diagnosis of diffuse infiltrative lung disease
  — Diagnostic sensitivity of 95%*
  — Distinguishes
    • Sarcoidosis
    • Pulmonary fibrosis (fibrosing alveolitis)
    • Lymphangitis carcinomatosa
    • Lymphangioleiomyomatosis
    • Hypersensitivity pneumonitis
    • Histiocytosis X
2 Prognosis and follow-up of diffuse infiltrative lung disease
  — Quantifies severity
  — Distinguishes active from irreversible fibrosis (ground glass)
  — Confirms number of lobes involved
3 Early diagnosis of CXR-negative disorders (e.g. in AIDS)
  — *P. carinii* pneumonia
  — Invasive aspergillosis
  — Pulmonary Kaposi's

* i.e. with 100% sensitivity for biopsy; CXR is only 80%

INVASIVE DIAGNOSTIC TESTS

Indications for invasive diagnosis of pulmonary infiltrates
1 Percutaneous needle aspiration
  — Cavitating infiltrates
  — Peripheral infiltrates
2 Bronchoscopy
  — Infiltrate of presumed infective etiology
  — Infiltrate of presumed neoplastic etiology
3 Bronchoalveolar lavage
  — Presumed opportunistic infection*
  — Cytology of peripheral infiltrates
4 Open lung biopsy: histopathology required, e.g.
  — Drug-induced lung fibrosis
  — Radiation pneumonitis

* May also require open lung biopsy

Indications for open lung biopsy in pulmonary fibrosis
1 Young age (< 60 years)
2 Atypical CXR or high-resolution CT
  — Nodular, patchy, adenopathy, effusion, failure

NB: *Clubbing* is consistent with an idiopathic etiology, and is thus *not* an indication for biopsy

SLEEP STUDIES

Indications for sleep studies
1 Suspected sleep apnea (p. 341)
  — Loud snoring plus daytime somnolence
  — Cor pulmonale, central cyanosis
  — Observed apneas

2 Unexplained progressive clinical deterioration in a patient with chronic obstructive airways disease

Measurements made during sleep studies
1 Measurement of sleep stages (3 h sleep required)
  — EEG
  — Submental EMG
  — Bilateral electro-oculograms*
2 Airflow measurement
  — Nasal/oral thermistors
  — CO_2 sensor or pneumotachography
  — Airway pressure (CPAP study)
3 Respiratory effort measurement
  — Chest/abdominal strain gauges
  — Surface EMG of respiratory muscles
  — Esophageal balloon (pleural pressure changes)
4 Arterial blood gases
  — Skin oximetry
5 ECG
  — Detects rate/rhythm disturbances linked to apnea

* To detect bilateral conjugate eye movements during REM sleep

MANAGING RESPIRATORY DISEASE

ASTHMA

Unexpected death in acute asthma: risk factors
1 Recent discharge from hospital
2 Frequent use of Emergency Room
3 Underutilization of long-term preventive medicine, and overdependence on inhaled sympathomimetics
4 IV administration of aminophylline in patients already on maintenance oral theophylline
5 Undiagnosed pneumothorax (affects up to 2% of hospitalized asthmatics)
6 Failure to refer the patient to intensive care for ventilation *before* he/she arrests

Considerations in assessing asthma severity
1 Patient's assessment of severity
  Request for admission by patient or family
2 Previous admission(s) for stabilization
3 History of steroid requirement, esp. if recent reduction
4 Rapid symptomatic development (labile disease)
5 Insufficient lung function to use usual inhalers
6 Iatrogenic factors
  — Inappropriate sedation
  — Precipitation by aspirin or β-blockers

Clinical criteria favoring hospitalization in acute asthma
1 General demeanor
  — Difficulty speaking (can't complete a sentence? PEFR < 50%)
  — Sweaty, anxious, irritable
  — Exhausted; confused; sitting forward
  — Late afternoon or evening presentation
2 Vital signs
  — Tachycardia > 150/min
  — Tachypnea > 28/min

— Forced expiratory time > 4 sec
— Blood pressure
 • Paradox* > 20 mmHg
 • Pulsus paradoxus (i.e. palpable paradox)
 • Hypotension (ominous)
3 Signs of respiratory distress
 — Stridor, audible wheezing
 — Accessory muscle use (e.g. sternomastoids)
 — Intercostal recession (chest wall indrawing)
 — Tracheal tug (descends on inspiration)
4 Signs of ventilatory failure
 — Central cyanosis
 — Sleepiness
 — 'Quiet' (grossly hyperexpanded) chest: implies PEFR < 35%
5 Pulmonary function tests
 — PEFR < 200 L/min
 — FEV_1 < 1 L *or* too incapacitated to perform adequately
 — $PaCO_2$ > 40 mmHg (*or* PaO_2 < 60 mmHg *or* acidosis)
6 CXR
 — Pneumothorax
7 ECG
 — P pulmonale ± right ventricular strain

NB: Presence of one or more of these signs on presentation may justify admission; persistence of any sign following bronchodilators makes admission mandatory
* Defined as systolic drop of > 12 mmHg on inspiration

Clinical criteria defining good asthma control
1 Negligible nocturnal symptoms
2 No severe acute attacks
3 Normal exercise tolerance and daily activities
4 Normal PEFR
5 Infrequent use of inhaled β_2-agonist

Sequential approach to the young patient with asthma
1 Occasional mild symptoms
 — Inhaled short-acting β_2-agonist (e.g. salbutamol)
2 Frequent (> twice-weekly) episodes? Add in
 — Prophylactic inhaled sodium cromoglicate (if ≥ 5 years old)
 — Low-dose inhaled steroids (beclometasone, budesonide, fluticasone)
3 Still symptomatic?
 — Add inhaled long-acting β_2-agonist (salmeterol, formoterol), *or*
 — Add low-dose oral theophylline (250 mg b.d.) *if* cost is limiting, *or*
 — Higher-dose inhaled steroids, *or*
 — Leukotriene pathway modifiers
4 Severe acute attacks (irrespective of usual control)
 — Short-term oral steroids (if ambulant)
 — IV salbutamol (emergency room)

Factors to exclude in refractory asthma
1 Poor compliance with preventive medication
2 Poor technique with inhaler therapy
3 Persistent exposure to allergens, occupational irritants, or smoking
4 Misdiagnosis (e.g. left ventricular failure, chronic bronchitis, vocal cord dysfunction)

Side-effects of inhaled steroids
1 Hoarseness
 — Due to laryngeal myopathy*
2 Oropharyngeal thrush
 — esp. Elderly patients
 — Commoner if given more than twice daily

* Hence, may contraindicate use in singers

Prophylaxis of exercise-induced asthma
1 Pre-exercise
 — Inhaled β_2-agonist (5–10 min prior)
 — Inhaled sodium cromoglicate or nedocromil sodium
2 Regular prophylaxis
 — Inhaled low-dose steroids
 — Oral leukotriene receptor antagonists

BETA-AGONIST THERAPY

Therapeutic interventions of proven value in chronic obstructive lung disease
1 Short-term value
 — β_2-agonists *and/or* anticholinergics
 — Oral steroids
2 Long-term value
 — Smoking cessation
 — Supplemental oxygen therapy
 — Lung reduction surgery in severe emphysema

Physiologic benefits of β_2-agonists
1 Bronchodilatation
2 Cholinergic inhibition
3 Increased mucociliary clearance
4 Suppression of inflammatory mediator release

Clinical status of long-acting β_2-agonists
1 High therapeutic:toxic ratio
2 Taken by inhaler twice daily
3 Always prescribed together with inhaled steroids

Adverse effects of β_2-agonists
1 Tremor, palpitations
2 Headache, muscle cramps
3 Hypokalemia* → arrhythmias
4 Precipitation of angina
5 Tolerance‡ → rebound bronchoconstriction
6 Over-reliance¶ → increased mortality

* Especially with intravenous β_2-agonist
‡ Especially with long-term β_2-agonist
¶ Increased frequency of inhaled β_2-agonist indicates a need to up the dose of regular inhaled steroids

LEUKOTRIENE PATHWAY-MODIFYING DRUGS

Therapeutic effects of leukotriene pathway blockade
1 Reduced airway wall edema
2 Reduced bronchial mucus production
3 Bronchodilatation

Indications for leukotriene pathway-modifying therapy
1 Aspirin-induced asthma*
2 Extrinsic asthma (exercise- or cold-induced)

3 Poor compliance with inhaler therapy
4 Allergic rhinitis
5 Corticosteroid-sparing in severe asthma

* Associated with nasal polyps

PRINCIPLES OF VENTILATORY SUPPORT

Varieties of ventilatory support
1 Non-invasive ventilation (NIV)
   — Volume-cycled
   — Pressure-cycled (BiPAP)
   — Continuous positive airways pressure (CPAP)
2 Mechanical (endotracheal intubation) ventilation

Indications for mechanical ventilation
1 Inability to achieve $PaO_2 > 55$ mmHg or O_2 saturation $> 88\%$ despite supplemental oxygen and other support
2 Progressive respiratory acidosis and/or respiratory muscle fatigue despite maximum therapy
3 Inability to clear secretions or protect airway
4 Impairment of consciousness
5 Cardiopulmonary arrest
6 Hemodynamic instability

Neurological precipitants of respiratory failure
1 Neuromuscular
   — Myasthenia gravis
   — Polymyositis, myotonic dystrophy
2 Neuropathy
   — Guillain–Barré syndrome
   — Diphtheria, acute intermittent porphyria
3 Anterior horn cell disease
   — Polio
   — Motor neuron disease
4 Spinal cord lesion
   — Trauma
   — Tumor; demyelination
5 Brainstem
   — Cerebrovascular accident
   — Encephalitis; polio; tumor; demyelination

OXYGEN THERAPY

Varieties of oxygen delivery systems
1 Nasal cannulae (24% O_2 = 2 L/min)
2 Venturi mask
3 Partial rebreathing mask

Complications of oxygen therapy
1 Neonates
   — Retinopathy
   — Closure of ductus arteriosus*
2 Patients with $PaO_2 > 60$ mmHg *and* $PaCO_2 > 40$ mmHg
   — Ventilatory depression (CO_2 retention)
3 Bleomycin or paraquat-treated patients
   — Worsening of lung toxicity

* Which can be a problem in complex ductus-dependent congenital heart diatheses

Indications for long-term low-flow oxygen therapy
1 Prerequisites
   — Severe chronic obstructive lung disease
   — Cessation of smoking for at least 6 months
2 Severe chronic hypoxemia with
   — $PaO_2 < 55$ mmHg on room air; *or*
   — If PaO_2 55–59 mmHg: presence of edema, polycythemia, P pulmonale on ECG, or hematocrit $> 55\%$
3 Controversial
   — End-stage non-obstructive lung disease
   — Cancer

Benefits of long-term oxygen therapy in chronic lung disease
1 Subjective relief from dyspnea
2 Improved exercise tolerance
3 Reduced pulmonary artery pressure
4 Fewer hospital admissions
5 Prolonged survival

Treatment modalities in obstructive sleep apnea
1 Weight loss (usually > 10 kg needed)
2 Nocturnal nasal CPAP*
3 Alternative treatments for mild disease
   — Dental prostheses
   — Uvulopharyngoplasty
   — Mandibular advancement surgery
   — Tracheostomy

* Includes BiPAP, 'smart' CPAP

TREATING PNEUMONIA

Poor prognosticators in community-acquired pneumonia
1 Tachypnea > 30/min
2 Altered consciousness
3 Systolic BP < 90 mmHg
4 Advanced age
5 Coexisting disease (cancer, CNS, liver, kidney)
6 Nursing home resident

Presumptive management of pneumonia in adults
1 Ambulatory patients *without* cardiopulmonary disease or other susceptibility
   — Macrolide (erythromycin, clarithromycin, etc.) or doxycycline
2 Ambulatory patients *with* cardiopulmonary disease or other susceptibility
   — β-lactam *plus* macrolide or doxycycline; *or*
   — Antipneumococcal fluoroquinolone (e.g. levofloxacin, moxifloxacin) alone
3 Inpatients, not in intensive care, *no* cardiopulmonary disease or susceptibility
   — Macrolide alone, *or*
   — β-lactam plus doxycycline, *or*
   — Antipneumococcal fluoroquinolone alone
4 Inpatients, not in intensive care, *with* cardiopulmonary disease or susceptibility
   — β-lactam *plus* macrolide or doxycycline
   — Antipneumococcal fluoroquinolone alone

5 Inpatients in intensive care *without* risk factors for *Pseudomonas* spp.
— β-lactam *plus* macrolide
6 Inpatients in intensive care *with* risk factors for *Pseudomonas* spp.
— Antipseudomonal β-lactam (imipenem/ meropenem, or piperacillin/tazobactam) *plus* aminoglycoside *plus* macrolide

Risk factors for penicillin-resistant *Streptococcus pneumoniae* (PRSP)
1 Age > 65
2 β-lactam therapy within the last 3 months
3 Alcoholism or immunosuppressive illness
4 Exposure to a child in a daycare center
5 Multiple medical comorbidities

PRSP drug of choice in high-grade resistance*
1 Vancomycin
2 Linezolid
3 Antipneumococcal fluoroquinolone
— Levofloxacin, moxifloxacin, gemifloxacin

* MIC > 2.0

TREATMENT OF ALTITUDE SICKNESS

Pathogenesis of acute mountain sickness (AMS)
1 Altitude-induced *hypoxemia*
2 *Respiratory alkalosis* limits ventilatory response to hypoxia*
3 *Pulmonary edema* due to high pulmonary artery pressures
4 *Cerebral edema* causes the typical AMS symptoms (treat with dexamethasone)

* Limits ventilatory response to hypoxemia, i.e. until acclimatization occurs with reduction of extracellular fluid bicarbonate levels

Prevention of acute mountain sickness
1 Physical factors in prevention of AMS
— Slow ascent; immediate descent if symptoms develop
2 Medical prophylaxis (NB: adjunctive only to above measures)
— Acetazolamide 250 mg b.d. from 48 h preascent
— Slow-release nifedipine 20 mg q 8 h during ascent

LUNG TRANSPLANTATION

Eligibility criteria for lung transplantation
1 End-stage lung disease
2 No other organ failure or systemic disease limiting lifespan
3 Age
— Single-lung transplant: < 65
— Double-lung transplant: < 60
— Heart–lung transplant: < 55

4 No suppurative lung disease remaining after transplant*
5 *Heart–lung transplants*‡ may be considered in cystic fibrosis (once $FEV_1 < 35\%$, FVC < 40%) or severe primary pulmonary hypertension (e.g. Eisenmenger's syndrome)

* Suppuration (e.g. bilateral bronchiectasis) contraindicates single-lung transplant due to inevitable contamination by remaining lung. Non-suppurative indications such as pulmonary fibrosis or α_1-antitrypsin deficiency are favored
‡ Heart–lung transplants en bloc are technically easier than double-lung procedures, since the latter require tracheal anastomosis

Problems with lung transplantation
1 Infection
— CMV, *P. carinii*
— *Aspergillus, Candida* spp.
2 Rejection
— Acute (< 6 months post-transplant)
— Obliterative bronchiolitis (= chronic rejection)
• esp. Heart–lung transplants ($\rightarrow$ up to 40%)*
3 Technical concerns
— Bronchial dehiscence/stenosis
• esp. Single-lung transplants
— Prior thoracic surgery or pleurodesis (relative contraindications)
4 Expense
— Initial procedure *plus* follow-up care
5 Shortage of donor organs

* Rejection rates may be reduced to 10% via use of tacrolimus, sirolimus, mycophenolate mofetil

Timing of problems after lung transplantation
1 First month
— Surgical complications
2 First month until first year
— Infection
3 After first year
— Bronchiolitis obliterans

UNDERSTANDING RESPIRATORY DISEASE

CYSTIC FIBROSIS

Pathogenesis of cystic fibrosis (CF)
1 Mutation of transmembrane conductance regulator (CFTR)
2 CFTR mutation causes defective chloride (Cl^-) transport, which in turn causes increased sodium (Na^+) and water resorption from duct and broncial lumen
3 Thick, tenacious secretions and sputum result, leading to high frequencies of *Pseudomonas* spp. superinfection*
4 Point mutation of phenylalanine at position 508 (F_{508}), the ATP-binding site, is the underlying defect in 70%; the other 30% of cases are due to hundreds of mutations
5 The heterozygote frequency of this mutation (about 1 in 40) has been suggested to reflect evolutionary

selection due to increased resistance to *Vibrio cholerae*

6 Severe phenotypes (meconium ileus, pancreatic insufficiency) usually imply 2 defective alleles (e.g. F_{508} homozygotes)

* Either *Ps. aeruginosa* or *Ps. cepacia*

Clinical features of immotile cilia syndrome
1 Genetic etiology; includes Kartagener's (in 50%)
2 Other manifestations include otitis media, nasal polyposis and infertility (esp. in males: 95%)
3 Affected females may develop salpingitis, but usually remain fertile (as in cystic fibrosis)
4 Electron microscopy confirms ultrastructural defect of dynein arms in bronchial/nasal cilia and in sperm
5 Young's syndrome (chronic sinopulmonary disease with azoospermia) has been linked to the Q1291H mutation

Therapeutic approaches to cystic fibrosis
1 Amiloride
— ↓ Na^+ reabsorption → ↓ sputum viscosity
2 High-dose ibuprofen
— Reduces lung destruction by reducing inflammation
3 Mucolytics
— incl. Inhaled DNases or α_1-antitrypsin
4 Transplanting damaged organ
— e.g. Lung transplant
5 CFTR gene therapy
— esp. Using adenovirus-like vectors (investigational)

SARCOIDOSIS

Main features distinguishing chronic from acute sarcoidosis
1 Age of presentation
— Older (> 30 years) patients
2 CXR
— Pulmonary infiltrates
— No hilar adenopathy
3 Skin
— Lupus pernio common
— Erythema nodosum unusual
4 Mikulicz syndrome (parotidomegaly and facial palsy)
— Common
5 Therapeutic response
— Steroid-resistant
6 Prognosis
— Poor

Cardiac manifestations of sarcoidosis
1 Heart block: first-degree/RBBB/complete heart block
2 Arrhythmias: SVT/VT/ventricular ectopic beats
3 Mitral valve disease
4 Pericarditis
5 Congestive cardiac failure
6 Sudden death

Indicators of disease activity in sarcoidosis
1 Symptoms
2 Investigations of organ involvement, e.g. lung
— CXR
— DL_{CO}
3 Bronchoalveolar lavage
— Increased overall cellularity
— Up to 40% lymphocytes (predominantly T_H)
— ↓ IgG:albumin ratio (cf. allergic alveolitis)
4 ^{67}Gallium scan
— A sensitive index of disease activity
— Extrapulmonary uptake (parotid, nodes) supports diagnosis but does *not* exclude lymphoma
5 Serum angiotensin-converting enzyme (ACE)
— Elevated in 70% of patients with active (acute) disease*
— Useful in monitoring response to steroids
6 Other laboratory associations
— Serum and/or urinary calcium (if elevated)
— Hypergammaglobulinemia (polyclonal)
— Lymphopenia (relative excess of T_S cells; cf. BAL)

* But *not* specific for diagnosis (see below); serum lysozyme and transcobalamin II are similar indices of disease activity, but less sensitive

Indications for corticosteroids in sarcoidosis
1 Intractable constitutional symptoms
2 Progressive lung parenchymal disease
3 Hypercalcemia* and/or persisting hypercalciuria
4 Hypersplenism
5 Vital organ involvement
— Heart
— CNS
— Eye

* May also respond to chloroquine

LUNG INFECTIONS

Predispositions to specific pulmonary infections
1 Tuberculosis (incl. reactivation)
— Silicosis
— Alcoholism
— Gastrectomy or jejunoileal bypass
— Active measles; uncontrolled diabetes mellitus
— Iatrogenic immunosuppression
2 *Mycobacterium kansasii/avium–intracellulare*
— Pre-existing lung disease
3 Anaerobic infections (abscess, aspiration pneumonia)
— Obtunded consciousness; anesthesia, alcoholism
— Poor dental hygiene
— Achalasia, scleroderma, Riley–Day syndrome
4 *Klebsiella* spp.
— Alcoholism, derelict lifestyle
5 *Ps. aeruginosa*
S. aureus
— Cystic fibrosis (bronchial colonization)

6 *Ps. pyocyanea*
   — Humidifier/ventilator therapy
7 *Nocardia asteroides*
   — Pulmonary alveolar proteinosis
   — Chronic granulomatous disease of childhood
8 *S. aureus*
   — Recent viral URTI (esp. influenza)
9 *P. carinii*
   Cytomegalovirus
   — Immunosuppression: transplant or AIDS
10 Aspergilloma
   — Old tuberculous cavities
   — Emphysematous bullae
   — Apical cavities in ankylosing spondylitis
   — Cystic fibrosis
   — Sarcoidosis
11 *Moraxella catarrhalis*
   — Chronic obstructive lung disease

Diagnosis of Legionnaires' disease
1 Direct fluorescent antibody (on lung biopsy, pleural fluid, sputum, BAL)
2 *Culture* of lung biopsy or pleural fluid in medium containing charcoal yeast-enriched (CYE) agar with alphaketoglutarate or cysteine/iron in 5% CO_2 (low yield)
3 Serology (indirect fluorescent antibody)
   — Four-fold rise to > 1:128 (usually takes ≥ 2 weeks)
   — Single titre of > 1:256 infection at any stage
4 Urine *Legionella* antigen (fastest test)

ATYPICAL PNEUMONIA

The atypical pneumonias: which ones are they?
1 Mycoplasma (*M. pneumoniae*)
2 Chlamydia
3 Legionnaires' disease (*L. pneumophila*)
4 Viral pneumonias

Clinical aspects of *Mycoplasma* pneumonia
1 Occurrence
   — Slowly spreading epidemics
   — Long incubation period, insidious onset
2 Course
   — Initial URTI transforms to LRTI
   — Family members often also affected
   — Clinical relapse following treatment often occurs
3 Extrapulmonary manifestations
   — Arthralgias/-itis
   — Headaches, meningism ± aseptic meningitis
   — Substernal discomfort (tracheobronchitis)
   — 'Cold' autoimmune hemolysis ± anemia
   — Ear pain due to bullous or hemorrhagic myringitis*
   — Erythema multiforme
   — Myopericarditis
4 Diagnosis
   — Routine sputum non-diagnostic
   — Throat swab may (eventually) yield positive cultures
   — Definitive diagnosis established by serology (CFT)

— Sensitive to macrolides, doxycycline, new-generation quinolones

* Classical but rare

Distinguishing features of psittacosis
1 History
   — Avian exposure
2 Symptoms
   — Epistaxis
   — Photophobia
   — Thrombophlebitis
   — Myalgias, confusion, stupor
3 Signs
   — Splenomegaly (± anicteric hepatomegaly)
   — Horder's spots (may simulate rose spots of typhoid)
   — Proteinuria
4 Investigations
   — Positive serology (CFT)*
   — Transbronchial biopsy → cytoplasmic inclusions (LCL bodies) within macrophages

* Even low-titer generally suffices for diagnosis in acute phase

Distinguishing features of Q ('query') fever
1 Distinction from other rickettsioses
   — Not transmitted from arthropods
   — No rash
   — Negative Weil–Felix reaction
2 Pleuritic chest pain
3 Weight loss (may be dramatic)
4 Granulomatous hepatitis (→ about 20%)
5 Culture-negative endocarditis (usually de novo) requiring valve replacement (typically aortic)

Clinical spectrum of Legionnaires' disease
1 Commoner in
   — Smokers
   — Debilitated patients
   — Males aged about 50–60 years
   — Moderate (about 30 g/day) alcohol intake
2 Transmission
   — No documented person-to-person spread
   — Nosocomial transmission not infrequent
   — Cooling towers may be disease reservoir
3 Distinguishing clinical features
   — Severe pneumonia with high fever, rigors
   — Encephalopathy ± headache
   — Gastrointestinal upset
   — Transient azotemia; hemoproteinuria
4 Investigations
   — Hyponatremia (SIADH); also → other pneumonias
   — Hypophosphatemia
   — Transient liver function test abnormalities
   — Negative routine cultures
5 Management
   — IV fluids if hypovolemic (diarrhea, sweats)
   — Electrolyte homeostasis
   — Erythromycin 2–4 g/day IV ± rifampicin 600 mg/day (continue for 2 weeks, even though defervescence occurs within 48 h)
   — PEEP if in respiratory failure (→ 10–20%)

ASPERGILLUS-RELATED LUNG DISEASE

Spectrum of *Aspergillus*-related pulmonary disease
1 Allergic bronchopulmonary aspergillosis
   — Treat with steroids
2 Aspergilloma ('fungus ball')
   — Treat conservatively or surgically
3 Invasive aspergillosis
   — Usually affects immunocompromised patients
   — Treat urgently with IV amphotericin B
   — Mortality approaches 95% in transplant patients
4 Chronic necrotizing aspergillosis
5 Hypersensitivity pneumonitis

Diagnosis of allergic bronchopulmonary aspergillosis (ABPA)
1 Asthma
2 Central bronchiectasis
3 Upper lobe pulmonary infiltrates on CXR
4 Eosinophilia > 1000/mL
5 Antibodies* and skin prick‡ positive for *Aspergillus fumigatus*
6 Elevated total serum IgE (> 2000 ng/mL)

* Often negative in *invasive aspergillosis*, which is diagnosed by lung biopsy or by serum/urine Aspergillus antigen detection
‡ Often negative in *aspergilloma*

PATHOGENESIS OF RESPIRATORY DISEASE

Childhood sequelae of cigarette smoke exposure
1 Sudden infant death syndrome (SIDS)
2 Chronic serous otitis media (glue ear)
3 Asthma
4 Lower respiratory tract infections
5 Impaired growth of lung function

Temporal sequence of events following smoking cessation
1 Heart rate and blood pressure
   — Normal within 20 min of last cigarette
2 Oxyhemoglobin and carbon monoxide levels
   — Normal within 8 h of last cigarette
3 Nicotine levels
   — Normal within 48 h of last cigarette
   — Physical craving maximal 3 days after last cigarette
   — Psychological craving is maximal 3 weeks after last cigarette
4 Myocardial infarction risk
   — Drops to 50% of smoker's risk 5 years after last cigarette
5 Lung cancer risk
   — Drops to 50% of smoker's risk 10 years after last cigarette

Pathogenesis of atopic asthma
1 Commoner in clean westernized environments
2 Up to ten times higher prevalence in some countries than others
3 Closely related to allergic rhinitis and eczema
4 Closely related to strong family history of atopy

Pathogenesis of emphysema
1 Protease–antiprotease imbalance in alveolar epithelial lining fluid causes proteolytic destruction of alveolae, thus reducing pulmonary gas-exchanging interface
2 Cigarette smoke efficiently inactivates the key antiprotease, α_1-antitrypsin (α_1AT), thus predisposing to emphysema
3 Free radical production from activated neutrophils (e.g. in chronic inflammation) may also contribute to damage
4 2% of emphysema patients have a detectable reduction in circulating α_1AT, reflecting a genetic mutation (ZZ) which causes impaired α_1AT release after hepatic synthesis
5 The extent to which heterozygotes (MZ) are predisposed to cigarette-induced emphysema is unclear
6 α_1AT augmentation therapy is being evaluated in α_1AT-deficient patients

CLINICAL FEATURES OF RESPIRATORY DISORDERS

Hypersensitivity pneumonitis*: making the diagnosis
1 Clinical
   — Recurrent dyspnea 4–6 h after antigen exposure
   — Dry cough; typically *no* wheezing
   — Fevers, progressive weight loss
   — Occurs *less* commonly in smokers
2 CXR
   — Mid and lower zone mottling (in acute phase)
   — Upper zone mottling (in chronic fibrosis)
3 Lung function tests
   — Restrictive (transient in acute phase)
4 Blood gases
   — Low PaO_2 and $PaCO_2$
   Diffusion capacity
   — Low DL_{CO}
5 Precipitins
   — Do *not* indicate pathogenicity‡
   — Do *not* correlate with disease activity
   — Tend to *exclude* diagnosis if negative
6 Immune profile
   — Total serum IgE levels typically *normal*
   — Eosinophilia *absent*
7 Bronchoalveolar lavage
   — Lymphocytosis
   — ↑ IgG:albumin ratio
8 Transbronchial biopsy
   — Granulomata related to airways
   — Bronchiolitis, mononuclear infiltrate
9 Inhalation provocation (the definitive diagnostic test)
   — Improvement on cessation of exposure
   — Relapse on rechallenge

* Extrinsic allergic alveolitis
‡ Exception: budgerigar exposure

Clinical features of yellow-nail syndrome
1 Usually presents in old age
2 Greenish-yellow nail discoloration and dystrophy

3 Associated with recurrent pleural effusions, peripheral lymphedema, myxedema

Clinical features of pulmonary alveolar proteinosis
1 Protean clinical manifestations, variable prognosis
2 Sputum → PAS-positive lipoprotein in epithelial cells
3 CXR → diffuse infiltrates, perihilar 'rosette' with normal heart size
4 Often complicated by opportunistic infection, esp. *Nocardia* (which may in turn metastasize to brain)
5 Whole lung lavage is the only therapeutic option of proven value

Clinical features of idiopathic pulmonary hemosiderosis
1 Age of onset < 20 years
2 Sputum → hemosiderin-laden macrophages
3 Presents with hemoptysis ± iron-deficiency anemia
4 Diffuse (predominantly basal) infiltrates on CXR
5 No renal disease; negative immunofluorescence and anti-GBM Ab (cf. Goodpasture's)
6 Disease activity is proportionate to the DL_{CO}

ADULT RESPIRATORY DISTRESS SYNDROME (ARDS)

Diagnostic criteria for adult respiratory distress syndrome
1 History
  — Previously normal lung function
  — Acute respiratory distress after a precipitating event
2 CXR
  — Diffuse infiltrates (sparing apices, costophrenic angles)
3 Blood gases
  — PaO_2 < 60 mmHg despite FiO_2 ≥ 60% (due to shunting)
  — $PaCO_2$ normal or low
  — Arterial-alveolar (A-a) oxygen gradient > 25
4 Pulmonary investigations
  — Reduced pulmonary compliance ('stiff lungs')
  — Pulmonary hypertension (> 30/15 mmHg) usual
  — Pulmonary wedge pressure normal (< 18 mmHg)
  — Thoracic compliance < 30 mL/cm H_2O
5 Therapy
  — Assisted ventilation (volume-cycled, patient-initiated) using positive end-expiratory pressure (PEEP) to increase the functional residual capacity (and hence increase compliance, thereby reducing intrapulmonary shunting)

Common antecedents of adult respiratory distress syndrome
1 Sepsis (incl. Gram-negative bacteremia, Sin nombre virus)
2 Aspiration (incl. near-drowning)
3 Inhalation (smoke, chlorine)
4 Multiple trauma
5 Massive transfusion

NB: ARDS *may* also occur in neutropenic patients even though neutrophils are implicated in the pathogenesis of ARDS

Treatment modalities in ARDS
1 Ventilation using permissive hypercapnia and limiting airway pressure
2 Prone ventilation
3 Steroids in late stage to reduce fibrosis
4 Exogenous surfactant (experimental)

REVIEWING THE LITERATURE: RESPIRATORY DISEASE

15.1 Paggiaro PL et al (1998) Multicentre randomised placebo-controlled trial of inhaled fluticasone propionate in patients with chronic obstructive pulmonary disease. Lancet 351: 773–780

Schuh S et al (2000) A comparison of inhaled fluticasone and oral prednisone for children with severe acute asthma. N Engl J Med 343: 689–694

Two studies examining the utility of inhaled corticosteroids. The first showed a small but significant improvement in COAD symptoms following 6 months' usage, without much toxicity. However, the second study concluded that inhaled steroids are not appropriate for severe acute asthma, and that oral steroids should be used instead.

15.2 Fahey T et al (1998) Quantitative systematic review of randomised controlled trials comparing antibiotic with placebo for acute cough in adults. Br Med J 316: 906–910

Meta-analysis of nine published trials, concluding that no benefit of routine antibiotic usage for acute cough was detectable, and that any (undetectable) benefit was outweighed by the side-effects.

15.3 Kon OM et al (1998) Randomized, dose-ranging, placebo-controlled study of chimeric antibody to CD4 (keliximab) in chronic severe asthma. Lancet 352: 1109–1113

Milgrom H et al (1999) Treatment of allergic asthma with monoclonal anti-IgE antibody. N Engl J Med 341: 1966–1973

Two studies assessing the promise of immunomodulatory antibody therapy in the treatment of asthma. In the earlier study, 22 patients were randomized; a significant clinical improvement in asthma parameters was apparent in those receiving 3 mg/kg of anti-CD4 antibody, suggesting the efficacy of T-cell-modulatory treatment. The later study of 106 asthmatic patients confirmed a decline in serum IgE levels associated with reduced steroid requirement in the antibody-treated group.

15.4 Antonelli M et al (1998) A comparison of noninvasive positive-pressure ventilation and conventional mechanical ventilation in patients with acute respiratory failure. N Engl J Med 339: 429–435

Plant PK et al (2000) Early use of non-invasive ventilation for acute exacerbations of chronic obstructive pulmonary disease on general respiratory wards: a multicentre randomized controlled trial. Lancet 355: 1931–1935

Two studies examining the therapeutic use of non-invasive positive-pressure ventilation in the setting of threatened or actual respiratory failure. In the former study, a small randomized comparison of 32 patients in acute respiratory failure indicated that non-invasive ventilation was as effective as endotracheal intubation, and associated with shorter stays in intensive care. In the latter study, 236 patients with decompensated chronic airways disease were randomized to conventional treatment or additional non-invasive ventilation; the latter group enjoyed better symptom control and reduced mortality.

15.5 Acute Respiratory Distress Syndrome Network (2000) Ventilation with lower tidal volumes as compared with traditional tidal volumes for acute lung injury and the acute respiratory distress syndrome. N Engl J Med 342: 1301–1308

Randomized study of 861 patients which was stopped early due to improved survival associated with the use of lower ventilatory tidal volumes and limiting airway pressures.

15.6 Sciurba FC et al (1996) Improvement in pulmonary function and elastic recoil after lung-reduction surgery for diffuse emphysema. N Engl J Med 334: 1095–1099

Geddes D et al (2000) Effect of lung-volume-reduction surgery in patients with severe emphysema. N Engl J Med 343: 239–245

Two studies attesting to the efficacy of (judicious) lung reduction surgery in relieving symptoms, but not mortality, in patients with severe emphysema.

15.7 National Emphysema Treatment Trial Research Group (2001) Patients at high risk of death after lung-volume-reduction surgery. N Engl J Med 345: 1075–1083

Randomized study of 1033 patients, showing high postoperative mortality in those patients with low FEV_1 or impaired diffusing capacity.15.8   Wong CA et al (1997) Inhaled corticosteroid use and bone mineral density in patients with asthma. Lancet 355: 1399–1403

15.8 Cumming RG et al (1997) Use of inhaled corticosteroids and the risk of cataracts. N Engl J Med 337: 8–14

Population-based study of 3654 people including 370 taking inhaled steroids; a strong dose-related association between inhaled steroids and cataracts was confirmed.

15.9 Wong CA et al (1997) Inhaled corticosteroid use and bone mineral density in patients with asthma. Lancet 355: 1399–1403

Dose-response analysis of 196 asthmatics, showing an inverse relationship between cumulative inhaled steroid dose and bone density.

15.10 Ratjen F et al (2001) Effect of inhaled tobramycin on early *Pseudomonas aeruginosa* colonization in patients with cystic fibrosis. Lancet 358: 177–178

Twice-daily inhalation of tobramycin eradicated *Ps. aeruginosa* in 14 of 15 patients with cystic fibrosis.

CHAPTER 16

Rheumatology

Physical examination protocol 16.1   You are asked to examine a patient with rheumatoid arthritis

Eyes:
scleritis, nodules
scleromalacia perforans
cataract (steroids)
retinopathy (chloroquine)
Schirmer's test

Hoarseness, stridor
Mouth – thrush (steroids)
stomatitis (gold); sicca
TMJ crepitus
Pinna antihelix – tophi
Scalp – psoriasis

Shoulders: range of movement
Crepitus on passive motion

Ulnar forearm: nodules/tophi
Elbows: active/passive range

Wrist: passive movements

Palms up:
palmar erythema, Raynaud's
thenar wasting
distal pinprick sensation
carpal tunnel repair scar
Tinel's sign

Nail changes (psoriatic)

Assess joint function:
MCP extension/abduction
grip strength; make fist
thumb abduction/opposition
use pen, do up buttons

Assess disease activity:
palpate synovial thickening
(? tender)
flexor tendon crepitus
nodules, vasculitis, clubbing

Characterize deformities:
hands palms-down; identify
sites of swelling and wasting
Look for ulnar drift, subluxation,
Z-deformity
Assess volar mobility of ulnar
styloid

Neck:
range of movement
occipital nodule

Chest:
rales, rubs, effusions
mitral/aortic incompetence
loud P_2
scoliosis, sacral edema/nodules

Skin:
purpura, petechiae
rash (? gold, D-pen)

Hepatosplenomegaly
Lymphadenopathy
Palpable kidneys (amyloid)

Hips:
passive movements
quadriceps wasting
proximal weakness
leg shortening

Knee:
varus/valgus deformity
synovial thickening
patellar tap/bulge
Baker's cyst
ligamentous integrity
range of motion

Foot/ankle:
dorsi-/plantarflexion
hallux valgus, cock-up toes
MTP head tenderness
subtalar joint: in-/eversion
midtarsal: rotation, ab-/adduction

Leg ulcers; edema
Neuropathy, long tract signs

Fever
Urinalysis

Introduce yourself
Position the patient (sitting up)
Obtain adequate exposure

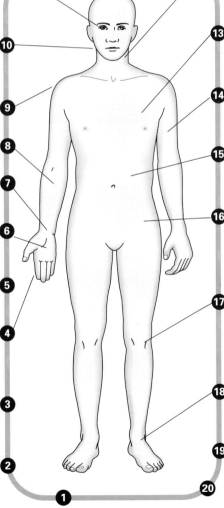

Physical examination protocol 16.2 You are asked to examine a young man with chronic low back pain

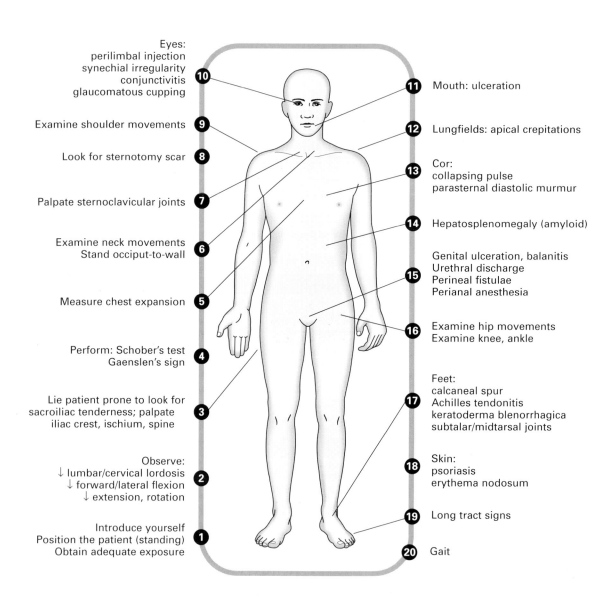

Eyes:
perilimbal injection
synechial irregularity
conjunctivitis
glaucomatous cupping — **10**

Examine shoulder movements — **9**

Look for sternotomy scar — **8**

Palpate sternoclavicular joints — **7**

Examine neck movements
Stand occiput-to-wall — **6**

Measure chest expansion — **5**

Perform: Schober's test
Gaenslen's sign — **4**

Lie patient prone to look for
sacroiliac tenderness; palpate
iliac crest, ischium, spine — **3**

Observe:
↓ lumbar/cervical lordosis
↓ forward/lateral flexion
↓ extension, rotation — **2**

Introduce yourself
Position the patient (standing)
Obtain adequate exposure — **1**

11 Mouth: ulceration

12 Lungfields: apical crepitations

13 Cor:
collapsing pulse
parasternal diastolic murmur

14 Hepatosplenomegaly (amyloid)

15 Genital ulceration, balanitis
Urethral discharge
Perineal fistulae
Perianal anesthesia

16 Examine hip movements
Examine knee, ankle

17 Feet:
calcaneal spur
Achilles tendonitis
keratoderma blenorrhagica
subtalar/midtarsal joints

18 Skin:
psoriasis
erythema nodosum

19 Long tract signs

20 Gait

Diagnostic pathway 16.1 This patient has unusual hands. What sort of process do you think is responsible?

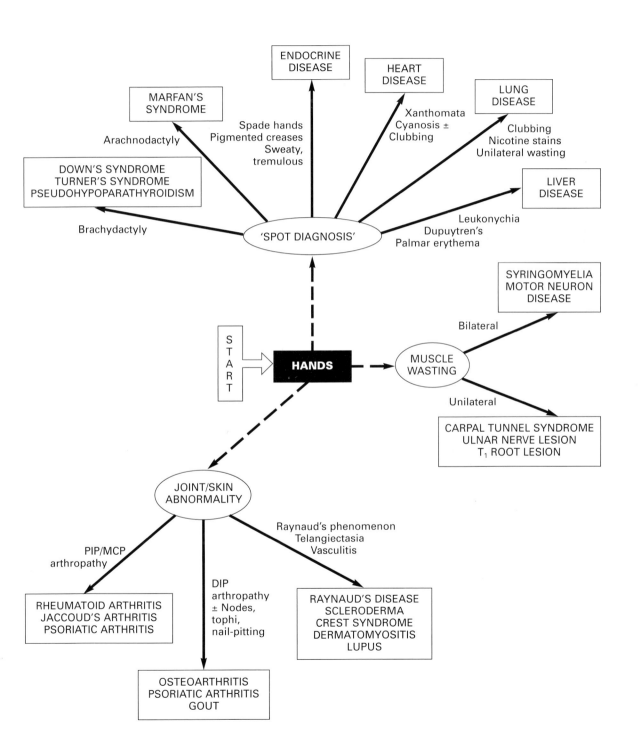

COMMON AND CLASSIC RHEUMATOLOGIC PROBLEMS

Common rheumatologic problems in clinical practice
1 Low back pain
2 Chronic osteoarthritis
3 NSAID complications

Classic rheumatologic problems in clinical exams
1 Rheumatoid hands
2 Tophaceous gout
3 Seronegative spondyloarthropathy

RHEUMATOLOGIC EMERGENCIES

Therapeutic emergencies in rheumatic disease
1 Atlantoaxial subluxation
— Tends to affect RA patients on long-term steroids
— R_x: surgical decompression and fusion (if symptomatic)
2 Temporal arteritis
— Draw blood for ESR as soon as diagnosis suspected
— R_x: prednisone 20–60 mg/day (high dose if eye disease)
— Commence treatment as soon as ESR drawn*
3 Septic arthritis
— Drain joint, Gram-stain, culture, sensitivity
— R_x: intravenous antibiotics
4 Vasculitic complications
— Mononeuritis multiplex
— Digital gangrene, bowel infarction
— R_x: high-dose steroids, cytotoxic drugs
5 Iridocyclitis
— Complicates seronegative arthropathies (*not* RA)
— R_x: mydriatics, topical/systemic steroids
Episcleritis
— Complicates RA (*not* seronegative arthropathies)
— R_x: topical steroids, NSAIDs, or systemic steroids
6 Iatrogenic: GI bleed, blood dyscrasia, adrenal dysfunction
— Identify and cease offending medication
— R_x: supportive

* Biopsy results unaffected by up to 48 h of steroids

CLINICAL ASSESSMENT OF RHEUMATOLOGIC DISORDERS

Clinical assessment of joint function: modified ARA criteria
1 ARA I
— Normal joint function (= no disease)
2 ARA II
— Adequate function despite symptoms (= early disease)
3 ARA III
— Reduced function, but self-care possible (= disease)
4 ARA IV
— Self-care precluded by dysfunction (= severe disease)

Systematic characterization of joint dysfunction
1 Dysfunction
— Loss of normal joint function
2 Disability
— Impairment of an activity by joint dysfunction
3 Handicap
— Effect of joint dysfunction on fulfilment of a role

Chronic arthritis: assessment of daily functional capacity
1 Mobility
— Getting out of bed
— Floor to chair; chair to bed
— Negotiating stairs
— Using public transport; shopping
2 Ability to wash
— Using toilet
— Shaving, brushing teeth, cutting nails
— Bathing
3 Dressing
— Using buttons and zips
— Doing up laces; putting on shoes, socks
— Combing hair
4 Feeding
— Preparing food; making tea
— Using cutlery; administering medications
— Chewing; eating apples, swallowing
5 Housework
— Turning taps, keys, dials
— Making beds; using telephone
— Hanging washing

DIAGNOSTIC PATTERNS IN CLINICAL RHEUMATOLOGY

Patterns of joint involvement in rheumatic disease
1 Rheumatoid arthritis (F:M = 3:1)
— MCPs, PIPs, wrists
— Knees, ankles
— Lateral MTPs, subtalar/midtarsal joints
— Cervical spine, incl. atlantoaxial joint
— TMJs (pain on chewing); cricoarytenoids (hoarseness)
2 Osteoarthritis (F:M = 3:1)
— DIPs and PIPs
— Base of thumb (first carpometacarpal joint)
— Knees, hips
— First MTP joint (involvement may be asymptomatic)
— Lumbosacral spine (i.e. apophyseal joints)
3 Seronegative spondyloarthropathies (M > F)
— Hips, knees, ankles (asymmetric, oligoarticular)
— Sacroiliac joints
— Spondylitis: often begins at thoracolumbar junction
4 Gout (M:F = 8:1)
— First MTP joint (at onset in 75%; eventually → 90%)
— Ankles and tarsal bones

— Knees, elbows (incl. olecranon bursa)
— DIPs and PIPs (much less commonly)

Key factors predisposing to osteoarthritis of specific joints
1 Hand
   — Bad genes (e.g. collagen gene 2A mutation)
2 Knee
   — Trauma
   — Obesity*
3 Hip
   — Abnormal joint shape

* Note that obesity has also been linked to osteoarthritis of the hands

Nodes and nodules in rheumatic disease
1 Heberden's nodes (DIP osteophytes in primary OA)
   Bouchard's nodes (PIP osteophytes in primary OA)
2 Rheumatoid nodules
3 Gouty tophi (DIPs, PIPs, elbows, ears, heels)
4 Xanthomata

Differential diagnosis of morning stiffness
1 Rheumatoid arthritis
   — Difficulty doing up buttons etc.
   — May improve with nocturnal NSAID suppositories
2 Ankylosing spondylitis
   — Low back pain/stiffness radiating to buttocks and thighs
   — Improved with exercise, NSAIDs
3 Polymyalgia rheumatica
   — Difficulty getting out of bed
   — *Marked* diurnal variation*
4 Osteoarthritis
   — Short duration of stiffness (< 15 min)
   — Pain may be worsened by prolonged use
5 Myxedema

* May be asymptomatic by evening (cf. rotator cuff syndrome)

Differential diagnoses of miscellaneous presentations
1 Young patient with joint deformity
   — Hemophilia (if male)
   — Juvenile chronic arthritis
   — Syringomyelia, Riley–Day (i.e. Charcot joint)
2 Charcot's joints
   — Common: diabetes mellitus ($\rightarrow$ foot)
   — Rare:
     • Tabes dorsalis ($\rightarrow$ knee)
     • Syringomyelia ($\rightarrow$ shoulder, elbow)
     • Leprosy (lepromatous)
     • Overzealous administration of intra-articular steroids
3 Acute monarthritis
   — Septic
   — Seronegative (incl. 'reactive')
   — Hemarthrosis (± trauma)
   — Crystal-induced
     • (Pseudo) gout
     • Triamcinolone*
4 Transient polyarthritis
   — SLE
   — Rheumatic fever, SBE, serum sickness

— Parainfectious (e.g. hepatitis B, gonorrhea)
— Reiter's syndrome, 'reactive' arthritides
— Henoch–Schönlein purpura
5 Arthropathy affecting DIPs
   — Primary (familial) osteoarthritis
   — Psoriatic arthritis
   — Other arthropathies (*if* extensive)
     • Juvenile chronic arthritis; RA
     • Gout
     • Sarcoidosis
     • Hemochromatosis
     • Multicentric reticulohistiocytosis
6 Sternoclavicular arthritis
   — Ankylosing spondylitis
   — Narcotic addiction
   — Tietze's syndrome
7 Chondrocalcinosis
   — Old age
   — Joint trauma (e.g. menisceal injury of knee)
   — Familial
   — Gout, OA, RA, Paget's
   — Metabolic predisposition
     • Hyperparathyroidism; hypophosphatasia
     • Hemochromatosis; ochronosis
     • Acromegaly; myxedema
     • Wilson's disease

* Typically causes arthritis a few hours after joint injection

Clinical patterns suggesting misdiagnosis
1 'Osteoarthritis' with MCP (esp. 2nd and 3rd) involvement ± chondrocalcinosis on X-ray
   — Hemochromatosis
   — Wilson's disease
2 'Psoriatic arthritis' with pustular skin lesions and/or prominent eye involvement
   — Reiter's syndrome
   'Psoriatic arthritis' with positive rheumatoid factor
   — Rheumatoid arthritis (i.e. with psoriasis)
3 'Ankylosing spondylitis' with negative HLA-B27 in a female
   — Psoriatic arthritis
   — Inflammatory bowel disease
4 Post-diarrheal 'reactive arthritis' followed by development of mucocutaneous lesion
   — Reiter's syndrome
   — Inflammatory bowel disease

Characteristics of benign (mechanical) back pain
1 Symptoms
   — Previous similar episode(s)
   — Sudden onset
2 Examination
   — Asymmetrical or uniradicular findings
   — Abnormal femoral stretch/straight leg raise

EXAMINATION OF SPECIFIC JOINTS

Examination of the hip
1 Check for leg *shortening*
   — e.g. Collapsed femoral head in OA
2 Test *movements*
   — Flexion, abduction, rotation

3 Test for fixed flexion deformity of the hip (*Thomas's test*)
  — With the patient supine, flex the contralateral hip to straighten lumbar spine (tilting pelvis to neutral)
  — Flexion of ipsilateral hip? = fixed flexion deformity
4 Look for *Trendelenburg sign* (downward tilt of contralateral pelvis when weight-bearing on affected hip)
  → Severe joint or (esp. if bilateral) neuromuscular disease

Differential diagnosis of elbow lesions
1 Rheumatoid nodule
2 Gouty tophus
3 Olecranon bursa (e.g. due to gout, trauma)
4 Synovial cyst (different location to above)
5 Skin lesions
  — Tendon xanthoma
  — Pseudoxanthoma elasticum
  — Psoriasis
  — Subcutaneous calcification in CREST syndrome

Clinical diagnosis of shoulder pain
1 All movements restricted (incl. passive abduction, rotation)
  — *Articular/capsular disease*
    • 'Frozen shoulder' (adhesive capsulitis)
    • Rheumatoid arthritis
    • Other synovitis (e.g. septic arthritis)
2 Active abduction/rotation only restricted (passive normal)
  — *Rotator cuff injury* (→ 'painful arc')
    • Supraspinatus tendinitis
    • Infraspinatus tendinitis: pain on active external rotation
    • Subscapularis tendinitis: pain on active internal rotation
    • Bicipital tendinitis: local tenderness, pain on supination

REPETITIVE STRAIN INJURY (RSI)

Clinical spectrum of repetitive strain injury
1 Tendonitis; tenosynovitis (de Quervain's, trigger finger, rotator cuff)
2 Epicondylitis (lateral or medial)
3 Ganglion cyst
4 Carpal/ulnar/radial tunnel syndromes
5 Thoracic outlet syndrome

Clinical tests for evaluating RSI
1 Tinel's test
  — Tapping the medial (ulnar) nerve causes paresthesiae
2 Cozen's test
  — Wrist extension with pronated forearm causes lateral epicondylar pain
3 Phalen's test
  — Keeping dorsal hand surfaces together, flexing wrists 90° for 60 sec causes paresthesiae in median nerve distribution (index and middle fingers)
4 Finkelstein's test
  — With the thumb against the palm, and the fingers flexed over the thumb, and with the hand held in ulnar deviation, pain occurring at the radial styloid indicates tendonitis of abductor pollicis longus and/or extensor pollicis
5 Adson's maneuver
  — With the jaw forward, shoulder hyperextension leads to paresthesiae associated with radial pulse weakening
6 Spurling's test
  — With the neck extended 20°, downward pressure applied to the top of the skull causes pain down the arm

Common clinical features of RSI
1 Usually unilateral
2 Pain most often affects hand, shoulder girdle, and neck
3 Common symptoms
  — Proximal muscular 'tightness'
  — Weakness of handgrip
  — Hand numbness and/or paresthesiae
4 *Not* associated with muscle wasting
  No objective reproducible neurological deficit
5 Best treated by continuing normal limb activity

CHARACTERISTICS OF SPECIFIC SYNDROMES

Adhesive capsulitis ('frozen shoulder'): course and therapy
1 *Pain* usually worsens within the first year of onset
2 *Function* usually improves over the first 2 years
3 > 50% of patients are left with some residual dysfunction
4 Best managed with gentle active movements

Carpal tunnel syndrome: physical findings
1 Numbness (± pain) of the first three digits
  — Sensory loss involves only the medial half* of middle or ring finger
  — 'Flick test': subjective relief of discomfort by downward flicking of the hand when awoken at night
2 Weakness
  — Thumb opposition and abduction
  — Wasting of thenar eminence
3 Provocative bedside tests
  — Positive Tinel's sign
  — Positive Phalen's test‡
  — Direct pressure over median nerve
  — Median nerve sensory loss after tourniquet applied
4 Predisposing stigmata, e.g.
  — Rheumatoid arthritis, pregnancy (common)
  — Acromegaly, myxedema (in exams)

* cf. proximal C6/7 nerve root lesion (e.g. due to coexisting cervical spondylosis): sensory loss involves entire finger
‡ Numbness/pain reproduced by flexing wrists for 1 min

RHEUMATOID ARTHRITIS (RA)

Clinical assessment of disease activity
1 History
  — Presence of constitutional symptoms
  — Duration of morning stiffness
  — Recent involvement of new joints
  — Recent reduction in range of joint movement
2 Physical examination
  — Number of *tender* swollen joints
  — Degree of soft-tissue swelling/tenderness
  — Ring size at proximal interphalangeal joints
  — Grip strength
  — Walking time for given distance

Differential diagnosis of impaired hand function in RA
1 Active disease
  — Synovitis
  — Tendinitis
2 Joint deformity
3 Tendon rupture
4 Carpal tunnel syndrome
5 Mononeuritis
6 Cervical vertebral compression
  — T1 nerve root
  — Spinal cord

Differential diagnosis of impaired walking in RA
1 Active disease
  — Metatarsal head involvement esp.
2 Inactive disease
  — Joint deformity, muscle contractures
3 Muscle wasting
  — Secondary to synovitis/deformity/steroids
4 Spastic paraparesis
  — Cervical myelopathy
5 Peripheral nerve lesions
  — Neuropathy, mononeuritis multiplex

Diseases that may mimic rheumatoid arthritis
1 Psoriatic arthritis
  — Must be rheumatoid factor negative
2 Juvenile chronic arthritis
  — Polyarticular RF+ subtype
3 Rheumatic fever
  — Arthritis typically spares neck and PIP joints
  Post-rheumatic fever (Jaccoud's) arthritis
4 Collagen diseases
  — SLE, MCTD, scleroderma
5 Other
  — Relapsing polychondritis
  — Multicentric reticulohistiocytosis
  — Erosive osteoarthritis
  — Calcium pyrophosphate deposition disease

Rheumatoid arthritis or osteoarthritis? Some comparisons
1 RA — Predominant DIP involvement rare
  OA — Predominant MCP involvement rare
2 RA — Disease → ulnar deviation at MCPs
  OA — Disease → first carpometacarpal joint involvement
3 RA — Tender dorsally subluxed ulnar styloid ('piano key')
  OA — Tenderness of first carpometacarpal joint
4 RA — Elbow → ↓ extension (ulnar–humeral joint disease)
  OA — Elbow → ↓ supination (radiohumeral involvement)
5 RA — First sign of neck involvement is ↓ rotation
  OA — First sign of neck involvement is ↓ lateral flexion

DISEASE MECHANISMS IN RHEUMATOID ARTHRITIS

Mechanisms of splenomegaly in rheumatoid arthritis
1 Primary disease manifestation (normal neutrophil count)
2 Felty's syndrome (↓ neutrophil count)
3 Sjögren's syndrome
4 Amyloidosis

Mechanisms of muscle wasting in rheumatoid arthritis
1 Systemic hypercatabolism
  — Wasting parallels weight loss
2 Disuse atrophy
3 Inflammatory (vasculitic) myositis
4 Neuropathic
  — Vasculitis
  — Entrapment
  — Splint-induced nerve compression (shouldn't happen)
5 Iatrogenic
  — Corticosteroid myopathy
  — Polymyositis/myasthenia gravis due to penicillamine

Mechanical basis of rheumatoid deformities
1 *Rupture* of flexor/extensor tendons
  — Indicated by loss of active (but not passive) movements beginning in one finger and progressing (without treatment) to involve all
  — Therapy = repair ruptured tendon, wrist synovectomy, + excision of ulnar head to prevent further rupture
2 Ulnar deviation
  — Subluxation of extensor tendons at MCP joints due to synovitic capsular ligamentous stretching
3 Swan-neck deformity
  — PIP joint hyperextension and compensatory DIP joint flexion due to interossei contractures and/or shortening of extensor tendon(s)
4 Boutonnière deformity
  — PIP fixed flexion contracture (with DIP hyperextension) due to division of extensor hood with volar slipping (± detachment and rupture) of extensor tendon from middle phalanx
5 Mallet finger deformity
  — Stretching or rupture of the extensor insertion into the dorsum of the terminal phalanx

6 Z-deformity of the thumb
  — MCP flexion and IP hyperextension due to prolapse of metacarpal head between the long and short extensor tendons, or to rupture of the thumb flexor
7 'Piano-key' sign
  — Hypermobility of a dorsally subluxated ulnar styloid due to laxity of the radioulnar joint (often painful)

Pathogenesis of anemia in rheumatoid arthritis
1 Active inflammatory ('chronic') disease*
2 Felty's syndrome
3 Iatrogenic
  — Aspirin/NSAID-induced GI bleeding‡
  — Gold/penicillamine-induced hypoplastic anemia
  — Sulfasalazine-induced hemolysis or folate deficiency

* NB: Anemia reflects disease *activity,* not *chronicity*
‡ Parenteral iron may cause arthritic 'flare'

COMPLICATIONS OF RHEUMATOID ARTHRITIS

Classical stigmata of rheumatoid vasculitis
1 Skin infarcts
2 Episcleritis
3 Neuropathy

Renal disorders in rheumatoid arthritis
1 Amyloidosis (nephrosis)
2 Renal tubular acidosis (in Sjögren's syndrome)
3 Analgesic nephropathy
4 NSAID-induced (usually benign) renal disease*, e.g.
  — Interstitial nephritis (→ hematuria ± proteinuria)
  — Nephrosis (rare)
5 Other iatrogenic renal syndromes
  — Transient reversible proteinuria (gold, penicillamine)
  — Nephrosis due to gold, penicillamine
  — Goodpasture's syndrome due to penicillamine

* NB: *Glomerular* disease as a primary disease manifestation of RA is quite rare

Pulmonary manifestations of rheumatoid arthritis
1 Pleural disease (pleurisy, effusions)
2 Fibrosing alveolitis, interstitial fibrosis
3 Bronchiolitis obliterans (→ acute, often fatal, lung syndrome)
4 Pulmonary arteritis/hypertension
5 Nodules; may lead to
  — Cavitation
  — Bronchopleural fistulae
  — Caplan's syndrome
6 Stridor due to
  — Cricoarytenoid arthritis
  — Nodule on vocal cords
7 Recurrent lower respiratory tract infections (Sjögren's)
8 Iatrogenic
  — Asthma (salicylates)
  — Allergic/fibrosing alveolitis (gold)
  — Goodpasture's (D-penicillamine)
  — Interstitial fibrosis (methotrexate, chlorambucil)

Rheumatoid complications with male predilection
1 'Rheumatoid lung' (fibrosis, effusions, nodules, pleurisy)
2 Accelerated vasculitis (e.g. → mononeuritis multiplex)
3 Mitral valvular regurgitation*

* Commoner post-mortem than aortic regurgitation, but *rarely* of clinical significance (unlike aortic regurgitation)

Diagnosis of Felty's syndrome
1 Defining criteria
  — Seropositive rheumatoid arthritis, *plus*
  — Splenomegaly, *plus*
  — Neutropenia
2 Frequent concomitants
  — Serious infections
  — Leg ulcers (vasculitic)
  — Mononeuritis multiplex
  — Anemia, thrombocytopenia
  — Lymphadenopathy, hepatomegaly
  — Sjögren's syndrome
  — Pigmentation, weight loss
3 Laboratory clues
  — Thrombocytopenia despite active disease
  — Hypocomplementemia
  — Positive ANA, high-titre RF (IgM)
4 Response to medical therapy
  — Leukocyte count may (paradoxically) improve after gold
5 Response to splenectomy
  — Arthritis not affected
  — Leukopenia usually improves at least temporarily
  — Infections may increase in frequency or severity

Bad prognostic indicators in rheumatoid arthritis
1 History
  — Male sex
  — Insidious onset
  — Polyarticular presentation
  — Marked (> 10%) weight loss
  — Disability within 1 year of onset
2 Signs
  — Fever; nodules; necrotizing scleritis
  — Lung fibrosis; neuropathy
  — Lymphadenopathy, splenomegaly (± Felty's/Sjögren's)
  — Purpura (any cause)
3 Complications
  — Early onset (< 3 years) of erosions
  — Development of amyloidosis
4 Routine laboratory testing
  — Marked normochromic anemia
  — Thrombocytosis; eosinophilia (unless gold-induced)
  — Hypoalbuminemia, polyclonal gammopathy
  — Markedly elevated ESR/acute phase reactants
5 Specific tests
  — Markedly elevated rheumatoid factor (IgM)
  — Positive neutrophil-specific ANA
  — Cryoglobulinemia
  — HLA-DR3 or -DR4 (research use only)

Prevalence of Raynaud's in autoimmune diseases
1 Scleroderma   — 95%
2 Sjogren's
  Systemic lupus   } — 25%
  Dermatomyositis
3 Rheumatoid arthritis — 5%

CRYSTAL ARTHROPATHIES

Presentations of calcium pyrophosphate deposition disease
1 Asymptomatic X-ray chondrocalcinosis — 30%
2 Pseudogout ($\rightarrow$ knee, wrist)   — 30%
3 Accelerated symmetric osteoarthritis — 30%
4 Pseudorheumatoid arthritis   — 5%
5 Pseudoneuropathic (Charcot) arthritis — rare

Clinical spectrum of abnormal hydroxyapatite deposition
1 Supraspinatus tendinitis
2 Periarthritis in chronic hemodialysis
3 Milwaukee shoulder (destructive crystal arthritis)
4 Calcinosis associated with scleroderma, dermatomyositis
5 Myositis ossificans
6 Repeated articular steroid injections into small finger joints

SERONEGATIVE SPONDYLOARTHROPATHIES

Ankylosing spondylitis: maneuvers on clinical examination
1 Chest expansion
   — If < 5 cm, indicates costovertebral involvement
2 Schober's test
   — Positive if full lumbar flexion fails to increase by > 5 cm the distance between L5 and a point 15 cm above
   — Indicates lumbar disease
3 Occiput to wall
   — Positive if failure of approximation
   — Indicates loss of cervicothoracic lordosis
4 Straight leg raising
   — Indicates malingering if normal in patient complaining of impaired forward flexion
5 Examination of peripheral joints, esp. hips and sternoclavicular joints

Potential complications of ankylosing spondylitis
1 HLA-B27 covariables
   — Enthesopathy
     • Plantar fasciitis
     • Achilles tendinitis
   — Anterior uveitis
   — Chronic prostatitis
2 Chest
   — Chest pain due to costovertebral joint disease
   — Aortic incompetence (due to aortitis*)
   — Pericarditis; cardiac conduction defects

— Restrictive lung function
   • Impaired chest wall excursion
   • Apical pulmonary fibrosis
3 Cauda equina syndrome
4 Amyloidosis
5 Leukemia (esp. CGL), bone sarcomas
   — If previously treated with spinal irradiation

* cf. RA, where valve dysfunction arises due to valvulitis or nodules

Ankylosing spondylitis in females
1 Neck involvement and peripheral arthritis more common
2 Extra-articular manifestations more common
3 Radiological changes milder
4 True incidence may be underestimated

Clinical patterns of psoriatic arthritis
1 Oligoarticular asymmetric type (70%)
   — 'Sausage' digits = flexor tendon sheath effusions*
   — Indicate underlying dactylitis
2 Distal interphalangeal joint type (15%)
   — Accompanies psoriatic nails
     • Pitting, hyperkeratosis, onycholysis
3 Pseudorheumatoid type
   — Seronegative; affects males and females equally
   — Arthritis severity varies with skin disease
4 Ankylosing spondylitis-type
   — HLA-B27+ in 75% (less common than AS/Reiter's)
5 Arthritis mutilans
   — Often associated with sacroiliitis
   — 'Telescoping' digits
   — 'Opera-glass' deformity (may be painless)
   — X-ray: 'pencil-in-cup' appearance

* Also found in Reiter's syndrome

Rheumatic aspects of inflammatory bowel disease (IBD)
1 A *non-deforming asymmetric arthritis*, principally affecting knees, ankles and PIPs, occurs in 15%
2 This peripheral arthritis occurs at least 6 months following onset of bowel disease. Its severity reflects that of IBD; colectomy abolishes it
3 *Erythema nodosum, uveitis, mouth ulcers* and *pyoderma* occur in association with peripheral arthritis in IBD
4 *Spondylitis/sacroiliitis* occurs in 5%, may predate onset of bowel symptoms, and is associated with HLA-B27. It is independent of IBD activity and unaffected by colectomy; no sex predilection
5 Arthritis and spondylitis in *Whipple's disease* remits with appropriate antibiotics and has *no* HLA association

Differential diagnosis of genital and oral ulceration
1 Reiter's syndrome; Behçet's syndrome
2 Crohn's disease
3 Pemphigus
4 Erythema multiforme
5 Syphilis, herpes simplex
6 Strachan's (orogenital) syndrome

Reiter's vs Behçet's syndrome: the clinical distinction
1 Reiter's
  — Male:female = 10:1
  — Painless ulcers
  — Predominant ocular manifestation: conjunctivitis
  — Long-term ocular disability rare
  — Long-term joint disability frequent ($\to$ 50%; often mild)
  — Spondylitis/sacroiliitis frequent
  — HLA association: B27
  — Infection seems important in pathogenesis
  — R_x: NSAIDs
2 Behçet's
  — Male:female = 2:1
  — Painful ulcers
  — Predominant ocular manifestation: uveitis
  — Long-term ocular disability almost invariable
  — Long-term joint disability rare
  — Spondylitis/sacroiliitis uncommon
  — HLA associations: B51 (plus B12; B5 in eye disease, esp. Japanese; colitis)
  — Racial/genetic factors seem important in pathogenesis
  — R_x: immunosuppressives (e.g. CSA, azathioprine)

Clinical spectrum of Behçet's syndrome
1 Mouth ulceration (98%)
2 Genital ulceration*
3 Skin lesions
  — Erythema nodosum*
  — Thrombophlebitis (in 30%; $\to$ sterile pustules at venepuncture sites)
4 Eye disease (esp. in males, Japanese; HLA-B5 in 80%)
  — Uveitis $\to$ pain, photophobia, blurred vision
  — Hypopyon; conjunctivitis, scleritis, phthisis bulbi
  — Retinal venulitis $\to$ 'battlefield' fundus
  — Optic neuritis, CRV occlusion
5 CNS disease (30%)
  — Aseptic meningitis
  — TIA-like episodes
  — Cranial nerve palsies
6 Colitis (in 30%; associated with HLA-B5)
  — May lead to perforation
  — Clinically overlaps with inflammatory bowel disease

NB: Spondylitis/sacroiliitis, when present, are linked to HLA-B27
* Associated with non-deforming arthritis

OCULAR SEQUELAE OF RHEUMATIC DISEASES

Differential diagnosis of painful red eye
1 Episcleritis
  — Focal hyperemia
  — Cornea clear
  — Pupil normal
  — Vision normal
2 Scleritis
  — Focal or diffuse hyperemia
  — Cornea usually clear
  — Pupil normal
  — Vision normal or mildly reduced
3 Angle-closure glaucoma
  — Diffuse hyperemia
  — Cornea very cloudy
  — Pupil dilated and unreactive
  — Vision severely reduced
4 Acute anterior uveitis
  — Diffuse hyperemia
  — Cornea slightly cloudy
  — Pupil constricted and poorly reactive
  — Vision mildly reduced
5 Superficial keratitis
  — Diffuse hyperemia
  — Cornea very cloudy
  — Pupil normal
  — Vision moderately reduced

Uveitis: etiological categorization
1 Seronegative arthritides (incl. inflammatory bowel disease)
  — *Severe* in
    • Behçet's
    • Juvenile chronic arthritis (ANA+, pauciarticular)
  — *Common* in
    • Ankylosing spondylitis
    • Reiter's syndrome (conjunctivitis commoner)
  — *Rare* in psoriatic arthropathy
2 Infection
  — Toxoplasmosis, toxocara
  — Leptospirosis, syphilis, TB, brucellosis, gonorrhea
3 Sarcoidosis
4 Vogt–Koyanagi syndrome
  $\to$ Chronic uveitis, recurrent aseptic meningitis, vitiligo
5 Idiopathic (60%) ± HLA-B27

Anterior vs posterior uveitis
1 Anterior uveitis (iritis)
  — Uniocular (acute) presentation usual
  — Painful red eye
    • Circumcorneal ('ciliary') hyperemia
    • Photophobia
    • Discharge
  — Visual acuity unaffected *unless* complicated by
    • Vitreous inflammation (iridocyclitis, hypopyon)
    • Corneal opacification (band keratopathy)
    • Cataracts, glaucoma (esp. if topical steroids used)
  — Slit-lamp examination: posterior synechiae
  — Signs of chronicity
    • Miosis
    • Keratopathy
    • Cataracts
    • Glaucoma
  — R_x: *Topical* steroids; mydriatics*
2 Posterior uveitis (choroidoretinitis)
  — Binocular (chronic) presentation usual
  — Painless white eye
  — Reduced visual acuity
    • Vitreous debris ('floaters')
    • Macular edema
    • Retinopathy

— Fluorescein angiography: retinal venous leakage
— R$_x$: *Systemic* steroids, ciclosporin; azathioprine

* Prevent formation of posterior synechiae

Ocular manifestations of rheumatoid arthritis
1 Keratoconjunctivitis sicca (in 20–30%)
2 Scleral disease
   — Episcleritis (hyperemia): good prognosis, sclera heals
   — Scleritis: intermediate prognosis, sclera scars
   — Scleromalacia perforans: poor prognosis, sclera sloughs
3 Scleral nodules and/or vasculitis
4 Iatrogenic
   — Corneal opacity, pigmentary retinopathy (chloroquine)
   — Cataracts (steroids)

Differential diagnosis of band keratopathy
1 Juvenile chronic arthritis (ANA+, RF–, pauciarticular type)
2 Long-standing hyperparathyroidism
3 Long-standing renal failure
4 Long-standing sarcoidosis
5 Long-term chloroquine treatment*

* NB: Corneal microdeposits also occur with amiodarone or chlorpromazine

Ocular complications of corticosteroid therapy
1 Herpes simplex keratitis ($\rightarrow$ *topical* steroids)
2 Papilledema (benign intracranial hypertension)
3 Cataract (p. 260)
4 Glaucoma

(p. 260)

INVESTIGATING RHEUMATIC DISEASES

SEROLOGIC ASSESSMENT OF RHEUMATIC DISEASE

The acute phase reactants
1 10–100× ↑ in inflammatory conditions*
   — C-reactive protein
   — Serum amyloid-A (SAA) component
2 2–10× ↑ in inflammatory conditions
   — α_1AT, α_1 antichymotrypsin, α_1 acid glycoprotein
   — C_3 (C_4, C_9); $C_{1\text{-INH}}$
   — Fibrinogen, haptoglobin
   — Plasminogen, α_2 antiplasmin
   — Factors V, VIII; AT III
   — Ferritin, ceruloplasmin
3 No change in inflammatory conditions
   — Serum amyloid P
   — Prothrombin
   — α_2 Macroglobulin
4 Decreased in inflammatory conditions
   — Albumin, prealbumin
   — Transferrin
   — Transthyretin, TBG
   — Factor XII

* Increased in RA/JCA, normal in SLE; rise quickly (within 6–10 h of inflammatory insult) unlike, say, fibrinogen (24–48 h)

Clinical utility of C-reactive protein estimations
1 Correlates more closely than ESR with
   — Radiographic progression of joint damage
   — Disease response to gold/penicillamine (in RA)
2 Useful in monitoring activity of
   — Ankylosing spondylitis
   — Juvenile chronic arthritis
3 Helpful in distinguishing infective episodes* in
   — SLE
   — Sicca syndrome
4 Grossly elevated values may aid in distinguishing
   — Rheumatoid arthritis (from SLE)
   — Crohn's disease (from ulcerative colitis)
   — Bacterial meningitis (from viral)
   — Pyelonephritis (from cystitis)

* ↑↑ CRP in infection; normal in active disease

Rheumatoid factors: clinical correlations
1 RA latex (human IgG)
   — Most sensitive test
2 Rose–Waaler (rabbit IgG)
   — Most specific test
3 Marked elevation in RA
   — Rheumatoid lung disease
   — Felty's, Sjögren's
4 Marked elevation in non-rheumatic conditions
   — SBE
   — Myeloma
   — Cryoglobulinemia

Grossly elevated ESR in rheumatoid arthritis
1 Highly active synovitis
2 Extra-articular vasculitis
3 Development of amyloidosis
4 Sjögren's syndrome
5 Septic arthritis

RADIOLOGICAL ASSESSMENT OF RHEUMATIC DISEASE

Classical X-ray signs of common rheumatic disorders
1 Rheumatoid arthritis
   — Cortical erosions in MCPs, ulnar styloid, carpals*
   — Early: soft-tissue swelling, juxta-articular osteoporosis
   — Late: joint (incl. atlantoaxial) subluxation, deformity
2 Primary (familial) osteoarthritis
   — Osteophyte formation
   — Subchondral sclerosis (no periarticular osteoporosis)
   — Joint space narrowing; loose bodies
   — Sparing of metacarpophalangeal joints
3 Chondrocalcinosis: calcification of cartilage in
   — Knee, wrist
   — Symphysis pubis
   — Intervertebral discs
4 Reiter's syndrome
   — Periostitis contiguous with affected joints
   — Calcaneal spurs
   — Asymmetric erosions (sparing hands) and sacroiliitis

5 Charcot (neuropathic) joint
   — Both sides exhibit destructive changes and
     sclerosis
   — Loose bodies; soft tissue swelling; no
     osteoporosis

* Most diagnostic sign

Differential diagnosis of radiographic erosions in hands
1 Rheumatoid arthritis
2 Gout
3 Psoriatic arthritis
4 Sarcoidosis
5 Miscellaneous
   — Gaucher's
   — Albright's (polyostotic fibrous dysplasia)
   — Osteitis fibrosa cystica ('brown tumors')
   — Aneurysmal bone cyst, non-ossifying fibroma

The abnormal spinal radiograph: features and diagnosis
1 Ankylosing spondylitis
   — Vertebral 'squaring'
   — Syndesmophyte formation (→ 'bamboo spine')
   — Romanus lesion (erosion of anterosuperior
     vertebra)
   — Apophyseal joint fusion
   — Sacroiliac joint erosion, sclerosis or fusion
   — Hip joint erosions
2 DISH (diffuse idiopathic skeletal hyperostosis; =
  Forestier's)
   — Heavy ossification of paraspinal ligaments
   — Olecranon and/or calcaneal spurs
   — Preservation of disc height
   — Normal sacroiliac joints
3 Pott's disease (spinal TB)
   — Gibbus (acute anterior angulation)
   — Paraspinal mass
   — Narrowing of disc space
   — Vertebral collapse (often affects contiguous
     vertebrae)
4 Metastatic carcinoma
   — Obliteration of pedicle in PA view
   — Discrete lytic (and/or sclerotic) spinal lesions
   — Multiple levels of vertebral collapse
5 (Old) Scheuermann's disease (adolescent
  osteochondritis)
   — Residual signs of vertebral epiphyseal
     osteochondritis
6 Straight back syndrome (± marfanoid habitus)
   — Marked reduction of AP chest diameter on
     lateral CXR

Differential diagnosis of sacroiliitis
1 Ankylosing spondylitis
2 Other seronegative arthritides
   — Psoriatic
   — Reiter's
   — Juvenile chronic arthritis
3 Inflammatory bowel disease, 'reactive'
  spondyloarthritis
4 Infection
   — Septic arthritis
   — TB
   — Brucellosis

5 Recurrent polyserositis (familial Mediterranean
  fever)
6 Ochronosis

Atlantoaxial subluxation: diagnosis and management
1 Pathogenesis
   — Odontoid erosion
   — Ligamentous destruction
2 Occurrence
   — Rheumatoid arthritis
   — Juvenile chronic arthritis
   — Ankylosing spondylitis
3 Diagnosis: lateral flexion (+ extension) cervical
  spine X-ray
   — Odontoid peg > 2.5 mm displaced on atlas
   — MRI: may show inflammatory mass
4 Management if symptomatic
   — If positive MRI scan, proceed to surgery
     • Transoral anterior approach, *plus*
     • Posterior cervical fusion
5 Management if asymptomatic
   — Cervical collar when driving
   — Check for atlantoaxial subluxation prior to
     anesthesia
   — Choose spinal rather than general anesthesia

INVASIVE ASSESSMENT OF JOINT DISEASE

Indications for joint aspiration
1 Diagnosis
   — Septic arthritis
   — Crystal synovitis
2 Therapy
   — Massive effusion interfering with joint
     function
3 Diagnosis and therapy
   — Hemarthrosis (± coagulation cover)

Indications for joint injection
1 Diagnosis
   — Arthrogram for suspected meniscal (knee)
     tears
   — Arthrogram for suspected (ruptured) Baker's
     cyst
2 Therapeutic
   — Intra-articular corticosteroids
   — 'Medical synovectomy' (^{90}yttrium)

Indications for diagnostic arthroscopy
1 Unexplained monarthritis
2 Suspected injury (e.g. → meniscus, cruciates)
3 Histologic diagnosis sought (e.g. villonodular
  synovitis)

Important diagnoses on synovial biopsy
1 Tuberculous arthritis
2 (Pigmented) villonodular synovitis
3 Amyloidosis
4 Ochronosis (alkaptonuria)
5 Synovial tumours (e.g. hemangioma)

ANALYSIS OF SYNOVIAL FLUID

Non-inflammatory effusions: characteristics and causes
1 Characteristics
  — Synovial fluid white cell count $< 2 \times 10^9$/L
  — High viscosity
  — Negative fibrin clot
2 Causes
  — Osteoarthritis
  — Post-traumatic
  — Sympathetic (e.g. adjacent to osteomyelitis)
  — Myxedema
  — Amyloidosis
  — Sickle-cell disease
  — Hypertrophic pulmonary osteoarthropathy

Synovial fluid leukocyte counts in health and disease
1 Normal
  — $< 0.2 \times 10^9$/L
2 'Non-inflammatory' synovitis (e.g. osteoarthritis)
  — $< 2.0 \times 10^9$/L; 10–30% polymorphs
3 Inflammatory synovitis
  — Septic arthritis
    • $5–500 \times 10^9$/L (av. 50×10^9/L)
    • 80-100% polymorphs
  — Gout
    • $2–200 \times 10^9$/L (av. 15×10^9/L)
    • 60–95% polymorphs
  — Reiter's syndrome
    • $2-50 \times 10^9$/L (av. 20×10^9/L)
    • 50–90% polymorphs
  — Rheumatoid arthritis
    • $2–100 \times 10^9$/L (av. 10×10^9/L)
    • 50–75% polymorphs

Other joint fluid abnormalities
1 ↓ Glucose level
  — Septic arthritis
  — Reiter's syndrome
  — Rheumatoid arthritis (*also* low in RA effusions)
2 Complement levels
  — ↑ In Reiter's syndrome
  — ↓ In RA, SLE, gout, sepsis*
3 Cytology
  — Phagocytosed leukocytes
    • Reiter's syndrome
  — 'Ragocytes'
    • Rheumatoid arthritis
  — Hemosiderin-laden *macrophages*
    • Recurrent hemarthroses
  — Hemosiderin-laden *synovial* cells
    • Hemochromatosis

* NB: *Plasma* complement levels may be similarly low in active SLE, but elevated in active rheumatoid arthritis. Hence, synovial:serum complement ratio is typically < 10% in RA without systemic vasculitis. When RA is complicated by systemic vasculitis, however, plasma complement levels are usually also low

Differential diagnosis of hemarthrosis
1 Hemophilia
2 Major trauma (e.g. fracture communicating with joint)
  Minor trauma in anticoagulated patient

3 Joint tumors, incl. pigmented villonodular synovitis
4 Charcot joint; arthritis mutilans
5 Calcium pyrophosphate deposition disease
6 'Traumatic tap'*

* Distinguish from true hemarthrosis by centrifuging aspirate and demonstrating absent xanthochromia

Crystal arthropathies: findings on joint aspiration
1 Gout
  — Needle-shaped urate crystals
  — Strongly negative birefringence (polarized microscopy)
  — Angle of extinction: parallel
  — Crystals may → non-inflamed joints in gouty patients
2 Pseudogout
  — Rhomboid-shaped pyrophosphate crystals
  — Weakly positive birefringence
  — Angle of extinction: oblique
3 Rheumatoid arthritis may mimic crystal synovitis due to cholesterol crystals in chronic effusions
4 Hydroxyapatite crystals may be seen on electron microscopy in OA or other arthritides, especially if bone destruction
5 Post-steroid injection flare (4–12 h later) due to steroid crystals

HLA IN RHEUMATIC DISEASE

Relative indications for tissue typing in rheumatic disease
1 Older male child (11–16 years) with oligoarthritis, if diagnosis of ankylosing spondylitis is neither certain nor unlikely
  — B27-positive
    • 90% risk of ankylosing spondylitis
    • ↓ Risk of chronic anterior uveitis
  — B27-negative
    • 15% probability of ankylosing spondylitis
    • ↑ Risk of chronic anterior uveitis
2 Controversial
  — DR3 screening to predict patients at increased risk of renal toxicity from gold/penicillamine

NB: *No* absolute – or routine – indications currently exist

HLA associations in rheumatoid arthritis
1 DR4
  — ↑ Incidence of (seropositive) disease
2 DR3
  — ↑ Incidence of *strongly* seropositive (aggressive) RA
  — ↑ Incidence of major side-effects (esp. proteinuria, cytopenia) from gold, penicillamine
  — ↑ Incidence of Sjögren's syndrome (which may be linked to either of the above two trends)
3 DR2
  — ↓ Incidence of disease
  — ↑ Incidence of stomatitis due to gold therapy

GENERAL MEASURES IN RHEUMATIC DISORDERS

Rationâle of exercise in joint disease
1 To maintain or restore muscle strength around joint
2 To maintain or restore range of joint movement
3 To prevent or minimize periarticular osteoporosis

Principles of occupational therapy in rheumatic disease
1 Provision of appliances to reduce joint strain
   — Work splints (for wrists)
   — Removable splints (for unstable knees)
   — Cervical collars (hard or soft)
2 Provision of appliances to improve function
   — Special shoes and insoles, non-slip mats
   — Walking sticks, wheelchairs, walking frames
   — Shopping cart
3 Home visits to adapt house for activities of daily living
   — Toilet aids, handrails, electric toothbrush
   — Tap turners, electric can opener, large-handled cutlery
   — Bookrest, page-turner, push-button phone

Principles of physiotherapy in rheumatoid arthritis
1 *Night splinting* to rest knees, wrists in position of function
   Serial splinting to reverse early deformities*
2 *Passive exercises* to maintain range of joint movement
   Isometric exercises to maintain muscle power
   Active exercises to maintain power and range of movement
3 Facilitation of exercise using
   — Ultrasound
   — Heat
   — Hydrotherapy

* e.g. knee flexion; bedrest may exacerbate deformity in active disease

How to treat nerve/tendon compression in rheumatoid arthritis
1 **S**plinting (esp. wrist or knee)
2 **S**ystemic treatment (e.g. gold)
3 **S**teroid injection (soluble preparation → ↓ risk of neurolysis)
4 **S**ynovectomy (esp. wrist or knee)
5 **S**urgical decompression

Effects of posture or physiotherapy on ankylosing spondylitis
1 *No* effect on rate of ankylosis
2 *Mild* reduction in pain
3 *Major* reduction in disability*

* e.g. eventual ankylosis → erect, not kyphotic, posture

Points to consider in NSAID prescribing
1 NSAIDs may improve joint *function* by reducing pain and inflammation; they do not reverse the arthropathy
2 The maximal tolerated dose of any given NSAID should be prescribed before being discarded as ineffective
3 Several NSAIDs may need to be tried to find the best one. In general, different NSAIDs should *not* be combined
4 Patients at high risk of NSAID-induced gastritis may be prescribed prophylactic omeprazole. Standard-risk patients should be prescribed lower-risk NSAIDs (e.g. ibuprofen, COX-2 inhibitors) to be taken after meals
5 Paracetamol may be the most cost-effective NSAID
6 Topical NSAIDs appear to have some activity, but their place in routine management remains uncertain

Non-steroidal anti-inflammatory drugs: toxicity
1 Gastrointestinal (esp. with high-dose aspirin, indometacin)
   — Dyspepsia, gastritis, ulceration*
2 CNS (esp. with indometacin)
   — Headache, confusion, dizziness
3 Blood dyscrasias (esp. with phenylbutazone‡)
   — Aplastic anemia, agranulocytosis, thrombocytopenia
4 Nephrotoxicity
   — Precipitation of acute renal failure
   — Edema (sodium retention); nephrosis
   — Papillary necrosis
   — Interstitial nephritis
5 Other: bullous dermatoses, hepatitis, aseptic meningitis

* Sulindac and ibuprofen are probably the least ulcerogenic of these drugs. In general, however, patient tolerance of any one drug is unpredictable
‡ Phenylbutazone now *only* indicated for refractory ankylosing spondylitis

Aspirin as first-line therapy
1 Juvenile chronic arthritis
2 Rheumatic fever
3 Rheumatoid arthritis
   Seronegative spondyloarthropathies (not AS)
   Soft tissue rheumatism
   — In USA
4 Osteoid osteoma

NB: The association of aspirin with Reye's syndrome makes monitoring mandatory in children younger than 12 requiring aspirin therapy

Predispositions to aspirin hepatotoxicity
1 Juvenile chronic arthritis
2 Reiter's syndrome
3 Chronic active hepatitis
4 Rheumatic fever
5 SLE

Presentations of aspirin sensitivity
1 Urticaria, bronchospasm, anaphylaxis
2 Pyrexia of unknown origin
3 Pneumonitis
4 Pancreatitis
5 Proctocolitis
6 Ulceration of the esophagus

Aspirin toxicity: the clinical spectrum
1 Anti-inflammatory action requires daily dosage of 2–4 g/day
2 Gastrointestinal intolerance is main cause of non-compliance
3 Tinnitus and vertigo are dose-related toxicities which may be clinically useful in regulating drug dosage. Hearing loss may necessitate treatment cessation; salicylate levels and/or audiograms may be useful in monitoring
4 Iron-deficiency anemia may occur in the absence of gastrointestinal symptoms; hypoprothrombinemia rare
5 High-dose regimens are uricosuric, whereas low-dose administration may lead to hyperuricemia and gout
6 Hepatotoxicity manifests as asymptomatic transaminase elevation which often normalizes if drug continued; it occurs more commonly in young patients

SELECTIVE CYCLOOXYGENASE-2 (COX-2) INHIBITORS

Physiological distinction between COX-1 and COX-2
1 COX-1
   — Constitutively synthesized in gastrointestinal epithelium
   — Stimulates prostaglandin E_2 and PGI_2 (prostacyclin) synthesis
   — Responsible for housekeeping functions: gastroprotection, platelet aggregation, renal function
   — Inhibition causes NSAID gastritis, hemorrhage*, nephrotoxicity
2 COX-2
   — Synthesis induced by proinflammatory stimuli
   — Expressed in brain, colorectal epithelium
   — Responsible for inflammation, pain, fever

* On the other hand, also responsible for the therapeutic antiplatelet effect of low-dose aspirin

Non-selective NSAIDs vs COX-2 inhibitors
1 Non-selective NSAIDs
   — COX-1 inhibition: piroxicam > indometacin > naproxen > diclofenac > ibuprofen*
2 COX-2 inhibitors
   — Celecoxib, rofecoxib, meloxicam

* Corresponds roughly to gastrotoxicity (this can be ameliorated by omeprazole prophylaxis)

SLOW-ACTING ANTIRHEUMATIC DRUGS (SAARDs)

Drugs used as SAARDs
1 Sulfasalazine
2 Methotrexate
3 Hydroxychloroquine
4 Gold: parenteral or oral (auranofin)
5 D-penicillamine
6 Azathioprine
7 Ciclosporin
8 TNF antagonists (e.g. etanercept)

Diseases treatable with remittive drug therapy
1 Gold
   — Rheumatoid arthritis
   — Sjögren's syndrome
      • Higher incidence of drug reactions
      • Sicca syndrome alone may not respond
   — Psoriatic arthritis
   — Juvenile chronic arthritis
   — Pemphigus (steroid-sparing)
2 D-Penicillamine
   — Rheumatoid arthritis
   — Cystinuria → proteinuria in 25%
   — Wilson's disease → proteinuria in 5%
   — Psoriatic arthritis
   — Heavy metal poisoning
3 Chloroquine
   — SLE (esp. joint and skin involvement)
   — Juvenile chronic arthritis
   — Rheumatoid arthritis
   — *Contraindicated* in psoriatic arthritis
4 Sulfasalazine
   — Rheumatoid arthritis
   — Seronegative spondyloarthropathies

Indications for methotrexate in non-malignant disease
1 Rheumatoid arthritis*
2 Juvenile chronic arthritis
3 Psoriasis‡
4 Crohn's disease

* Effective in 70% and better tolerated than the other SAARDs (5-year continuation rate > 50%, whereas only 20% for other SAARDs)
‡ Hepatotoxicity may be dose-limiting

Gold: toxicity
1 Pruritic rash
   — Occurs in 30% of treated patients
   — May mimic lichen planus, pityriasis rosea

— Frequently preceded by peripheral eosinophilia
— Aurothiomalate (IMI) > triethylphosphine gold (oral)
2 Gastrointestinal
   — Stomatitis, mouth ulcers
   — Diarrhea (triethylphosphine gold)
3 Leukopenia, thrombocytopenia
   — An absolute indication for treatment cessation
   — Heavy metal chelators may be indicated if acute
4 Proteinuria
   — Occurs in 5% of treated patients
   — If < 1 g/day, drug may be cautiously reintroduced *after* normalization of protein excretion
   — If > 1 g/day, cease gold therapy indefinitely
5 Nephrosis
   — Occurs in 1% of treated patients
   — Recovery may take 18 months
6 Rare:
   — Fibrosing alveolitis
   — Enterocolitis, cholestasis
   — Neuropathy

D-Penicillamine: toxicity

1 Loss of taste, anorexia, nausea
   — Occurs in 25%
   — Improves with continued treatment
2 Proteinuria (25%), nephrosis (5%)
3 Thrombocytopenia (10%)
4 Early rash (10%) in first month: may reintroduce R_x
   Wrinkly skin (elastosis serpiginosa perforans)
   Late (pemphigus-like) rash in 5%; if severe, cease R_x
5 Rare
   — SLE, myasthenia gravis, polymyositis
   — Goodpasture-like syndrome
6 Lack of efficacy (25%)
   — Similar incidence to gold
   — More likely if previously unresponsive to gold

TREATING RHEUMATOID ARTHRITIS

Rheumatoid arthritis: indications for remittive therapy

1 Symptomatic young patients (esp. females) with polyarticular disease and high levels of rheumatoid factor
2 Radiological erosions developing in the first year of disease
3 Troublesome symptoms despite NSAIDs for 6 months
4 Extra-articular disease affecting vital organ function

Prescribing strategy in rheumatoid arthritis

1 First-line therapy: symptomatic treatment only
   — NSAIDs
   — Aspirin 3–4 g/day (popular in USA only)
2 Remittive drugs ($\rightarrow \downarrow$ erosions)
   — Methotrexate (oral weekly dose: 7.5–10 mg)
   — Gold (intramuscular or oral)
   — D-Penicillamine (oral)
   — Sulfasalazine (oral)
   — (Hydroxy)chloroquine (oral)

3 Failure of conventional remittive drugs?
   — Cytotoxics (azathioprine, cyclophosphamide)
   — Systemic corticosteroids

NB: Nocturnal slow-release NSAIDs (oral or suppositories) may help minimize morning stiffness in RA

Relative efficacy of remittive drugs

1 High efficacy
   — Methotrexate
   — Sodium aurothiomalate
2 Intermediate efficacy
   — Penicillamine
   — Sulfasalazine*
3 Mild efficacy
   — Antimalarials
   — Triethylphosphine gold

* But often used before other drugs due to good tolerance

Relative toxicity of remittive drugs

1 High toxicity
   — Sodium aurothiomalate
2 Intermediate toxicity
   — Penicillamine
   — Methotrexate*
3 Mild toxicity
   — Sulfasalazine
   — Triethylphosphine gold
   — Antimalarials

* Patients should avoid alcohol (due to risk of liver toxicity) and take supplementary folate

Indications for systemic steroids in rheumatoid arthritis

1 Development of stridor
2 Necrotizing scleritis
3 Pleuropericarditis
4 Other signs of extra-articular vasculitis threatening vital organ function (e.g. mononeuritis multiplex)
5 Persistent arthritis despite adequate trial of SAARDs

SYSTEMIC STEROIDS IN RHEUMATIC DISEASE

Prescribing steroids in rheumatoid arthritis

1 Uncommonly indicated; if necessary, treatment should be aimed at a specific goal (i.e. a temporizing measure only)
2 Treatment should be low-dose: 5–7.5 mg prednisone/day max.
3 To minimize adrenal suppression, use a single a.m. dose only
4 Alternate-day steroids don't work in RA; if symptoms appear well-controlled on alternate-day steroids, then the patient probably doesn't need steroids at all

Potency and toxicity of various corticosteroids

1 30 mg cortisone acetate
   = 25 mg hydrocortisone
   = 5 mg (methyl)prednis(ol)one, triamcinolone
   = 1 mg dexamethasone, betamethasone

2 Hydrocortisone causes sodium retention; hence, useful in adrenal replacement therapy, but not otherwise
3 Triamcinolone, given systemically, is the most myopathic of the corticosteroids; therefore only used topically
4 Prednisone is a prodrug; hence, in severe liver disease, better to use prednisolone (the active metabolite)

ACTH or prednisone? Pros and cons of ACTH therapy

1 Disadvantages of ACTH
   — Expensive
   — Painful (daily intramuscular injections)
   — Difficult to adjust or taper dosage
   — Greater salt/fluid retention than prednisone (reflecting greater mineralocorticoid effect)
   — Pigmentation; bruising; severe allergic reactions
2 Advantages of ACTH
   — For juvenile chronic arthritis patients
      → ↓ Growth stunting
   — For hospitalized patients with inflammatory arthritis
      → No adrenal suppression (hence, easy to stop)
   — For polymyositis/dermatomyositis/multiple sclerosis
      → ↓ Muscle wasting (androgen effect)
   — For post-menopausal female patients
      → ↓ Osteoporosis (↑ androstenedione → ↑ estrone)

INTRA-ARTICULAR STEROIDS

Potential indications for intra-articular steroids

1 Systemic treatment contraindicated (e.g. blood dyscrasia)
2 Systemic treatment inadequate to control inflammation at one or more joints (incl. Baker's cyst)
3 Troublesome oligoarticular inflammation not warranting systemic therapy (e.g. in seronegative arthropathy)
4 To mobilize (and reduce deformity) in rehabilitation
5 Rapid analgesia required

Intra-articular steroids: which joints?

1 Common
   — Knee, shoulder
2 Less often
   — Ankle, elbow, fingers
3 Rare
   — Hip

Intra-articular steroid therapy: potential morbidity

1 Crystal-induced synovitis (a 'flare' of pain and swelling a few hours after injection; esp. with triamcinolone)
2 Charcot-like arthropathy (i.e. severe joint destruction, though probably *not* due to loss of pain sensation)
3 Cushing's syndrome
4 Septic arthritis, *or*
   Suppression of inflammatory signs (e.g. in septic arthritis complicating RA)

ANTIMALARIALS IN RHEUMATIC DISEASE

Potential hazards of antimalarial chemotherapy

1 Chloroquine is avoided in psoriatic arthritis due to the risk of a pustular exacerbation (which may be indistinguishable from keratoderma blenorrhagica of Reiter's syndrome)
2 Chloroquine should not be administered in full dosage to SLE patients with porphyria cutanea tarda. If the drug is prescribed in this context, the patient should be phlebotomized on at least two prior occasions and the drug given in low-dose twice-weekly schedule
3 Oculotoxicity includes cycloplegia (→ transient blurring) and corneal microdeposits (rarely culminating in band keratopathy) in addition to the well-known retinopathy

Features of chloroquine retinopathy

1 Occurrence is commoner with
   — Renal impairment
   — SLE
   — Concomitant probenecid therapy
   — Daily dosage > 150 mg *base* per day*
   — Chloroquine (than with hydroxychloroquine)
2 Occurrence *cannot* be predicted by onset of visual symptoms (more commonly due to presbyopia or cycloplegia)
3 Best (monthly) screening tests are
   — Observation of the foveal reflex
   — Charting the pericentral visual fields to a red object using an Amsler chart (paracentral scotoma is the first sign)
4 Baseline slit-lamp examination is recommended, plus further examinations every 4–6 months in the event of any symptoms
5 The classic 'bull's eye' macula may supervene despite early cessation of therapy

* i.e. > 250 mg chloroquine phosphate/sulfate or 400 mg hydroxychloroquine

THE HYPERURICEMIC PATIENT

Etiology of hyperuricemia in childhood

1 Associated with gout in childhood
   — HGPRT deficiency (Lesch–Nyhan syndrome)
   — PRPP synthetase overactivity
2 Not associated with gout in childhood
   — Acute leukemia (→ lymphoblastic, post-chemo)
   — Chronic hemolysis (e.g. sickle-cell disease)
   — Lead poisoning
   — Von Gierke's; Gaucher's
   — Severe diabetes mellitus, hypertriglyceridemia

Management aspects of gout and hyperuricemia

1 Modalities available for treating acute gouty arthritis
   — Colchicine (traditional remedy; major GI toxicity)
   — NSAIDs (now more popular than colchicine)
   — Joint aspiration
   — Intra-articular corticosteroids

2 Modalities available for long-term gout prophylaxis
   — Allopurinol
   — Uricosurics: probenecid, sulfinpyrazone
3 Drugs inhibiting uricosurics (avoid in gouty patients)
   — Thiazides
   — Ethambutol
   — Low-dose salicylate
   — Ciclosporin

Exclusive indications for allopurinol administration
1 Tophaceous gout, *or* gouty bony erosions
2 Recurrent troublesome acute gouty attacks
3 Recurrent urate calculi, *or*
   Recurrent oxalate calculi with hyperuricosuria
4 Prevention of uric acid nephropathy in patients at risk for tumor lysis syndrome prechemotherapy
5 *Massive* urate overproduction (> 7.2 mmol/24 h urine) despite low-purine alcohol-free diet, esp. if family history of renal disease
6 Lesch–Nyhan syndrome

NB: Asymptomatic hyperuricemia or uncomplicated gout are *not* indications for maintenance allopurinol

Allopurinol: toxicity
1 Major hypersensitivity reactions (toxic epidermal necrolysis, vasculitis, eosinophilia) may be heralded by rash or fever
2 Major reactions are commoner in renal impairment and/or diuretic therapy, and may lead to renal failure
3 Hepatotoxicity is an uncommon but serious sequela
4 Ampicillin rashes are more frequent
5 Allopurinol potentiates
   — 6MP, azathioprine (four-fold)
   — Warfarin (weak effect)

OPERATIVE OPTIONS IN JOINT DISEASE

Rheumatoid arthritis: the place of surgery
1 Resection of metatarsal heads
   — For forefoot pain due to MTP subluxation
2 Total articular arthroplasty
   — Ideal for hip
3 Excision arthroplasty
   — Excision of radial head in severe erosive elbow arthritis
   — Resection of distal ulna as part of wrist synovectomy
4 Synovectomy (improves symptoms for about 2 years)
   — Knee: for refractory Baker's cyst
   — Wrist: for refractory nodular tenosynovitis
5 Miscellaneous
   — Silastic MCP joint replacement (deformity recurs)
   — Immediate tendon reanastomosis for rupture
   — Posterior cervical fusion for atlantoaxial subluxation
   — Decompression of entrapment neuropathies
   — Splenectomy in Felty's syndrome

Total hip replacement: indications and complications
1 Indications
   — Patient > 50 with unrelieved severe hip arthritis
   — *Any* patient with permanent loss of hip mobility (< 45° flexion, < 10° abduction) leading to reduced activity
2 Complications
   — Implant loosening
   — Infection of bone–cement interface
   — Metal sensitivity (→ loosening)
   — Mechanical failure
   — Post-operative thromboembolism despite prophylaxis

Arthrodesis or osteotomy? Clinical considerations
1 Arthrodesis
   — Favored joints: wrist; ankle (subtalar joint only)
   — Less popular: knee, hip, tarsal, 1st MCP
   — Best for young (20–30 years) patients
   — Best for monarthritis (↓ mobility less significant)
   — Preferred to osteotomy if joint architecture destroyed
2 Osteotomy
   — Favored joints: hip, knee
   — Best for patients younger than 50
   — Best for painful stable joints (↑ mobility not a priority)
   — Preferred to arthrodesis if X-ray confirms asymmetrical disruption of joint architecture

Anesthetic considerations in patients with rheumatic disease
1 Rheumatoid arthritis
   — If cervical spine X-ray shows atlantoaxial subluxation and/or odontoid erosion in an asymptomatic patient, use soft collar and spinal anesthesia
   — If atlantoaxial subluxation or odontoid erosion occurs in a patient with symptoms of cord compression, assess with MRI and consider cervical spine surgery *prior* to elective operation
   — If temporomandibular joint disease evident, anticipate difficult endotracheal intubation (though rarely a major problem in RA; cf. in JCA)
2 Ankylosing spondylitis
   — Lower cervical spondylosis and/or TMJ disease may make intubation difficult
   — Costovertebral involvement may restrict ventilation
3 Juvenile chronic arthritis
   — Intubation may be difficult due to micrognathia

Patient selection for 'medical synovectomy'*
1 Most effective for recurrent inflammatory knee effusions
2 Any risk of pregnancy is an absolute contraindication
3 Youth is a relative contraindication (risk of leukemogenesis)
4 Ideally, the joint to be injected should be devoid of gross synovial thickening or severe destructive changes

5 Adequate rest, physiotherapy, drugs, and intra-articular steroids should precede use of medical synovectomy

* i.e. intra-articular instillation of, say ^{90}yttrium

PAGET'S DISEASE

Treatable causes of pain in Paget's disease
1 Osteoarthritis (hip, knee) due to limb deformity
2 Pseudogout
3 Nerve entrapment
4 Microfractures due to cortical expansion
5 Pathological fracture
   — Disease-related
   — Supervening osteosarcoma
   — Diphosphonate use

Indications for commencement of specific chemotherapy
1 Serum alkaline phosphatase > 1000 U/L
2 Severe bone pain unresponsive to conservative measures
3 Intractable angina or heart failure (if due to Paget's)
4 Progressive deformity of weight-bearing long bones or skull base, esp. in relatively young patients
   Osteolytic lesions affecting long bones, esp. if painful
5 Hypercalcemia (precipitated by immobilization or trauma) and/or radio-opaque renal calculi
6 Neurological sequelae
   — Spinal cord compression
   — Peripheral nerve entrapment
   — Visual failure due to macular degeneration
   — Progressive deafness accompanied by tinnitus

Drug treatment: relative indications and contraindications
1 Calcitonin
   — Indications
     • Severe bone pain requiring rapid relief
     • Painful osteolytic lesions
     • Hypercalcemia/symptomatic hypercalciuria
     • Failure or toxicity of alternative therapy
   — Contraindications
     • Resistance due to neutralizing antibodies
     • Unsuitability of parenteral administration; expense
2 Bisphosphonates (clodronate, pamidronate, etidronate)
   — Indications
     • Predominant skull involvement
     • Mild to moderate bone pain
     • Incomplete clinical/biochemical response to calcitonin
   — Contraindications
     • Severe bone pain (may be worsened)
     • Development of fractures*
     • Known (pre-existing) osteolytic lesions
     • Development of diarrhea while on treatment

* With etidronate only

UNDERSTANDING RHEUMATIC DISEASE

POLYMYALGIA RHEUMATICA

Diagnostic criteria for polymyalgia rheumatica (PMR)
1 Major criteria
   — Age > 50 (usually > 65)
   — ESR > 50 mm/h
   — Bilateral shoulder/pelvic girdle morning stiffness > 1 h duration
   — Response to low-dose (~ 15 mg/day prednisone) steroids
2 Minor criteria
   — Weight loss, night sweats, fever; depression
   — Symmetrical proximal arm muscle tenderness
   — ↑ Alkaline phosphatase/GGT, ↓ Hb
   — Positive joint scintigraphy*
   — Normal CPK, EMG, muscle biopsy

* i.e. synovitis, but *no* myositis or vasculitis/arteritis, in 'pure' PMR

Exclusion of coexisting temporal arteritis
1 50% of temporal arteritis patients have symptoms of PMR
2 50% of *all* PMR patients (± symptoms of temporal arteritis) will have giant-cell arteritis on temporal artery biopsy
3 10–20% of patients with *clinically pure* PMR will be found to have temporal arteritis on biopsy
4 False-negative biopsies may occur due to 'skip lesions' (i.e. the *abnormal* arterial segments) causing sampling error; for a 2 cm biopsy, however, false-negative rate is < 5%
5 Height of initial ESR *does not* predict disease severity or likelihood of complications
6 With proper management, the diagnosis of giant-cell arteritis is *not* associated with reduced life expectancy

INFLAMMATION AND INFECTION

Proinflammatory cytokines in joint disease
1 Interleukin-6
2 Interleukin-1β, tumor necrosis factor-α
3 Interferon-γ
4 Transforming growth factor-β

Infections commonly associated with arthritis
1 *Staphylococcus aureus*, esp. in intravenous drug abusers
2 *S. albus*, esp. in prosthetic joints
3 *Salmonella* spp., esp. in hyposplenic patients*
4 *Haemophilus influenzae*, esp. in children
5 *Neisseria gonorrheae*, esp. in young women
6 Lyme disease (spirochetal etiology)

* Causes osteomyelitis or spondylitis

Infections commonly associated with arthralgias
1 Associated with arthralgias alone
   — Influenza A

— Coxsackie B, EBV, mumps
— Mycoplasmas
— Brucellosis

2 Associated with arthralgias ± arthritis
— Hepatitis B
— Rubella (incl. rubella vaccine)
— Parvovirus
— Alphaviruses (arboviruses)
  • Ross River, Sindbis, Chikungunya, Barmah Forest
— Disseminated gonococcal infection

Reactive arthritis: occurrence and manifestations

1 Etiology
— Postdysenteric
  • *Shigella flexneri*
  • *Salmonella* spp.
  • *Yersinia enterocolitica*
  • *Campylobacter jejuni*
— Venereal: *Chlamydia trachomatis*
2 Symptoms
— Knee and ankle pain 1–3 weeks following infection
— Enthesopathy (tenosynovitis, plantar fasciitis)
— Low back pain
3 Urethritis may occur with post-dysenteric syndrome
— e.g. In prepubertal children
4 Joint fluid is sterile
5 The initial episode generally settles over about 3 months
6 Long-term prognosis is good, but 50% will have recurrence

Rheumatologic manifestations of HIV infection

1 Seronegative spondyloarthropathy
— Heel pain, enthesopathy
— Remains associated with HLA-B27
— Tends to be more severe than in HIV-negative disease
2 Septic arthritis
— Typically affects axial joints
— Pathogen may be transferred by sex or needles
3 AIDS-associated arthritis
— Often very painful
— Lower-limb oligoarthritis or symmetric polyarthritis
— Synovial fluid: 'non-inflammatory' profile (p. 369)

OTHER ARTHROPATHIES

Juvenile chronic arthritis: a working classification

1 Systemic onset ('Still's disease')
— RF–, ANA–
— Age of onset < 16 years
— Quotidian fever usual ± ↑ WCC
— Non-pruritic rash, Koebner phenomenon (p. 393)
— ± Polyserositis, hepatosplenomegaly, adenopathy
— 50% → polyarticular disease, 50% remit
— Acute phase associated with significant mortality
— Commonest cause of death is amyloidosis

2 Polyarticular non-systemic ('juvenile rheumatoid arthritis')
— RF+ (100%) ANA+ (75%)
— 90% female
— Late childhood onset → severe adult disease
3 Pauciarticular disease (→ knee) and/or chronic uveitis (50%)
— RF–, ANA+ (50%)
— 90% female, early childhood onset
— Major joint disability unusual
— Severe eye disease common
4 Pauciarticular disease (→ hip), sacroiliitis, acute uveitis (10%)
— RF–, ANA–, HLA-B27+ (75%)
— 90% male
— May progress to typical ankylosing spondylitis

Clinical aspects of miscellaneous arthropathies

1 Jaccoud's (post-rheumatic fever) arthropathy
— Moderately severe rheumatic heart disease
— History of severe or prolonged rheumatic fever
— Mildly symptomatic but deforming arthropathy
— Reducible ulnar deviation and PIP hyperextension
— Good hand function despite extent of deformity
— No erosive or destructive changes on X-ray
— Rheumatoid factor negative
2 Palindromic rheumatism
— Equal incidence in males and females
— Asymptomatic between exacerbations
— Typically affects hand, wrists, carpal tunnel
— 90% rheumatoid factor negative at diagnosis
— May evolve to typical RA (and become seropositive)
3 Relapsing polychondritis
— Associated with autoimmune disease in 30%
— Fever, arthralgias, episcleritis, swollen floppy ears
— Nasal septum involvement/collapse ('saddle nose')
— Laryngeal disease → hoarseness, respiratory obstruction
— Tracheobronchial degeneration, sudden death
— Approx. 10% →
  • Aortic valvular incompetence/aneurysm
  • Mitral valve prolapse
— Responds to corticosteroid administration

Rheumatologic manifestations of sickle-cell disease

1 Gout
2 Sickle crisis →
— Lower limb arthralgias, myalgias
— Acute synovitis with non-inflammatory effusion
3 'Hand–foot' syndrome*
4 Secondary hemochromatotic arthropathy (transfusional)
5 Septic arthritis/osteomyelitis from *Salmonella* (hyposplenic)
6 Aseptic (avascular) necrosis

* Dactylitis due to periostitis, marrow expansion and/or infarction

AVASCULAR NECROSIS OF BONE

Avascular necrosis of the femoral head: predispositions

1 Primary (Perthes' disease: epiphyseal osteochondritis)
2 Local trauma
   — Slipped epiphysis (often bilateral in fat children)
   — Femoral neck fractures
   — Traumatic dislocation
3 Sickle-cell disease (including sickle trait)
4 Hypercoagulable states, e.g.
   — Hb C disease
   — Paroxysmal nocturnal hemoglobinuria
   — Nephrotic syndrome; pregnancy
5 SLE, rheumatoid arthritis
   Corticosteroid administration
   Renal transplantation
6 Alcoholism, cirrhosis, pancreatitis
7 Myxedema
8 Gaucher's disease
9 Caisson (decompression) disease; hyperbaric oxygen
10 Therapeutic irradiation

Diagnosing avascular necrosis of the femoral head

1 X-ray of abducted hip
   — Irregular femoral head, translucent band, sclerosis
2 ^{99m}Tc diphosphonate scan
   — Low isotope uptake (only useful post-trauma)
3 CT scan
   — Subchondral rarefaction
4 MRI
   — Clear definition of area of ischemic necrosis

REVIEWING THE LITERATURE: RHEUMATOLOGY

16.1 Cummings SR et al (1998) Endogenous hormones and the risk of hip and vertebral fractures among older women. N Engl J Med 339: 733–738

Cohort study of 271 women older than 65, showing that undetectable serum estradiol and elevated sex hormone binding globulin were predictive of hip and vertebral fracture.

16.2 Cassidy JD et al (2000) Effect of eliminating compensation for pain and suffering on the outcome of insurance claims for whiplash injury. N Engl J Med 342: 1179–1186

Study of 7462 whiplash victims before and after a change in the compensation law to a 'no-fault' policy that avoided payments for pain and suffering. The authors found that the prognosis of injuries improved significantly after the law reform.

16.3 Cherkin DC et al (1998) A comparison of physical therapy, chiropractic manipulation and provision of an educational booklet for the treatment of patients with low back pain. N Engl J Med 339: 1021–1029

Andersson GB et al (1999) A comparison of osteopathic spinal manipulation with standard care for patients with low back pain. N Engl J Med 341: 1426–1431

The former study of 321 patients showed a benefit, but debatable cost-effectiveness, of either physiotherapy or chiropractic. The second study of 178 patients showed comparable efficacy of osteopathy and medical therapies.

16.4 Vroomen PC et al (1999) Lack of effectiveness of bed rest for sciatica. N Engl J Med 340: 418–423

Randomized study of 183 patients with severe sciatica, showing that 'watchful waiting' was as effective as complete bed rest in resolving symptoms.

16.5 Hoffman JR et al (2000) Validity of a set of clinical criteria to rule out injury to the cervical spine in patients with blunt trauma. N Engl J Med 343: 94–99

Study of 34 069 patients from 21 centers, showing that cervical spine X-rays are not needed if (a) no midline neck tenderness, (b) no intoxication, (c) normal alertness, (d) no focal neurologic deficit, and (e) no distracting painful injury elsewhere.

16.6 Van der Windt DA et al (1998) Effectiveness of corticosteroid injections versus physiotherapy for treatment of painful stiff shoulder in primary care: randomised trial. Br Med J 317: 1292–1296

Small randomized study of 109 patients, showing that steroid injections were more effective than physiotherapy alone, particularly with respect to the speed of symptom relief. However, triamcinolone injections were associated with menstrual disturbances and facial flushing.

16.7 Kerrigan DC et al (1998) Knee osteoarthritis and high-heeled shoes. Lancet 351: 1399–1401

Measurement of knee torques in 20 women wearing their favorite stilettos confirmed 23% increased compressive forces at the patellofemoral joint and medial knee compartment, consistent with a role in osteoarthritis.

16.8 Steinbach G et al (2000) The effect of celecoxib, a cyclooxygenase-2 inhibitor, in familial adenomatous polyposis. N Engl J Med 342: 1946–1952

Placebo-controlled crossover study of 77 patients, showing that COX-2 inhibitors modestly (11–14%) reduced the size and number of new polyps, consistent with the proapoptotic effect of NSAIDs on gastrointestinal epithelium.

16.9 Lipsky PE et al (2000) Infliximab and methotrexate in the treatment of rheumatoid arthritis. N Engl J Med 343: 1594–1602

Bathon JM et al (2000) A comparison of etanercept and methotrexate in patients with early rheumatoid arthritis. N Engl J Med 343: 1586–1593

van den Bosch F et al (2000) Crohn's disease associated with spondyloarthropathy: effect of TNF-alpha blockade with infliximab on articular symptoms. Lancet 356: 1821–1822

Choi HK et al (2002) Methotrexate and mortality in patients with rheumatoid arthritis: a prospective study. Lancet 359: 1173–1177

The first two studies used inhibitors of the tumor necrosis factor signaling pathway, with the first showing efficacy when added to methotrexate in a cohort of refractory patients, and the second showing superiority to oral methotrexate. The third shows that the same strategy is effective in seronegative spondyloarthritides. Unexpectedly, the fourth study showed a significant survival benefit associated with methotrexate therapy of RA due to reduced cardiovascular mortality.

16.10 Bombardier C et al (2000) Comparison of upper gastrointestinal toxicity of rofecoxib and naproxen in patients with rheumatoid arthritis. N Engl J Med 343: 1520–1528

Randomized study of 8076 rheumatoid patients, showing that the COX2 inhibitor caused significantly less gut rot than did the notorious naproxen.

CHAPTER 17

Sexual and reproductive medicine

Physical examination protocol 17.1   You are asked to examine a patient who has been referred to the Reproductive Medicine clinic

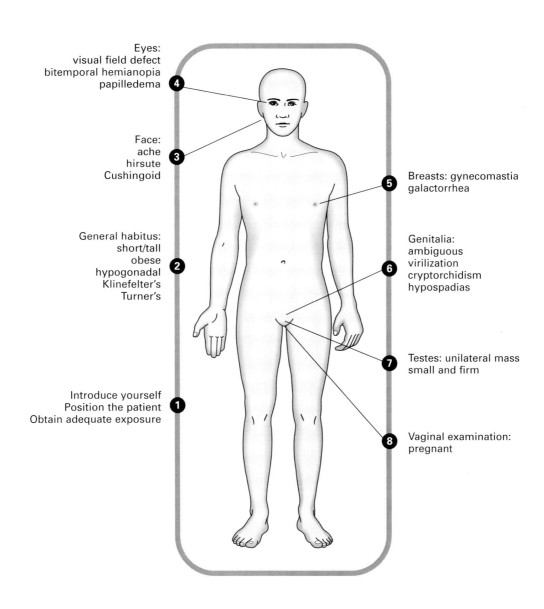

Eyes:
visual field defect
bitemporal hemianopia
papilledema
4

Face:
ache
hirsute
Cushingoid
3

Breasts: gynecomastia
galactorrhea
5

General habitus:
short/tall
obese
hypogonadal
Klinefelter's
Turner's
2

Genitalia:
ambiguous
virilization
cryptorchidism
hypospadias
6

Testes: unilateral mass
small and firm
7

Introduce yourself
Position the patient
Obtain adequate exposure
1

Vaginal examination:
pregnant
8

COMMON AND CLASSIC SEX-RELATED PROBLEMS

Common sexual or reproductive problems in clinical practice
1 Venereal diseases
2 Infertility or impotence
3 Menopausal or premenstrual symptoms

Classic sexual or reproductive problems in clinical exams
1 Benign neoplasms of the prostate or endometrium
2 Thromboembolic complications of oral contraceptives
3 Pre-eclampsia

SEXUAL AND REPRODUCTIVE EMERGENCIES

Assessment and management of priapism
1 Definition: penile erection lasting more than 6 h
2 Causes
 — 'Artificial' erection due to impotence treatment (p. 386)*
 — Disease (e.g. chronic myeloid leukemia, sickle cell, myeloma)
3 Management
 — Call the urologist; then observe as he/she aspirates 50 mL blood from each corpus cavernosum using a 19 G butterfly needle
 — Monitor the blood pressure and heart rate
 — If the erection returns despite aspiration, assist the urologist in diluting phenylephrine 1 mg in 5 mL normal saline, and observe as he/she injects 1 mL of this solution through the same butterfly needle
 — Repeat further cycles of aspiration and/or injection as needed
 — Firmly compress the bleeding site following needle withdrawal until hemostasis is achieved
4 Treat any underlying disease

* Esp. intracavernosal (injectable) treatments

CLINICAL ASPECTS OF SEXUAL AND REPRODUCTIVE DISORDERS

Prolactinomas: clinical presentations in females
1 Galactorrhea (in 50% *only**)
2 Hypogonadism‡ ($\downarrow$ FSH/LH)
 — Reduced libido
 — Amenorrhea due to ovulatory failure
 — Infertility: regular anovulatory menstrual cycles
3 Dysfunctional uterine bleeding
4 Visual field defect (in 5%)
 — If macroadenoma present (in 30%)
5 Osteoporosis
 — If *long-term* reduction of E_2 results

* Conversely, most cases of non-puerperal lactation do *not* have $\uparrow$ prolactin
‡ Indication for active treatment

Distinguishing features of prolactinomas in males
1 Less common; later age of presentation
2 Galactorrhea distinctly unusual
3 Hypogonadism in 90%: impotence, obesity, infertility
4 Visual symptoms common due to high frequency (80%) of macroadenomas (usually associated with $\uparrow\uparrow$ prolactin)

Diseases associated with gynecomastia
1 Paraneoplastic β-HCG production
 — Testicular germ cell tumor, choriocarcinoma
 — Adrenal tumors
2 Primary or secondary hypogonadism
 Androgen insensitivity syndromes
3 Systemic disease
 — Chronic liver disease/cirrhosis
 — Thyrotoxicosis
 — Renal failure ± hemodialysis
4 Drugs (p. 387)

Headaches associated with bilateral testicular enlargement?
1 Mumps
2 FSH-secreting pituitary adenoma

Indications for formal investigation of the hirsute patient
1 Sudden onset of hirsuties
2 Virilization
3 Cushing's syndrome
4 Serum testosterone > 6 nmol/L
5 Serum prolactin > 1500 U/L

ABNORMAL SEXUAL DEVELOPMENT

Differential diagnosis of cryptorchidism
1 Hypothalamic disease
 — e.g. Kallmann's syndrome ($\downarrow$ GnRH)
2 Pituitary disease
 — e.g. Anencephaly ($\downarrow$ LH)
3 Testicular (Leydig cell) insufficiency
 — 5-α-reductase deficiency ($\downarrow$ DHT)
 — 3-β-dehydrogenase deficiency ($\downarrow$ testosterone)
4 Testicular (Sertoli cell) insufficiency
 — e.g. Hernia uteri inguinalis ($\downarrow$ AMH)
5 Spermatic cord defects
 — e.g. Testicular feminization (androgen resistance)

Phenotypes of abnormal sexual development
1 Klinefelter's syndrome
 — Karyotype: XXY (due to chromosomal non-disjunction)
 — Eunuchoid male with small firm (hyalinized) testes
2 Turner's syndrome
 — Karyotype: XO (due to chromosomal non-disjunction)
 — Prepubertal female with streak (vestigial) ovaries

3 True hermaphroditism
— Karyotype: XX/XY (due to dizygotic fusion)
— Ambiguous genitalia with ovary + testis (or ovotestis)
4 Male pseudohermaphroditism: *androgen insensitivity syndrome* (complete or partial)
— Formerly designated 'testicular feminization'
— Due to mutations affecting androgen receptors
— Karyotype: XY (X-linked defective androgen receptor)
— ↑ LH, testosterone levels (end-organ insensitivity)
— Physical features
  • 'Normal' breasts
  • Short vagina (absent uterus/oviducts)
  • ↓↓ Axillary/genital hair
  • Clitoromegaly, 'bulging groins'
— Presents with
  • Inguinal herniae (containing testes)
  • Primary amenorrhea in adolescence/adulthood
— R_x: Castrate after puberty (prevents gonad neoplasia)
5 Male pseudohermaphroditism: *5-α-reductase deficiency*
— Karyotype: XY (autosomal recessive, but signs → males)
— Failure to activate testosterone to dihydrotestosterone
— Causes 'penis-at twelve' syndrome: masculinization occurs at puberty due to ↑↑ testosterone secretion
— Prepubertal phenotype: male with hypospadias, epispadias or vagina, impalpable prostate, cryptorchidism, micropenis
6 Female pseudohermaphroditism
— Karyotype: XX
— Seen in congenital adrenal hyperplasia: 21-hydroxylase, 11-β-hydroxylase or 3-β-dehydrogenase deficiency
— *Partial* enzyme defects may manifest only with hirsutism or menstrual irregularities

Rationâle of investigating suspected precocious puberty
1 To prevent premature closure of bony epiphyses
2 To confirm treatable etiologies
— Congenital adrenal hyperplasia
— Gonadal tumors
— Pituitary tumors
3 To avoid psychological damage in precocious infants

When to investigate suspected precocious puberty
1 Boys younger than 7 with any sign of puberty
2 Boys with any sign of early puberty in the absence of testicular enlargement
3 Girls younger than 6 with breast development or pubic hair
4 Boys younger than 9, or girls younger than 8, with signs of early puberty associated with a rapid increase in linear growth
5 Boys or girls of any age with signs of early puberty appropriate for the opposite sex

TESTING OF SEXUAL AND REPRODUCTIVE DISORDERS

Predominant estrogens in the human life cycle
1 E_1 (estrone)
— Post-menopausal
2 E_2 (estradiol)
— Child-bearing years
3 E_3 (estriol)
— Pregnancy
— Fetal life

Approach to investigation of amenorrhea
1 Measure urinary HCG to exclude pregnancy
2 ↑ FSH
— Proceed to karyotyping if 'primary' amenorrhea
— Consider diagnosis of premature menopause
3 ↓ FSH: perform
— Serum prolactin
— Thyroid function tests (esp. TSH)
— Skull X-ray + coronal CT/visual field mapping
4 ↓ FSH and ↑ LH: perform GnRH stimulation to confirm Stein–Leventhal syndrome (→ exaggerated LH response)
5 ↑ Testosterone: consider
— Testicular feminization
— 5-α-reductase deficiency*

* cf. 17-ketoreductase deficiency → ↓ testosterone

Laboratory features of anorexia nervosa
1 ↓ FSH/LH/17β-estradiol/DHEA
2 Normal serum prolactin
3 'Sick euthyroid'
 Delayed peak following TRH and GnRH stimulation
4 ↑ GH/ACTH/cortisol
5 Hyposthenuria

Hirsutism: clinical and laboratory characterization
1 Exclude racial or familial causes
2 Exclude hypothyroidism, anorexia nervosa, Cushing's, ovarian or adrenal tumors, congenital adrenal hyperplasia
3 Exclude drug-induced causes
— Phenytoin
— Minoxidil, diazoxide
— Steroids, ciclosporin; androgens, danazol
4 ↑ Plasma DHEA/urinary 17-ketosteroids
— Adrenal origin (e.g. tumor)
 ↑ ACTH-inducible rise in 17-hydroxyprogesterone
— Late-onset 21-hydroxylase deficiency
5 ↑↑ Testosterone, normal DHEA
— Ovarian origin (e.g. Sertoli–Leydig cell tumor*)
6 LH:FSH > 2.5 *plus*
 ↑ Free testosterone
— Polycystic ovary (Stein–Leventhal) syndrome; see below

* 'Arrhenoblastoma' (term no longer used)

Gonadotrophic characterization of amenorrhea
1 ↑ FSH
— Ovarian failure (1°/2°)
2 ↑ LH, normal FSH
— Polycystic ovary (Stein–Leventhal) syndrome
3 ↑ LH, normal FSH
— Pregnancy
4 ↓ FSH, ↓ LH
— Hypopituitarism
5 ↓ FSH, ↑ prolactin
— Hyperprolactinemia + prolactinoma

Differential diagnosis of hyperprolactinemia
1 Pregnancy or puerperium
2 Pituitary tumor
3 Myxedema
4 Renal failure
5 Drugs, esp. phenothiazines

Elevated prolactin levels: quantitative significance
1 Plasma prolactin > 5000 mU/L (200 ng/mL)
— Prolactinoma (diagnostic)
2 Plasma prolactin < 1500 mU/L
— Non-prolactinoma hyperprolactinemia
3 Intermediate levels
— Prolactinoma (consistent)
— 'Pseudoprolactinoma'*

* 'Non-functioning' pituitary tumor compressing pituitary stalk

Investigating infertility in the menstruating female
1 Check ovulation
— Chart basal body temperature for several months
— Measure mid-luteal phase serum progesterone
2 Serum prolactin
3 Laparoscopy in secretory phase with diagnostic curettage
— Diagnosis
• Endometriosis
• Polycystic ovaries
• Unruptured luteinized follicles
— Therapy
• Hydrotubation (tubal insufflation)

Features of polycystic ovary (Stein–Leventhal) syndrome
1 Symptoms due to abnormal metabolism of
— Androgens (and related steroid hormones)
— Insulin (resistance; hyperinsulinemia)
2 Common symptoms
— Progressive hirsutism (often since adolescence)
— Irregular periods (± infertility, amenorrhea)
— Weight gain, obesity (due to hyperinsulinemia)
3 Supportive investigations
— Abnormal glucose tolerance test
• Subclinical insulin resistance common
— Abnormal pelvic ultrasound*
• Polycystic ovaries (4–8 mm diameter) in 80%
— Abnormal lipids
• esp. ↓ HDL_2
4 Sex hormones
— ↑ Free testosterone > 5 nmol/L (→ acne, alopecia, hirsuties)
— ↑ Plasma LH (→ amenorrhea)
— LH:FSH ratio > 2.5

* NB: The sonographic finding of polycystic ovaries is non-specific (i.e. found in up to 20% of 'normal' women, as well as in other hyperandrogenic anovulatory conditions) and hence of little diagnostic value. It is also insensitive, being false-negative in 10–20% of women with polycystic ovaries

Consequences of hyperinsulinemia in polycystic ovary syndrome
1 IGF-1-dependent ovarian thecal hyperplasia, leading to increased LH, followed by anovulation, followed by increased androgen activity
2 Inhibition of hepatic synthesis of IGFBP1, leading to increased free IGF-1, leading in turn to ovarian thecal hyperplasia
3 Inhibition of hepatic synthesis of SHBG, potentiating the increase in free androgen levels

Investigation of males with abnormal sexual phenotype
1 Small (firm) testes, hypogonadal, ↑ FSH
— Karyotype (?Klinefelter's)
2 Small testes, virilized
— 17-OH-progesterone (?congenital adrenal hyperplasia)
3 Normal testicular size, ↑ FSH
— Irreversible azoospermia (e.g. tubular hyalinization)
4 Normal testicular size, azoospermia, normal FSH
— Varicocele
— Epididymal/vas obstruction (e.g. Young's syndrome)
5 Normal testicular size, azoospermia, ↓ FSH
— Exclude pituitary tumor
6 Absent pubic hair*
— Investigate for gonadal failure

* cf. females: absent pubic hair implies *adrenal* failure

Criteria for normal semen analysis
1 Ejaculate volume:	2–5 mL	
2 pH:	7.2–7.8	
3 Number:	$30–200 \times 10^6$/mL*	
4 Motility:	90% active forward progression after 30 min	
	60% active forward progression after 3 h	
5 Morphology:	50% normal oval shapes	
6 White cell count:	< 1 million/mL	

NB: Evaluate three times over a 6–12 week period before concluding azoospermia
* Number may drop during (hot) summer; 'contraceptive' azoospermia may also be inducible by weekly testosterone injections

TREATING SEXUAL AND REPRODUCTIVE DISORDERS

INFERTILITY TREATMENT

Pathogeneses of infertility
1 Oligospermia	—	30%
2 Female hormonal dysfunction	—	30%
3 Tubal disease	—	20%
4 Uterine disease	—	10%

5 Cervical disease   —   3%
6 Unidentifiable causes   —   5%

Prime indications for assisted reproduction*
1 Tubal disease
   — Main indication for IVF
2 Endometriosis
3 Male subfertility
   — Main indication for GIFT

* Certain diagnoses must be *excluded* (e.g. hyperprolactinemia)

'Test-tube' pregnancies: what's the success rate?*
1 Extracorporeal fertilization
   — In vitro fertilization (IVF)‡
     • Embryos cultured to 4–8 cell stage, then
       replaced
     • 15% deliveries per operation
2 Intrafallopian transfer
   — Gamete intrafallopian transfer (GIFT)
     • 20% deliveries per operation
   — Zygote intrafallopian transfer (ZIFT)
     • 24% deliveries per operation

* NB: The most critical factor determining success is the *number*
of eggs (or embryos) transferred, not the therapeutic technique.
Keep in mind that the natural fecundity rate is only 25%
‡ 30% embryos harbor lethal chromosomal anomalies

Factors reducing probability of successful assisted pregnancy
1 Asymmetrical, poorly defined blastomeres
2 Advanced age of egg donor
3 Parental smoking (either partner)

Infertility treatment in polycystic ovary syndrome
1 Fertility drugs, e.g.
   — Clomifene
   — Pulsatile (stimulatory) GnRH therapy
2 Treatment of insulin resistance (hyperinsulinemia
   → ↑ ovarian androgens)
   — Metformin, glitazones
3 Ovarian cyst electrocautery
   — Performed at laparoscopy

Complications of fertility drug therapy
1 Multiple pregnancy
2 Increased miscarriage rate
3 Ovarian hyperstimulation syndrome
   — Massive ovarian enlargement (stromal edema)
   — Third-space fluid accumulation*
   — Severity parallels ↑ plasma estradiol
   — Renin levels also elevated
   — Increased risk in polycystic ovary syndrome

* Ascites, pleural and pericardial effusions – occasionally fatal

Therapeutic options in endometriosis
1 Danazol (synthetic androgen)*
2 Progestogens (e.g. norethisterone,
   medroxyprogesterone)
3 Gestrinone (an antiprogestogen and weak androgen)
4 GnRH agonists‡
5 Surgical ablation

* Duration of treatment limited by hyperlipidemia
‡ Duration of treatment limited by bone demineralization

ORAL CONTRACEPTIVES

Beneficial effects of combined oral contraceptives
1 Contraception (incl. fewer ectopic pregnancies;
   cf. IUDs)
2 Less dysmenorrhea or menorrhagia; less
   endometriosis
3 Less benign breast disease
4 Fewer follicular and luteal ovarian cysts
5 Lower risk of endometrial and ovarian cancer

Patient evaluation prior to (estrogenic) oral contraception
1 Past history of neoplasia
   — Breast cancer
   — Endometrial cancer
   — Hydatidiform mole
   — Uterine leiomyomata (fibroids)
   — Hepatic tumors
   — Prolactinoma
2 History of disorder worsening during pregnancy
   — Pruritus
   — Jaundice
   — Herpes gestationis (*not* a viral infection)
   — Otosclerosis
3 History of vascular disorder
   — Thromboembolism
   — Cardio- or cerebrovascular condition
   — Hypertension (incl. pulmonary)
   — Cigarette smoking
   — Migraine (esp. 'classical', focal, basilar)
4 Examination
   — Weight, urinalysis, blood pressure
   — Breasts, liver, fundi
   — Vaginal examination
5 Baseline investigations
   — Cervical smear
   — Urine HCG
   — Serum lipids (fasting)
   — Liver function tests
   — ECG if indicated

Drug interactions with oral contraceptives (OCs)
1 Drugs reducing OC efficacy due to hepatic enzyme
   induction
   — Rifampicin (contraindicated in OC users);
     griseofulvin
   — Phenytoin, carbamazepine, barbiturates
2 Drugs antagonizing OCs due to ↓ enterohepatic
   recirculation
   — Tetracycline, ampicillin, purgatives
3 Hepatic enzyme inhibition by OCs → potentiation of
   — Imipramine
   — Barbiturates
   — Chlordiazepoxide; pethidine
4 Reduction of epileptic threshold by OCs (i.e. seizure
   activity may worsen despite increased
   anticonvulsant levels)

Pharmacologic strategies for opposing estrogen
1 Antiestrogens (e.g. tamoxifen)
   — Compete for binding of estrogen receptors
   — May have some (weak) estrogenic effects

2 Progestogens (e.g. norethisterone, megestrol)
— Enhance hypothalamic negative feedback on estrogen
3 Androgens (esp. danazol)
— Suppress HPA axis by reducing GnRH pulses
4 Aromatase inhibitors (e.g. aminoglutethimide)
— Prevent peripheral production of active estrogen metabolites
5 GnRH agonists
— Downregulate LH/FSH receptors if used continuously, thus suppressing estrogen release from ovary
— May cause initial 'flare' of estrogen release

GONADOTROPIN-RELEASING HORMONE THERAPIES

Classification and mechanisms of GnRH therapies
1 GnRH agonists
— e.g. LHRH agonists
• Buserelin, goserelin
• Leuprorelin
— Stimulate gonadotropin (FSH/LH) secretion
— *Pulsatile* therapy → ↑ gonadal hormone secretion (i.e. simulates physiologic GnRH action)
— *Continuous* therapy* → ↓ gonadal hormone secretion (via downregulation of GnRH receptors)
2 GnRH antagonists (investigational)
— Competitively inhibits GnRH by binding receptors
— Do *not* cause LH/FSH secretion
— Advantages
• Immediate effect (cf. agonist suppression)
• No 'flare' of neoplastic disease activity

* e.g. given by depot intramuscular injection

Indications for pulsatile (stimulatory) GnRH therapy
1 Anovulatory infertility (any cause)*
— e.g. Prior to egg harvest for assisted reproduction
2 Hypogonadotropic hypogonadism (e.g. Kallmann's)
— e.g. For initiation of puberty

* Alternatives to GnRH analogs include clomifene, HMG (human menopausal gonadotropin) and HCG

Indications for continuous (suppressive) GnRH therapy
1 Females
— Endometriosis
— Polycystic ovary syndrome
— Uterine fibroids, dysfunctional uterine bleeding
— Premenopausal breast cancer (adjuvant, metastatic)
2 Male
— Metastatic prostate cancer
3 Both sexes
— Contraception (potentially)
— Precocious puberty (if hypergonadotropic)

Problems with suppressive GnRH therapy
1 Expense
2 Hot flushes, loss of libido (both sexes)
3 Bone demineralization
— Density falls 2–5% every 6 months
— May be reversible on periodic cessation

SEX HORMONE REPLACEMENT THERAPY

Physiologic effects of estrogen
1 Menstruation
2 Vaginal cornification
3 Cervical mucus formation
4 Breast development
5 Axillary hair

Absolute indications for estrogen replacement
1 Gonadal dysgenesis
2 Premature menopause*
3 Post-menopausal females at *high* risk for coronary events, but *no* risk factors for thrombosis, or for breast or endometrial cancer

* e.g. premature ovarian failure, Wertheim's hysterectomy

Benefits of post-menopausal low-dose estrogen replacement
1 Improvement of vasomotor instability (hot flushes)
2 Prevention/reversal of atrophic vaginitis
3 Reduced morbidity and mortality from osteoporotic fractures
4 Reduced morbidity from coronary artery disease*
— 15% ↓ LDL
— 15% ↑ HDL_2
— ↓ Lp(a)
5 Reduced incidence of Alzheimer's dementia
6 Possible reduction in colonic adenomatous polyps and cancers

* But HRT does *not* appear effective in secondary prevention of myocardial infarction, and may even increase risks in the first year post-infarct due to prothrombotic effects; nor does it appear to reduce stroke

Neoplastic hazards of hormone replacement
1 Endometrial cancer (due to unopposed E_2)*
— Absolute risk 1% per year; relative risk about six-fold
— Risk reduced by concomitant progestogen therapy‡
2 Hepatic adenoma (due to E_2)
— Prone to intraperitoneal hemorrhage
3 Breast cancer
— Long-term estrogens slightly increase risk
— Progestogens may further increase risk

* Risk also increased with long-term adjuvant tamoxifen therapy
‡ Similar protective effect of combined therapy claimed for ovarian cancer

Potentially beneficial effects of DHEA* supplementation
1 Increased free serum IGF-1 levels‡
2 Decreased plasminogen activator inhibitor-1 (PAI-1)
3 Increased bone density
4 Protective against neurotoxins and depression

* The androgenic adrenal steroid dehydroepiandrosterone
‡ Insulin-like growth factor-1, the anabolic mediator of growth hormone action

Hazards of exogenous androgen therapy
1 Acne, weight gain (increased muscle)
2 Testicular atrophy, azoospermia
3 Erythrocytosis, thrombocytosis
4 Precipitation or worsening of sleep apnea
5 Hepatotoxicity: peliosis hepatis (hemorrhagic liver cysts), cholestasis, hepatic adenomas or carcinomas*
6 Dyslipidemia: $\uparrow$ LDL, $\downarrow$ HDL$_2$
7 Increased libido and aggression
8 Psychological dependence

* Occurs with alkylated androgens; rare with testosterone

MIFEPRISTONE (RU 486; 'MORNING AFTER' PILL)

Varieties of emergency contraception
1 Post-coital high-dose hormone administration (80% efficacy)
2 Post-coital insertion of an intrauterine device (IUD; 99% effective)

Abortifacient drugs
1 Antiprogestins
   — Oral mifepristone
2 Prostaglandin E$_1$ agonists:
   — Oral or vaginal misoprostol ($\pm$ oral tamoxifen)
   — Vaginal gemeprost
3 Trophoblast toxins
   — Oral or IM methotrexate*

* Followed a few days later by vaginal misoprostol

Effects of mifepristone*
1 Blocks progesterone (and glucocorticoid) receptors
2 Induces endometrial sloughing
3 Softens the cervix
4 Disinhibits endometrial contraction
5 Teratogenicity uncertain

* A semisynthetic steroid similar to norethisterone; weakly antiandrogenic

Potential indications for mifepristone
1 Termination of early ($\leq$ 9 weeks) pregnancy*
   — i.e. 'Abortion pill'
   — May obviate suction termination and anesthesia
   — Single dose (600 mg) effective in ~ 75%; addition of 1 mg gemeprost pessary increases efficacy to 95%‡
2 Facilitation of protracted labor
   — i.e. May help avoid Cesarean
3 Dilatation and softening of cervix to expedite
   — Endometrial biopsy, D&C
   — Difficult IUD insertion
4 Unproven indications
   — Cushing's disease, adrenal tumors
   — Glaucoma
   — Meningioma
   — Breast cancer
   — Endometriosis

* Sometimes combined for this purpose with the antiulcerogenic prostaglandin misoprostol; do not confuse the two when treating ulcers
‡ NB: Appropriate clinic observation, instruction and follow-up is essential; 1% require emergency transfusion or evacuation, while ~ 30% need opiates

Contraindications to mifepristone as abortifacient
1 Absolute contraindications
   — Pregnancy unproven
   — Adrenal insufficiency (incl. steroid use)
   — Bleeding diathesis
   — Unwillingness to proceed to suction termination if medical abortion unsuccessful or incomplete
2 Relative contraindications
   — Heavy smoking > 35 years, cardiovascular disease
   — Renal failure; asthma
   — Alcohol abuse, liver failure
   — Current (last week) aspirin/NSAID use
3 Avoid due to lack of efficacy
   — Ectopic pregnancy

Alternative methods of post-coital contraception*
1 High-dose ethinylestradiol (or other estrogen)
   — Effective, but nauseating
2 Short-course estrogen/progestogen oral contraceptive
   — Two 'full-dose' tablets (ethinylestradiol 100 μg + levonorgestrel 500 μg) repeated 12 h later
   — 2% still become pregnant
3 Danazol
   — Less effective than estrogens
4 Prompt insertion of copper IUD
   — May be recommended only to mothers

NB: None of the above treatments are quite as effective emergency contraceptives as mifepristone
* Within 72 h; not referred to as 'abortion' since implantation has not occurred

MALE SEXUAL DYSFUNCTION

Precoitus treatment of premature ejaculation
1 Clomipramine 100 mg
2 Sertraline (an SSRI) 50 mg
3 Clonidine 100 μg

Iatrogenic causes of retrograde ejaculation
1 Transurethral prostatectomy
2 α-blockers

Iatrogenic causes of anorgasmia
1 Naloxone
2 SSRIs

Drugs causing impotence
1 Hormones
   — Estrogens
   — Antiandrogens (e.g. cyproterone, finasteride)
2 Cardioactive drugs
   — β-blockers, calcium blockers, ACE inhibitors
   — Diuretics, esp. spironolactone, thiazides

— Fibrate hypolipidemics, esp. clofibrate, gemfibrozil
— Digoxin
3 Psychoactive drugs
— Phenothiazines (exception: olanzapine), haloperidol, risperidone
— Antidepressants: SSRIs, MAOIs, tricyclics
— Anticonvulsants: carbamazepine, phenytoin
— Anxiolytics: benzodiazepines
— Antiparkinsonians: L-DOPA
— Mood stabilizers: lithium
4 H_2-receptor antagonists
— esp. Cimetidine > ranitidine, famotidine
5 Antirheumatics
— Indometacin, allopurinol
6 Metabolic inhibitors
— Disulfiram
7 Anticancer drugs
— Cytotoxic chemotherapy
— Opiates
8 Recreational drugs
— Nicotine (smoking)
— Alcohol
— Marijuana, heroin

Organic causes of impotence to exclude pretreatment
1 Diabetes or peripheral vascular disease
2 Liver disease (esp. alcoholic) or renal failure
3 Neurologic disease (e.g. stroke, multiple sclerosis)
4 Hypogonadism
5 Sickle cell disease

Treatment options in impotence
1 Exclusion of iatrogenic or secondary causes
2 Psychosexual (counselling and/or behavioral) therapies
3 Sildenafil (Viagra, a phosphodiesterase inhibitor)
4 Transurethral or intracavernosal alprostadil*
5 Testosterone skin patches or injections (if hypogonadal)
6 Prolactin (if low libido but not hypogonadal)
7 Vacuum devices (if alprostadil injections fail)
8 Penile prostheses (e.g. for Peyronie's): silicone or inflatable

* Prostaglandin E_1 analog, associated with risk of priapism. Other injectables include papaverine, phentolamine and VIP

Contraindications to sildenafil (Viagra) treatment
1 Concomitant ingestion of organic nitrates (e.g. glyceryl trinitrate spray, oral isosorbide dinitrate) incl. 'recreational' amyl nitrate*
2 Unstable angina, cardiac failure, or recent history of myocardial infarction or stroke‡
3 Hepatic impairment
4 Retinal degeneration
5 Peyronie's disease (fibrotic penile deformity)
6 Priapism predisposition (e.g. sickle cell disease)
7 CYP 3A4 inhibitors¶
— Ritonavir therapy (*also* inhibits CYP 2C9)
— Erythromycin, ketoconazole, other HIV protease inhibitors

* Combination of these medications can trigger catastrophic hypotension; *any* cause of pre-existing hypotension is also a contraindication

‡ Treadmill testing may be indicated prior to prescription, as may first-dose post-ingestion monitoring of blood pressure
¶ Sildenafil is metabolized by the cytochrome P_{450} enzymes CYP 3A4 and 2C9. If using with (say) erythromycin, begin with low-dose (25 mg) sildenafil

THERAPY OF FEMALE SEX AND GYNECOLOGIC DISORDERS

Treatment options in idiopathic hirsutism
1 Mild hirsutism
— Reassurance
2 Moderate hirsutism, pregnancy desired
— Shaving, waxing, depilatory creams, electrolysis
3 Moderate hirsutism, pregnancy not desired
— Combined oral contraceptive (causes ovarian suppression)
• Reduces free testosterone by increasing SHBG and reducing LH
— GnRH analogs (cause ovarian suppression)
• Best for polycystic ovary syndrome and ovarian hyperandrogenism
4 Severe hirsutism, pregnancy desired
— Dexamethasone 0.25 mg nocte*
• Reduces ACTH → ↓ adrenal androgens
5 Severe hirsutism, pregnancy not desired
— Spironolactone; cyproterone acetate
• Block interaction of DHT with androgen receptor
— Finasteride
• Blocks 5-α-reductase
6 Polycystic ovary syndrome
— Octreotide

* But *not* indicated *unless* specific defect in adrenal biosynthesis identified

Treatment options in premenstrual syndrome
1 $GABA_A$ receptor agonists (e.g. alprazolam)
2 SSRIs: fluoxetine, sertraline

Treatment options in menorrhagia
1 NSAIDs (e.g. mefenamic acid)
2 Antifibrinolytic therapy (tranexamic acid)
3 Intrauterine progestogens (levonorgestrel)
4 Short-term treatments
— Danazol, gestrinone (androgenic side-effects)
— GnRH analogs (osteoporotic side-effects)
5 Iron supplements (adjunctive only)
6 Surgery: D&C, hysterectomy

UNDERSTANDING SEXUAL & REPRODUCTIVE DISORDERS

PREGNANCY

Physiologic changes during pregnancy
1 Cardiovascular changes*
— Increased cardiac output (↑ heart rate/stroke volume)
• Ventricular hypertrophy
— Increased blood volume (→ hemodilution, ↓ Hb)
• S_3, systolic ejection murmur

— Decreased peripheral resistance
  • ↑ Pulse pressure
— Aortic unfolding
  • Inverted T wave in $V_{2/3}$
2 Respiratory changes
— Increased tidal volume (progesterone effect)
— Decreased residual volume (diaphragm elevation)
3 Renal changes
— Increased renal blood flow and GFR
— Increased tubular reabsorption
— Decreased plasma urea/creatinine
4 Genitourinary changes
— Uterine enlargement
  • Myometrial cell hypertrophy (E_2 effect)
  • Increased blood supply (1–1.5 L/min)
— Collecting tract dilatation (progesterone effect)
  • Bladder relaxation
  • Ureteric reflux, stasis, infection
— Frequency of micturition
  • Increased urine production (early)
  • Uterine compression of bladder (late)
5 Endocrine changes
— Adrenocortical hyperfunction
  • Increased ACTH *and* cortisol
  • Increased renin (esp. 1st trimester)
— Hypothalamic hyperfunction
  • Increased oxytocin release (posterior pituitary)
— Anterior pituitary changes
  • Increased prolactin, placental lactogen (HPL)
  • Reduced FSH/LH (due to ↑ E_2, progesterone)
  • Reduced growth hormone (due to ↑ HPL)

* Reflect increased oxygenation requirement

Diseases often improved by pregnancy
1 Rheumatoid arthritis*
2 Graves' disease
3 Sarcoidosis
4 Migraine
5 Chronic renal failure

* But prone to 'flare' in puerperium

Diseases often worse in pregnancy
1 Diabetes mellitus
— Glucose intolerance
— Microvascular disease
2 Diabetes insipidus
— Pituitary
— Nephrogenic
3 Nerve entrapment syndromes
— Carpal tunnel*
— Meralgia paresthetica
4 Intracranial lesions (may enlarge)
— Pituitary macroadenoma, esp. prolactinoma
— Suprasellar meningioma
— Arteriovenous malformation
5 Infections
— Viruses: varicella, measles, polio, influenza, HCV
— Malaria (increased post-partum susceptibility)
6 Miscellaneous
— SLE, esp. with antiphospholipid syndrome or renal disease
— Epilepsy

— Sickle-cell anemia
— Cardiovascular disorders (p. 65)

* Note that this may also *respond* to hormone replacement therapy in post-menopausal women

Effects of pregnancy on multiple sclerosis
1 Improves during 3rd trimester
2 Worsens during first 3 months post-partum

Factors implicated in recurrent miscarriages
1 Poor oocyte quality (e.g. age-related)
— Tends to be more important than implantation failure
2 LH hypersecretion (mid to late cycle)
— incl. Polycystic ovary syndrome
— Impairs fertilization
3 Antiphospholipid antibodies
4 Low prostacyclin:thromboxane ratio
5 Chromosomal abnormalities

IATROGENIC SEXUAL AND REPRODUCTIVE DYSFUNCTION

Major drug classes causing male sexual dysfunction*
1 Alcohol/narcotic addiction
2 Estrogens, corticosteroids
3 Antiandrogens: flutamide, cyproterone acetate, ketoconazole
4 Antiandrogenic side-effects: spironolactone, cimetidine, digitalis
5 Antihypertensives: methyldopa, propranolol
6 Phenothiazines, tricyclics

* Loss of libido; impotence; ejaculatory impairment; hypogonadism; infertility

Clinical relevance of anabolic steroids
1 Include
— Nandrolone decanoate, stanozolol
2 Established use
— Aplastic anemia (→ erythropoiesis)
3 Commonest use
— Bodybuilding amongst athletes (illicit)
4 Hazards
— Testosterone suppression (testis atrophy, impotence)
— Liver tumors (hepatoma, angiosarcoma)

Drug-induced gynecomastia and/or galactorrhea
1 Gynecomastia alone (± impotence); normal prolactin
— Alcohol (± chronic liver disease)
— Estrogens; androgens, progestogens (→ estrogens)
— Antiandrogens
  • Cyproterone acetate, flutamide
  • Spironolactone
  • Cimetidine
— Weak estrogens
  • Digitoxin
  • Ketoconazole

2 Gynecomastia and/or galactorrhea ($\uparrow$ prolactin)
   — Methyldopa, reserpine
   — Heroin, morphine, marijuana
   — Tricyclics, haloperidol, phenothiazines

Drug-induced azoospermia: causes

1 Cytotoxics (esp. MOPP, alkylators)
2 Sex steroids (incl. high-dose androgens; $\rightarrow \downarrow$ FSH)
3 'Anti-androgens'
   — Danazol etc. ($\rightarrow \downarrow$ LH $\rightarrow \downarrow$ testosterone)
   — Cimetidine
   — Spironolactone
4 Sulfasalazine
5 Colchicine, phenytoin, nitrofurantoin; major tranquillizers
6 Alcohol, marijuana

Sexual morbidity of cancer treatment

1 Hysterectomy
   — Infertility
2 Radical prostatectomy
   — Impotence; infertility
3 Mastectomy, intestinal stoma
   — Disturbed sexual self-image
   — Impaired libido
4 Pelvic interstitial radiation
   — Vaginal fibrosis, dyspareunia
5 Abdominoperineal resection, cystectomy
   — Impotence (exclude depression)
6 Para-aortic lymphadenectomy
   — Retrograde ejaculation
7 Oophorectomy, menopausal induction
   — Loss of libido, lubrication difficulties
8 Drugs inhibiting libido or sexual responsiveness
   — Hormonal agents
   — Cytotoxic drugs
   — Narcotics, hypnotics, antidepressants

Infertility following cancer chemotherapy

1 Chemotherapy for testicular germ cell tumors
   — Patients may be oligospermic pretreatment
   — Virtually *all* become infertile during chemotherapy*
   — 80% show partial recovery within 18 months
2 Leukemias and lymphomas
   — High-dose *intermittent* treatment causes less sterility
   — Long-term maintenance therapy (incl. oral alkylating agents) is associated with high incidence of sterility

* cf. Gestational trophoblastic tumors: patients *rarely* sterilized by therapy

REVIEWING THE LITERATURE: SEXUAL AND REPRODUCTIVE MEDICINE

17.1 Lee MM et al (1997) Measurements of serum Mullerian inhibiting substance in the evaluation of children with nonpalpable gonads. N Engl J Med 336: 1480–1486

Study of 65 virilized children with non-palpable gonads, showing a clearcut predictive significance of serum MIS elevation for the presence of testicular tissue. MIS was more sensitive, but just as specific, as testosterone for the prediction of testicular tissue.

17.2 Schobel HP et al (1996) Pre-eclampsia – a state of sympathetic overactivity. N Engl J Med 335: 1480–1485

Study of sympathetic nerve activity in nine pre-eclampsia patients compared with 21 control women, showing that sympathetic vasoconstrictor activity contributes significantly to the pathogenesis.

17.3 Thomson AJ et al (1998) Randomised trial of nitric oxide donor versus prostaglandin for cervical ripening before first-trimester termination of pregnancy. Lancet 352: 1093–1096

Study of 66 primigravidae showing that isosorbide mononitrate pretreatment of first-trimester terminations was associated with fewer side-effects than prostaglandins alone.

17.4 Pastuszak AL et al (1998) Use of misoprostol during pregnancy and Mobius syndrome in infants. N Engl J Med 338: 1881–1885

The prostaglandin E_1 analog misoprostol was found to be associated with an increased incidence of congenital facial paralysis (Moebius syndrome) following unsuccessful termination attempts, in this case-control analysis of 96 Moebius infants.

17.5 Stolk EA et al (2000) Cost utility analysis of sildenafil compared with papaverine-phentolamine injections. Br Med J 320: 1165–1168

Dutch study of 169 individuals of both sexes, suggesting that sildenafil is cost-effective (approx. US $6000/QALY).

17.6 Wyatt KM et al (1999) Efficacy of vitamin B6 in the treatment of premenstrual syndrome. Br Med J 318: 1375–1381

Systematic review of nine studies enrolling 940 patients, concluding that pyridoxine supplements of up to 100 mg/day appear useful in reducing symptoms of premenstrual depression and other premenstrual symptoms.

17.7 Schellenberg R et al (2001) Treatment for the premenstrual syndrome with agnus castus fruit extract: prospective, randomized, placebo-controlled study. Br Med J 322: 134–137

Improvement of PMS symptoms was documented in 52% of 170 patients given the fruit extract, compared with 24% of controls.

17.8 Hernandez-Diaz S et al (2000) Folic acid antagonists during pregnancy and the risk of birth defects. N Engl J Med 343: 1608–1614

Longitudinal case-control study of 3870 patients, showing that multiple folate antagonists (e.g. trimethoprim, triamterene, phenytoin, carbamazepine, phenobarbital) caused birth defects including not only neural tube abnormalities but also cardiovascular, oral cleft and urinary tract anomalies.

17.9 Jick H et al (2000) Risk of venous thromboembolism among users of third generation oral contraceptives: cohort and case-control studies. Br Med J 321: 1190–1195

Kemmeren JM et al (2001) Third generation oral contraceptives and risk of venous thrombosis: meta-analysis. Br Med J 323: 131–134

Two analyses concluding that third-generation oral contraceptives pose a higher risk of thrombosis than do earlier models.

17.10 Bhattacharya S et al (2001) Conventional in-vitro fertilisation versus intracytoplasmic sperm injection for the treatment of non-male-factor infertility. Lancet 357: 2075–2079

Study of 415 couples, showing no advantage of ICSI over conventional IVF.

CHAPTER 18

Skin disease

Physical examination protocol 18.1   You are asked to examine a patient who has recently developed a rash

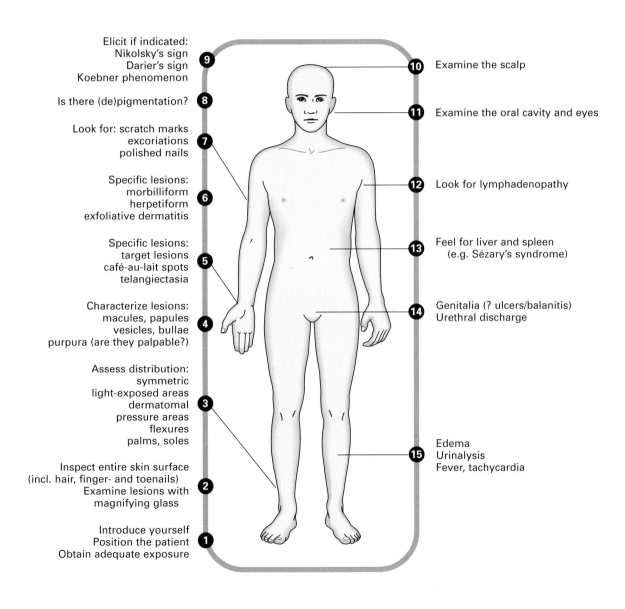

Elicit if indicated:
Nikolsky's sign
Darier's sign
Koebner phenomenon

9

Is there (de)pigmentation?

8

Look for: scratch marks
excoriations
polished nails

7

Specific lesions:
morbilliform
herpetiform
exfoliative dermatitis

6

Specific lesions:
target lesions
café-au-lait spots
telangiectasia

5

Characterize lesions:
macules, papules
vesicles, bullae
purpura (are they palpable?)

4

Assess distribution:
symmetric
light-exposed areas
dermatomal
pressure areas
flexures
palms, soles

3

Inspect entire skin surface
(incl. hair, finger- and toenails)
Examine lesions with
magnifying glass

2

Introduce yourself
Position the patient
Obtain adequate exposure

1

10   Examine the scalp

11   Examine the oral cavity and eyes

12   Look for lymphadenopathy

13   Feel for liver and spleen
(e.g. Sézary's syndrome)

14   Genitalia (? ulcers/balanitis)
Urethral discharge

15   Edema
Urinalysis
Fever, tachycardia

Diagnostic pathway 18.1   This patient has a 'spot diagnosis' – what is it?

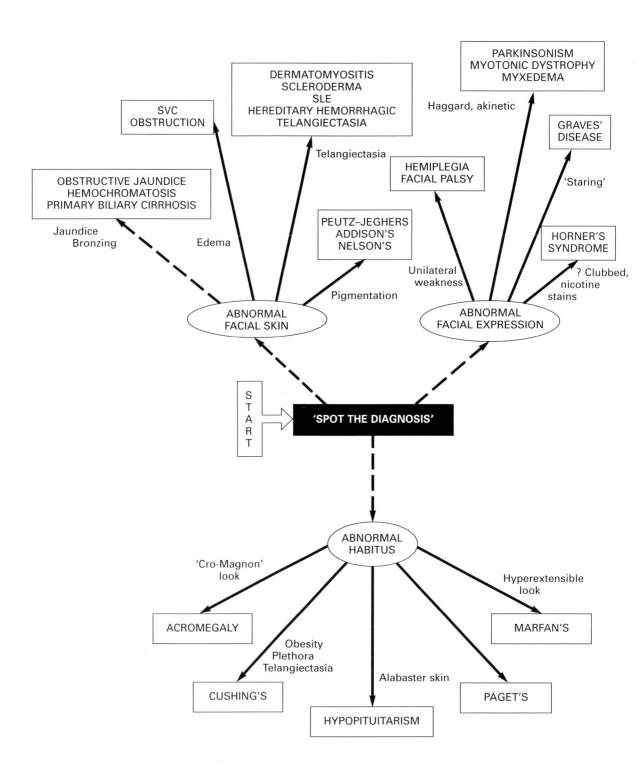

COMMON AND CLASSIC SKIN DISORDERS

Common dermatologic problems in clinical practice
1 Psoriasis
2 Eczema
3 Acne

Classic dermatologic problems in clinical exams
1 Purpura
2 Psoriasis with arthropathy
3 Bullous dermatoses

DERMATOLOGIC EMERGENCIES

Management of extensive full-thickness burns
1 Fluid resuscitation with crystalloids (sodium-salt solutions)
2 Treatment of inhalation injury (e.g. with 100% oxygen)
3 Topical 1% silver sulfadiazine (antimicrobial prophylaxis)
4 Skin cleaning with chlorhexidine; tetanus prophylaxis
5 Sterile gauze dressing (except face and neck)
6 Wound excision and skin grafting as early as possible
7 Recombinant human growth hormone*
8 Grafting of ex vivo-cultured autologous keratinocytes

* Accelerates graft site re-epithelialization, and hence regrafting

CLINICAL ASSESSMENT OF SKIN DISEASE

Eponymous signs of skin disease
1 Nikolsky's sign →
 • Pemphigus (esp. foliaceous)
 • Porphyria (PCT, EP, VP)
 • Staph scalded skin syndrome
 — Denotes palpable shear-inducible separation of stratum corneum from underlying epidermis → blister formation
2 Darier's sign →
 • Urticaria pigmentosa
 — Denotes whealing of macule on rubbing
3 Koebner phenomenon →
 • Psoriasis
 • Still's disease
 • Lichen planus
 • Viral warts
 — Denotes skin lesions on areas of local trauma (e.g. scratches) due to papillary layer disruption

Skin rashes: diagnostic checklist for examinations
1 Purpuric
 — Vasculitis (is it palpable?)
 — Hematological (dependent distribution?)
2 Blistering
 — Vesicobullous
 • Pemphigus, bullous pemphigoid

 • Dermatitis herpetiformis (vesicular)
 • Porphyria cutanea tarda
 — Pustular
3 Exfoliative (scaly) or plaque-like
 — Psoriasis
 — Lymphoma (esp. T cell)
4 Suggesting systemic disease, e.g.
 — Herpes zoster
 — Eruptive xanthomata
 — Pretibial myxedema
 — Erythema nodosum
 — Acanthosis nigricans
5 Secondary syphilis (never hurts to mention)
6 Drug eruption (always mention)

Clinical patterns in skin disease
1 Asymmetric
 — Fungal
 — Contact dermatitis
 — Zoster (dermatomal)
2 Widespread symmetrical maculopapular
 — Drug eruption
 — Exanthem
3 Palms and soles
 — Erythema multiforme, Stevens–Johnson
 — Reiter's; pustular psoriasis
 — Secondary syphilis
 — Toxic shock; atopic eczema; 'pink disease'
4 Flexures
 — Psoriasis
 — Seborrheic dermatitis
 — Fungal, eczema, intertrigo
5 Limbs
 — Flexor aspects
 • Eczema
 • Lichen planus
 • Bullous pemphigoid
 — Extensor aspects
 • Psoriasis
 • Erythema multiforme
 • Dermatitis herpetiformis
6 Pruritic
 — Lichen planus
 — Dermatitis herpetiformis
 — Drug eruptions
 — Eczema, contact dermatitis, scabies

Symptoms and signs of melanoma
1 Common
 — Primary skin lesion: suspicious if A, B, C, D
 • *A*symmetric shape
 • *B*order irregularity
 • *C*olor variegated (incl. black)
 • *D*iameter > 6 mm
 — Spread to regional lymph nodes
 — Cerebral metastases, meningeal carcinomatosis
 — Pulmonary metastases
 — Skin metastases (may be indolent)
2 Classical
 — Hepatomegaly and unilateral scleral icterus (i.e. liver metastases from retinal primary; glass eye)

SKIN LESIONS OF GENERAL MEDICAL SIGNIFICANCE

Medical conditions associated with pruritus
1 Obstructive jaundice (e.g. PBC)
2 Chronic renal failure
3 Polycythemia rubra vera ('aquagenic')*
4 Hodgkin's disease; also CLL, lung cancer
5 Thyrotoxicosis; hypothyroidism
6 Estrogens: pregnancy, oral contraceptives
7 Parasitic infestations, esp. trichinosis
8 Drugs, esp. narcotic abuse

* NB: Exclude iron deficiency

Erythema nodosum: associated underlying conditions
1 **S**arcoidosis
2 **S**ulfonamides (and other drugs)
3 **S**treptococci (and TB, leprosy, toxoplasmosis)
4 Inflammatory bowel disease

Miscellaneous erythemas: diagnostic significance
1 Erythema induratum
   — Tuberculosis
2 Erythema ab igne
   — Myxedema, neuropathy
3 Erythema marginatum
   — Truncal rash in rheumatic fever
4 Erythema gyratum repens
   — Internal malignancy
5 Necrolytic migratory erythema
   — Glucagonoma

FACIAL RASHES

The central facial rash: diagnostic possibilities
1 SLE
2 Acne rosacea
3 Lupus pernio
4 Dermatomyositis
5 Porphyria cutanea tarda
6 Secondary syphilis

Differential diagnosis of facial telangiectases
1 Scleroderma
2 Hereditary hemorrhagic telangiectasia
3 Chronic liver disease (spider nevi)
4 Carcinoid syndrome
5 Ataxia telangiectasia (involve conjunctiva also)

Photosensitive skin rashes: predispositions
1 SLE
2 Porphyrias
   — Cutanea tarda
   — Erythropoietic
3 DNA repair deficiencies
   — Bloom's syndrome
   — Xeroderma pigmentosum, Cockayne's syndrome
4 Pre-existing dermatosis
   — Rosacea; atopic dermatitis

   — Pellagra, Hartnup disease
   — Dermatomyositis, lupus
5 Drugs
   — Chlortetracycline
   — Chlorpropamide
   — Chlorpromazine

Differential diagnosis of sun-induced red weals
1 Polymorphic light eruption
2 Systemic lupus erythematosus
3 Erythropoietic protoporphyria
4 Solar urticaria

DISORDERS OF PIGMENTATION

Likely causes of diffuse hyperpigmentation in short cases
1 ACTH
   — Addison's disease
   — ACTH-secreting tumor
   — Nelson's syndrome
2 Chronic renal failure
3 Hemochromatosis
4 Primary biliary cirrhosis
5 Porphyria cutanea tarda
6 Drug-induced (e.g. busulfan)

Differential diagnosis of discrete hypopigmented areas
1 Vitiligo
2 Tinea versicolor
3 Tuberculoid leprosy
4 'Ash-leaf macules' of tuberous sclerosis
5 Morphea (localized patches of scleroderma)

SKIN APPENDAGES

Diagnostic features of the fingernails in systemic disease
1 Clubbing, nicotine stains
   — Lung cancer
2 Pitting
   — Psoriasis
3 Subungual splinters
   — Infective endocarditis
4 Telangiectasia, nailfold infarcts
   — Collagen diseases
5 'Half-and-half' (Lindsay's) nails
   — Renal failure
6 Leukonychia
   — Hypoalbuminemia (esp. liver disease)
7 Koilonychia (spoon nails)
   — Chronic iron deficiency
8 Onycholysis
   — Thyrotoxicosis
9 Yellow nails
   — Lymphatic hypoplasia (+ chylous effusions)
10 Blue lunules
   — Wilson's disease

11 Periungual fibromata
— Tuberous sclerosis
12 Candida
— Hypoparathyroidism

Etiological significance of splinter hemorrhages
1 Trauma
2 Infective endocarditis
3 Trichinosis (transverse splinters)

INVESTIGATING SKIN DISEASE

Immunological aids to clinical dermatology
1 Pemphigus vulgaris
— Serum antibodies to intercellular cement (70%)
— Direct fluorescence
• Epidermal staining with IgG, C_3
2 Pemphigoid (bullous or cicatricial), herpes gestationis
— Serum antibodies to basement membrane (60%)
— Direct fluorescence
• Linear IgG and/or C_3 at dermoepidermal junction (i.e. subepidermal)
3 Dermatitis herpetiformis
— ± Serum reticulin antibodies (25%)
— Direct fluorescence
• IgA in dermal papillae*
4 SLE
— Direct fluorescence
• Linear IgM, IgG or C_3 at dermoepidermal junction* (= 'lupus band')
Discoid LE
— Direct fluorescence
• Negative in normal skin (cf. SLE)
5 Erythema multiforme
— Direct immunofluorescence
• Negative in affected skin

* In both normal and affected skin

Diagnostic procedures in dermatologic disease
1 Wood's lamp (black light)
— Vitiligo
— Ash-leaf macules of tuberous sclerosis
2 Dark-field examination
— Syphilis
3 Tzanck preparation
— Distinguishes herpes simplex from folliculitis
— Distinguishes pemphigus from pemphigoid
4 20% potassium hydroxide (KOH) preparation
— Superficial fungal infections
5 Patch test
— Contact dermatitis
6 Skin scrapings
— Fungal infection, scabies
7 Punch biopsy
— Histopathologic corroboration (e.g. neoplasia)
— Culture (deep mycosis, bacteria, mycobacteria)
— Immunofluorescence (lupus, pemphigoid)

The bullous dermatoses: how to tell them apart
1 Pemphigus vulgaris
— Mucosal involvement typical, esp
• Recurrent oral ulceration
• Conjunctivitis
• Genital, nasal, scalp or umbilical ulceration
— Age of onset 40–60
— Bullae are small, flaccid, fragile (rarely intact)
— Present as erosions and heal without scarring
— Histology → 'acantholytic' cells
— Autoimmune association
— Often requires *massive* steroid doses (120–240 mg prednisone/day)
— Rarely remits spontaneously; 'malignant' course
2 Bullous pemphigoid
— Mucosal involvement rare
— Mainly affects flexor aspects of extremities
— 80% patients > 70 years old
— Bullae are large, tense, non-fragile
— *No* acantholytic cells
— May respond to relatively low doses of steroid (e.g. 40 mg prednisone/day)
— May remit spontaneously; often self-limiting
3 Cicatricial (benign mucous membrane) pemphigoid
— Primarily affects conjunctivae, mouth, pharynx
— Classically afflicts middle-aged women
— Tense blisters → prominent atrophic scars
— May → entropion, symblepharon, dysphagia
— Requires long-term corticosteroid therapy
4 Dermatitis herpetiformis
— Typically manifests with (herpetiform) vesicles
— May affect scapulae, sacrum, scalp, and extensor aspects of knees, elbows; buttocks
— Associated with pruritus, eosinophilia, intestinal villous atrophy, and HLA B8/DRw3
— May respond to
• Dapsone (short-term)
• Gluten-free diet (long-term)
— May be aggravated by iodine ingestion
5 Porphyria cutanea tarda
— Atrophic scars on light-exposed regions
— Facial hypertrichosis; pigmentation
6 Acquired epidermolysis bullosa
— Atrophic scarring
— Associated with amyloidosis, malignancy
7 Pellagra
— Light-exposed regions → 'Casal's necklace'

Staging and management of malignant melanoma
1 Breslow thickness (depth of invasion) 1 mm
— i.e. Confined to superficial dermis
— Good prognosis (90% cure)
— Excise with 1 cm margin
2 Breslow thickness 1–2 mm
— Moderate prognosis
— (Re-)excise with 2 cm margin
3 Breslow thickness > 2 mm
— i.e. Invading subcutaneous fat
— Poor prognosis (20% cure only)
— Re-excise with 3 cm margin
4 Clinically suspicious regional nodes *or* > 3 mm thick 1°
— Check CXR and LFTs
— Proceed to en bloc dissection if negative

MANAGING SKIN DISEASE

DRUG ERUPTIONS

Immune mechanisms of drug-induced skin reactions
1 Type I reaction (urticaria)
Common causes
— Penicillin, sulfonamides
— Aspirin
— Sera, contrast media
2 Type II reaction (cytotoxic), e.g. ITP
Common causes
— Quinine
— Methyldopa
— Gold
3 Type III reaction (vasculitis), e.g. drug-induced lupus
Common causes
— Hydralazine, procainamide
— Sulfonamides
— Penicillin
4 Type IV reaction (contact dermatitis)
Common causes
— Topical antihistamines
— Topical neomycin

Clinical patterns of drug-induced skin reactions
1 Toxic epidermal necrolysis
— β-lactams, allopurinol
— Phenytoin, barbiturates, carbamazepine, etc.
2 Erythema multiforme (± Stevens–Johnson; see below)
— Sulfonamides (sulfasalazine, co-trimoxazole)
— NSAIDs, esp. phenylbutazone*, piroxicam
— Anticonvulsants, esp. carbamazepine
— Allopurinol
— Steroids (!)
3 Erythroderma
— Gold
4 Fixed drug eruption
— Barbiturates
— Phenolphthalein (in laxatives)
5 Serum sickness-like reactions (morbilliform, urticarial)
— β-lactams, β-blockers
— IV/IM proteins (serum, vaccines, streptokinase)
6 Small-vessel vasculitis (palpable purpura, esp. on legs)
— Penicillins, sulfonamides
— Allopurinol
— Thiazides, phenytoin, propylthiouracil

Physical signs signifying severe drug eruptions
1 Fever, tachycardia, hypotension
2 Lymphadenopathy, arthritis
3 Glossitis, mucositis, facial involvement
4 Blistering, positive Nikolsky's sign
5 Confluent erythema ('red man')
6 Palpable purpura, skin necrosis

Clinical spectrum of drug-induced bullous disease
1 Erythema multiforme
— e.g. Co-trimoxazole
2 Photosensitization, e.g.
— Psoralens
— Demeclocycline
— Nalidixic acid
3 Porphyria cutanea tarda, e.g.
— Oral contraceptives
— Diethylstilbestrol (in prostate cancer)
4 Fixed drug eruption (→ hands, feet, penis), e.g.
— Quinine: in tonic water
— Phenolphthalein: in laxatives
5 Following coma → skin necrosis
— e.g. Barbiturates
6 Pemphigus-like rash
— Penicillamine
7 Pemphigoid-like rash
— e.g. Furosemide (frusemide)
8 Pellagra-like rash
— Isoniazid
9 Vasculitis → hemorrhagic bullae
— e.g. Allopurinol*

* Esp. in renal failure and/or concomitant diuretic therapy

Distinguishing features of Stevens–Johnson syndrome*
1 Systemic illness (fever, arthralgias)
2 Purulent or pseudomembranous conjunctivitis with corneal ulceration/perforation or symblepharon
3 Buccal ulcers, bullous stomatitis ± genital/anal ulcers
Acute bloodstained crusting of swollen lips

* = Erythema multiforme affecting mucous membranes

Drug eruptions: miscellaneous characteristics
1 Rashes due to drug sensitivity are classically
— Symmetrical
— Truncal
— Pruritic
— Associated with eosinophilia
2 Sensitization to drugs occurs
— Most frequently with *topical* use
— Least frequently with *oral* use
3 Drug rashes are distinctly *unlikely* with
— Digoxin
— Erythromycin
— Benzodiazepines
— Hormones, vitamins

Conditions predisposing to ampicillin rashes
1 Infectious mononucleosis (EBV)
2 CMV infection
3 Chronic lymphocytic leukemia
4 Concurrent allopurinol treatment

THERAPEUTIC APPROACHES TO SKIN DISEASE

Common measures in the management of drug eruptions
1 Withdraw suspected offending drug(s)
2 Emollients

3 Topical steroids
4 Oral antihistamines

Dermatoses responsive to topical steroids
1 Eczema*
2 Psoriasis
3 Seborrheic dermatitis

* May also respond to topical doxepin

Relative potency of topical steroids
1 High potency
   — Betamethasone dipropionate
2 Intermediate potency
   — Betamethasone valerate
   — Triamcinolone acetonide
3 Mild potency
   — Hydrocortisone valerate
   — Triamcinolone hexacetonide
4 Least potency
   — Hydrocortisone base (1%)

Treatment modalities in psoriasis
1 Coal tar baths, dithranol
2 Steroids (topical)
3 Topical calcipotriol (> calcitriol, tacalcitol)
4 PUVA plus psoralens *or* narrow-band ultraviolet B
5 Methotrexate
6 Etretinate
7 Ciclosporin, tacrolimus, or mycophenolate mofetil
8 Systemic steroids

Fungal nail infections
1 Onychomycoses
   — Caused by dermatophytes (e.g. *Trichophyton rubrum*)
   — Treat with topical tioconazole or amorolfine, or with oral terbinafine
2 Paronychia
   — Caused by *Candida* spp.
   — Treat with terbinafine cream and/or oral itraconazole

Refractory fungal infection of nails?
1 Psoriasis
2 Contact irritants; trauma
3 Haven't treated for long enough (takes months)*

* Hence, always confirm diagnosis by nail analysis to ensure optimal drug therapy

Antineoplastic efficacy of synthetic retinoids
1 Regression of preneoplastic lesions
   — Oral leukoplakia
   — Senile keratoses (incl. transplant-associated)
2 ↓ Tumors in xeroderma pigmentosum patients
3 Mycosis fungoides (some responses)
4 Acute promyelocytic leukemia

Medical treatment of androgenetic alopecia*
1 Two licensed treatments
   — Topical minoxidil 2%
   — Oral finasteride (a 5-α-reductase inhibitor that prevents conversion of testosterone to its active metabolite dihydrotestosterone)

2 Minoxidil
   — 15% achieve 'cosmetically significant' regrowth of hair, 50% have delayed progression of hair loss
   Finasteride
   — 30–45% achieve 'cosmetically significant' regrowth of hair, 50% have delayed progression of hair loss
3 Effects are more marked at the occipital vertex than in the frontotemporal region
4 With finasteride, loss of libido and impotence occur in 2%

* Note that homozygotes for 5-α-reductase II deficiency do *not* develop androgenetic alopecia

UNDERSTANDING SKIN DISEASE

ULTRAVIOLET RADIATION

Radiation types triggering various photodermatoses
1 Visible light
   — Cutaneous porphyrias
2 UV-A
   — Polymorphic light eruption
   — Drug-induced photosensitization
   — Cutaneous porphyrias
3 UV-B
   — Lupus erythematosus
   — Herpes labialis
   — Vitiligo or albinism
   — Xeroderma pigmentosum

Medical consequences of ultraviolet radiation
1 UV-A (320–400 nm, long-wavelength UV, 'black light')
   — Low energy, high skin penetration
   — Responsible for tanning (not burning); used in tanning lamps
   — Present in solar radiation all day
   — Acute exposure implicated in pathogenesis of
     • Photosensitive drug eruptions
     • Porphyria rashes
   — Chronic exposure is implicated in
     • Skin aging
     • Melanoma*
   — High-dose UV-A + psoralen sensitizers (PUVA: for psoriasis, mycosis fungoides) cause
     • Skin SCCs (incl. penis and scrotum)
     • Melanoma (see Ref. 18.1)
2 UV-B (290–320 nm, medium-wavelength UV)
   — High energy, high skin penetration
   — Attenuated by ozone layer
   — Essential for endogenous vitamin D_3 production
   — Absorbed by PABA-containing sunscreens
   — Present in solar radiation mainly 1000–1500 h
   — Acute exposure causes
     • Sunburn (erythema)
     • Snow blindness (keratitis)
   — Chronic exposure is implicated in
     • Non-melanoma skin cancers (SCCs, BCCs)
     • Cataract

— May reduce immune surveillance and thus predispose to
  • Squamous cancers (HPV)
  • Leprosy, leishmaniasis
  • Reactivation of herpes simplex
3 UV-C (200–290 nm, short-wavelength UV)
  — High energy, low skin penetration
  — Used in sterilizing lamps
  — May cause sunburn in climbers ($\downarrow$ ozone; doesn't reach to sea level)
  — May cause cataracts in experimental models

* Melanoma is associated with sunburn episodes, but relationship may be indirect; ocular melanoma has *no* relationship to UV

Therapeutic utility of PUVA
1 Psoriasis
2 Atopic eczema
3 Vitiligo
4 Mycosis fungoides

Therapeutic utility of narrow-band ultraviolet B
1 Psoriasis
2 Refractory atopic eczema (steroid-sparing)
3 Cutaneous porphyria
4 Pityriasis lichenoides
5 Polymorphic light eruptions, actinic prurigo, solar urticaria

THE SKIN AND CANCER

Classical cutaneous complications of cancer
1 Skin infiltration
  — Metastases (e.g. breast cancer, melanoma)
  — Kaposi's sarcoma
  — Histiocytosis X
2 Erythroderma
  — Sézary syndrome, mycosis fungoides
3 Excoriations (pruritus)
  — Hodgkin's disease, polycythemia vera
4 Herpes zoster
  — esp. Myeloma, lymphoma, CLL
5 Dermatomyositis* (esp. steroid-resistant variant)
  — e.g. Ovarian/gastric/lung cancer
6 Radiotherapy effects
  — Early: erythema, desquamation
  — Late: atrophy, fibrosis, telangiectasia
7 Acanthosis nigricans (widespread, mucosal, pruritic)
  — Gastrointestinal adenocarcinomas, esp. gastric
8 Thrombophlebitis migrans
  — Mucin-secreting adenocarcinomas, esp. pancreas
9 Necrolytic migratory erythema
  — Glucagonoma
10 Systemic nodular panniculitis (Weber–Christian)
  — Pancreatic acinar cell carcinoma
  Acute febrile neutrophilic dermatosis (Sweet's)
  — Acute myeloid leukemia
11 Xanthomatosis
  — Multiple myeloma
12 Post-proctoscopic periorbital purpura; 'pinch' purpura
  — Myeloma with supervening amyloidosis

13 Erythema gyratum repens
  Hypertrichosis lanuginosa ('malignant down')
  Bullous pyoderma gangrenosum
  — Not associated with any *specific* tumor type
14 Pemphigoid
  Psoriatic exacerbations
  Erythema multiforme
  Bowen's disease
  — Association with cancer *unproven*

* Associated with cancer in 15% cases; cf. polymyositis 9%

Inherited syndromes predisposing to non-melanoma skin cancer
1 Xeroderma pigmentosum
2 Basal cell nevus (Gorlin's) syndrome
3 Epidermodysplasia verruciformis
4 Albinism

Inherited cancer syndromes with skin signs
1 Peutz–Jeghers syndrome (lip/buccal freckling)
  — Gut polyps (mainly hamartomas)
2 Von Recklinghausen's disease
  — Schwannomas, pheochromocytoma
3 Gardner's syndrome
  — Osteomas, colorectal Ca
4 Cronkhite–Canada syndrome
  — Gut hamartomas and carcinomas
5 Cowden's disease (multiple hamartomas)
  — Thyroid and breast cancers
6 Muir–Torre syndrome (sebaceous tumors)
  — Proximal colonic and genitourinary carcinomas
7 Tylosis (palmar–plantar hyperkeratosis)
  — Esophageal cancer
8 Mucosal neuromatosis (MEN2b)
  — Intestinal ganglioneuromas, pheo-, Ca thyroid

Diseases reduced by circumcision
1 HIV/AIDS
2 Herpes simplex genitalis
3 Cervix cancer (i.e. in partner)
4 Penile cancer
5 Urinary tract infection
6 Phimosis

URTICARIA

Urticarial problems in clinical practice
1 Ordinary urticaria
  — May be IgE-mediated (e.g. reactions to insects)
  — May *also* be non-immunologically mediated
    • Histamine-containing foodstuffs (e.g. frozen tuna)
    • Arachidonic acid pathway inhibitors (e.g. aspirin)
    • Mast-cell degranulation (e.g. opiates)
  — Topical therapy generally ineffective; oral antihistamines or exclusion diets may help
2 Chronic urticaria
  — Defined as recurrent (> 3 months) pruritic lesions (< 24 h duration)
  — May be accompanied by arthralgias, adenopathy, abdominal pain

— Mediated by histamine, *not* IgE; prick tests –
— Precipitating dietary factor identifiable in 25%
— Plasmapheresis or histamine antagonists may be useful; steroids contraindicated

3 Cholinergic urticaria
— Affects head/upper trunk, esp. young patients
— Transient painful pruritic lesions with 'blush'
— Rapid skin cooling may abort an attack

4 Cold urticaria: *familial*
— Autosomal dominant; presents in infancy
— Rash may appear *hours* after cold exposure
— Associated fever, arthralgias, leukocytosis

5 Cold urticaria: *acquired*
— Rash occurs within *minutes* of skin contact with cold water or ice (diagnostic test)
— Syncope may ensue, may cause sudden death in young people (drowning)

6 Solar urticaria
— Weal occurs within 1–3 min of sun exposure
— Localized to sun-exposed areas
— Differential diagnosis: SLE, drug reactions

7 Pressure urticaria
— Affects pressure areas (e.g. feet, buttocks, back)
— Tender swelling 2–12 h after pressure injury

8 Scratch urticaria (delayed dermographism)
— Redness, weals, itch occur hours after scratching
— Distinct from *simple dermographism*, which affects 5% of people and is *not* pruritic

9 Vasculitic urticaria
— Serious condition, may be life-threatening
— Painful non-pruritic lesions lasting > 24 h
— ± Fever, abdominal pain, arthritis, nephritis
— Hypocomplementemia (C_3, C_4, THC), ↑ ESR

10 Angioneurotic edema
— → Mucocutaneous junctions: lips, eyes, penis
— Large tender swellings, often pruritic
— Glottal edema may be a complication, esp. when angioedema occurs with anaphylaxis

NB: Urticaria does *not* occur in association with hereditary angioedema (C1-INH deficiency)

SKIN SYNDROMES

Sweet's syndrome: acute febrile neutrophilic dermatosis

1 Manifests with tender erythematous skin plaques (esp. head and neck, arms) plus fever and neutrophilia
2 Also → arthritis, conjunctivitis, mouth ulcers, proteinuria
3 20% of patients have a malignancy (e.g. acute leukemia); such patients have more severe skin lesions and cytopenias
4 Symptoms are generally steroid-responsive, and may resolve within 2–3 months in patients without malignancy

The dysplastic nevus ('B-K mole') syndrome: features

1 Nevi typically 5–15 mm in diameter
2 Characterized by irregular borders and variegated color
3 Mainly affects trunk, but also sun-deprived areas
4 Often > 100 in number
5 Continue to appear after age 35
6 Histology
— Melanocytic hyperplasia
— Cytologic atypia
— Spindle-shaped melanocyte 'nests'
— Lymphocytic superficial dermal infiltrates
7 Autosomal dominant transmission
8 Risk of developing melanoma approaches 100% in DNS patients with positive family history of melanoma

Skin syndromes in HIV-infected patients

1 Kaposi's sarcoma
2 Opportunistic infections
— Herpes zoster (early event)
— Oral hairy leukoplakia (?EBV/*Candida*)
— Molluscum contagiosum
— Norwegian (severe) scabies, fungal infections
— (Myco)bacterial infections, incl. folliculitis
— Bacillary angiomatosis*
— Syphilis (primary or secondary)
— Chronic (> 4 weeks) ulcerating herpes simplex‡
3 Pathogen-non-specific skin presentations
— Acute exanthem (at seroconversion)
— Xerosis (dry skin): itchy, lichenified
— Seborrheic dermatitis (esp. scalp)
— Psoriasiform rashes (± Reiter's syndrome)
— Morbilliform rash with co-trimoxazole (in 70%)

* Responds to erythromycin; ? due to cat-scratch bacillus
‡ Occurs late; an AIDS-defining event

Target antigens in autoimmune bullous diseases

1 Pemphigus vulgaris
— Desmoglein 3
2 Pemphigus foliaceous
— Desmoglein 1
3 Paraneoplastic pemphigus
— Desmoplakins I/II
4 Epidermolysis bullosa
— Collagen type VII
5 Bullous pemphigoid
— Bullous pemphigoid antigen I
6 Cicatricial pemphigoid, herpes gestationis
— Bullous pemphigoid antigen II

REVIEWING THE LITERATURE: SKIN DISEASE

18.1 Chaudhari U et al (2001) Efficacy and safety of infliximab monotherapy for plaque-type psoriasis: a randomized trial. Lancet 357: 1842–1847

Placebo-controlled randomized comparison of two dose levels of a monoclonal antibody against tumor necrosis factor-alpha, showing good responses at both infliximab dose levels.

18.2 Mease PJ et al 2000 Etanercept in the treatment of psoriatic arthritis and psoriasis: a randomised trial. Lancet 356: 385–390

Randomized trial of 60 patients with this tumor necrosis factor receptor antagonist demonstrated significant improvements in both the arthritis (87% vs 23% control) and the skin lesions (26% vs 0% improved).

18.3 Marcil I, Stern RS (2001) Squamous-cell cancer of the skin in patients given PUVA and ciclosporin: nested cohort crossover study. Lancet 358: 1042–1045

Nested cohort crossover study of 28 psoriasis patients, showing that ciclosporin increases the risk of squamous cell skin cancer in patients previously treated with PUVA.

18.4 Stern S et al (1997) Malignant melanoma in patients treated for psoriasis with methoxalen (psoralen) and ultraviolet A radiation (PUVA). N Engl J Med 336: 1041–1045

Prospective cohort study of 1380 PUVA patients showing an increase in melanoma frequency beginning 15 years after the first treatment.

18.5 Matilainen V et al (2000) Early androgenetic alopecia as a marker of insulin resistance. Lancet 356: 1165–1166

Case-control study (154 cases) showing that males who began to lose their hair before age 35 were at strikingly increased risk of hyperinsulinemia, hypertension, obesity, and hyperlipidemia. Other studies have suggested an increased risk of prostate cancer associated with this phenotype.

18.6 Drago F et al (1997) Human herpesvirus 7 in pityriasis rosea. Lancet 349: 1367–1369

Interesting one-off PCR-based study of 12 pityriasis rosea patients, showing presence of HHV-7 DNA in all plasma and skin samples of cases, but none in the plasma or skin of controls.

18.7 Reynolds NJ et al (2001) Narrow-band ultraviolet B and broad-band ultraviolet A phototherapy in adult atopic eczema. Lancet 357: 2012–2016

Randomized comparison of narrow-band UVB (an effective psoriasis therapy), UVA phototherapy, or visible light, showing a significant improvement in refractory eczema for those patients receiving UVB therapy.

CHAPTER 19

Statistics, screening, epidemiology, evidence-based medicine, preventive medicine and clinical trials

Common problems confounding interpretation of clinical trials

1 Small numbers
2 Inadequate controls*
3 Lack of endpoint definition
4 Insufficient long-term follow-up
5 Publication bias towards positive studies
6 Unstated criteria for patient exclusion/attrition
7 Inadequate statistical power (> significance) of results

* Including inadequate blinding, uncompensated placebo effects

There are *no* emergencies in the world of statistics and evidence-based medicine; this is one of the career attractions of being a dedicated EBM nerd.

Evolution of clinical research from clinical assessment

1 Case-control study
— Evolved from clinical history-taking
2 Cohort study
— Evolved from clinical follow-up
3 Randomized controlled study
— Evolved from clinical treatment

Strengths and weaknesses of epidemiological studies

1 *Case-control* studies
— Advantages
• Cheap and quick
• Relatively few participants required
• Suitable for rare diseases and/or long-latency diseases
• Can assess multiple risk factors or exposures
— Disadvantages
• Difficult to select control group (selection bias, unreliable history)
2 *Cohort* studies
— Advantages
• Minimal bias
• Measures incidence as well as relative risk

— Disadvantages
• Large number of participants needed
• Long follow-up required
• High attrition rate usual
• Expensive and slow

Top ten worldwide causes of health disability

1 Cigarette-induced diseases
2 Diarrheal disease*
3 Depression
4 Perinatal morbidity
5 Tuberculosis
6 Motor vehicle accidents
7 Malaria
8 Sexually transmitted diseases (including HIV)
9 Violence (including war)
10 Congenital disorders

* Usually due to lack of clean drinking water

Measures quantifying the utility of diagnostic tests

1 Sensitivity
— Percentage of people detected who (in fact) have the disorder
— = 100% – false-negative percentage
2 Specificity
— Percentage of people excluded who (in fact) don't have the disorder
— = 100% – false-positive percentage
3 Positive predictive value*
— Extent to which a positive test correctly indicates the presence of the disorder
— = % detected/% recalled
4 Likelihood ratio*
— Extent to which a positive test is more likely to be found in someone with the disorder compared to someone without the disorder

* Negative test significances can be similarly characterized (e.g. by the negative predictive value)

Factors supporting the causality of a statistical association*

1 Strength of the association (e.g. low p value), *plus*
2 Sensitivity, specificity, reproducibility of the association
3 Dose-response gradient demonstrated
4 Appropriate temporal relationship
5 Scientific plausibility

* Hill's criteria; can be applied, for example, to the pathogenicity or otherwise of an association of a microbe with a disease

Parametric vs non-parametric statistical tests

1 Parametric tests
   — Assume that the data are sampled from a particular form of distribution (e.g. normal distribution)
   — More powerful than non-parametric tests; hence, preferable to use if possible
2 Non-parametric tests
   — Do not assume that the data are sampled from any particular form of distribution; hence, tend to be less powerful than parametric tests

Which statistical test to use?

1 To compare two sets of data from a single sample
   — Parametric: Paired *t* test
   — Non-parametric: Wilcoxon matched pairs test
2 To compare two unrelated data sets from a single sample
   — Parametric: Unpaired *t* test
   — Non-parametric: Mann–Whitney test
3 To test the null hypothesis that, in two or more independent samples, the distribution of a given continuous variable is the same
   — Parametric: χ^2
   — Non-parametric: Fisher's exact test
4 To test the strength of a linear association between two continuous variables
   — Parametric: Pearson's *r* correlation coefficient
   — Non-parametric: Spearman's r_σ rank correlation coefficient

CANCER SCREENING

General principles of cancer screening

1 *Effectiveness* of a screening test depends on
   — The availability of *effective treatment*
   — The ability to identify (and test) *high-risk groups*
2 The most effective screening test in current use is the *Pap (cervical) smear*
3 *Mammography* of women aged 50–70 reduces breast cancer-specific mortality by 20–30%

Sources of bias in evaluating cancer screening tests

1 *Lead time bias*
   — By detecting disease at an earlier (presymptomatic) stage, subsequent survival is spuriously prolonged when compared with a symptomatic cohort
2 *Length time bias*
   — By instituting mass screening programs, a relative excess of patients with *indolent* disease will be detected initially (since at any one time the *prevalence* of slowly-growing tumors will tend to be greater, even if the *incidence* of aggressive tumors is similar), leading to an illusory survival improvement in the screened cohort

Colorectal cancer: recommendations for 'high-risk' screening

1 Ulcerative colitis (pancolitis > 10 years' duration, *or* left-sided colitis > 20 years' duration)
   — 6-monthly sigmoidoscopy + annual colonoscopy with multiple biopsies
   — Proctocolectomy is indicated if high-grade dysplasia
2 Familial adenomatous polyposis (FAP): first-degree relative
   — Children have 50% chance of inheriting disease
   — Annual flexible sigmoidoscopy after age 15
   — Extend to 3-yearly sigmoidoscopy if clear at age 35
   — Genetic screening (5q- mutation) may be useful
   — Prophylactic surgery if polyps develop
3 Hereditary non-polyposis colorectal cancer (HNPCC)
   — Lynch syndrome I (site-specific Ca colon)
   — Lynch syndrome II (cancer family syndrome, with additional cancers of endometrium, ovary, etc.)
   — Annual fecal occult blood testing from age 25
   — 2-yearly colonoscopy from age 30
4 Patients with previous adenoma(s) or carcinoma
   — Colonoscopy every 3–5 years; occult blood testing has a purely supplementary role in follow-up here
5 First-degree relative of patient with colorectal cancer
   — Annual fecal occult blood testing from age 40
   — ± Flexible sigmoidoscopy every 5 years
   — Positive occult blood? Colonoscopy

Fecal occult blood testing in standard-risk patients

1 2–5% of tests performed in standard-risk subjects will be positive, and of these 75% will have no abnormality
   — i.e. False-positive rate for polyp/Ca detection is 75%
   — False-positive rate for Ca detection alone is ~ 95%
   — These rates translate into many unnecessary tests
2 20% of cancers appear never to bleed
   — i.e. False-negative rate for Ca detection is > 20%
   — False-negative rate for polyp detection is much higher
3 Less than 1% of screened standard-risk subjects will have a carcinoma. Tumors detected in this way are twice as likely to be Duke's stage A or B than are symptomatic tumors
4 Annual screening of standard-risk subjects *may* reduce cancer-specific mortality. Hence, annual occult blood testing + digital rectal exam (?± 10-yearly sigmoidoscopy) *may* be justifiable after age 50
5 The *cost-effectiveness* of fecal occult blood screening remains unproven

False-positive and -negative fecal occult blood tests

1 *False-negatives* may arise due to
   — Sampling error; or delay in test development
   — Proximal site of bleeding
   — Vitamin C ingestion

2 *False-positives* may arise due to
— Red meat, iron tablets
— Aspirin, other NSAIDs

Asymptomatic mammographic lesions meriting biopsy
1 Mass lesion
— May be stellate ± spiculated margins
2 'Suspicious' microcalcifications
— Linear
— Branching

* May indicate intraductal carcinoma accompanying invasive tumors

Common causes of false-positive mammograms*
1 Fat necrosis (e.g. post-traumatic)
2 Fibrocystic disease
3 Scarring
— Post-surgical (e.g. lumpectomy)
— Post-irradiation

Investigation and management of the abnormal cervical smear
1 Mild-to-moderate dyskaryosis
— Repeat smear in 6 months (± endocervical curettage)
2 Two further smears → mild dyskaryosis, *or*
One further smear → moderate dyskaryosis, *or*
Severe dyskaryosis (once)
— Proceed to colposcopy and punch-directed biopsy
3 Minor cervical intraepithelial neoplasia (CIN grade I–II)
— Cryocoagulation/cold coagulation
4 CIN III (localized, or upper limits undefinable)
— Cone biopsy (large loop excision of transformation zone) using diathermy loop
CIN III involving most of cervix or → vaginal fornix
— CO_2 laser photovaporization
5 Invasive SCC cervix
— Hysterectomy or radiotherapy

Early detection of prostate cancer*
1 Elevated PSA (if > 4 ng/mL; but *esp.* if > 10 ng/mL)
2 Transrectal ultrasound ± needle biopsy
3 Digital rectal examination (less sensitive than PSA)

* Too non-specific and insensitive to justify routine screening; these measures only reliably detect tumors > 0.5 cm diameter. Annual rectal examination after age 50 (± PSA before) is reasonable but *not* proven effective

MANAGEMENT ASPECTS OF EVIDENCE-BASED MEDICINE

Parameters for quantifying interventional efficacy
1 Numbers (of patients) needed to treat/screen to avoid one death (or other outcome)
2 Relative reduction in disease-specific mortality or morbidity (per intervention or interval)
3 Absolute reduction in mortality or morbidiy (per intervention or interval)

Number needed to treat (NNT) or screen: clinical significance
1 Quantifies the degree of benefit of a therapeutic intervention by estimating the number of patients who have to be treated to prevent one stated adverse outcome
2 Represents the reciprocal of the absolute risk reduction. For example, if drug A gives a 12% benefit rate compared to drug B's 8%, then the absolute risk reduction is 4% (1/25), making the NNT 25
3 Particularly useful in placebo-controlled trials, but 'placebo effect' needs to be factored out.

How to prevent cancer
1 Lung cancer and other cigarette-induced neoplasms
— Stop smoking
2 Skin cancer
— ↓ UV-B exposure
3 Hepatoma
— Hepatitis B vaccination
4 SCC cervix
— Condom and diaphragm usage
5 Oral cancer
— Vitamin A, cessation of betel-nut ingestion
6 Penile cancer
— Circumcision

CLINICAL TRIALS

Points to discuss with patients prior to trial enrolment
1 Prognosis with and without treatment
2 Probability of therapeutic benefit (cure, complete or partial remission, disease-free interval, symptoms)
3 Risks of infertility/teratogenicity/premature menopause; availability of sperm banking
4 Likely severity of alopecia; availability of wig-making
5 Likely severity and duration of nausea; prophylactic drugs
6 Need for allopurinol (in hematologic malignancies)
7 Requirement for regular blood tests
8 Urgent significance of fever or bruising/bleeding
9 Rationâle of clinical trials and informed consent
10 Long-term risk of second malignancy, esp. in good-prognosis disease treated with alkylating agents ± radiotherapy

Clinical assessment of the cancer patient commencing on trial
1 Assessment and documentation of disease extent
— Measurement (and/or photography) of visible lesions
— Radiographic corroboration
— Measurement of tumor markers
— Invasive staging *if* stage-specific therapy exists
2 Assessment of vital organ function
— Left ventricular function (pre-doxorubicin)
— Lung function (pre-bleomycin)
— Renal function (pre-platinum)
3 Assessment of immune status (in leukemia, transplantation)
— CXR, tuberculin test
— Viral (CMV, HSV, hepatitis B) and toxoplasma serology

4 Assessment of venous access
— Consideration of an implantable infusion port/catheter
5 Assessment of psychological adjustment to disease, and to disease- and treatment-related disability

Levels of evidence on which to base clinical decision-making
1 Level I evidence
— Ia: based on meta-analysis of pooled data from many randomized controlled trials
— Ib: based on at least one randomized controlled trial
2 Level II evidence
— Based on at least one well-designed unrandomized controlled trial
3 Level III evidence
— Based on descriptive studies (e.g. case-control studies), comparative or retrospective data
4 Level IV evidence
— Based on expert opinions and consensus committees, or case series studies, in the absence of any of the above data

Types of clinical drug trial
1 *Phase 1 study*
— Toxicologic dose-finding study which determines maximum tolerated dose (i.e. side-effects) in heavily pretreated, poor-prognosis patients
2 *Phase 2 study*
— Using doses found 'safe' in the phase 1 study, patients with various tumor types are treated to determine the drug's anticancer activity when used alone
3 *Phase 3 study*
— Sensitive tumor types identified by the phase 2 study are treated with the new drug in a prospective randomized comparison with standard treatment

UNDERSTANDING EVIDENCE-BASED MEDICINE

TOXIC OCCUPATIONAL EXPOSURES

Diseases due to occupational exposure to toxic agents
1 Asbestosis
2 Occupational asthma, industrial bronchitis
3 Hearing loss (noise-induced)
4 Contact dermatitis
5 Solvent poisoning
6 Lead poisoning (acute or chronic)
7 Toxic hepatitis
8 Silicosis
9 Miscellaneous poisoning
— Pesticides, carbon monoxide

Malignancies inducible by toxic workplace exposure
1 Mesothelioma, lung cancer
— Asbestos

2 Bladder cancer
— *p*-aminodiphenyl, benzidine, naphthalene dyes
3 Leukemia
— Ionizing radiation, benzene
4 Nasal sinus carcinoma
— Chromium, nickel, wood dust
5 Hepatoma
— Vinyl chloride monomer
6 Scrotal/skin cancer (e.g. in chimney sweeps)
— Aromatic hydrocarbons (e.g. in coal, creosote)

EPIDEMIOLOGIC BASIS OF CANCER

Cell kinetics in tumor evolution
1 Tumor too small to be detected by sensitive screening tests
— 1 mm tumor diameter
— Roughly equivalent to 10^6 tumor cells
— Represents approximately 20 tumor cell doublings
2 Tumor too small to be symptomatic; detectable by screening
— 1 cm tumor diameter (~ 1 g tumor burden)
— Roughly equivalent to 10^9 tumor cells
— Represents approximately 30 tumor cell doublings
3 Tumor clinically evident; advanced disease, usually incurable
— 1 kg total tumor burden
— Roughly equivalent to 10^{12} tumor cells
— Represents approximately 40 tumor cell doublings

Incidence of malignant disease: the commonest cancers*
1 Western-world males
— Lung cancer (25% all cancers, 40% cancer mortality)
— Colorectal cancer (10–15% cancers, similar mortality)
— Prostate cancer (10% cancers, similar mortality)
2 Western-world females
— Breast cancer (25% cancers, 15% mortality)
— Colorectal cancer (10–15% cancers, similar mortality)
— Lung cancer (10% cancers, and rising: 15% mortality)
3 Commonest malignancies in Third World populations
— Gastric cancer (commonest malignancy world-wide)
— Esophageal and oral cancer
— Hepatoma
— SCC cervix

* Excluding non-melanomatous skin cancer

Malignancies changing in incidence
1 Cancers increasing in frequency
— Lung cancer (in Third World, and in women)
— Mesothelioma
— Melanoma
— Hepatoma

— Early-onset (< 35-years-old) SCC cervix
— Kaposi's sarcoma
— Testicular tumors
— Lymphoma (esp. 1° cerebral)
2 Cancers declining in frequency
— Gastric cancer
— Lung cancer (in Western middle-class males)

Geographical clustering of various cancers

1 Hepatoma — Mozambique, South-East Asia
2 Gastric cancer — Japan, Chile, China, Russia
3 Oral cancer — India, South-East Asia
4 Esophageal cancer — Iran, Turkey, Afghanistan, China
5 Nasopharynx cancer — South China, Eskimos
6 Skin cancer — Australia
7 SCC cervix — Chile, Latin America, Asia
8 Penile cancer — Uganda

Dietary factors implicated in carcinogenesis

1 Betel-nut tobacco chewing
  Alcohol, incl. mouthwashes } — Oral cancer
2 Alcohol and tobacco
  Opium; dietary deficiencies } — Esophageal cancer
  Bracken fern (in Japanese)
3 Salted fish — Nasopharyngeal Ca
4 Aflatoxin — Hepatoma
5 Overnutrition (obesity) — Endometrial/ gallbladder Ca

Major risk factors for various cancers

1 Breast
— Affected first-degree relative(s), esp. premenopausal
— *BRCA1* (or *2*) mutations (e.g. in Ashkenazi Jews)
— Late age of first full-term pregnancy
2 Endometrial
— Prolonged exogenous estrogen administration
— Obesity, nulliparity, high social class
3 Cervix
— Early and/or promiscuous sexual activity (HPV)
— Smoking
— HLA DQw3
4 Hepatoma
— Macronodular cirrhosis
  • HBV, HCV*
  • Hemochromatosis
  • α_1-antitrypsin deficiency
— Alcohol, aflatoxin, anabolic steroids
Hepatic adenoma
— Estrogens
Angiosarcoma
— Thorotrast, arsenic, vinyl chloride monomer
5 Gallbladder
— Gallstones (chronic cholecystitis); obesity
— Porcelain (calcified) gallbladder
6 Bile ducts
— Inflammatory bowel disease
— *Clonorchis sinensis* infestation
7 Colorectal
— Familial polyposis; villous adenoma
— Inflammatory bowel disease, esp. ulcerative colitis

— Affected first-degree relative(s); Gardner's syndrome
8 Esophageal (SCC)
— Cigarettes, alcohol; corrosive ingestion
— Pickled vegetables
— Achalasia, celiac disease, Plummer–Vinson syndrome
— Tylosis (palmar–plantar hyperkeratosis: rare)
Esophageal (adenocarcinoma)
— Barrett's (columnar) esophagus
— Chronic severe esophageal reflux
9 Lung
— Cigarettes (incl. passive smoking)
— Asbestos‡ (synergy with cigarettes for both lung and laryngeal Ca)
— Radon (emits α-particles)
— Scars (predispose to adenocarcinoma)
— Scleroderma (predisposes to alveolar cell carcinoma)
10 Mesothelioma
— Asbestos: 'blue' (crocidolite) > white (chrysotile¶) > brown (amosite) > black (anthophyllite)
11 Bladder (TCC) and other urothelial cancers (ureteric, renal pelvis)
— Male sex; past history of bladder cancer
— Aromatic dye/naphthalene (arylamine) exposure (e.g. dye, rubber, textile workers)
— Cigarettes, analgesics, cyclophosphamide
— Low fluid intake
Bladder (SCC)
— *Schistosoma hematobium* infestation
12 Thyroid
— Low-dose (< 2000 rad) external beam irradiation
— Multinodular goiter
— Gardner's/Cowden's/Verner's syndromes
13 Lymphoma
— Radiotherapy, chemotherapy
— Sjögren's syndrome (also → pseudolymphoma)
Leukemia, esp. AML
— Chemotherapy, radiation therapy
— DNA repair deficiencies
— Ionizing radiation, incl. ?radon exposure
— Miscellaneous mutagens (e.g. benzene)
14 Osteosarcoma
— Paget's disease
— Osteogenesis imperfecta
— Familial retinoblastoma
15 Testicular tumors
— Cryptorchidism
— Testicular feminization syndrome
16 Melanoma
— Dysplastic nevus syndrome
— Repeated childhood sunburn§
17 Lip cancer
— Smoking
— Solar exposure
18 Ovarian tumors, esp. granulosa cell
— Clomifene fertility stimulation
19 Gastric (MALT) lymphoma *and* gastric cancer
— *Helicobacter pylori*

* May also be associated with hepatoma in non-cirrhotics
‡ Note that asbestos-related *neoplasms*, including mesothelioma, may occur at lower exposures than asbestosis. Hence, asbestos-

exposed individuals have an increased risk of lung cancer even in the absence of radiographic pulmonary fibrosis
¶ Crocidolite induces mesotheliomas four times more potently than does chrysotile. However, all asbestos forms appear equally potent in inducing lung cancer; hence, chrysotile is the most important variety of asbestos in epidemiological terms, since it accounts for 95% of world production
§ May reflect genetic UV sensitivity rather than a causal event; *no* relationship with retinal melanoma

Malignancies associated with cigarette smoking
1 Lung cancer
   — SCC > SCLC > large-cell > adenoCa > alveolar cell*
2 Squamous cell carcinomas of mouth *and* larynx *and* esophagus‡
3 Transitional cell carcinoma of bladder *and* renal pelvis
4 Pancreatic adenocarcinoma
5 SCC cervix¶
6 Colorectal cancer

* cf. mesothelioma: *not* associated with smoking
‡ cf. nasopharyngeal carcinoma: *not* associated with either smoking or alcohol ingestion. Note also that 'smokeless' tobacco is also a potent cause of oral cancer
¶ Association may be environmental rather than causal

Malignancies associated with alcohol ingestion
1 Upper aerodigestive cancers: mouth, pharynx, larynx, esophagus (beer and spirits)
2 Liver
3 ?Breast ?rectum (beer)

Viruses implicated in tumorigenesis
1 Epstein-Barr virus (EBV)
   — Endemic Burkitt's lymphoma
   — Immunoblastic lymphoma
   — Primary cerebral lymphoma (if immunosuppressed)
   — Hodgkin's disease
   — Nasal T cell lymphoma (lethal midline granuloma)
   — Nasopharyngeal carcinoma
2 Hepatitis B
   — Hepatocellular carcinoma
3 Hepatitis C
   — Hepatocellular carcinoma
   — Mixed cryoglobulinemia type II, evolving to non-Hodgkin's lymphoma
4 HPV serotypes 16* (50%); 18‡ (20%); 31 and 45 (10%); and 25 others (20%)
   — Squamous cell carcinoma (SCC) of the cervix
   — Also implicated in penile, vulvar¶ and (some) anal carcinomas (SCC)
5 HPV serotypes 5, 8
   — Skin SCCs in renal transplant patients
   — Epidermodysplasia verruciformis
6 HTLV-I and II
   — T-cell leukemia/lymphoma
7 HHV8 (replication promoted by HIV-1)
   — Kaposi's sarcoma

* Seropositivity for HPV-16 increases risk of cervix cancer development by 15-fold
‡ Prognosis is poorer for HPV-18 than for HPV-16-associated early-stage Ca cervix
¶ But older females with keratinizing vulvar cancers represent an HPV-negative pathogenesis

19.1 LeLorier J et al (1997) Discrepancies between meta-analyses and subsequent large randomized, controlled trials. N Engl J Med 337: 536–542

Comparison of 19 meta-analyses and 12 large randomized studies addressing the same issues, showing poor correlation between the two research modalities.

19.2 Tramer MR et al (1997) Impact of covert duplicate publication on meta-analysis: a case study. Br Med J 315: 635–640

Analysis of 84 studies on the efficacy of the antiemetic drug ondansetron, showing that 17% of the studies and 28% of the patient data were duplicated between publications – thereby biasing the conclusions of meta-analyses that inadvertently include all these inputs.

19.3 Stern JM, Simes JR (1997) Publication bias: evidence of delayed publication in a cohort study of clinical research projects. Br Med J 315: 640–644

Analysis of 748 studies, confirming the widely held suspicion that manuscripts boasting positive results are more often and more quickly accepted for publication. Moreover, studies with indefinite results had an even lower rate of acceptance than did negative studies.

19.4 Yuan J et al (1999) *Helicobacter pylori* infection and risk of gastric cancer in Shanghai, China. Cancer Epidemiol Biomarkers Prev 8: 621–624

Case-control study of 188 gastric cancer patients and 548 controls, showing a 4-fold risk for gastric cancer conferred by *H. pylori* seropositivity.

19.5 Michaud DS et al (1999) Fluid intake and the risk of bladder cancer in men. N Engl J Med 340: 1390–1397

Reduced fluid intake and micturition was found to be associated with increased risk of bladder cancer in this case-control study, supporting the uro-contact theory of pathogenesis.

19.6 Narod SA et al (1998) Oral contraceptives and the risk of hereditary ovarian cancer. N Engl J Med 339: 424–428

Both *BRCA1* and *BRCA2* mutation carriers exhibited 50–60% decreased incidence of ovarian cancer if oral contraceptives had been taken in the past.

19.7 Lagergren J et al (1999) Symptomatic gastroesophageal reflux as a risk factor for esophageal adenocarcinoma. N Engl J Med 340: 825–831

Swedish case-control study of 820 controls, 167 patients with esophageal SCC, 262 with adenocarcinoma of the gastric cardia, and 189 with esophageal gastric adenocarcinoma. A history of long-standing severe reflux was associated with a 44-fold increased risk of esophageal adenocarcinoma, compared with a 4-fold increase for adenocarcinoma of the gastric cardia and no increase for esophageal SCC.

19.8 Neumann F et al (2001) Treatment of *Chlamydia pneumoniae* infection with roxithromycin and effect on neointima proliferation after coronary stent placement (ISAR-3). Lancet 357: 2085–2089

Meurice T et al (2001) Effect of ACE inhibitors on angiographic restenosis after coronary stenting (PARIS). Lancet 357: 1321–1324

Two randomized double-blind placebo-controlled studies of post-PTCA inhibition linked to elaborate theories of pathogenesis – but both therapeutically negative.

19.9　Jick H et al (2000) Statins and the risk of dementia. Lancet 356: 1627–1631

Reid IR et al (2001) Effect of pravastatin on frequency of fracture in the LIPID study: secondary analysis of a randomized controlled trial. Lancet 357: 509–512

Two analyses of the possible extracardiac benefits of statins, confirming a protective association with cognition (in the former) but failing to confirm a bone-strengthening effect (in the latter).

19.10　Pignone M et al (2000) Use of lipid lowering drugs for primary prevention of coronary heart disease: meta-analysis of randomized trials. Br Med J 321: 983–986

LIPID Study Group (2002) Longterm effectiveness and safety of pravastatin in 9014 patients with coronary heart disease and average cholesterol concentrations. Lancet 359: 1379–1387

The first paper showed that statin therapy reduced coronary events but not overall mortality when administered to patients without a cardiovascular history, whereas the second paper showed that patients with a cardiac history benefited from statins (including survival benefit) even if their cholesterol levels were normal.

19.11　Terry P et al (2001) Fatty fish consumption and risk of prostate cancer. Lancet 357: 1764–1765

In this study, a two- to three-fold increased risk of prostate cancer was found in individuals not eating fish.

19.12　Bonithon-Kopp C et al (2000) Calcium and fibre supplementation in prevention of colorectal adenoma recurrence. Lancet 356: 1300–1306

Randomized study of 665 colorectal adenoma patients, showing a slightly increased (i.e. not decreased) risk of adenoma recurrence in patients on ispaghula husk fiber supplements.

Further Reading

1 BEST GENERAL TEXTBOOK: Weatherall DJ et al (eds) *Oxford Textbook of Medicine*
Like expensive and weighty stethoscopes, expensive and weighty textbooks are not a prerequisite for passing medical exams. Owning one decent reference book can make life easier, however. This massive 4376-page compendium has a sort of classic ageless quality to it, and the editors have purged some of the errors and imbalances of earlier editions. Altogether, the most comprehensive and globally applicable textbook of medicine.

2 BEST MCQs: **MKSAP** (Medical knowledge self-assessment program)
For candidates who need a 'quiz-show' format to sustain their interest in the lead-up to an exam, this American Medical Association publication is good (it includes excellent state-of-the-art summaries of each subspecialty in addition to the self-assessment questions) – provided that either you or your library can afford it. If not, look for other publications which feature detailed and authoritative answers.

3 BEST JOURNAL: *New England Journal of Medicine*
The *NEJM* and the *Lancet* are the only two general medical journals containing original articles worth perusing on a regular basis; the former is more influential and politically correct, the latter more quirky and interesting. Dozens of other journals (original and review) are worth auditing, however, if you can find the time.

4 BEST SUBSPECIALTY TEXTS

Cancer
Short and readable:
UICC Manual of Clinical Oncology. Springer, Berlin
Reference:
De Vita VT et al (eds) *Cancer: Principles and Practice of Oncology*. Lippincott, Philadelphia

Cardiology
Short and readable:
Schlamt RC, Hurst JW *Handbook of the Heart*. McGraw-Hill, New York
Reference:
Braunwald E (ed) *Heart Disease*. Saunders, Philadelphia

Endocrinology
Short and readable:
Besser GM, Thorner MG *Clinical Endocrinology*. Times Mirror, New York
Reference:
De Groot L (ed) *Endocrinology*. Saunders, Philadelphia

Gastroenterology
Short and readable:
Christensen J *Bedside Logic in Diagnostic Gastroenterology*. Churchill Livingstone, Edinburgh

Reference:
Sleisenger MH et al (eds) *Gastrointestinal Disease*. Saunders, Philadelphia

Hematologic disease
Short and readable:
Hoffbrand AV, Pettit JE *Essential Hematology*. Blackwell, Oxford
Reference:
Lee RG et al *Wintrobe's Clinical Hematology*. Lea & Febiger, Philadelphia

HIV-related disease
Short and readable:
Masci JR *Outpatient Management of HIV infection*. CRC Press, New York
Reference:
Merigan TC, Bartlett JG, Bolognesi D (eds) *Textbook of AIDS medicine*. Lippincott, Williams & Wilkins, Philadelphia

Immunology, autoimmune disease and transplantation
Short and readable:
Male D *Immunology: an Illustrated Outline*. Mosby, London
Reference:
Samter M (ed) *Immunologic Diseases*. Little, Brown, Boston

Infectious disease
Short and readable:
Grist NR et al *Diseases of Infection*. OUP, Oxford
Reference:
Gorbach SL et al (eds) *Infectious Diseases*. Saunders, Philadelphia

Metabolic and nutritional disorders
Short and readable:
Wilson G *Clinical Genetics: a Short Course*. Wiley-Liss, New York
Stanbury JB et al (eds) *The Metabolic Basis of Inherited Disease*. McGraw-Hill, New York

Neurology
Short and readable:
Wilkinson I *Essential Neurology*. Blackwell, Oxford
Reference:
Swash M, Oxbury J *Clinical Neurology*. Churchill Livingstone, Edinburgh

Palliative care, rehabilitation and gerontology
Reference:
Doyle D, Hanke G, Macdonald N (eds) *Oxford Textbook of Palliative Medicine*. OUP, Oxford
Hazzard WR et al (eds) *Principles of Geriatric Medicine and Gerontology*. McGraw-Hill, New York

Pharmacology and toxicology
Short and readable:
Neal MJ *Medical Pharmacology at a Glance*. Blackwell, Oxford
Goodman LS, Gilman AG et al *The Pharmacological Basis of Therapeutics*. Macmillan, New York

Psychiatry and addiction
Short and readable:
Burns AS et al *MCQs and Short Notes in Psychiatry*. Wright, Bristol
Reference:
Kaplan HI, Sadock BS *Comprehensive Textbook of Psychiatry*. Williams & Wilkins, Baltimore

Renal and urologic disease
Short and readable:
Whitworth JA, Lawrence JR *Textbook of Renal Disease*. Churchill Livingstone, Edinburgh

Respiratory disease
Short and readable:
Flenley DC *Respiratory Medicine*. Baillière Tindall, London
Reference:
Brewis R et al (eds) *Respiratory Medicine*. Baillière Tindall.

Rheumatology
Short and readable:
Moll JMH *Manual of Rheumatology*. Churchill Livingstone, Edinburgh

Reference:
Katz WZ *Diagnosis and Management of Rheumatic Diseases*. Lippincott, Philadelphia

Sexual and reproductive medicine
Short and readable:
Maurice WL *Sexual Medicine in Primary Care*. Mosby, St Louis
Reference:
Yen SC, Jaffe RB (eds) *Reproductive Endocrinology: Physiology, Pathophysiology, and Clinical Management*. Saunders, Philadelphia

Skin disease
Short and readable:
Fitzpatrick TB et al *Color Atlas and Synopsis of Clinical Dermatology*. McGraw-Hill, New York
Reference:
Rook A et al (eds) *Textbook of Dermatology*. Blackwell, Oxford

Statistics, epidemiology and clinical trials
Short and readable:
Sackett DL, Haynes B, Tugwell P, Guyatt GH *Clinical Epidemiology: a Basic Science for Clinical Medicine*. Lippincott, Williams & Wilkins, Philadelphia
Reference:
Friedman LM, Furberg C, Demets DL *Fundamentals of Clinical Trials*. Springer, Berlin

5 BEST BOOK FOR PASSING MEDICAL EXAMS:
.... I'm afraid I'll have to leave this one up to you.

Abbreviations

A_2	aortic component of second heart sound
AA	Alcoholics Anonymous
A-a	alveolar-arterial (oxygen)
Ab	antibody
ABPA	allergic bronchopulmonary aspergillosis
ABVD	*Adriamycin* (doxorubicin), *bleomycin, vinblastine, dactinomycin*
ACE	angiotensin-converting enzyme
AChRAb	acetylcholine receptor antibody
ACTH	adrenocorticotrophic hormone
AD	autosomal dominant
ADH	antidiuretic hormone (vasopressin)
ADP	adenosine diphosphate
AER	auditory evoked response
AF	atrial fibrillation
AFB	acid-fast bacilli
AFP/αFP	α-fetoprotein
Ag	antigen
AI	aortic incompetence
AIDS	acquired immunodeficiency syndrome
AIHA	autoimmune hemolytic anemia
a.k.a.	also known as
ALA	aminolevulinic acid
ALL	acute lymphoblastic leukemia
ALT	alanine aminotransferase (SGPT)
AMH	anti-Müllerian hormone
AMI	acute myocardial infarction
AML	acute myelocytic leukemia
AMOL	acute myelomonocytic leukemia
ANA	antinuclear antibody
ANCA	antineutrophil cytoplasmic antibodies
Ang	angiotensin
ANLL	acute non-lymphocytic leukemia
ANP	atrial natriuretic peptide
AP	anteroposterior
APC	adenomatous polyposis coli (gene, locus) *or* aspirin–phenacetin–caffeine *or* antigen-presenting cell
APCC	activated prothrombin complex concentrate
AP(M)L	acute promyelocytic leukemia
APSAC	anistreplase (anisoylated plasminogen streptokinase activator complex)
APTT	activated partial thromboplastin time
APUD	amine precursor uptake and decarboxylation
AR	autosomal recessive, *or* androgen receptor *or* aortic regurgitation
ARA	American Rheumatology Association
ara-C	cytosine arabinoside
ARC	AIDS-related complex
ARDS	adult respiratory distress syndrome
AS	ankylosing spondylitis *or* aortic stenosis
ASD	atrial septal defect
ASO	antistreptolysin O (titer)
AST	aspartate aminotransferase (SGOT)
AT	antitrypsin
ATG	antithymocyte globulin
AT-III	antithrombin III
atm	atmospheres (pressure)
ATN	acute tubular necrosis
ATP	adenosine triphosphate
ATRA	all-*trans*-retinoic acid
AV	atrioventricular, arteriovenous
AVM	arteriovenous malformation
AVR	aortic valve replacement
AXR	abdominal X-ray
AZT	zidovudine (= azidothymidine)
b.d.	twice-daily (dosage)
BAL	bronchoalveolar lavage, *or* dimercaprol
BAO	basal acid output
BCC	basal cell carcinoma
BCG	bacillus Calmette–Guérin
BCNU	1,3-bis(2-chloroethyl)-*l*-nitrosourea (carmustine)
BJP	Bence-Jones protein
BNP	B-type natriuretic peptide
BP	blood pressure
BPH	benign prostatic hypertrophy
BSP	bromsulfthalein
BuDR	bromodeoxuridine
BUN	blood urea nitrogen
C1–7(8)	cervical vertebrae (nerve root)
C_1-INH	C_1-esterase inhibitor
$C_{3,4}$(etc.)	complement components
Ca	cancer
Ca^{2+}	calcium
CABG	coronary artery bypass graft
c-*abl*	cellular oncogene *abl*
CAH	chronic active hepatitis, *or* congenital adrenal hyperplasia
cALLA	common ALL-antigen
cAMP	cyclic adenosine monophosphate
CAPD	chronic ambulatory peritoneal dialysis
CCF	congestive cardiac failure
CCK	cholecystokinin
CCl_4	carbon tetrachloride
CCU	coronary care unit
CD	cellular determinant
CDCA	chenodeoxycholic acid
CEA	carcinoembryonic antigen
cf.	confer (compare, contrast)
CFT	complement fixation test
CFTR	cystic fibrosis transmembrane conductance regulator
CGDC	chronic granulomatous disease of childhood
CGL	chronic granulocytic leukemia (= CML)
CH_{50}	total hemolytic complement
CHAD	cold hemagglutinin disease
CHOP	*cyclophosphamide, hydroxydaunorubicin (doxorubicin, Adriamycin), Oncovin (vincristine), prednisone*

CJD	Creutzfeldt–Jakob disease
CK	creatine kinase
Cl⁻	chloride ion
CLL	chronic lymphocytic leukemia
CMC	chronic mucocutaneous candidiasis
CML	chronic myeloid (granulocytic) leukemia
CMML	chronic myelomonocytic leukemia
CMT	Charcot–Marie–Tooth disease
CMV	cytomegalovirus
c-*myc*	cellular oncogene *myc*
CN	cranial nerve(s), *or* cyanide
CNS	central nervous system
COAD	chronic obstructive airways disease
Con-A	Concanavalin A
c-*onc*	cellular oncogene
CPAP	continuous positive airways pressure
CPK	creatine phosphokinase
CPR	cardiopulmonary resuscitation
c.p.s.	cycles per second
CRA	central retinal artery
CREST	*c*alcinosis, *R*aynaud's, *e*sophageal dysfunction, *s*clerodactyly and *t*elangiectasia (syndrome)
CRF	chronic renal failure
CRH	corticotrophin-releasing hormone
CRP	C-reactive protein
CRV	central retinal vein
CSA	ciclosporin (A)
CSF	cerebrospinal fluid, *or* colony-stimulating factor
CSM	carotid sinus massage
CT	computed tomography
CTS	carpal tunnel syndrome
CVA	cerebrovascular accident
CVP	central venous pressure, *or* chlorambucil, *v*incristine, *p*rednisone
CXR	chest X-ray
2-D	two-dimensional (real-time)
D&C	dilatation and curettage
DAT	direct antiglobulin (Coombs') test
DCA	dichloroacetate
DDAVP	de-amino D-arginine vasopressin ('desmopressin')
DD$_x$	differential diagnosis
DES	diethylstilbestrol
DF-2	'dysgonic fermenter' 2 (*C. canimorsus*)
DFA	diffuse fibrosing alveolitis
DFO	desferrioxamine
DHCC	dihydroxycholecalciferol
DHEA	dehydroepiandrosterone
DHFR	dihydrofolate reductase
DHT	dihydrotestosterone
DIC	disseminated intravascular coagulation
DIP	distal interphalangeal joint
DISIDA	disopropyl iminodiacetic acid (cf. HIDA)
DIT	di-iodotyrosine
DKA	diabetic ketoacidosis
DL$_{CO}$	diffusing capacity to carbon monoxide (transfer factor)
DM	diabetes mellitus, *or* dystrophia myotonica
DNA	deoxyribonucleic acid
DNCB	dinitrochlorobenzene
DNS	dysplastic nevus syndrome

2,3-DPG	2,3-diphosphoglycerate
dsDNA	double-stranded deoxyribonucleic acid
DTs	delirium tremens
DTH	delayed-type hypersensitivity
DU	duodenal ulcer
DVT	deep venous thrombosis
D$_x$	diagnosis
EACA	epsilonaminocaproic acid
EB(V)	Epstein–Barr (virus)
ECG	electrocardiogram (a.k.a. EKG)
ECHO	enteric cytopathic human orphan (virus)
ECOG	Eastern Cooperative Oncology Group
EDTA	ethylenediaminetetraammonium
EEG	electroencephalogram
ELISA	enzyme-linked immunosorbent assay
EM	electron microscopy, *or* erythema multiforme
EMA	epithelial membrane antigen
EMG	electromyography
EN	erythema nodosum
ENT	ear, nose and throat
EP	erythropoietic protoporphyria
EPG	electrophoretogram
EPS	electrophysiologic studies
ER	estrogen receptor, *or* endoplasmic reticulum, *or* emergency room
ERCP	endoscopic retrograde cholangiopancreatogram
esp.	especially
ESR	erythrocyte sedimentation rate
EUA	examination under anesthesia
F VIII$_c$	coagulant moiety of factor eight
Fab	antibody fragments
FAB	French–American–British (classification)
5-FC	flucytosine
FDPs	fibrin degradation products
Fe	iron
FEV$_1$	forced expiratory volume in 1 second
FFP	fresh frozen plasma
FiO$_2$	concentration of inspired oxygen
FMF	familial Mediterranean fever
FNA	fine needle aspiration
FSH	follicle-stimulating hormone
FTA-ABS	fluorescent treponemal antibody absorption test
FTI	free thyroxine index
5-FU	5-fluorouracil
FVC	forced vital capacity
GABA	γ-aminobutyric acid
GBM	glomerular basement membrane
GBS	Guillain–Barré syndrome
GFR	glomerular filtration rate
GGT	γ-glutamyl transpeptidase
GH(RF)	growth hormone (releasing factor)
GH(RH)	growth hormone (releasing hormone)
GHPS	gated heart pool scan
GI(T)	gastrointestinal (tract)
GIFT	gamete intrafallopian transfer
GIP	glucose-dependent insulinotrophic polypeptide ('gastric inhibitory polypeptide')
GN	glomerulonephritis
GnRH	gonadotrophin-releasing hormone
G6PD	glucose-6-phosphate dehydrogenase

GTT	glucose tolerance test	IBD	inflammatory bowel disease
GU	gastric ulcer	IBS	irritable bowel syndrome
GVHD	graft-versus-host disease	ICU	intensive care unit (a.k.a. ITU)
Gy	Gray (100 rad)	IDDM	insulin-dependent diabetes mellitus
h	hour(s)	IDL	intermediate density lipoproteins
HAART	highly active antiretroviral therapy	IEPG	immunoelectrophoretogram
HAV	hepatitis A virus	IF	immunofluorescence
HB	heart block	IFA	indirect fluorescent antibody
Hb	hemoglobin	IFN	interferon
HbA$_{1c}$	glycosylated hemoglobin	Ig	immunoglobulin
HBcAg	hepatitis B core antigen	IGF-1	insulin-like growth factor I (somatomedin C)
HBeAg	hepatitis B 'e' antigen		
HbO$_2$	oxyhemoglobin	IGFBP1	insulin-like growth factor binding protein 1
HBsAg	hepatitis B surface antigen	IHC	idiopathic hemochromatosis
HbSC	sickle-C hemoglobin	IHD	ischemic heart disease
HbSS	(homozygous) sickle-cell hemoglobin	IL-1	interleukin-1
HBV	hepatitis B virus	IM(I)	intramuscular (injection)
HCC	(25) hydroxycholecalciferol *or* hepatocellular carcinoma	IMP	inosine-5'-monophosphate
		INH	isoniazid
(β)HCG	human chorionic gonadotrophin (beta-subunit)	INR	international normalized (coagulation) ratio
HCl	hydrochloric acid	IP	interphalangeal (joint), *or* intraperitoneal
HCL	hairy cell leukemia	iPTH	immunoreactive parathyroid hormone
HCO$_3^-$	bicarbonate	IQ	intelligence quotient
HCV	hepatitis C virus	ITP	idiopathic thrombocytopenic purpura
HD	Hodgkin's disease, *or* Huntington's disease	ITT	insulin tolerance test
		IUD	intrauterine device
HDL	high-density lipoprotein	IV	interventricular
HDV	hepatitis D virus (δ particle)	IV(I)	intravenous (injection)
HEV	hepatitis E virus	IVC	inferior vena cava
HGPRT	hypoxanthine-guanine phosphoribosyl transferase	IVF	in vitro fertilization
		IVP	intravenous pyelogram
HHV	human herpesvirus	JCA	juvenile chronic arthritis
HI	*Haemophilus influenzae*	JVP	jugular venous pressure
(5)-HIAA	hydroxyindoleacetic acid	K$^+$	potassium
HIDA	hydroxyiminodiacetic acid (^{99m}Tc-labelled)	LAD	left axis deviation, *or* leukocyte adhesion deficiency
HIT	heparin-induced thrombocytopenia	LAHB	left anterior hemiblock
HIV	human immunodeficiency virus	LBBB	left bundle branch block
HLA	human leukocyte antigen	LCAT	lecithin-choline acyltransferase
HOCM	hypertrophic (± obstructive) cardiomyopathy	LDL	low-density lipoprotein
		L-DOPA	*levo-d*ihyd*r*ox*y*phen*y*l*a*lanine
HPA	hypothalamopituitary axis	LE	lupus erythematosus
HPL	human placental lactogen	LES	lower esophageal sphincter
HPO	hypertrophic pulmonary osteoarthropathy	LFTs	liver function tests
		LGV	lymphogranuloma venereum
HPT	hyperparathyroidism	LH	luteinizing hormone
HPV	human papillomavirus	LHRH	luteinizing hormone releasing hormone
HR	heart rate	LIF	leukemia inhibitory factor
HRT	hormone replacement therapy	LMN	lower motor neuron
HS	hereditary spherocytosis *or* herpes simplex *or* heart sounds	LP	lumbar puncture
		LPHB	left posterior hemiblock
HSP	heat-shock protein, *or* Henoch–Schönlein purpura	LRTI	lower respiratory tract infection
		LV(H)	left ventricle (hypertrophy)
HSV	herpes simplex virus, *or* highly selective vagotomy	LVF	left ventricular failure
		MALT	mucosa-associated lymphoid tissue
5-HT	5-hydroxytryptamine (serotonin)	MAO	maximal acid output
HTLV	human T cell leukemia virus	MAO(I)	monoamine oxidase (inhibitor)
HTN	hypertension	MBC	minimal bactericidal concentration
H-V	His-ventricle	MCHC	mean corpuscular hemoglobin concentration
H-X	histiocytosis X		
HZ	herpes zoster	MCP	metacarpophalangeal (joint)
^{131}I	radioiodine	MCQ	multiple choice question
IAT	indirect antiglobulin (Coombs') test	MCT	medullary carcinoma of the thyroid

MCTD	mixed connective tissue disease
MCV	mean corpuscular volume
MDP	manic-depressive psychosis
M:E	myeloid:erythroid (ratio)
MEN	multiple endocrine neoplasia
MESNA	sodium-2-mercaptoethanesulfonite
MF	myelofibrosis, *or* mycosis fungoides
MH	malignant hyperthermia
MHC	major histocompatibility complex
MI	myocardial infarction, *or* mitral incompetence
MIBG	metaiodobenzylguanidine
MIC	minimal inhibitory concentration
MIF	migration inhibitory factor
min	minutes
MLC	mixed lymphocyte culture
MND	motor neuron disease
MOPP	*mustine* (nitrogen mustard), *Oncovin* (vincristine), *procarbazine*, *prednisone*
6-MP	6-mercaptopurine
MR	mitral regurgitation
MRC	Medical Research Council (UK)
MRCP	magnetic resonance cholangiopancreatography
MRI	magnetic resonance imaging
mRNA	messenger RNA
MRSA	methicillin-resistant *Staph. aureus*
MS	mitral stenosis, *or* multiple sclerosis
MSU	midstream urine (specimen)
MTP	metatarsophalangeal (joint)
MVAC	*methotrexate*, *vinblastine*, *Adriamycin* (doxorubicin), *cisplatin*
MVP	mitral valve prolapse
N	normal
Na^+	sodium
NAD	nicotinamide adenine dinucleotide
NADH	nicotinamide
NAP	neutrophil alkaline phosphatase (score)
NB	note well
NBT	nitroblue tetrazolium
NHL	non-Hodgkin's lymphoma
NK	natural killer
NMR	nuclear magnetic resonance
NP59	^{131}I-6-β-iodomethyl-19-norcholesterol
NSAIDs	non-steroidal antiinflammatory drugs
NSU	non-specific (-gonococcal) urethritis
OA	osteoarthritis
OC	oral contraceptive
OCG	oral cholecystogram
OPSI	overwhelming post-splenectomy infection
OX (2, 19, K)	Weil–Felix reactions
P_2	pulmonary component of second heart sound
PA	pernicious anemia, *or* posteroanterior
PABA	para-aminobenzoic acid
$PaCO_2$	arterial partial pressure of carbon dioxide
PAI	plasminogen activator inhibitor
PAN	polyarteritis nodosa
P_AO_2	alveolar partial pressure of oxygen
P_aO_2	arterial partial pressure of oxygen
PAS	periodic acid-Schiff, *or* p-aminosalicylic acid

PBC	primary biliary cirrhosis
PBG	porphobilinogen
PCK	polycystic kidneys
PCNA	proliferating cell nuclear antigen
PCP	phenycyclidine ('angel dust')
PCR	polymerase chain reaction
PCT	porphyria cutanea tarda
PCV	packed cell volume (hematocrit)
PCWP	pulmonary capillary wedge pressure
PDA	patent ductus arteriosus
PDGF	platelet-derived growth factor
PE	pulmonary embolism
PEEP	positive end-expiratory pressure (ventilation)
PEFR	peak expiratory flow rate
PERLA	pupils equal, react to light and accommodation
PET	positron emission tomography
PGI_2	prostacyclin
Ph^1	Philadelphia (chromosome)
PHA	phytohemagglutinin
PI	prothrombin index (see INR) *or* pulmonary incompetence
PICA	posterior inferior cerebellar artery (lateral medullary) syndrome
PID	pelvic inflammatory disease
PIP	proximal interphalangeal joint
PiZZ	phenotype for homozygous $α_1AT$ deficiency
PLAP	placental alkaline phosphatase
PMR	polymyalgia rheumatica
PNH	paroxysmal nocturnal hemoglobinuria
p.o.	orally
POEMS	*polyneuropathy*, *organomegaly*, *endocrinopathy*, *M spike*, *skin changes*
PP	pancreatic polypeptide
PR	per rectum, *or* progesterone receptor
p.r.n.	as necessary
prob.	probably
PRPP	phosphoribosyl-1-pyrophosphate
PRV	polycythemia rubra vera
PS	pulmonary stenosis
PSA	prostate-specific antigen
PT	prothrombin time
PTC	percutaneous transhepatic cholangiogram
PTCA	percutaneous transluminal coronary angioplasty
PTH	parathyroid hormone
PTHrP	parathyroid hormone-related peptide
PTTK	partial thromboplastin time (with kaolin)
PTU	propylthiouracil
PUO	pyrexia (fever) of unknown origin
PUVA	psoralens/ultraviolet light (UV-A wavelength)
PV	per vagina
PVB	*cisplatin*, *vinblastine*, *bleomycin*
q (4 h)	every (4 hours)
q.i.d.	four times daily
Q-T_c	corrected Q-T interval
q.v.	which sees (i.e. discussed elsewhere)
RA	rheumatoid arthritis, *or* right atrium
RBBB	right bundle branch block

RBC	red blood cell	TLC	total lung capacity
RBF	renal blood flow	TMJ	temporomandibular joint
RDW	red-cell distribution width (anisocytosis)	TNF	tumor necrosis factor
REM	rapid eye movement	TNM	tumor/nodes/metastases (staging system)
RF	rheumatoid factor	tPA	tissue plasminogen activator
RIA	radioimmunoassay	TPHA	treponema pallidum hemagglutination
RIBA	radioimmunoblot assay	TPI	treponema pallidum immobilization (test)
RNA	ribonucleic acid		
RNP	ribonucleoprotein	TPN	total parenteral nutrition
RPGN	rapidly progressive glomerulonephritis	TRH	thyrotrophin-releasing hormone
RPR	rapid plasma reagin (syphilis test)	T_s	suppressor T cell
RSV	respiratory syncytial virus	TS	tricuspid stenosis
RTA	renal tubular acidosis, or road traffic accident	TSH	thyroid-stimulating hormone (thyrotrophin)
RV(H)	right ventricle (hypertrophy)	TSI	thyroid-stimulating immunoglobulin
R_x	treatment	TT	thrombin time
SAP	serum alkaline phosphatase	TTP	thrombotic thrombocytopenic purpura
SBE	subacute bacterial endocarditis	TURP	transurethral resection of the prostate gland
SC	subcutaneous		
SCA	sickle-cell anemia	TWAR	epidemic pneumonia, named after first two isolates: TW-183 and AR-39
SCC	squamous cell carcinoma		
SCID	severe combined immunodeficiency	TXA_2	thromboxane A_2
SCLC	small-cell lung cancer	U2 (-6)	spliceosomal molecule
sec	seconds	UDCA	ursodeoxycholic acid
SHBG	sex hormone binding globulin	UDP	uridine diphosphate
SIADH	syndrome of inappropriate ADH secretion	UMN	upper motor neuron
		URTI	upper respiratory tract infection
SIDS	sudden infant death syndrome	UTI	urinary tract infection
SK	streptokinase	UV	ultraviolet
SLE	systemic lupus erythematosus	VC	vital capacity
Sm	Smith (antigen, antibody)	V_D	volume of distribution
spp.	species	VD	venereal disease
SRS-A	slow-reacting substance of anaphylaxis	VDRL	Venereal Disease Research Laboratory (test)
ssDNA	single-stranded DNA		
SSER	somatosensory evoked response	VEB	ventricular ectopic (premature) beat
SSPE	subacute sclerosing panencephalitis	VER	visual evoked response
SSRI	selective serotonin reuptake inhibitor	VF	ventricular fibrillation
SVC	superior vena cava	VIP	vasoactive intestinal peptide
SVT	supraventricular tachycardia	VLDL	very low density lipoprotein
SXR	skull X-ray	V/Q	ventilation perfusion
$t_{1/2}$	half-life	VMA	vanillylmandelic acid
T2–12	thoracic vertebrae nos 2–12	VP	variegate porphyria
TB	tuberculosis	VSD	ventricular septal defect
TBG	thyroid-binding globulin	VT	ventricular tachycardia
Tc	technetium (^{99m}Tc = isotopic Tc)	VWD	von Willebrand's disease
TC	transcobalamin	VWF	von Willebrand factor
TCC	transitional cell carcinoma	WAS	Wiskott–Aldrich syndrome
t.d.s.	thrice daily	WBC	white blood cell
TdT	terminal deoxytransferase	WCC	white cell count
TF	transferrin	WDLL	well-differentiated lymphocytic lymphoma
TFTs	thyroid function tests		
TG	triglyceride	WHO	World Health Organization
6-TG	6-thioguanine	WPW	Wolff–Parkinson–White (syndrome)
TGB	thyroglobulin	WR	Wassermann reagent (test)
T_H	helper T cell	XD	X-linked dominant
THC	total hemolytic complement, or tetrahydrocannabinol	XR	X-linked recessive
		YMDD	amino acids tyrosine/methionine/aspartate/aspartate
TI	tricuspid incompetence		
TIA	transient ischemic attack	ZES	Zollinger–Ellison syndrome
TIBC	total iron-binding capacity		

Index